PRACTICAL EMERGENCY MEDICINE

EDITED BY

Ian Greaves
Consultant in Emergency Medicine
British Army

Graham Johnson
Consultant in Emergency Medicine
St James's University Hospital, Leeds

ARNOLD

A member of the Hodder Headline Group
LONDON

First published in Great Britain in 2002 by
Arnold, a member of the Hodder Headline Group,
338 Euston Road, London NW1 3BH

http://www.arnoldpublishers.com

Distributed in the United States of America by
Oxford University Press Inc.,
198 Madison Avenue, New York, NY10016
Oxford is a registered trademark of Oxford University Press

British Library Cataloguing in Publication Data
A catalogue record for this book is available from the British Library

Library of Congress Cataloging-in-Publication Data
A catalog record for this book is available from the Library of Congress

ISBN 0 340 80619 2

1 2 3 4 5 6 7 8 9 10

Publisher: Joanna Koster
Project Editor: James Rabson
Production Controller: Bryan Eccleshall
Cover Design: Terry Griffiths

Typeset in 9.5/12 pt Palatino by
Charon Tec Pvt. Ltd, Chennai, India
Printed and bound in Malta by Gutenberg Press Ltd

What do you think about this book? Or any other Arnold title?
Please send your comments to feedback.arnold@hodder.co.uk

PRACTICAL EMERGENCY
MEDICINE

CONTENTS

PREFACE

There are plenty of books about emergency medicine (or accident & emergency medicine) so why have we written another one?

Practical Emergency Medicine has been written to fulfil a particular need that no other currently available book addresses. There are many excellent 'pocketbooks' and there are a number of excellent highly referenced definitive multi-volume texts but no other medium-sized, profusely illustrated introductory textbook is currently available. *Practical Emergency Medicine* has been designed to fill this gap.

This book is designed principally for senior house officers seeking an introduction to the specialty and a source of information during their early months in the emergency department, although it also contains more than enough material to be used as a reference by registrars and more senior staff. Because of the range of topics it covers, general practitioners will also find it useful.

The text has been designed to be attractive and easy to read with maximum use of tables, key points, summary boxes and two-colour text. The information is presented in a manner intended to illuminate rather than overwhelm. We hope that readers will enjoy reading it as much as we have enjoyed preparing it.

This is the first edition of *Practical Emergency Medicine* and if any reader notices any sins of omission or commission, we would be most grateful if these could be brought to our attention for correction in the future.

Emergency medicine has a breadth and variety unmatched in any other specialty: we hope that this book conveys its fascination and becomes a valued aid in improving patient management.

Ian Greaves
Graham Johnson

ACKNOWLEDGEMENTS

Many people have directly and indirectly contributed to the production of this book. Both editors wish to thank their families, to whom this book is dedicated, without whose support and patience 'yet another book' would never have been completed.

We would like to thank Nick Dunton and Lucy Strachan from Arnold for their patience and technical support and Geoffrey Smalldon for his assistance in the early stages of this project. Our clinical colleagues have been generous with their advice and help with illustrations and our sincere thanks are due to them.

Mr Gavalas would like to thank Dr Kessoris, Mr P. Tekkis and Dr A. Challiner for their contributions.

We would also like to thank the Resuscitation Council (UK) for permission to reproduce the algorithms for management of adult and paediatric cardiac arrest.

The publishers would like to thank the authors and publishers of the following sources for permission to reproduce illustrations in this book:

Figures 2.1, 4.8(a), 4.8(b), 22.6, 23.2, 23.5, 23.8, 23.9, 23.10, 24.4, 29.2, 39.2 and 39.5: reproduced with permission from David V. Skinner and Fiona Whimster (eds), *Trauma*, published by Arnold, London, 1999.

Figures 8.1, 8.2, 8.3 and 8.4: redrawn from Karen A. Illingworth and Karen H. Simpson, *Anaesthesia and Analgesia in Emergency Medicine*, 1st edition, published by Oxford University Press, 1996.

Figures 14.2, 14.4 and 40.11: reproduced with permission from Peter Armstrong and Martin L. Wastie (eds), *Concise Textbook of Radiology*, published by Arnold, London, 2000.

Figures 23.3, 23.4, 23.6, 25.4, 28.1, 29.8, 39.10 and 42.4: reproduced with permission from Ian Greaves and Keith Porter (eds), *Pre-hospital Medicine*, published by Arnold, London, 1999.

Figures 25.5 and 35.1: reproduced with permission from R.C.G. Russell, Norman S. Williams and Christopher J.K. Bulstrode (eds), *Bailey & Love's Short Practice of Surgery*, 23rd edition, published by Arnold, London, 2000.

Figure 27.15: reproduced with permission from Neil Watson, *Hand Injuries and Infections*, published by Gower Medical Publishing Ltd, London, 1986.

Figure 11.22: reproduced with permission from Stephen Westaby and John Odell (eds), *Cardiothoracic Trauma*, published by Arnold, London, 1999.

Figures 24.9, 25.2, 25.6, 25.10, 25.17, 25.22, 26.1, 26.6, 26.9, 26.12 and 31.2: reproduced with permission from Louis Solomon, David J. Warwick and Selvadurai Nayagam (eds), *Apley's System of Orthopaedics and Fractures*, 8th edition, published by Arnold, London, 2001.

Figures 36.1, 36.2, 36.4, 36.5 and 36.6: reproduced with permission from Narciss Okhravi, *Manual of Primary Eye Care*, published by Butterworth-Heinemann, a division of Reed Educational & Professional Publishing Ltd, Oxford, 1999.

Figures 28.2, 28.3, 28.4, 28.5 and 28.6: reproduced with permission from Settle, J.A.D., *Burns: The First Five Days*, published by Smith and Nephew Pharmaceuticals Ltd, 1986.

Figures 30.1 and 30.2: reproduced with permission from Ronald Marks, *Roxburgh's Common Skin Disorders*, 16th edition, published by Arnold, London, 1994.

Figure 42.7: reproduced from *Report on the Accident to Boeing 737-400 G-OBME near Kegworth, Leicestershire on 8 January 1989*, Department of Transport. Crown copyright material is reproduced with the permission of the Controller of HMSO and the Queen's Printer for Scotland.

Figure 42.1: reproduced from *Investigation into the Clapham Junction Railway Accident*, Department of Transport, by permission of the Metropolitan Police Service.

For

Julia, Thomas and Owen

And my parents
Margaret and Bob Greaves
IG

Clare, Hannah, Mark and Christopher

And my parents
Margaret and John Johnson
GJ

CONTRIBUTORS

Ian Greaves MRCP(UK) FFAEM RAMC
Consultant in Emergency Medicine
British Army

Adrian A. Boyle MRCP
Specialist Registrar in Emergency Medicine
East Anglian Rotation

Andrew S. Brett MRCP
Consultant in Emergency Medicine
Channel Islands

Kieran Cunningham MRCPI
Specialist Registrar in Emergency Medicine
Mersey Rotation

Peter Dyer FRCS
Consultant Maxillofacial Surgeon
Royal Preston Hospital

Manolis C. Gavalas FRCS FFAEM
Consultant in Emergency Medicine
University College Hospital, London

Graham Johnson FRCS FFAEM
Consultant in Emergency Medicine
St James's University Hospital, Leeds

Tajek B. Hassan MRCP(UK) FFAEM
Consultant in Emergency Medicine
Leeds General Infirmary

Michael A. Howell FRCS FFAEM
Consultant in Emergency Medicine
Royal Navy

Rod McKenzie MRCP(UK)
Specialist Registrar in Emergency Medicine
East Anglia Rotation

Clifford J. Mann MRCP(UK) FFAEM
Consultant in Emergency Medicine
Taunton & Somerset Hospital, Taunton

Robert J. Russell MRCP(UK)
Specialist Registrar in Emergency Medicine
British Army

PART ONE

BASIC PRINCIPLES

CHAPTER ONE

CLINICAL ASSESSMENT AND DOCUMENTATION

- Introduction
- History taking
- Mechanism of injury

- Examination
- Documentation
- Further reading

INTRODUCTION

The skills of taking a history and performing a clinical examination are the most important components of the accurate assessment that is a prerequisite for correct diagnosis and appropriate treatment. Whilst in the relative calm and unhurried environment of a ward a doctor can usually take a detailed history and perform a complete examination before initiating treatment, medical staff in emergency departments often have to act rapidly in order to preserve life and prevent disability. Even in patients with non-life-threatening injuries or illness, pressures of work in busy departments dictate that only a brief assessment needed to define a plan of investigation and treatment is carried out. Within this space of time it is not only important to obtain information relevant to the patient's condition but a doctor–patient relationship needs to be established in which the doctor demonstrates that he is competent, caring and trustworthy. Documenting the clinical findings and subsequent investigation and treatment appropriately and in a concise format is also a skill that is new to a doctor starting work in an emergency department.

This chapter examines the three areas of history taking, examination and documentation in relation to emergency department work. Each patient in each department requires a different approach but certain principles underlie safe and effective emergency medical care and these are emphasized.

HISTORY TAKING

The time and workload pressures in an emergency department determine that a more focused clinical history is obtained. More detail can be added later when this is required. The important components of an emergency department history can be remembered with the aid of the mnemonic AMPLE (Table 1.1).

Often a complete history is not available from the patient and other witnesses to the illness or accident should be interviewed. The most important of these is the paramedic who has transported a patient from the scene of their accident or illness. They can give vital information on the mechanism of injury (Fig. 1.1) that forms one part of the diagnostic jigsaw in the multiply injured patient.

Table 1.1: The AMPLE history

A	Allergies
M	Medication
P	Past illness
L	Last ate or drank
E	Events and environment of injury or illness

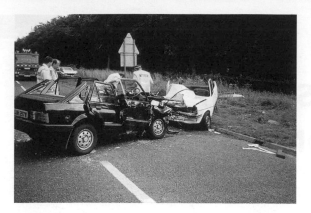

Figure 1.1: A high-energy frontal road traffic accident.

Similarly in the comatose patient, clues to diagnoses such as self-poisoning, hypothermia and carbon monoxide poisoning can be obtained from the ambulance service staff. The ambulance staff are, however, busy and if the correct questions are not asked early, vital information will be lost. The patient's friends and relatives are often not only witness to the accident or illness but may be able to give more information on a patient's general medical background.

Listen to what the paramedics have to tell you.

Additional details are often provided by or can be obtained from the patient's general practitioner. There may have been a recent contact with the patient which is relevant to the emergency department or details of past medical history or medication that are important to the assessment and treatment of the patient. It is vital that the history obtained and documented by the triage nurse is carefully checked. Other aspects of the case may be brought to light, and at other times variations in the explanation of injury may lead to the suspicion of child abuse.

ALLERGIES

Allergy may be the cause of a patient's presentation to the emergency department or may influence the choice of treatment of their condition. The patient may be able to give a clear history of previous allergic reactions but on occasions warning

bracelets, pre-existing hospital records or history from the general practitioner or relatives may be the only clue.

MEDICATIONS

Care should be taken to examine and document the medications being taken by a patient. These are not uncommonly the cause of the patient's presenting complaint or may indicate intercurrent disease or influence the physiological response to injury or illness. In conditions for which another doctor has already initiated treatment, the response to treatment may be helpful in determining further therapy.

PAST ILLNESS

The past medical history should be determined, as the presenting complaint may be a new manifestation of an established disease. Previous episodes of similar symptoms and their course and subsequent investigation and treatment may give clues to the nature of the current episode.

LAST MEAL

The time and content of the last meal or drink may determine the timing of treatment, particularly general anaesthesia. Many traumatic and non-traumatic emergencies result in gastric stasis and therefore carry a risk of vomiting and aspiration if the patient's level of consciousness is reduced. Measures to prevent this, for example by decompressing the stomach with a nasogastric tube, may be necessary.

EVENTS AND ENVIRONMENT

Whether the patient is presenting with an illness or injury the important components of the history are 'what happened and when?' In the first instance it is advisable to pose an open question allowing the patient to describe the circumstances of their illness or injury and the evolution of their symptoms. This can then be followed by a series of closed questions designed to search for specific features of the history of diagnostic importance to the doctor such as the radiation of pain, sweating and nausea which often accompanies ischaemic cardiac pain.

Pain is the commonest presenting complaint in an emergency department yet due to its subjective nature it is a difficult symptom to assess. In determining severity, a visual analogue score may provide a more objective measure of severity and a baseline to help assess the effect of intervention to reduce pain. The type of pain may be described by a number of adjectives but the site, radiation and factors that exacerbate and relieve the pain will give important diagnostic clues. The effect of analgesics taken or administered prior to arrival in the department may also give an indication of severity.

MECHANISM OF INJURY

An understanding of the mechanism of injury will help predict the pattern of injury that will be found on subsequent examination and investigation.

This applies both to relatively minor injury when the patient will usually be able to provide the required information (Table 1.2) but also to major injury when a reliable description of the mechanism of injury can often only be obtained from emergency services staff present at the scene of the accident (Table 1.3).

A set of mechanisms of injury which predict serious injury (Table 1.4) are also recognized and when these are present, the doctor should be aware of the possibility of serious occult injury in an apparently well patient.

EXAMINATION (FIG. 1.2)

The assessment of injury or illness in the history will allow the examination to be focused on specific areas and systems for important positive and negative findings. It is rarely necessary to examine the patient completely other than in major injury when an absolutely comprehensive examination is in order to ensure that no injury is missed.

Table 1.2: Some mechanisms of injury and related patterns of injury

Inversion injury of ankle	Lateral ligament injury
	Fracture of lateral malleolus
	Bimalleolar fracture
Flexion rotation injury to knee	Tibial collateral ligament injury
	Medial meniscus tear
	Anterior cruciate rupture
Fall on outstretched hand	Greenstick fracture radius
	Colles' fracture
	Fracture of radial head
	Fracture of neck of humerus

Table 1.3: Injuries associated with specific mechanisms of injury

Fall from height	Fractures of both calcanei
	Pelvic fracture
	Thoracolumbar spinal fracture
Frontal impact road accident	Facial injuries
	Fracture sternum with blunt myocardial injury
	Fracture dislocation of hip
	Patellar fracture
Side impact car passenger	Spinal injury
	Side of impact chest injury
	Side of impact abdominal injury

Table 1.4: Mechanisms of injury associated with life-threatening injury

| Road traffic impact > 40 mph |
| Fall greater than 2 m |
| Ejection from vehicle |
| Death in vehicle |
| Pedestrian collision speed greater than 30 mph |

The process of examination starts at the first contact with the patient and important information can be gleaned from the patient's appearance and the way questions are answered. In all patients in whom a serious illness or injury may exist an initial assessment often called the primary survey is carried out (Chapter 4). An appropriate response

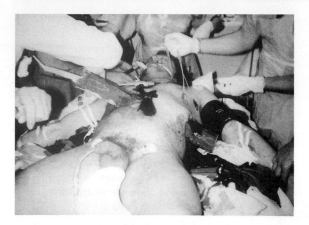

Figure 1.2: Examining the victim of major multi-system trauma.

to questions indicates that the patient has a clear airway, a good respiratory effort allowing them to talk and good cerebral perfusion allowing an alert mental state and orientated and appropriate responses. In the seriously ill or injured patient the detection of any life-threatening abnormality should be followed by attempts to correct it before the assessment moves on.

Prior to the patient being seen by the doctor, the nursing staff will have often recorded a number of observations. These will usually be the baseline observations of pulse, temperature and blood pressure but will vary from case to case. In children a record of weight is vital to the correct calculation of drug doses. The Glasgow Coma Score (p. 31) may also be recorded where there is actual or potential impairment of conscious level. Increasingly, a pulse oximeter reading is provided though in interpreting this it is important to know the amount of oxygen the patient was breathing at the time and appreciate the limitations of the technique.

Examination of many emergency department patients involves assessment of musculoskeletal injuries. New senior house officers in emergency departments often have little experience of these injuries and as a result misdiagnosis and inappropriate treatment are not uncommon. Each limb injury should be examined by looking, feeling and moving.

Limb injuries — look, feel and move.

The injury should first be inspected for bruising, swelling and deformity. Wounds, both old and new, are also noted. Then the area should be palpated to localize tenderness and to assess circulation and nerve supply distal to the injury. Finally, movement should be assessed: initially active movement by the patient to determine the range of movement that can be achieved, followed by passive to detect abnormal movement as a result of major ligamentous injury.

DOCUMENTATION

Good-quality clinical care requires good note-keeping. The ability to produce accurate yet concise documentation is an essential skill in emergency medicine. Patients may return to the department with unresolved problems and are then seen by other doctors. Without accurate notes of previous attendances, continuity of care is further hampered. The records may also be needed several years later in order to defend an allegation of medical negligence or provide evidence in criminal proceedings. Accurate records are therefore beneficial for both the patient and the doctor. Certain features are essential (Table 1.5) and are common to all cases but the actual content of the record will obviously largely vary with the content of the consultation.

A large number of abbreviations are used in emergency department records (Table 1.6) and these may vary from department to department. Although sometimes humorous at the time, remarks and abbreviations that are insulting to patients should be omitted as the doctor may later be called to account for them.

Various proformas have been produced in order to encourage accurate record-keeping in particular types of cases. These are particularly helpful in ensuring complete data collection in complex cases such as multiple injuries (Fig. 1.3); however, when printed on separate sheets these are often difficult to store and become separated from the patient's main record. All such inclusions should be securely attached to the patient's main record.

While it is self-evident that all important positive findings are recorded, it is also important to document potentially important negative findings.

Table 1.5: Essential features of emergency department records

Each entry is legible, timed and signed with the writer's name also printed.
The notes should contain the history, examination, diagnosis, treatment and arrangements for further treatment.
Discussions with and referrals to other doctors should be documented, including the other doctor's name.
The investigations and their results should be noted.
Recognized abbreviations are acceptable. However, write RIGHT and LEFT in full.

Table 1.6: Commonly used abbreviations

BID	Brought in dead
DID	Died in department
DNB	Digital (or ring) block
DOA	Dead on arrival
FB	Foreign body
FDP	Flexor digitorum profundus
FDS	Flexor digitorum superficialis
FPL	Flexor pollicis longus
FOOSH	Fall on outstretched hand
GCS	Glasgow Coma Score
HIA	Head injury advice
LoC	Loss of consciousness
NV	Neurovascular
PERL	Pupils equal and reacting to light
POP	Plaster of Paris
RoS	Removal of sutures
SS	Steristrip
TRIN	To return if necessary

Under most legal systems something that was not documented was not done. However, the production of many pages of meticulous notes about every patient with a minor injury will delay the care of other patients and frustrate a colleague who subsequently has to review the patient.

Anatomical outlines are also available for use in indicating the location of injuries and are particularly valuable in the subsequent completion of police statements (Fig. 1.3). Information initially recorded in words ('a 2-cm laceration over the right eye...') should never be transcribed to a visual record on such an anatomical chart.

Examples of the application of these principles with good-quality documentation for patients with an acute myocardial infarction (Fig. 1.4), a minor head injury (Fig. 1.5) and a hand laceration (Fig. 1.6) are given below. Positive and negative findings which affect decision making with respect to investigation, diagnosis and treatment are included.

The assessment of a patient with chest pain is focused on identifying life-threatening conditions that benefit from immediate treatment, principally acute myocardial infarction (Fig. 1.4). The nature, duration and distribution of the pain are noted with a search for symptoms that commonly accompany cardiac pain, such as sweating and nausea. Examination focuses on situations that might complicate acute myocardial infarction or other potential diagnoses. Results of investigations are documented as is the treatment administered. It is particularly important to document the time thrombolysis was started for subsequent audit.

The objective in the head-injured patient is to identify the seriously injured patient and a group of apparently well patients who are at increased risk of the subsequent development of an intracranial haematoma. In assessment of a head injury, the history will elicit the mechanism of injury, duration of loss of consciousness and the development of symptoms such as headache and vomiting since the injury. Certain mechanisms of injury (falls) are associated with a higher incidence of intracranial haemorrhage than others (road traffic accidents). Specific factors in the past medical history such as anticoagulation or a further recent injury may influence management. It is often necessary to elicit information from friends, bystanders and observers.

The examination should include a description of the local signs of injury to the head, such as a scalp laceration or haematoma, and their position. The Glasgow Coma Score (recorded as its E, M and V components if not normal), the pupillary reactions and the presence of any focal motor neurological signs are noted. A meticulous neurological examination will add no further information and will only delay management. The investigations performed (particularly skull X-ray) and their results are noted. If a decision is made to discharge the patient, the identity of the person who will be responsible for them after discharge should be recorded, as should the nature of the instructions given regarding return to hospital.

Name _____ Age/D.O.B. _____ Date _____ Time of arrival _____

Address _____ A/E No: _____

CAUSE	TYPE OF INJURY	DETAILS OF RTA	PROTECTIVE DEVICES
FALL > 2m ☐	BLUNT ☐	PEDAL CYCLIST ☐	SEAT BELT ☐
FALL < 2m ☐	PENETRATING ☐	MOTOR CYCLIST ☐	CHILD RESTRAINT ☐
RTA ☐	CHEST CRUSH ☐	PILLION ☐	HELMET ☐
ASSAULT ☐	BURN ☐	VEHICLE DRIVER ☐	AIRBAG ☐
STABBING ☐	INHALATION ☐	FRONT PASSENGER ☐	NONE ☐
SPORT ☐	INTRUSTION ☐	BACK PASSENGER ☐	MODE OF ARRIVAL
COLLAPSE ☐	EJECTED ☐	PEDESTRIAN ☐	AMBULANCE ☐
NAI ☐	TRAPPED ☐	SPEED MPH _____	HELICOPTER ☐
OTHER (STATE) ☐	ANY OTHER ☐ DEATH INVOLVED	OTHER (STATE)	CAR ☐
_____		_____	OTHER ☐

PRIMARY SURVEY

ASSESSMENT

AIRWAY ☐
☐ Normal   Gag Y/N
☐ Unconscious
☐ Facial fractures

CERVICAL SPINE
☐ Normal   ☐ Suspect injury   ☐ Firm collar   ☐ In line traction

BREATHING ☐
RR ON ARRIVAL.........................../min
☐ Trauma   (blunt/penetrating)
☐ Pneumothorax (open / closed / tension)
☐ Haemothorax
☐ Flail segment

CIRCULATION ☐
SYSTOLIC BP ON ARRIVAL...............mmHg
☐ Haemorrhage
   ☐ External
   ☐ Internal   ☐ Chest
                  ☐ Abdomen
                  ☐ Pelvis

PALE ☐   SWEATING ☐   RESTLESS ☐   CYANOSED ☐   APPEARANCE NORMAL ☐

RESUSCITATION

☐ Spontaneous
☐ *Mask/mask + airway*   _ _ _ % O²
☐ Ventilated   ☐ ETT - size _ _ _
☐ N-G tube

☐ Chest drain
   Left   Right
   Size _ _ _ _   *Size _ _ _ _ _*

IV (1)-*site* _ _ _ _   *Size* _ _ _ _ _
IV (2)-*site* _ _ _ _   *Size* _ _ _ _ _
Blood ordered   ☐ 0 Neg
Time ____ hrs   ☐ Grouped
                ☐ X-match
                ☐ G + S
☐ Pressure dressings
☐ Arterial blood gases
☐ ECG monitor

DYSFUNCTION*
** G.C.S. on Arrival _____
○ Alert
○ Respond to Command
○ Responds to Pain
○ Unresponsive
  Pupils Equal? Y/N

○ Spinal Care / Stabilisation
  Splint (state type)

INVESTIGATIONS   tick box ☑

BLOOD TAKEN   FBC ☐   U&E ☐   X-MATCH ☐   AMYLASE ☐   UNITS @ _____

PORTABLE X-RAYS: LATERAL ☐   CHEST ☐   PELVIS ☐   @ _____
                   C-SPINE   URINE

ECG (12 lead)   @ _____   Catheter Inserted Time _____ Size _____
BLOOD GASES   @ _____   Residual Volume _____ mls

TO: CT SCAN -   HEAD ☐   CHEST ☐   ABDO ☐   SPINE ☐   @ _____ RETURN @ _____
TO ULTRA SOUND - ABDO ☐   CHEST ☐   @ _____ RETURN @ _____
TO X-RAY -   HEAD ☐   CHEST ☐   ABDO ☐   PELVIS ☐ @ _____ RETURN @ _____
                  SPINE ☐   LIMB ☐   @ _____ RETURN @ _____

FLUID INPUT

IV SITE 1			IV SITE 2			IV OTHER			RUNNING TOTAL
TIME	FLUID	VOLUME	TIME	FLUID	VOLUME	TIME	FLUID	VOLUME	
						COMPLETED PRE-HOSPITAL FLUIDS			

Figure 1.3: Trauma chart.

Accident & Emergency

	DRUG	DOSAGE	ROUTE	PRESCRIBED BY	GIVEN BY	TIME
M E D I C A T I O N						

TETANUS TOXOID	Covered / not covered	Tetanus toxoid booster given **Y/N**

			DATE	
	Frequency of Recorungs		TIME	

COMA SCALE

Eyes Open	4	Spontaneously			Eyes closed by swelling = C
	3	To speech			
	2	To pain			
	1	None			
Best verbal response	5	Orientated			Endotracheal tube or tracheostomy = T
	4	Confused			
	3	Innapropriate Words			
	2	Incomprehensible sounds			
	1	None			
Best motor response	6	Obeys commands			Usually record the best arm response
	5	Localised pain			
	4	Withdraws to pain			
	3	Flexion to pain			
	2	Extends to pain			
	1	None			

TOTAL:-

Pupil Scale (m.m.): • 1, • 2, ● 3, ● 4, ● 5, ● 6, ● 7, ● 8

Blood pressure and Pulse rate: 240 230 220 210 200 190 180 170 160 150 140 130 120 110 100 90 80 70 60 50 40 30

Respiration 20 10

Temperature °C: 41 40 39 38 37 36 35 34 33 32 31

PUPILS	right	Size			+ reacts
		Reaction			− no reaction
	left	Size			c. eye closed by swelling
		Reaction			

LIMB MOVEMENT

ARMS	Normal power		
	Mild weakness		
	Severe weakness		
	Spastic flexion		
	Extension		
	No response		
LEGS	Normal power		
	Mild weakness		
	Severe weakness		
	Extension		
	No response		

Record right (R) and left (L) separately if there is a difference between the two sides

PHA.M.R.21

FLUID OUTPUT					
URINE OUTPUT		**OTHER**			**RUNNING TOTAL**
TIME	VOLUME	TIME	VOLUME	TYPE	

REFERRALS

		Grade	Time	
			Called	Arrived
	Anaesthetiest			
	Gen. surgeons			
	Orthopaedic			
	Neurosurg.			
	Thoracic			
	Plastic			
	Max. fac.			
	Other			

Figure 1.3: *(Continued).*

SECONDARY SURVEY								
Examined	Head	Neck	Chest	Abdo	Pelvis	T/L Spine	UL	LL
Yes/No								

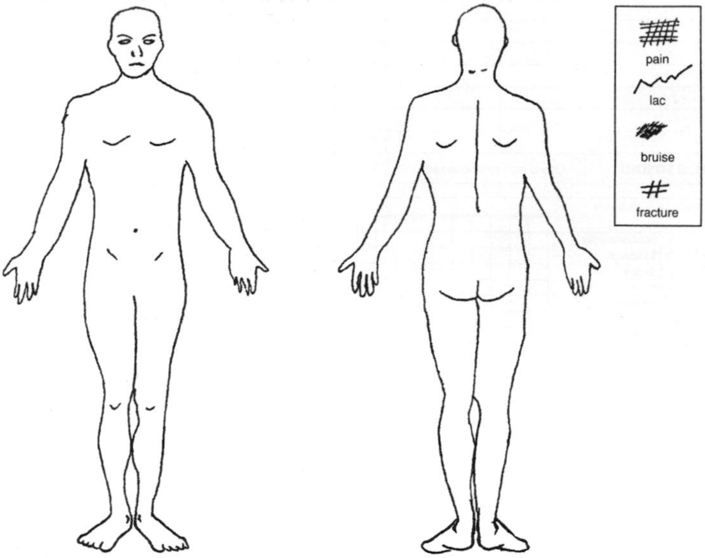

pain

lac

bruise

fracture

Significant PMH:

Medication (incl. steroids):

Allergies

NEXT OF KIN	IDENTIFIED Y N	CONTACTED Y N

NAME _____ RELATIONSHIP _____
ADDRESS _____
_____ PHONE NO _____

PROPERTY WITH PATIENT ☐ RELATIVE ☐ FRIEND ☐ POLICE ☐
VALUABLES IN SAFE ☐ ID BRACELET ☐

DESTINATION FROM A & E

○ Ward (Specify)_____ Time _____ ○ C T Scan Time _____
○ I T U Time _____ ○ Transfer (Specify) Time _____
○ Theatre Ortho/General Time _____ ○ Died Time _____

NURSING NOTES

PRT46

Figure 1.3: *(Continued).*

```
JONES 0439
61y male
1hour crushing central chest pain radiating neck and left arm
Sweaty, SoB, Vomited x1
Known angina 3 years
GTN – no relief

Other fit and well      No allergies
Meds GTN only
Smokes 20/day
Family history negative

O/E
Pale Sweaty
P 76    BP 145/80    JVP normal    HS I+II+0
Chest clear
No oedema
ECG Acute anteroseptal myocardial infarct

Plan   Aspirin 300 mg oral
       Diamorphine 5 mg IV
       Metoclopramide 10mg IV
       Streptokinase 1.5 megaunits in 1 h (0500h)
       Refer Medicine (0510h)
                                Sally Jones
                                JONES
```

Figure 1.4: Sample documentation for chest pain.

```
SMITH 1029
23y male
Playing football – clash of heads 1 h ago
LoC < 30 s Not vomited. Local headache
Normally fit and well. No other injuries

O/E
GCS 15  PERL  Neuro intact
Right parietal scalp haematoma

For SXR

DS 1115
SXR NBI
Diagnosis  Minor head injury
Home with head injury instructions (with wife)
TRIN
Discharge 1120h
                                David Smith
                                SMITH
```

Figure 1.5: Sample documentation for a patient with minor head injury.

Most injuries presenting to emergency departments occur to the limbs. The nature and time of injury should be recorded. Whether the patient is right- or left-handed is pertinent as even minor injuries to a dominant limb in the elderly can reduce their ability to live independently. In assessing a hand injury it is vital to document the position of any wounds and the results of a systematic examination of each tendon and nerve which may be affected by the injury.

```
DAVIES 1232
Laceration to right (non-dominant) wrist with glass 2 h ago.
Tripped and fell through window
No other injuries

Tet. Immune

O/E

3 cm laceration transverse palmar aspect right wrist

Palmaris longus tendon visible divided

FDS  intact all 4 digits
FDP  intact all 4 digits
FPL  intact

Median nerve sensory – reduced
               motor – no contraction

Ulnar nerve motor and sensory intact
DD and elevate
X-ray – ?FB

DAVIES
1320

X-ray – no FB
Refer Hands for exploration and repair median nerve (1325 h)
                                Peter Davies
                                DAVIES
```

Figure 1.6: Sample documentation for patient with a hand injury.

Table 1.7: Variability of fracture patterns with age

Shoulder	Elderly	Fracture neck of humerus
	Young adults	Fracture clavicle
Elbow	Adults	Fracture radial head
	Children	Supracondylar fracture
Wrist	Elderly	Colles' fracture
	Young adults	Scaphoid fracture
	Children	Greenstick fracture of radius

Certain mechanisms of injury, such as a fall on an outstretched hand, can be associated with a variety of bony injuries at different levels of the limb in a range of age groups (Table 1.7).

FURTHER READING

Guly, H.R. (1996) *History Taking, Examination and Record keeping in Emergency Medicine*. Oxford University Press, Oxford.

CHAPTER TWO

INVESTIGATIONS IN EMERGENCY MEDICINE

- Introduction
- Radiology and imaging
- Haematology
- Biochemistry
- Microbiology

- Electrocardiography (ECG)
- Near-patient testing
- Other investigations
- Further reading

INTRODUCTION

Diagnosis in emergency departments, as in other areas of medical practice, is largely dependent on an adequate history and examination. Investigations should rarely play a major role and are not a substitute for good clinical technique. With the greater availability of more sophisticated tests, it is increasingly common to see patients submitted to a battery of investigations which are unlikely to alter clinical care within the emergency department. As in treatment decisions, the selection of appropriate investigations should be based on sound evidence that they are likely to aid the diagnosis and treatment of the patient. The use of unnecessary investigations costs the National Health Service money and causes delays to patient care.

The indiscriminate use of investigations is no substitute for a careful history and examination.

Therefore, in general, investigations should be limited to those that are likely to alter the immediate management of the patient. On occasions when an intravenous cannula has been inserted it is sensible to remove blood for routine tests to save the patient from receiving a further venepuncture. However, these samples can then either be sent with the patient to the ward or be despatched to

the laboratory but should not delay decisions on treatment. Other tests are either completely unnecessary or can be left to staff on the in-patient wards or in general practice to perform.

Improvements in technology have resulted in the ability to provide many tests at the patient's 'bedside'. Simple tests such as urinalysis and blood glucose estimation have been accepted practice for some time. Now many emergency departments are able to carry out a wider battery of tests including sensitive pregnancy tests, blood gas analysis and simple haematological and biochemical assays. Ready availability should not encourage exces-sive use.

The appropriate use of different types of investigation is now addressed under the broad headings of radiology and imaging, haematology, clinical chemistry, microbiology, electrocardiography and near-patient testing.

RADIOLOGY AND IMAGING

Most patients attending an emergency department will undergo a radiological investigation. Many expect to be X-rayed and may be dissatisfied if an X-ray is not requested. In order to expedite the care of patients with minor injuries many departments now train their triage nurses to request a limited range of X-rays prior to the patient being seen by a doctor. Diagnostic imaging is responsible for a major proportion of the population's radiation exposure and it is therefore appropriate that we try and limit radiological examinations to those that are necessary for the management of illness and injury. Some plain radiographs, such as lumbar and thoracic spine films, are associated with particularly large radiation doses.

> Always ask – will this X-ray alter my treatment?

Few junior doctors starting work in emergency departments have experience in interpreting radiographs and therefore missed abnormalities are common. Many radiology departments now have a 'hot reporting' service, which provides a report from the radiologist at the time the X-ray is performed. All hospitals should have a system whereby X-rays of patients discharged from the emergency department are subsequently checked by experienced radiologists. Any omissions of care can then be rectified by recalling the patient to the department.

Increasingly robust and easily applicable guidelines are being produced which can guide a doctor in making a decision about whether an X-ray is necessary. These aim to identify a group of patients needing an X-ray while reducing the numbers of X-rays performed. A well researched and proven example of these guidelines are the Ottowa ankle rules. In general, X-rays in trauma should only be performed where there is a history of significant injury which is accompanied by bone tenderness or significant bruising, swelling or loss of function. Examples of good X-ray requesting practice are included in the specific chapters. A good summary of indications for radiological examination is available in a booklet entitled 'Making the Best Use of a Department of Clinical Radiology' published by the Royal College of Radiologists (see Further Reading).

At the same time it has been recognized that certain X-rays are of little value, as they do not alter patient management even if they demonstrate a fracture. For example, nasal bone X-rays (Table 2.1) will not assess deformity, which is the main criterion for assessing whether a nasal injury needs further treatment.

In order to achieve the maximal benefit from a radiology department it is vital that relevant clinical information is provided on the request card so that the radiologist can understand the clinical problem that needs resolution. If there is doubt about whether a radiological examination is likely to be helpful or which type of investigation is appropriate, discussion with a radiologist may prevent a pointless X-ray being performed.

Table 2.1: Unnecessary X-rays

Nasal bone X-rays
Rib views for chest trauma
Lumbar spine X-rays in most young patients with atraumatic back pain
X-rays of the minor toes for injury when no deformity is present
Soft tissue neck X-rays for foreign body
Skull X-rays with persisting reduced level of consciousness (CT needed)
Erect abdominal films

Table 2.2: Indications for emergency ultrasound

Vaginal bleeding in pregnancy
Suspected deep venous thrombosis
Gynaecological pain
Possible ruptured abdominal aortic aneurysm
Irritable hip
Abdominal pain ?cholelithiasis
Scrotal pain
Radiolucent soft tissue foreign body

ULTRASOUND

Access to a good ultrasonography service is an increasingly important part of an emergency department's diagnostic capability (Table 2.2). Ultrasound has the advantage of being portable, which allows it to be brought to the patient when the patient is too sick to go to the X-ray department. It also does not involve exposing the patient to radiation. An experienced operator is, however, required if good diagnostic accuracy is to be achieved, and few hospitals can supply a staffed 24-hour service.

Most ultrasound investigations will be requested to investigate vaginal bleeding in pregnancy or pelvic pain in women. Increasingly, the investigation of suspected deep venous thrombosis is carried out with ultrasound though in some cases further investigation may still be needed even if the scan is normal.

In children with a clinical diagnosis of irritable hip, ultrasound can detect the presence of an effusion in the hip joint and guide its aspiration. The aspirated fluid can than be examined with microscopy and cultured. Symptomatic relief is often good simply from removal of the fluid. Torsion of the testis is largely a clinical diagnosis; however, where there is uncertainty ultrasound can detect other intrascrotal pathology and colour Doppler techniques can be used to assess the blood flow through the affected testis. In trauma of the testis, ultrasound can also detect the degree of injury and determine whether surgery is indicated for disruption of the tunica albuginea.

Focused abdominal sonography for trauma (FAST) is increasingly recognized as a simple rapid tool for the investigation of intra-abdominal bleeding in trauma. Like other ultrasound studies it relies on the skill and experience of the operator.

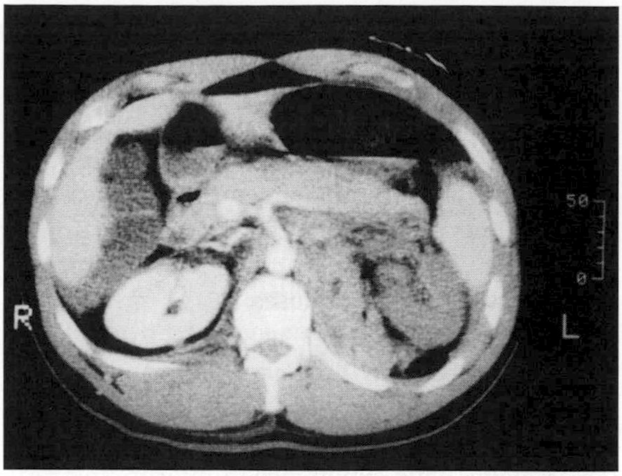

Figure 2.1: Abdominal CT scan showing a large retroperitoneal haematoma and non-perfusion of the left kidney. The patient had fallen on to his abdomen and avulsed the kidney from the renal artery.

COMPUTERIZED TOMOGRAPHY (CT)

CT scanning, especially of the head and the abdomen, is now more widely available than ever before (Fig. 2.1). Whilst it provides sensitive and specific diagnostic information, transfer of the patient to the CT suite is necessary. Radiation doses from the examination are substantial. Patients, especially those who have potentially sustained major injury, should not be transferred to the CT scanner unless they have protected airways and are haemodynamically normal. The decision to carry out a CT scan should therefore be made by a senior doctor.

Other early indications for the use of CT include the investigation of possible intracranial haemorrhage. In these case the request for a CT mandates further investigation (lumbar puncture) if the scan is normal.

CONTRAST RADIOGRAPHY

There are few immediate indications for contrast radiography in the emergency department. Generally, patients will be submitted to these investigations only after consultation with the relevant specialist. Radiation doses from investigations such as intravenous urography or arch aortography are particularly high.

HAEMATOLOGY

Requests for blood counts outnumber those for other blood investigations but rarely alter patient management. On occasions this investigation unexpectedly detects anaemia and will give some information regarding its cause. More commonly it is the white-cell count that attracts interest. The presence of a leucocytosis in patients with abdominal pain, particularly when appendicitis is suspected, is widely sought by junior surgeons but is of little help in diagnosis and decision making. A raised white-cell count should raise the doctor's index of suspicion that significant pathology is present but should not alone change decisions on treatment.

An increasing proportion of the population takes anticoagulant drugs for a wide variety of indications. They not uncommonly present to emergency departments with problems related to the medication, particularly excessive bleeding either from minor injuries or into normal tissues. There should therefore be a low threshold for checking the patient's international normalized ratio (INR) as many will be found to be over anticoagulated and will need referral back to their supervising clinic. The INR should be in the therapeutic range of 2.0–4.5.

Table 2.3: Patients at risk of disseminated intravascular coagulation

Trauma, particularly following massive transfusion
Severe sepsis
Post transfusion reaction
Near drowning

Other groups of patients requiring coagulation studies include those with liver disease and where disseminated intravascular coagulation is suspected (Table 2.3). In the early stages of resuscitation it is good practice to assess coagulation to establish a baseline against which subsequent estimates can be compared.

BIOCHEMISTRY

Urea and electrolyte analyses are often requested on patients as part of a diagnostic screen. Again these investigations rarely result in change of management, especially in previously fit patients with an acute illness. Blood sugar analyses from near-patient finger-prick testing are accurate and formal laboratory analysis adds little.

Serum amylase is a valuable investigation in that high levels are diagnostic of acute pancreatitis. However, in patients with chronic or acute relapsing pancreatitis the amylase level may remain normal. Amylase estimation also lacks sensitivity and specificity in the diagnosis of pancreatic trauma.

For patients who have taken overdoses, serum salicylate and paracetamol levels are valuable in determining treatment. There is, however, no value in taking these samples within 4 h of ingestion. Otherwise 'drug screening' is not routinely performed, as there is no potential benefit to the management of the patient. Similarly, estimations of serum ethanol levels, whilst popular in the United States, are not routinely performed and when required for forensic purposes should be taken by a police surgeon. Some departments provide standard 'breathalysers' for the rough assessment of the level of intoxication.

Arterial blood gas analysis has a valuable role to play in assessing the severity of illness in a number of groups of patients (Table 2.4). In interpreting the results of arterial blood gas analysis it is important

Table 2.4: Indications for arterial blood gas analysis

Post cardiac arrest
Diabetic ketoacidosis
Respiratory failure
Overdoses (tricyclics, salicylate)
Trauma in the head-injured patient
Renal failure

Table 2.5: Technical factors affecting results of blood gas analysis

Time from sampling to analysis
Presence of air in the syringe
Excessive volume of heparin in the syringe
Patient temperature

Table 2.6: Arterial blood gas analysis – pH values

If pH <7.35 acidosis is present
If pH >7.45 alkalosis is present

to consider the patient's status when the sample was taken, particularly the inspired concentration of oxygen and whether the patient was receiving ventilatory support. If the sample is analysed within 15 min by the laboratory, precautions such as packing the sample with ice can be avoided. Other technical considerations in sampling which may affect the results are listed in Table 2.5.

Sampling can be from either the radial, the brachial or the femoral artery. Radial artery sampling is painful for the patient and should be preceded by an Allen test to ensure that the hand is not totally dependent on the artery for blood supply. It is important to ensure that a minimum of 3 min of constant pressure is applied to the puncture site and that normal distal circulation resumes after removal of pressure. Because of the small size of the radial artery there is a much higher failure rate when this vessel is used for blood gas sampling. In shocked patients the femoral artery should be used unless there is an obvious contraindication.

In interpreting the results the first priority is to determine whether the patient has an acidosis or an alkalosis (Table 2.6). The partial pressure of oxygen (PaO_2) is then assessed but relative normality or abnormality can only be assessed with knowledge of the inspired oxygen concentration (Table 2.7). For example, a patient with a normal PaO_2 despite

Table 2.7: Normal values in arterial blood gas analysis

PaO_2	9.31–13.1 kPa (70–100 mmHg)
$PaCO_2$	4.5–6.0 kPa (34–45 mmHg)
Standard and actual bicarbonate	23–28 mmol l^{-1}
Base excess	0 ± 2.0 mmol l^{-1}

Table 2.8: Causes of metabolic acidosis

Lactic acidosis – shock, post-resuscitation
Renal failure
Diabetic ketoacidosis
Drugs – salicylates

Table 2.9: Causes of respiratory acidosis

Central respiratory depression – drugs, head injury
Upper or lower airway obstruction
Parenchymal pulmonary disease
Inadequate ventilatory mechanics –
    haemopneumothorax, Guillain–Barré syndrome

Table 2.10: Causes of metabolic alkalosis

Alkali ingestion
Repeated vomiting – pyloric stenosis

Table 2.11: Causes of respiratory alkalosis

Hyperventilation as a result of:
    Hypoxic drive
    Salicylate ingestion
    Anxiety
    Hyperventilation syndrome
    Therapeutic hyperventilation (in head injury)

Table 2.12: The alveolar–arterial oxygen gap

Alveolar–arterial oxygen gap =
    $(150 - 1.25 \times$ Measured $PaCO_2) - ($Measured $PaO_2)$

For a patient breathing room air
    Normal value   <10 mmHg in young patient
                          <20 mmHg in older patient

breathing a high inspired concentration of oxygen has a significant problem. In assessing patients with chronic respiratory disease it is important to remember that an abnormal result may not represent an acute deterioration but their normal condition.

The $PaCO_2$ represents the degree of alveolar ventilation. A high result suggests inadequate ventilation and a low result hyperventilation. The actual bicarbonate is derived from the pH and $PaCO_2$ whereas the standard bicarbonate is the value corrected for a normal $PaCO_2$ and temperature and therefore reflects metabolic changes. The base excess is also a derived value, which represents the buffering capacity.

In metabolic acidosis the pH is reduced and bicarbonate levels are low with a negative base excess and hyperventilation, resulting in a normal or reduced $PaCO_2$. Causes are given in Table 2.8.

In respiratory acidosis (Table 2.9) the pH is decreased and the $PaCO_2$ increased as a result of reduced alveolar ventilation. In some cases metabolic compensation allows the pH to remain normal despite the carbon dioxide retention. The bicarbonate levels rise and the base excess is positive.

In metabolic alkalosis there is an increase in plasma bicarbonate levels and a positive base excess either as a result of loss of acid from the gastrointestinal tract or from increased ingestion of alkalis (Table 2.10). The $PaCO_2$ may rise as the patient attempts to compensate by hypoventilation.

With respiratory alkalosis, hyperventilation has occurred as a result of one of a number of factors (Table 2.11). The $PaCO_2$ is therefore reduced and there is a compensatory reduction in bicarbonate levels with negative base excess.

It is not uncommon in critically injured or ill patients to see mixed pictures of blood gas abnormality. For example, following a prolonged cardiac arrest there is likely to be a mixture of respiratory acidosis as a result of carbon dioxide retention and metabolic acidosis as a result of a build-up of lactic acid.

Arterial blood gases are also of use in the assessment of suspected pulmonary embolism. The alveolar–arterial oxygen gap (Table 2.12) can be calculated from the results of a blood gas analysis with the patient breathing air. A widened gap is suggestive of pulmonary embolism. However, this information should not be relied on alone to determine whether to discharge the patient or refer them for further investigation and treatment.

MICROBIOLOGY

In most clinical conditions presenting to emergency departments, treatment cannot be delayed for the results of bacterial cultures. Antibiotics are therefore often prescribed on the basis of an informed guess as to the nature of the causative organism and its sensitivity to antibiotics. This, however, should not deter the doctor from taking samples for microbiological analysis prior to treatment. This is particularly important in septicaemia as once antibiotics have been administered, subsequent attempts to identify the causal organism may be unsuccessful.

Diagnosis of infection may be made by examining samples such as urine or fluid aspirated from a joint. Previously urine microscopy and Gram staining was a common examination in the evaluation of abdominal pain. As near-patient testing has improved, the microscope has been replaced by quantitative analysis of the contents of the urine, including protein, blood, leucocytes and nitrite. These tests accurately predict the results of urine microscopy in that samples negative for protein, blood and nitrite are also clear on microscopy. Routine microscopy can therefore be omitted in these cases.

Microscopic examination of fluid aspirated from a joint is helpful in the diagnosis of inflammatory arthropathies. Gram staining may detect organisms giving the diagnosis of septic arthritis. More commonly non-specific inflammatory reactions are seen, although when crystals are seen in the joint fluid the differential diagnosis is narrowed down to one of the crystal arthropathies.

ELECTROCARDIOGRAPHY (ECG)

Most obviously, ECG is used in the differential diagnosis of chest pain. It cannot be over-stressed that whilst a positive ECG may be diagnostic, a negative ECG cannot exclude the presence of an ischaemic cardiac process. It is important, especially in the presence of continuing symptoms suggestive of myocardial infarction, that the ECG is repeated regularly.

A normal ECG does not exclude ischaemic heart disease.

Table 2.13: Indications for performing an electrocardiograph (ECG)

Chest pain
Undiagnosed dyspnoea
Palpitations
Collapse of unknown cause
Overdoses of cardioactive drugs
Electric shock

As with X-rays, many junior doctors have little experience in interpreting ECGs and errors are not uncommonly made. Many modern machines contain diagnostic software and interpret the reading but, similarly to an X-ray report, responsibility for correct interpretation of the investigation rests with the doctor treating the patient. If there is any doubt, a senior opinion should be sought.

On occasions cardiac disease can present occultly, especially in the elderly. It is therefore wise to have a low threshold for performing this relatively cheap investigation, which causes no untoward side-effects (Table 2.13). Other than the changes of cardiac ischaemia the ECG will also be helpful in diagnosing cardiac dysrhythmias and acute pericarditis. More rarely electrolyte disturbances, pulmonary embolism, hypothermia, drug toxicity and intracerebral haemorrhage may cause characteristic changes in the ECG.

NEAR-PATIENT TESTING

Modern technology has allowed the analysis of blood and urine to be taken to the patient's bedside. This may include haematological and biochemical analysis and blood gas analysis, though in most departments these tests are still performed in the laboratory. Urine testing is a simple investigation, which can be performed rapidly within the emergency department. As noted above, modern dipstick tests include an analysis of urinary nitrites and leucocytes and are highly sensitive in the diagnosis of urinary infection. A normal dipstick test is strongly predictive of a normal microscopic examination and essentially rules out lower urinary tract infection in the differential diagnosis of abdominal pain. Urine analysis is a vital component of the investigation of a pyrexial child, although

Table 2.14: Conditions detected by urine testing

Urinary tract infection
Ureteric colic
Diabetes mellitus
Trauma to the urinary tract
Genitourinary malignancy

collecting specimens from infants requires the use of a 'U bag' and an inevitable degree of contamination of the specimen.

A list of conditions in which urine testing plays an important role in diagnosis in the emergency department is given in Table 2.14.

More recently, bedside kits to allow testing for cardiac enzymes and D-dimers have become available and it is likely that the next few years will see these assume a major role in the early diagnosis and exclusion of acute coronary syndromes and venous thromboembolic disease in the emergency department.

OTHER INVESTIGATIONS

The pregnancy test may be helpful in the differential diagnosis of abdominal pain in women and the management of the complications of pregnancy, such as ectopic pregnancy. Tests are now available as kits, which can be used in the emergency department. These are extremely sensitive and give a positive result within a few days of the patient's first missed period.

In carbon monoxide poisoning, carboxyhaemoglobin levels are a valuable aid to diagnosis. The presence of raised carboxyhaemoglobin levels indicates that the patient has been exposed to carbon monoxide. However, the level does not correlate well with the patient's clinical condition as a result of variations in the duration of exposure, time and treatment since removal from the gas. It is not therefore used in determining the need for treatment, particularly hyperbaric therapy (see Chapter 15).

FURTHER READING

Royal College of Radiologists (1993) *Making the Best Use of a Department of Clinical Radiology*. RCR, London.

CHAPTER THREE

COMMUNICATION

- Introduction
- Communications with the ambulance service
- General practitioners

- Referring patients to colleagues
- Breaking bad news
- Communicating with the police

INTRODUCTION

An emergency department is a unique environment in which to practise medicine. In a short space of time a doctor needs to assemble all the pieces of information available to formulate a differential diagnosis of a patient's condition and plan investigation and treatment. Often the information required for diagnosis is not available from the patient and other sources such as paramedics, friends and relatives need to be interviewed. The expertise needed to provide optimal treatment is often only achieved by integrating the efforts of a number of professions, both medical and non-medical. The emergency department doctor is pivotal in this process of integration of those involved in the past, present and future care of a patient and it is only by effective communication that optimal care will be achieved.

COMMUNICATIONS WITH THE AMBULANCE SERVICE

Good patient care requires a smooth transition of responsibility from prehospital care to the hospital environment. Local arrangements between the ambulance service and hospital will vary; however, some system for notifying the hospital in advance of the arrival of a seriously ill or injured patient is essential. This allows the hospital to assemble the personnel and resources needed to treat the patient. Most obviously this will consist of a trauma team.

In most areas, messages from the ambulance crew will be relayed through the ambulance control room. Unfortunately, this often leads to distortions and delays. It is preferable and increasingly common to have the ability to talk directly to the crew via radio or a cellular phone. Experimental schemes of transmitting video pictures back to the hospital are being assessed.

When the patient arrives in the department, the ambulance crew will often be under pressure to hand over the patient rapidly in order to release themselves for another call. The crew will have important information on the circumstances in which the patient was found, changes in their condition during the transfer to hospital and the treatment they have received. Failure to obtain that information early and effectively will lead to it being lost. The crew should also provide a patient report form with details of vital signs and the treatment administered (Fig. 3.1).

GENERAL PRACTITIONERS

The general practitioner (GP) provides the patient with access to medical services on a continuing basis. Communication is a two-way process and therefore consists of receiving and obtaining information from GPs about the patient and feeding back the results of consultations and investigations to help achieve continuity of care. The GP is often

Date: / /	Call time :	**East Anglian Ambulance NHS Trust**
Location	Arrival :	IN CONFIDENCE EAAT/ T 47444
	Depart :	**TRAUMA Patient Report Form**
	Hospital :	

Call sign:	Attendant:	Address
PATIENT M / F	Surname	Forename

d.o.b / /   **GP:**

Relevant Medication / PMH

Allergies

ASSESSMENT   Incident type:

History / Mechanism of Injury

Call Type:	□ 999	□ GP Urgent

Bystander Action:

Drugs □ Entonox   □ Failed Venous Access

Type	Dose	Box #	Route	Time
				:
				:
				:
				:
				:

Secondary Survey Injuries

If RTA:	□ Pedestrian	□ Motor cyclist
(√/×/?)	□ Driver	□ Front/ Rear Passenger
□ Airbag	□ Helmet	□ Seat belts

If Trapped, for how long:

□ Unconscious prior to arrival   □ Vomited
□ Fitting prior to arrival   □ Alcohol

PRIMARY SURVEY & INTERVENTION

Airway	□ Clear	□ Obstructed
□ OP	□ Nasal	□ ET Tube
□ Surgical	□ Suction	Oxygen _____%
C-spine	□ Normal	□ Manual Control
Breathing	□ Adequate	R □ Sounds □ L
	□ Ventilated	□ Chest drain
Circulation/	□ External	□ Possible Internal
Bleeding	□ None/ slight	□ Radial pulse (√/×)

IV fluid type:

L size:_____	Vol.	Time	Vol.	Time
R size:_____		:		:
Disability	□ A	□ V	□ P	□ U

C#   Closed Fracture
O#   Open Fracture   L   Laceration
B   Burn (shade area)   A   Abrasion
F   Foreign body   C   Contusion

□ ECG attached   Arrhythmia:

COMMENTS

SECONDARY SURVEY & MANAGEMENT

Time	:	:	:
Pulse (rate / regularity)			
Respiratory Rate			
Blood pressure	/	/	/
SpO$_2$ / Cap. refill (√/×)			
Response (GCS) Eye	__ /4	__ /4	__ /4
Verbal	__ /5	__ /5	__ /5
Motor	__ /6	__ /6	__ /6
Total	__ /15	__ /15	__ /15
or Response (AVPU)	A V P U	A V P U	A V P U
Trauma score			
Pain score	__ / 10	__ / 10	__ / 10
Skin colour / texture			
Skin temperature			

Pupils	R	L	R	L	R	L
Dilated	O	O	O	O	O	O
Normal	o	o	o	o	o	o
Constricted	°	°	°	°	°	°
React? (√/×)	□	□	□	□	□	□

GP letter attached □
Condition unchanged during transport □

PATIENT DISPOSAL		Time :
Hospital:	Other:	

Immobilisation

□ Spinal Board   □ Ex. Device   □ Frac straps
□ Box   □ Cx. Collar   □ Traction
□ Traction   Other:

Signed
By Staff Nurse / Midwife / Doctor on behalf of hospital

Signed
By Paramedic / Technician of EAAT

© A Ercole, SJ Butler EAAT 1998

Figure 3.1: An ambulance report form.

a vital source of information on the patient's past medical history, current medications and the circumstances surrounding an illness. Therefore it is often important to talk to the GP when one of their patients presents to the department.

Feeding back information to the GP can be achieved by a number of routes. Many modern emergency department computer systems have the facility to generate a letter giving brief details of the presenting complaint, investigation and treatment. For more complex cases this may be insufficient and further detail may need to be added to the letter or the GP contacted directly by telephone.

REFERRING PATIENTS TO COLLEAGUES

The ability to make a good referral to a colleague from a different specialty is a vital component of the skills needed to work effectively in an emergency department. Doing this well involves giving an impression that you are competent and have assessed the patient thoroughly. The information needed should be communicated succinctly and fluently.

Few people have the ability to summarize a complicated case instantly without at least a few moments of preparation. It is therefore always worth mentally rehearsing the way the case is to be presented. The referral should be succinct but comprehensive. A framework for this is given in Table 3.1. The referring doctor in particular must be clear about what is required of the doctor

receiving the referral (advice, an opinion or admission) and why that is necessary.

The time of the referral, and the name of the doctor to whom the patient has been referred, must be recorded in the notes; the grade of doctor should also be recorded.

BREAKING BAD NEWS

Death, major injury and serious illness can strike randomly and unpredictably. The relatives of patients called to an emergency department are often placed in a situation for which they are completely unprepared. Communicating with relatives is an important part of managing a patient but the suddenness and often tragic nature of the events presents special difficulties. Few doctors receive adequate training in breaking bad news. It is an unpleasant task for the medical and nursing staff but one that if done badly will add further distress both to the relatives and to the inexperienced staff responsible. Although there is no single correct way to perform this task, a number of general points should be considered (Table 3.2).

The relatives of deceased or seriously ill patients will usually be shown to a specially designated room where a senior nurse will look after them. This nurse will therefore have had some opportunity to get to know the relatives and assess their expectations.

Table 3.1: Framework for a referral

Introduce yourself and confirm the identity of the person you are talking to
Tell them what you want (advice, to see the patient, admit the patient)
Identify the patient and their age
Presenting complaint
Significant past history
Positive examination findings
Relevant results of investigation
Treatment given in emergency department
Diagnosis or differential diagnosis
What further investigation or treatment is required

Table 3.2: Breaking bad news

Prepare yourself, remove bloodstains, gloves, aprons and masks
Confirm the identity of the patient and the relatives
Find out about the relatives from the nurse who has sat with them
On entering the room position yourself close to the next of kin and at eye level
Introduce yourself, establish eye contact with everyone
Confirm the identity of the relatives and friends
Be honest and unambiguous. Clarify and repeat the news if necessary
Allow time for the relatives to react
Be empathic and concerned. Touch or hold the relative
Do not rush
Make yourself available for further questions later
Contact the coroner and GP

Table 3.3: Reactions to bad news

Denial
Anger
Guilt
Distress
Neutrality
Acceptance

Prior to entering a room to speak to relatives in these circumstances it is important to find out to whom you are to speak and what they may already know about their relative's condition. It is wise to sit close to the nearest relative and make eye contact whilst introducing yourself and confirm that you know their relationship to the patient. In such a stressful situation the relatives will only take in a small proportion of what is said to them. The patient's current condition should be explained early and in unambiguous terms. Use phrases such as 'I am sorry your husband has died'. Avoid using euphemisms such as 'we've lost him' or 'he has passed on'. These only produce periods of uncertainty and confusion. Similarly, trying to support the relatives by offering ideas such as 'at least he is at peace now' is inappropriate. The relatives feel only their loss and there is rarely any consolation in bereavement.

The initial intensity of the relatives' reaction is rarely what is anticipated and any one of a number of emotions may occur, alone or in combination (Table 3.3). Guilt, that some omission on the part of the nearest relative has resulted in the tragedy, is a common emotion and it is usually appropriate to provide reassurance that nothing would have changed the outcome. There will often also be questions about the mode of death and whether the patient was aware or suffered. In most emergency department situations with sudden death, it is often the case that the patient experienced no prior distress.

Always give the impression of having plenty of time, even if you do not. Allow periods of silence for the relatives to absorb the news and produce questions. Be prepared for questions concerning the possibility of organ donation and the procedures that are to be followed with respect to investigation of the death.

COMMUNICATING WITH THE POLICE

Emergency department work inevitably regularly interfaces with that of the police. Historically, the two have enjoyed good relations but on occasions this is strained by a perception that the police are trying to breach patient confidentiality and that the hospital is obstructing the police. The doctor's first duty is to his or her patient and confidentiality must be maintained, except in specific defined circumstances (Table 3.4). Following a road traffic accident the police are entitled to be told the patient's name, address, age and a brief description of the injuries and their consequences. In the event of the police requesting information in the investigation of a serious criminal offence (e.g. rape, murder) the matter should be dealt with between senior doctors and police officers.

Table 3.4: Revealing patient details to the police

With the patient's consent
Following a road traffic accident
When a patient is suspected of a serious criminal offence

APPROACH TO THE TRAUMA PATIENT

INTRODUCTION

Trauma is the leading cause of death in the first four decades of life. It is also responsible for maiming many young people in their most productive years. Historically, severe trauma has been poorly managed in the UK. When the Royal College of Surgeons of England studied trauma deaths in 1988 they found that up to a third of deaths were potentially avoidable and produced a series of recommendations for the future development of trauma management (Table 4.1). Patients were dying as a result of easily treatable conditions such as airway obstruction and tension pneumothorax, or because the presence of haemorrhage was either not recognized or inadequately treated.

In the 10 years since the report on the management of major injuries, the treatment of the severely injured has improved. One component of this improvement has been the introduction to the UK from America of the Advanced Trauma Life Support (ATLS) course. This teaches a didactic prioritized system of assessment and resuscitation of the patient in the first hour after injury (Table 4.2) which has now become the benchmark for the early management of patients with severe injury in the UK.

THE ATLS APPROACH

The assessment and management of the trauma patient requires the rapid identification and correction of life-threatening injuries. Attention is focused first on those conditions that are most rapidly fatal. Therefore the airway is opened and protected whilst immobilizing the cervical spine. Major life-threatening breathing abnormalities are identified and corrected. The presence of shock is sought, any bleeding controlled and intravenous fluid infusions started. A brief assessment of neurological status is performed and the patient is fully exposed but protected from hypothermia. This initial sequence of assessment and management is known as the primary survey (Table 4.3). The primary survey is regularly revisited to ensure that any interventions performed have corrected the problem and that there has been no deterioration.

The aim of the primary survey is to identify and correct immediately life-threatening conditions.

Once immediately life-threatening conditions have been treated and resuscitation commenced, a more detailed secondary survey is carried out to detect all the patient's injuries, no matter how

Table 4.1: Recommendations for the development of trauma services

Multidisciplinary team approach to the
  management of major injury
Increased consultant involvement in patient
  management
Improved training for ambulance crews
Adoption of Advanced Trauma Life Support
  courses
National audit of trauma outcome

Table 4.2: Assessment and management of the trauma patient

Primary survey
Resuscitation
Secondary survey
Re-evaluation
Transfer
Definitive care

Table 4.3: The primary survey

Airway with cervical spine control
Breathing
Circulation with haemorrhage control
Disability
Exposure and environment

minor. Even relatively minor injuries can result in life-long disability if not recognized and treated early. Assessment may be rendered difficult by the presence of other injuries or the use of drugs or alcohol that impair the patient's ability to co-operate with examination. Early screening radiographs are taken and monitoring devices used to give objective estimates of the patient's progress.

Primary survey and resuscitation take place simultaneously.

ORGANIZING A RESPONSE

The most critical period for any severely injured patient is the first 60 min from the time of injury – the so-called 'golden hour'. Within this time the patient should receive initial management at the scene of the accident from paramedics, be transported to a hospital capable of dealing with their injuries and be receiving definitive treatment for life-threatening injuries. The shorter the time to the initiation of definitive care, the better the survival rate.

The optimal management of the multiply injured patient is a complex task that requires a co-ordinated approach from a team of senior doctors experienced in the management of these patients. These cases should not be managed by unsupervised junior doctors. Most hospitals in the UK now have a formal response to trauma in the form of a trauma team. This usually consists of emergency, orthopaedic, anaesthetic and general surgical specialists who are summoned to the resuscitation room when a severely injured patient is being received or is expected. In the hospitals achieving the best results in trauma care, consultants are directly involved in providing this care at all times. At its most effective the trauma team works to a predefined plan of assessment and management under the control of a team leader.

Preparation for the arrival of the patient should involve the arrival of the members of the trauma team in the resuscitation room (Table 4.4). On the basis of information from the ambulance service it is often possible to anticipate which specialties will be required. A designated team leader should allocate areas of responsibility to each member of the trauma team but will ideally remain a 'hands-off' observer who directs the process of care. Other technicians and specialties may need to be alerted. Specifically, the radiographer, radiologist and the blood-bank technician will usually be required.

Each member of the team must take precautions to protect themselves against the spread of viral diseases such as human immunodeficiency virus (HIV) and hepatitis from the patient by blood contamination (Table 4.5). There is no time when a patient is received to attempt to assess the risk they pose to carers, and it should therefore be assumed that they carry viral diseases and appropriate protective precautions should be taken. Each member of a trauma team must be immunized against hepatitis B. All staff should also, as a minimum, wear gloves, an apron and eye protection and should be responsible for the safe disposal of any sharps they use.

Table 4.4: Composition of a trauma team

Emergency consultant, registrar and SHO
Orthopaedic consultant and registrar
General surgery registrar
Anaesthetic registrar or consultant

Table 4.5: Viral diseases with potential for transmission to healthcare workers

Hepatitis B
Hepatitis C
Human immunodeficiency virus (HIV)

THE PRIMARY SURVEY

The primary survey is a prioritized process of assessment and resuscitation. Once identified, each immediately life-threatening abnormality must be corrected before moving on with the assessment. If only a single doctor is present this is done sequentially; however, with multiple doctors acting under the control of a team leader, the process is accomplished more rapidly simultaneously.

> Any immediately life-threatening abnormality must be corrected before assessment continues.

AIRWAY WITH CERVICAL SPINE CONTROL

An occluded airway will kill a patient in 3 min. Some techniques used to open the airway also move the cervical spine. Although cervical spine injury is present in only a small percentage of patients with major injuries, movement of the cervical spine in opening the airway may damage a previously intact spinal cord rendering the patient paraplegic or quadriplegic.

The safest policy is therefore to assume a cervical spine injury is present in any patient until it can be proved otherwise. Therefore the cervical spine is immobilized, initially by manual in-line immobilization (Fig. 4.1) and later by a semi-rigid cervical collar with sandbags and head tapes (Fig. 4.2). This immobilization is left in place until a suitably experienced clinician, often with the help of a

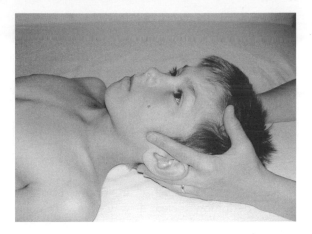

Figure 4.1: Manual inline cervical immobilization. Note that the ears are not covered in order to preserve the patient's hearing.

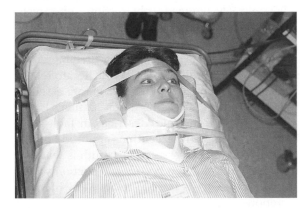

Figure 4.2: Cervical immobilization with collar sand bags and tape.

complete set of adequate X-rays, clears the cervical spine as normal.

> Adequate cervical control requires a well-fitting semi-rigid cervical collar, sandbags and head tapes. Manual in-line immobilization may be used instead of any or all of the above.

All traumatized patients should be given oxygen at the maximal concentration possible from the earliest point in their treatment. This requires the use of a well-fitting oxygen mask with a reservoir bag and the wall oxygen supply at $15 \, \mathrm{l \, min^{-1}}$. Oxygen masks without reservoir bags and devices such as nasal prongs are inadequate.

Assessment of airway patency is accomplished by speaking to the patient and then listening to air

Table 4.6: Airway management techniques

Removal of foreign bodies and suction
Simple airway manoeuvres – chin lift, jaw thrust
Airway adjuncts – oropharyngeal airway,
                         nasopharyngeal airway
Definitive airway – orotracheal intubation,
                      nasotracheal intubation,
                      needle or surgical
                      cricothyroidotomy

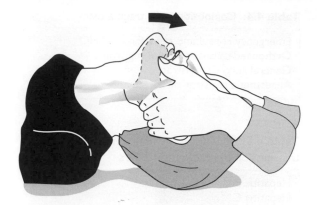

Figure 4.3: The jaw thrust manoeuvre.

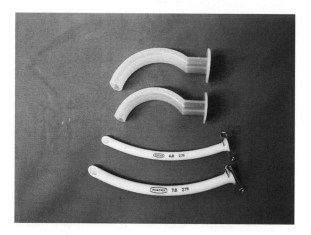

Figure 4.4: Oropharyngeal (Guedel) and nasopharyngeal airways.

movement. A patient who can vocalize normally has, by definition, a clear airway. One with noisy breathing has a partially obstructed airway and one who is not breathing may have a completely obstructed airway. Failure to manage airway obstruction adequately is a result of either failure to recognize that a problem exists or failure to relieve a recognized obstruction effectively. Although it is always wise to involve an anaesthetist in the management of airway problems, there may be some delay in their arriving. Once an airway problem is recognized, action to relieve it must start immediately. It is therefore essential that every doctor managing trauma patients is able to perform the techniques described in Table 4.6.

Initially, simple interventions are used and the response to these assessed. The mouth is searched for obstructing foreign bodies and suction with a Yankauer catheter is used to remove any blood or secretions.

If this fails to correct the airway obstruction simple airway manoeuvres are tried. The commonest cause of airway obstruction is the tongue occluding the airway by falling on to the posterior pharyngeal wall. Simple airway manoeuvres are designed to pull the tongue away from the pharyngeal wall. This is done by lifting the mandible forwards. Since the tongue is attached to the mandible the tongue will also be lifted forwards. Of the two techniques available jaw thrust is preferred, as it tends to move the cervical spine less than the chin lift manoeuvre. In jaw thrust fingers are placed behind the angles of the mandible and the jaw is pushed upwards. The patient is then reassessed to see if the manoeuvre has corrected the airway obstruction (Fig. 4.3).

If simple airway manoeuvres are unsuccessful or obstruction recurs when the airway manoeuvre is released, then the next step is to try simple airway adjuncts. These are the oropharyngeal (Guedel) and

nasopharngeal airways (Fig. 4.4). The former is more widely used though the latter is gaining increasing popularity.

The oropharyngeal airway is designed to fit over the tongue and keep the tongue off the posterior pharyngeal wall. It will normally only be of benefit in maintaining an improvement produced by one of the simple airway manoeuvres. The airway needs to be sized by measuring the length of the airway against the distance between the incisors and the angle of the jaw (Fig. 4.5). There are two methods of insertion. Most commonly the airway is initially inserted with its convex aspect towards the tongue. When the soft palate is reached it is rotated through 90° and inserted fully. Alternatively, the tongue is held down with either a tongue depressor or a laryngoscope blade and the airway inserted directly with its convex surface

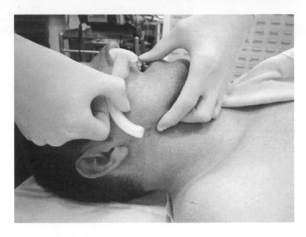

Figure 4.5: Sizing an oropharyngeal airway.

towards the palate. The airway may not be tolerated by patients who retain their protective airway reflexes and may provoke vomiting.

The nasopharyngeal airway is gaining popularity as it is better tolerated by patients and is particularly useful in cerebrally irritated patients when the mouth cannot be opened. However, its use should be avoided in patients with potential frontal basal skull fracture, where there is a risk of the airway passing through the cribriform plate into the cranium. Similarly to the oropharyngeal airway, it works by keeping the tongue off the posterior pharyngeal wall. The airway is sized by comparison with the nostril. The airway is lubricated and inserted into the nostril that appears largest. It should be remembered that the air passage through the nose passes directly backwards and not upwards to the nasal bridge. The airway is therefore passed gently backward using its curve to pass over the upper aspect of the soft palate and into the oropharynx. Prior to insertion, a safety pin is passed through the flange of the airway to prevent it being aspirated. Once inserted, the airway is reassessed to determine if the intervention has relieved the obstruction.

The next stage of the hierarchy of airway intervention is the provision of a definitive airway. This involves the insertion of a (usually cuffed) tube into the trachea. This may be carried out through the anatomical routes of the mouth (oral endotracheal intubation) or the nose (naso-endotracheal intubation). Alternatively, it may be necessary to surgically create a passage into the trachea. The recommended technique for this is cricothyroidotomy, which may involve the passage of a cannula

(needle cricothyroidotomy) or a tube (surgical cricothyroidotomy) through the cricothyroid membrane.

The commonest route for insertion of a definitive airway is oral endotracheal intubation. This often requires the use of muscle relaxant drugs by someone experienced in their use (usually an anaethetist) but on occasions it may be desirable to intubate the trachea in a deeply unconscious patient prior to the arrival of an anaesthetist. The technique is best learnt from an anaesthetist in theatre, having gained some familiarity with the equipment and technique by using an intubation manikin.

Naso-endotracheal intubation in trauma is performed blind in that the larynx is not visualized with a laryngoscope during the procedure. It has the advantage of causing less movement of the cervical spine and being better tolerated by patients who have not been anaesthetized. The tube is directed towards the laryngeal inlet by listening to the sounds of the patient's spontaneous respiration at the tip of the tube. Although there are many enthusiasts for this technique who successfully utilize it in the USA, it has failed to gain popularity in the UK and should not be practised by non-anaesthetists.

The surgical techniques for inserting a definitive airway are used when the airway cannot be opened by other means. This therefore often follows a failed attempt at endotracheal intubation. It is particularly useful when the larynx cannot be identified on laryngoscopy, as in major maxillofacial trauma, or when a tube cannot be passed through the laryngeal inlet, as in severe inhalation burns.

NEEDLE CRICOTHYROIDOTOMY

The simple technique of passage of a large-calibre intravenous cannula through the cricothyroid membrane into the airway allows the supply of some oxygen (Fig. 4.6). This is carried out by attaching the cannula to a wall oxygen supply by a piece of oxygen tubing. By cutting a side hole in the oxygen tubing and covering the hole for 1 s and uncovering it for 4 s, jet insufflation (but not ventilation) is performed. This buys time until an airway can be formally established. Although oxygen is insufflated, relatively little expiration of carbon dioxide occurs and the patient becomes increasingly hypercapnic.

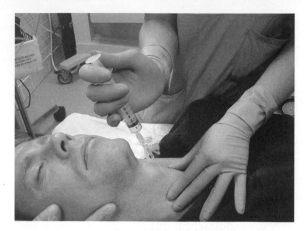

Figure 4.6: Needle cricothyroidotomy.

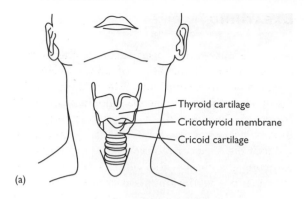

(a)

It is essential to remember that *needle* cricothyroidotomy will be ineffective when the threat to the airway is from major haemorrhage from facial injuries.

SURGICAL CRICOTHYROIDOTOMY

A more effective technique is to formally open the airway through an incision into the cricothyroid membrane. A tracheostomy tube (or even a size 6 endotracheal tube) can then be inserted through the incision to allow ventilation. In practice, this technique of surgical cricothyroidotomy often takes no longer than needle cricothyroidotomy. Formal surgical cricothyroidotomy will protect the airway from haemorrhage from above (Fig. 4.7).

CONFIRMING ENDOTRACHEAL TUBE PLACEMENT

Following insertion of a definitive airway it is vital to check the position of the tube (Table 4.7). Malpositioning of the tube in the oesophagus will rapidly result in hypoxia and death. Visualizing the tip of the tube passing through the vocal cords is an important component of this assessment. The chest movements should be assessed and the thorax auscultated to ensure equal air entry on both sides. Passage of the endotracheal tube too far through the vocal chords is most likely to intubate the right main bronchus which lies more vertically than the left. Unequal air entry is suggestive of

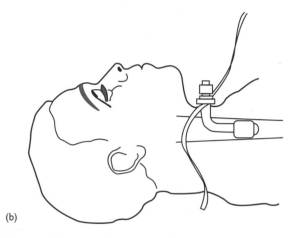

(b)

Figure 4.7: Surgical cricothyroidotomy.

Table 4.7: Confirming endotracheal placement

Auscultate over the lung apices and in the axillae
Auscultate over the epigastrium
Check for equal chest expansion
Apply end-tidal carbon dioxide detector

either endobronchial insertion of the tube or intrathoracic pathology. The endotracheal tube should be attached to an end-tidal carbon dioxide monitor. The presence of carbon dioxide in the expired gases is a strong indicator of correct tube placement. If a chest X-ray is subsequently taken, this can also be used to check that the tube has not inadvertently been inserted into the right or left main bronchus. Pulse oximetry will also give an objective assessment of the state of oxygenation and, following insertion of a definitive airway and ventilation with high concentrations of oxygen, saturation should be near 100%.

BREATHING

After the airway has been secured, attention is turned to the identification of immediately life-threatening chest conditions. Major chest injuries result in both hypovolaemia and hypoxia until corrected. The immediately life-threatening conditions are recognized by clinical examination without the need for radiology. The technique for assessing the chest is the same as in any clinical examination, but the limitations imposed by carrying out the examination in a noisy environment with a patient who is often unable to co-operate are accepted. The first stage is to look at the visible thorax for wounds, bruising and abrasion, and to assess the presence and symmetry of chest movement. Paradoxical respiratory movement suggestive of flail chest may also be seen. Palpate the chest for surgical emphysema and the position of the trachea. The chest is then percussed and auscultated for breath sounds and heart sounds. Added information may be obtained from looking at the jugular venous pulse.

The six immediately life-threatening conditions that may be detected and need treatment in the primary survey (Table 4.8) are described elsewhere. The methods of treatment are usually simple and consist of decompressing the pleural or pericardial spaces with either a chest drain or a needle, administering supplemental oxygen and initiating fluid replacement. The goal is the correction of hypoxia and hypovolaemia. Definitive treatment in the form of a thoracotomy to control bleeding may be necessary in a minority, but in most cases specialist involvement is not required.

CIRCULATION WITH HAEMORRHAGE CONTROL

Shock in a trauma patient is haemorrhagic until proven otherwise.

There are a number of causes of shock (Table 4.9) in a trauma patient, although it should be presumed that the cause is haemorrhage and hypovolaemia until proven otherwise. The failure to recognize a patient who is hypovolaemic as a result of haemorrhage and to provide adequate surgical control of bleeding was one of the main causes of avoidable

Table 4.8: Immediately life-threatening chest injuries detected in the primary survey

Airway obstruction
Tension pneumothorax
Open pneumothorax
Massive haemothorax
Flail chest
Cardiac tamponade

Table 4.9: Causes of shock in a trauma patient

Haemorrhagic
Non-haemorrhagic:
Cardiogenic
Neurogenic
Septic

death found in the Royal College of Surgeons report on the Management of Major Injuries. Again, assessment techniques in the primary survey are those of simple clinical examination. The pulse rate and volume are assessed. The adequacy of the peripheral circulation can be assessed by noting the capillary refill in the nail beds. More subtle factors such as changes in mental state also add to the diagnosis of shock, especially in its early stages when the more obvious clinical signs may be absent. Blood pressure is not an essential component of this assessment as it may only fall when the patient has already lost a third of their circulating blood volume. Hypovolaemia is better detected in its early stages before hypotension occurs, though the early signs are subtle. The physical signs of shock may be approximately correlated with the percentage loss of circulating blood volume (Table 4.10).

Increasing emphasis is placed on the control of haemorrhage in the management of shock (Table 4.11). While it is possible to normalize the haemodynamic variables by infusing large volumes of crystalloid or colloid solution, it is better to preserve the patient's own red cells by preventing further bleeding. The clinician must therefore formulate a differential diagnosis of potential sites of bleeding in the shocked patient and investigate appropriately. Haemorrhage control may be achieved simply by applying local pressure to a bleeding wound (the use of tourniquets or clips is frowned upon). However, the control of haemorrhage from a ruptured spleen needs a laparotomy and that from a major pulmonary vessel requires

Table 4.10: Classification of haemorrhagic shock

	Class I	Class II	Class III	Class IV
% Blood volume loss	0–15	15–30	30–40	>40
Pulse	<100	>100	>100	>100
Blood pressure	Normal	Reduced pulse pressure	Reduced	Reduced
Capillary refill	Normal	Delayed	Delayed	Delayed
Mental state	Anxious	Lethargic	Obtunded	Coma
Urine output	Normal	Reduced	Reduced	Anuric

Table 4.11: Locations of haemorrhage in the trauma patient

External
Internal:
   Thoracic
   Intra-abdominal/retroperitoneal
   Pelvic
   Multiple long bone fractures

a thoracotomy. The patient may therefore have to leave the resuscitation room to be taken to theatre for haemorrhage control as part of the primary survey.

Intravenous access is secured as part of the management of the circulation. The preferred method of venous access is with two wide-bore intravenous cannulae in the ante-cubital fossae. This has the advantage of providing high flow rates for fluid infusion without the complications associated with central venous access. Cannulation of the common femoral vein should be used if the upper limb veins cannot be used. If adequate veins are not accessed percutaneously, cutdown onto the long saphenous vein at the ankle (in an adult) or intra-osseous access (in a child) is attempted. Once access is gained, bloods are taken for routine analysis but most importantly to allow cross-matching of blood for transfusion. Central venous access has relatively little role as the catheters used are long and thin and therefore have a higher resistance to fluid flow. However, they may be useful for monitoring the heart's response to a fluid challenge in more complex shock situations.

The choice of intravenous fluid for infusion has until recently been controversial. However, there is now good evidence that crystalloid solutions such as Hartmann's solution or normal saline are preferable to synthetic colloids. The fluid should be warmed and given in boluses, following which the patient should be reassessed. Blood should be used early.

In most laboratories, blood will be provided as either fully cross-matched, type specific or O negative depending on the urgency of the request. O-negative blood (the universal donor) is available immediately from a fridge and is therefore used mostly when the patient is in extremis. Type-specific blood is of the same blood group as the patient's but the full battery of cross-matching tests has not been performed and the incidence of transfusion reaction, though still low, is therefore higher than for fully cross-matched blood. It is usually available in 10–15 min. Fully cross-matched blood usually takes 40–60 min to be available.

The diagnosis of non-haemorrhagic shock is based on a failure of the patient to respond to intravenous fluid infusion and the absence of an injury causing significant haemorrhage. In practice, it is not uncommon for shock in a multiply injured patient to have both haemorrhagic and non-haemorrhagic aetiology. A search should be made for an injury that might be associated with non-haemorrhagic shock, such as a cervical spinal cord injury or a precordial penetrating injury, which might be associated with a cardiac tamponade.

Neurogenic shock follows a cervical or high thoracic spinal injury that results in disruption of the thoracolumbar sympathetic outflow. There is therefore unopposed vagal action on the heart resulting in bradycardia and vasodilatation of the vascular tree as a result of loss of the sympathetic mediated vasoconstrictor tone. Central venous monitoring should be instituted to guide fluid infusion and any degree of hypovolaemia should be corrected first. Evidence of reduced organ perfusion is best judged by monitoring urinary output and, if present, should be corrected by the use of vasopressors by those experienced in their use.

Table 4.12: AVPU scale for level of consciousness

A	Alert
V	Responds to vocal stimulus
P	Responds to painful stimulus
U	Unresponsive

Table 4.13: The Glasgow Coma Scale

Eye opening	4	Spontaneous
	3	To voice
	2	To pain
	1	None
Motor response	6	Obeys commands
	5	Purposeful
	4	Withdrawal
	3	Flexion to pain
	2	Extension
	1	None
Verbal response	5	Alert and orientated
	4	Confused
	3	Inappropriate words
	2	Incomprehensible sounds
	1	None

Cardiogenic shock following trauma is usually the result of a pericardial tamponade or blunt myocardial injury. The treatment of these conditions is dealt with in Chapter 23. Septic shock as a result of injury does not occur until several hours later, and therefore will only be seen in an emergency department following late presentation or missed diagnosis.

DISABILITY (NEUROLOGICAL EVALUATION)

The mini-neurological examination in the primary survey consists of an assessment of conscious level and examination of the pupillary reactions. The use of the AVPU scale (Table 4.12) allows a rapid though rather crude assessment of conscious level. The Glasgow Coma Scale (Table 4.13) is more sensitive and provides a better baseline for subsequent re-evaluation. The pupillary sizes and their reaction to light are compared.

The objective of this is to provide a baseline assessment of neurological status against which subsequent assessments can be compared for improvement or deterioration. Specifically, the clinical signs of an expanding intracranial haematoma are sought.

The classic picture associated with the expansion of an intracranial haematoma is of deteriorating conscious level, an ipsilateral fixed dilated pupil and a contralateral hemiparesis. The latter two signs usually occur at a late stage when substantial deterioration in conscious level has already taken place. If good results are to be achieved by surgical evacuation for intracranial haematomata, the deterioration in the patient's condition should be detected before this.

EXPOSURE AND ENVIRONMENT

For assessment a trauma patient must be fully exposed by removing their clothes so that each part of them can be seen and assessed. However, this exposure renders them liable to hypothermia as they are cooled by the ambient temperature and occasionally by inadequately warmed intravenous fluids. Children are particularly at risk of hypothermia as a result of their high surface area to body weight ratio.

Precautions should therefore be taken and the patient covered with a warming blanket as soon as examination is complete. Intravenous fluids, particularly blood, should be given through a fluid-warming device.

At the end of the primary survey it is good practice to repeat the assessment paying particular attention to the effect of any interventions that have been carried out. If all is well the assessment can move on to a stage of further interventions and investigations. If, at any stage during the primary survey or subsequently, the patient shows signs of deterioration, a formal but brief reassessment of ABCDE is carried out until a cause is identified.

Any deterioration mandates reassessment of the whole primary survey from airway.

MONITORING, TUBES AND INITIAL RADIOGRAPHS

The procedures described in this section may be carried out at any point in the resuscitation, depending on the injuries found and the resources available.

Table 4.14: Monitoring severely injured patients

ECG
Pulse oximetry
Blood pressure – invasive or non-invasive
End-tidal carbon dioxide (if intubated)
Urine output
Central venous pressure

They are brought together at this point in that they are usually performed before the secondary survey is commenced.

The monitoring used on a severely injured patient (Table 4.14) should consist of a minimum of ECG, non-invasive blood pressure monitoring, pulse oximetry and recording of urinary output. The ECG will give an accurate reading of the pulse rate and rhythm. Non-invasive blood pressure monitoring gives regular readings that allow trends to be detected and responses to fluid boluses assessed. Care should be taken to avoid the temptation of relying too heavily on blood pressure readings, as the cardiovascular system can compensate well for blood loss and blood pressure may not fall till more than a third of the circulating volume has been lost.

The clinical detection of hypoxia is difficult. Many of the clinical signs are not present until late and are inconsistent. The pulse oximeter gives a continuous and non-invasive assessment of oxygen saturation. It measures the absorption of light by a capillary bed, estimating the ratio of oxygenated to deoxygenated haemoglobin in relation to the arterial pulse. The oxygen saturation is related to the arterial partial pressure of oxygen by a sigmoid curve that can be shifted by factors such as acidosis and temperature.

Although it gives important information there are a number of drawbacks to pulse oximetry. It is often difficult to obtain accurate readings from patients who are peripherally vasoconstricted by cold or hypovolaemia. Pulse oximetry will also give invalid readings in the presence of carbon monoxide poisoning. The oximeter does not give an index of ventilatory adequacy, and patients may be capable of maintaining good oxygen saturation despite inadequate ventilation if they are breathing high concentrations of oxygen. Ventilatory inadequacy may result in carbon dioxide retention, which causes raised intracranial pressure in the head-injured patient. Arterial blood gas analysis may therefore still be necessary and is desirable in many patients to confirm the information provided by the pulse oximeter and provide further data on pH and carbon dioxide levels.

The urinary output is a good way of assessing the perfusion of the capillary bed of a vital organ. As the patient bleeds, the kidneys are one of the first organs to experience a reduction in blood supply and oliguria results.

To assess urine output accurately a catheter should be inserted, having first confirmed by local and rectal examination that there is no evidence of urethral injury. Once the bladder has been emptied, timed collections into a urometer will allow an accurate assessment of urine output. Examination of the will also give diagnostic information on the presence of injury to the urinary tract. A urine output of more than $50\,\mathrm{ml\,h^{-1}}$ implies that the renal capillary bed is well perfused and that the patient has an adequate circulating blood volume. A lower output should raise the possibility of inadequate fluid resuscitation or continuing bleeding. Measures should be taken to investigate and correct these possibilities.

In an intubated patient monitoring of end-tidal carbon dioxide provides confirmation of successful tracheal intubation and alerts the team to the possibility of the tube being displaced. Many portable and fixed monitors have the capability to monitor carbon dioxide levels in the expired gases, and small disposable colorimetric devices are available which connect to the endotracheal tube.

In addition to the urinary catheter, a gastric tube should also be inserted. This provides diagnostic information on the presence of bleeding in the stomach. More importantly, it allows the stomach to be drained and therefore reduces the risk of vomiting and aspiration of gastric contents. In injured children, the stomach often distends with air and the presence of an acute gastric dilatation makes abdominal assessment difficult. Decompression of the stomach with a gastric tube is again beneficial. In any patient with a suspected midface or basal skull fracture the gastric tube should be inserted through the mouth. If the nasal route is used, the tube may be passed through the cribriform plate and into the cranial cavity.

The initial radiographs are taken in the resuscitation room and should not be allowed to interrupt the process of assessment and resuscitation. The pelvic

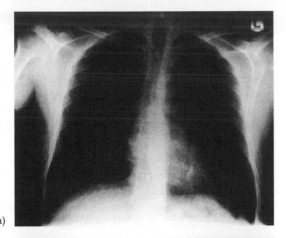

(a)

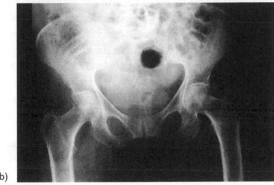

(b)

Figure 4.8: Primary survey X-rays. (a) Normal chest X-ray. (b) Normal pelvic X-ray.

and chest X-rays are important (Fig. 4.8) as they may detect significant injuries which require early management but which are difficult to detect clinically. A lateral cervical spine X-ray was formerly carried out at this stage, but as long as the patient's neck has been securely immobilized the findings on a lateral cervical spine film will not alter management in the first hour. The radiological assessment of the neck can therefore be safely deferred to a later time. Further radiography, particularly of extremity injuries, can also be delayed until the patient is sufficiently stable to leave the resuscitation room and all life-threatening injuries have been dealt with.

THE TRAUMA HISTORY

As in any medical assessment, the history plays an important role in diagnosis. In the multiply injured patient, life-saving interventions often have to be

Table 4.15: The AMPLE trauma history

A	Allergies
M	Medications
P	Past illnesses
L	Last ate and drank
E	Events and environment

Table 4.16: Events and environment

Blunt trauma:
Speed and direction of impact
Height of fall
Protective devices
Penetrating trauma:
Type of weapon
Direction of impact
Paramedic interventions
Exposure to cold, chemicals and radiation

made before the full history is known. Often the patient is unable to provide the history and many of its components, particularly relating to the mechanism of injury, will be obtained from witnesses to the accident and paramedics who attended the scene. The important components of the trauma history are easily remembered using the mnemonic AMPLE (Table 4.15).

The presence of allergies obviously affects the choice of medications administered to the patient. Many medications, particularly cardiac ones such as beta-blockers and diltiazem, can alter the cardiovascular response to haemorrhage. The medicines a patient takes can also give a clue as to the presence of intercurrent disease. Knowledge of a patient's past illnesses and operations can affect the way injuries are managed. Any major pre-existing illness increases the mortality rate following injury. The last meal eaten or the last drink is likely to be retained in the stomach, as gastric emptying is delayed following trauma. It is better to remove the contents from the stomach with a gastric tube than to attempt to suction them out of the lungs after aspiration has occurred.

The events and the environment in which the injury occurred are pieces of a jigsaw which when assembled with the examination and investigation findings allow us to gain a picture of all the patient's injuries and understand them in terms of the accident (Table 4.16). In blunt trauma, the energy and direction of the impact will help determine the injuries sustained. Protective devices such as seat belts and air bags may offset this. For example, in a frontal collision the driver may strike their head on and break the windscreen ('bulls eye the windscreen') and sustain facial fractures. They may also hit their chest on the steering wheel, causing a fracture of the sternum with myocardial contusion or an anterior flail chest. Finally, their knees are thrown against the dashboard, producing fractures of the patella and posterior fracture dislocation of the hip (Fig. 4.9). It is vital that assumptions about the likely injuries do not lead to other injuries being overlooked.

In penetrating injuries from a knife, the pattern of organ damage can be predicted by knowing the insertion point of the knife, how far it went in, and in what direction. In gunshot wounds the pattern of injury is less predictable. The path of the bullet is unpredictable. The type of weapon used may produce either high or low-energy transfer, and the severity of the wounds and tissue injury will be more severe in the former (see Chapter 29).

The environment in which the injury occurs is also important. A skier who falls and breaks their leg but is not found for several hours is likely to be hypothermic. Wounds sustained in agricultural surroundings are prone to infections such as gas gangrene and tetanus. More rarely, the victim of an accident may become contaminated with either chemicals or radioactivity. In these circumstances the doctors and nurses treating the patient should ensure that they do not become victims themselves. Patients should be decontaminated before treatment is initiated. In chemical incidents the help of the emergency services may be required to identify the substances involved and provide information on potential toxic effects and the treatment required.

THE SECONDARY SURVEY

Prior to conducting the secondary survey, all immediately life-threatening injuries should have been identified and treated. The secondary survey is a meticulous and methodical head-to-toe examination of the patient that should identify every injury. On occasions, the need to take the patient to theatre as part of the primary survey will result in the secondary survey taking place on an intensive care unit or a ward. It is vital that doctors working in these departments recognize this and conduct the necessary assessment. This will involve reassessment of many areas that have already been examined in the primary survey. A thorough neurological examination is also performed.

If an injury is missed at the initial presentation, delays in diagnosis lead to increased morbidity and mortality. Even relatively trivial injuries to the extremities can result in significant long-term problems if they are not identified and promptly treated. Further radiographs are performed as guided by the clinical examination. When required, analgesia should be given as intravenous opiates in small boluses titrated to achieve the desired effect. Consideration should also be given to tetanus and antibiotic prophylaxis.

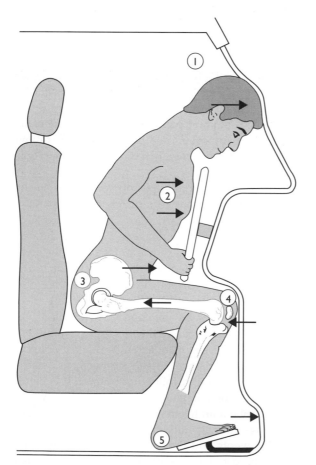

Figure 4.9: Frontal impact injuries. 1, Head and neck injuries; 2, chest injuries; 3, posterior hip dislocations; 4, knee injuries; 5, foot and ankle injuries with entrapment.

TRANSFER TO DEFINITIVE CARE

The decision to transfer a patient is based on the recognition that the patient's needs are greater than the capabilities of the initial hospital. Any transfer of a seriously injured patient is a time of high risk, whether the transfer is by ambulance to another hospital or simply along the corridor to an operating theatre, CT scanner or intensive care unit. During transfer, patients regularly experience periods of oxygen desaturation and hypotension. Displacement of endotracheal tubes, vascular access and other monitoring and treatment devices is common. Prior to any transfer all patients should have a protected airway, monitoring, and be accompanied by an experienced doctor with suitable equipment.

Most interhospital transfers in the UK are to neurosurgical units. In general, head-injured patients should be paralysed and intubated for the transfer and an experienced anaesthetist should accompany the patient. Any haemorrhage should be surgically controlled before the patient leaves the initial hospital, even if this means a laparotomy prior to the transfer. There must be direct consultation between the referring and receiving doctors.

OTHER CONSIDERATIONS

Major injury occurs randomly and relatives often arrive at hospital with little knowledge of the severity of the injury. The trauma team leader should ensure that the relatives are kept informed of the patient's progress, and as early as possible a senior doctor should discuss with them the nature of the injuries. In most cases the relatives will want to know a prognosis, though this is often difficult to make in the early stages. Where possible, and especially when the patient is a child, the relatives should be allowed access to the resuscitation room in the company of a nurse designated to support them and answer their questions. The relatives and friends may also be a useful source of information regarding the patient's past medical history.

Accurate documentation of the patient's assessment and treatment is vital, especially when care is transferred to another department or hospital. In many departments a trauma chart (Fig. 1.3) will be available which provides a suitable format in which to document the management of a seriously injured patient.

FURTHER READING

American College of Surgeons Committee on Trauma (1997) *Advanced Trauma Life Support*. American College of Surgeons, Chicago.

Driscoll, P., Gwinnutt, C. and Jimmerson, C. (1994) *Trauma Resuscitation – The Team Approach*. Palgrave, Basingstoke, Hants.

Royal College of Surgeons (1988) *Management of Major Injuries*. Royal College of Surgeons, London.

CHAPTER FIVE

WOUND MANAGEMENT

- Introduction
- Wound healing
- Principles of wound assessment and management

- Specific types of wound
- Further reading

INTRODUCTION

Approximately one in four emergency department attendances is for the treatment of wounds. Most wounds are of a minor nature but a few are life threatening and many may maim and disable. The correct management of wounds requires a careful assessment by history taking, examination and selective investigation, followed by the choice of appropriate treatment and, on occasions, continuing out-patient supervision. Inadequate management will encourage infection and poor healing, resulting in delayed healing, scarring and loss of function, thereby turning a minor injury into a major problem. Rarely, relatively minor wounds may cause life-threatening infections such as tetanus and gas gangrene.

This chapter outlines the principles of wound management by revising the process of wound healing and examining aspects of the history, examination and documentation of wounds. The general principles of investigation and treatment are then discussed, followed by specific discussion of the more difficult wound management problems that present to emergency departments.

WOUND HEALING

After haemostasis has occurred an acute inflammatory reaction takes place, with exudation and the migration to the wound area of phagocytic cells that remove necrotic tissue. Over the course of the next few days granulation tissue is formed in the wound and epithelial cells at the wound edges proliferate and start to cover the surface. Fibroblasts migrate into the granulation tissue and start to produce collagen. Over subsequent weeks and months the collagen becomes organized and the strength of the wound increases towards normal. The red scar fades to a white line as the vascularity of the wound returns to normal.

The main complication of wound healing is infection. The cause is usually multifactorial and will include contamination at the time of injury, delay in wound management, the presence of dead or devitalized tissue and inappropriate handling and closure of the wound. Infection results in delayed healing and the formation of unsatisfactory scars. Prevention is better than cure. Thoroughly toiletting a wound, handling the edges atraumatically and avoiding closure when the wound is contaminated are more effective than prescribing prophylactic antibiotics.

PRINCIPLES OF WOUND ASSESSMENT AND MANAGEMENT

In any injury the identification and treatment of life-threatening injuries and conditions should take precedence.

HISTORY

As with any injury, it is important to determine how, where and when a wound occurred. The mechanism of injury allows us to build up a picture of the types and magnitude of forces to which the patient has been exposed. It helps us to recognize which patients may have a serious underlying injury that may not be apparent on initial examination of the wound. Specific risks are associated with wounds occurring in certain environments, such as gas gangrene from agricultural injuries and the risk of leptospirosis in relation to wounds in sewer workers. Wounds sustained abroad may have greater significance, such as the potential for rabies from a dog bite in continental Europe. A prolonged time lapse before treatment of the injury will influence the infection risk and help determine whether it is justifiable to close a wound. In children, it is important always to be aware that a wound may not be the result of an accident. If the wound is not consistent with the explanation offered the matter must be pursued in line with local child protection guidelines.

Factors in the general medical history may influence the treatment of wounds. Patients on steroids sustain wounds easily and heal poorly. Minor wounds in ischaemic or anaesthetic tissues such as diabetic feet may eventually lead to loss of the limb. It is important always to determine a patient's tetanus status and provide the appropriate immunizations. In prescribing medication and applying dressings, a history of allergy is also required.

Tetanus toxoid 0.5 ml deep IM injection.

EXAMINATION AND DOCUMENTATION

The wound should be carefully examined and the examination findings documented. This is particularly important in cases where the wound is the result of an assault, as the doctor may subsequently be expected to provide a statement for the police or even to appear in court. The examination should, where relevant, search for potential underlying injuries to tendons, major nerves, vessels and vital organs. The wound, its size and its position should be carefully described. Certain terms are particularly useful in the description of wounds

Table 5.1: Terms used in describing wounds

Wound	A full-thickness breach in the skin or mucosa
Incised wound	A wound caused by a sharp object such as glass or a knife
Laceration	A wound caused by a blunt object. The skin is torn rather than cut
Penetrating wound	A wound usually from a fine object with a fine path of subcutaneous injury

(Table 5.1). It is often helpful to record the examination findings as a diagram in the notes.

PROPHYLAXIS

Any wound can act as the portal for entry for tetanus. The most important factor in tetanus prophylaxis is adequate management of the wound, with cleaning, debridement, removal of foreign bodies and, on occasions, delayed closure. All patients with wounds must therefore have their tetanus immunity checked. If they are not tetanus immune or there is uncertainty regarding their tetanus status, action must be taken to protect them (Table 5.2). Certain wounds, particularly those in which there has been a delay in presentation, those containing devitalized tissue and foreign bodies and contaminated wounds, are at higher risk of producing tetanus.

Cleaning and debridement are the most important techniques for preventing wound infection.

General antibiotic prophylaxis for wounds should be considered but is needed only in a minority of cases. The routine use of depot penicillin preparations for wounds only encourages the development of antibiotic resistance and is no longer accepted practice. Again, the most important factor in wound infection prophylaxis is adequate care of the wound, especially avoiding closure of potentially infected wounds. In the emergency department the main indications for antibiotic prophylaxis are bite wounds (human or animal), an underlying minor fracture (such as distal phalanx) in patients where bacteraemia might lead to

Table 5.2: Tetanus prophylaxis

Tetanus-prone wounds are:	
More than 6 hours old	
Infected wounds	
Puncture wounds	
Contaminated wounds or those with devitalized tissue	
For tetanus-prone wounds:	
If last booster or completed course < 10 years	No action
If last booster or completed course > 10 years	Toxoid booster and immunoglobulin
If not immunized or status unknown	Toxoid course plus immunoglobulin
Clean wounds:	
If last booster or completed course < 10 years	No action
If last booster or completed course > 10 years	Toxoid booster
If not immunized or status unknown	Toxoid course

Toxoid booster is 0.5 ml of tetanus toxoid given IM
Immunoglobulin is 250 IU of human tetanus immunoglobulin given IM to a different site from toxoid
Toxoid course is three monthly injections of 0.5 ml of tetanus toxoid

Table 5.3: Indications for antibiotic prophylaxis for wounds

Bite wounds
Open fracture or joint injury
Patient at risk of bacterial endocarditis
Contaminated puncture wounds
Leptospirosis risk

endocarditis, and puncture wounds from contaminated sources which cannot be fully cleaned. These are dealt with in more detail in Table 5.3.

Certain specific circumstances may demand prophylaxis. People sustaining wounds whilst working in sewers or where there are rats are at risk of contracting leptospirosis. The appropriate antibiotic prophylaxis is penicillin. In animal bite wounds sustained abroad the need for rabies prophylaxis should be considered. Advice in these cases should be sought from a consultant in communicable diseases. For needlestick injuries local protocols are established for the prevention of hepatitis B and for HIV prophylaxis. An outline of these is given later in this chapter.

INVESTIGATIONS

Investigations in relation to wounds are largely focused on the detection of an underlying bone or joint injury or a foreign body in the wound. X-rays should be used to detect underlying bone injury based on the mechanism of injury and local examination findings when a fracture seems likely. It should be remembered that any fracture detected in proximity to a wound is presumed to be an open fracture and will usually require formal surgical treatment, although fractures of the distal phalanx are generally considered to be an exception. Any penetrating wound in proximity to a joint should raise the possibility that the wound has penetrated the joint. A risk of septic arthritis therefore exists. X-rays taken of the joint may show intra-articular air; however, if there is any clinical suspicion of penetrating joint injury the patient should be referred for exploration of the wound with possible debridement and lavage.

One of the commonest errors in wound management that often results in litigation for medical negligence is failure to detect a retained foreign body (Fig. 5.1). Foreign bodies are often easily detectable by careful examination and exploration of the wound. Any possibility of a radio-opaque foreign body in a wound should lead to a request for an X-ray. Glass, metal, crockery and painted wood or plastic are all potentially radio-opaque. Fragments of teeth may sometimes be found in bite wounds from small animals such as cats, although they may also rarely occur in dog bites and hand wounds sustained in punching an adversary in the mouth. Radiolucent foreign

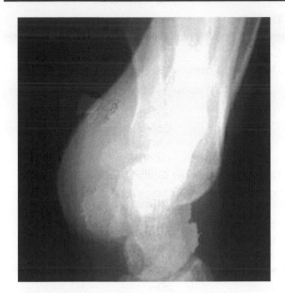

Figure 5.1: Radio-opaque glass foreign body in a hand wound.

bodies such as wood or thorns may be detected and localized with ultrasound.

Taking routine bacteriological swabs from a clean wound is of no value. If the wound is already infected a swab may be of value if the infection fails to respond to the first antibiotic prescribed; however, the organisms present in infected wounds are usually predictable and antibiotics can be prescribed rationally without the guidance of the microbiology department.

ANAESTHESIA

Adequate anaesthesia is an essential prerequisite not only to closing a wound but to allow adequate cleaning and debridement. It is certainly justifiable to anaesthetize a wound, or even in some cases the whole patient, with a general anaesthetic, just to clean a wound. Any combination of topical, locally and regionally injectable local anaesthetics or Entonox may be used. Local anaesthetics are covered elsewhere in this volume, but caution must always be exercised in relation to toxic doses. Local anaesthesia for large wounds is often limited by the maximum safe dose of the anaesthetic agent. Vasoconstrictors (such as adrenaline) or dilute solutions may be useful when large areas of wound have to be treated.

Maximum safe dose for lignocaine is 3 mg kg^{-1} body weight.

CLEANING AND DEBRIDEMENT

Debridement is the removal of devitalized tissue and foreign bodies from a wound. This is the most important step in adequate wound management, particularly in relation to the prevention of infection. All wounds presenting to emergency departments are by definition already contaminated. The patient should be placed in a room where there is adequate lighting and the appropriate surgical equipment should be used. Prior to commencing treatment the wound should be fully anaesthetized. The person treating the wound should be aware of the potential for transmission of infection from the patient and should take appropriate precautions.

Cleaning the wound generally requires the use of large volumes of fluid. This may be normal saline or even tap water. Disinfectant or antiseptic solutions such as povidone-iodine, chlorhexidine, cetrimide or hydrogen peroxide should be avoided as they are toxic to the cells. Using a syringe with a fine needle attached to irrigate a wound is a useful and effective technique, but spray may cause eye contamination and is a potential route of spread of viral infections.

Often simple irrigation with saline or water will be insufficient to remove all foreign material and contamination from the wound. Mechanical methods of cleaning then become necessary. In the first instance the use of a brush (e.g. a sterile toothbrush) may help, but often the only way of removing all contaminated material is to excise it using a scalpel. In some cases the most efficient way to debride an untidy contaminated wound is to excise the whole wound to healthy clean tissue, leaving incised edges which it may be justifiable to close primarily.

It is important to recognize the limitations of what is possible in an emergency department and to refer patients with large complex contaminated wounds for treatment by a surgeon in an operating theatre under a general anaesthetic. Extensive and prolonged explorations of wounds for foreign bodies should be avoided, especially in areas near major neurovascular structures. The treatment may do more harm than good. Blind probing of a wound for foreign bodies that have not been visualized or located on X-ray is almost invariably fruitless.

HAEMOSTASIS AND WOUND CLOSURE

Before wound closure is considered, active bleeding should have stopped. This will usually happen spontaneously. Elevation and the application of local pressure will aid the natural process of haemostasis. Following the application of pressure to a bleeding wound it should be left undisturbed for at least 5 min and the temptation to look and see if bleeding has stopped earlier should be resisted. Elevation of wounds, particularly on the extremities, is effective and is usually helped by a high arm sling or, for the lower limbs, by placing the patient on a trolley and tipping it to a head-down position.

If simple measures fail to control bleeding, other techniques, such as the injection of a local anaesthetic with a vasoconstrictor or the use of a haemostatic dressing, may help. If a single bleeding vessel is the source of blood loss, it can be isolated and tied off with an absorbable suture.

Prior to closing a wound, the balance of benefits and potential side-effects of closure should be assessed. If closure is not indicated at the time of presentation (primary closure), it is worth considering closing the wound several days (delayed primary closure) or even weeks later (secondary closure). Factors that should indicate and contraindicate primary wound closure are shown in Table 5.4. If there is any doubt regarding closure, it is always safer to leave the wound open, apply a dressing and bring the patient back for review 2 days later.

If a wound is suitable for primary closure, a suitable method then has to be chosen. There is currently a wide range of options and these are dealt with individually, although it is acceptable and good practice to combine more than one technique in a single wound.

Suture

Suturing is a surgical procedure and appropriate selection of wounds for suturing, good technique and aftercare are vital to achieving good healing with minimal scar formation. Prior to suturing the wound must be clean, dry, uncontaminated and anaesthetized. Almost always simple interrupted sutures are used. The commonly used suture sizes

Table 5.4: Factors influencing wound closure

Indications	Contraindications
Wound less than 6 hours old	More than 6 hours old
Clean	Contaminated
Incised. Tidy	Lacerated or contused. Untidy Contains devitalized tissue

Table 5.5: Preferred suture sizes and materials

	Adults	Children
Face	5/0	6/0
Scalp	3/0 absorbable	4/0 absorbable
Arm and forearm	4/0	5/0
Hand	5/0	5/0
Trunk	3/0	4/0
Lower limbs	3/0	4/0

Table 5.6: Guide times to suture removal

Face	5 days (4 for children)
Scalp	7 days if non-absorbable used
Arm and forearm	7 days
Hand	7 days
Trunk	10 days
Lower limbs	10 days (14 if extensor aspect of knee)

and materials used in each body region are shown in Table 5.5, and the lengths of time the sutures are left prior to removal are shown in Table 5.6.

For general skin use a monofilament, non-absorbable, synthetic suture such as nylon produces the best results. Braided non-synthetic sutures, such as silk, despite being easier to handle and knot, produce poorer scars and higher rates of wound infection. Absorbable sutures, such as catgut and Vicryl, are useful in tissues which heal well and where suture removal may be difficult, particularly in the scalp or the finger tips of children. Good technique requires the use of fine sutures with careful wound handling to minimize trauma to the wound edges and the minimum of tension. Only enough tension to appose the wound edges should be used. If apposition cannot be easily achieved it is better to delay wound closure until swelling has subsided and undertake delayed primary closure. Excessive tension on the sutures will promote further swelling and increase

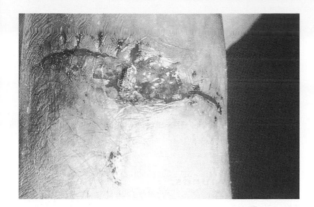

Figure 5.2: Poorly inserted sutures causing wound-edge ischaemia.

ischaemia at the wound edge, thereby delaying healing (Fig. 5.2).

Adhesive wound tapes

The use of wound tapes (Steristrips®) to close wounds is popular, as it does not require local anaesthetic. This technique is suitable for closing wounds on flat surfaces of the body where there is relatively little movement, such as the forehead. The tapes are also particularly useful where the skin is friable and the use of sutures would render the wound edge more ischaemic, as in pretibial laceration in an elderly person. They should not, however, be used in proximity to joints, and particularly not on the hands.

One risk of the use of wound tapes is that adequate cleaning and debridement will not be performed, as local anaesthetic is not used. This must be avoided and the wound anaesthetized if necessary for preparation. To achieve good adhesion of the strips the skin surrounding the wound must be dry, and the use of Benzoin Tincture (Tinct. Benz.) increases adhesion. The tapes are applied with the minimum amount of tension to achieve apposition of the wound edges, but with gaps between the tapes.

Tissue glue

The use of medical tissue adhesives has become increasingly popular, especially for the closure of lacerations in children. Good cosmetic results are generally achieved. Again local anaesthetic is not routinely used, but adequate wound preparation must still be performed. The wound edges are manually apposed and then glued together with interrupted spots of adhesive. Care needs to be taken around the faces of uncoopera-tive children to avoid overflow of the glue into the eyes. It is also easy for the doctor or nurse to become stuck to the patient! Tissue adhesives are not suitable for use near joints.

Staples

Surgical stapling guns have found some popularity, especially for the closure of scalp wounds. Again, they can generally be used without local anaesthesia. This is a quick but relatively expensive form of closure, especially as a staple remover needs to be provided.

Hair tying

A long-standing method of closing scalp wounds is to tie the hair across the wound to appose the edges. The knotted hair is cut off when the wound is healed. This is not recommended as a sole method of wound closure.

DRESSINGS

Some wounds, particularly those on the face or scalp, do not require dressing. If a dressing is to be applied there is a wide and bewildering array of materials to choose from. They are often better known by their trade names (Table 5.7). Local guidelines may be available to determine the choice of dressing. It is important to be aware that some patients are allergic to certain dressings and adhesives. In general the types of dressings used can be subdivided as follows.

Absorbent dressings and wound dressing pads

For most dry wounds all that is necessary is a dressing of sterile gauze or a low-adherence pad held in place by either a bandage or adhesive tape. Some dressings are manufactured from charcoal cloth to deodorize smelly wounds.

Tulle

These dressings are commonly used for a wide range of wounds to prevent adherence of the

Table 5.7: Types of dressings and their trade names

Absorbent dressings and wound dressing pads:	
Perforated film absorbent dressings	Melolin® Release®
Knitted viscose primary dressing	N-A dressing®
Charcoal cloth dressings	Actisorb Plus® Carbosorb®
Tulle:	
Paraffin gauze	Jelonet® Paratulle®
Chlorhexidine-impregnated tulle	Bactigras®
Framycetin-impregnated tulle	Sofra-Tulle®
Gels and colloids:	
Hydrogels	Kaltostat® Sorbsan®
Hydrocolloids	Granuflex® Comfeel®
Vapour-permeable films and membranes:	
Vapour-permeable adhesive film dressing	Opsite® Tegaderm®

wound to the dressing. In practice they will adhere to most moist wounds if left in place for more than a few days. The tulle is either impregnated with paraffin or medicated with chlorhexidine or framycetin. Generally, there appears to be little benefit in using the medicated tulle dressings, which can potentially provoke allergy and are significantly more expensive.

Gel and colloids

Although expensive, these dressings have achieved popularity because they can be left on moist wounds for periods of up to 7 days, thereby reducing the costs associated with regular redressing. They absorb some moisture from the wound to form a gel. They are thought to promote healing by maintaining a moist environment whilst absorbing excess fluid from the wound.

Vapour-permeable films and membranes

These are transparent and have the advantage of allowing the wound to be monitored in a sterile environment.

TYPES OF WOUND AND USE OF DRESSINGS

Other than recent wounds treated by primary closure, a number of more complicated wound management situations can occur, and with the advent of a number of new dressings there are a variety of treatment options.

Infected wounds

These require local cleaning and debridement of any residual necrotic or foreign material. A bacteriological swab may be helpful if at review the wound has not responded to the first-choice antibiotic. Gel and colloid dressings can absorb wound exudate and are easy to remove. Charcoal cloth-based dressings have the advantage of reducing the unpleasant smells from the wound.

Epithelializing wounds

Wounds undergoing epithelialization need an appropriate environment to encourage healing. Infrequent dressing changes will lead to conventional dressings drying out and, on removal of the dressing, avulsion of the healing cells. Hydrocolloid dressings provide a moist sealed area over the wound, do not adhere, and can be left intact between changes for up to a week.

Necrotic and sloughy wounds

Wounds containing dead tissue are best treated by the physical removal of slough and debridement. An alternative approach is to use a hydrocolloid to aid in the removal of slough and separation of necrotic tissue. The use of hypochlorite solutions is still defended by many but the toxicity of the solution to the tissues in the wound probably outweighs any benefit.

Granulating wounds

These require a moist environment but dressings should not damage the friable granulations when they are removed. Tulle dressings are acceptable, but again there are advantages to using a hydrocolloid.

Closed wounds

Such wounds have had their edges apposed, usually by suturing. In general a simple dry dressing is required to absorb any blood or exudate from the wound.

AFTERCARE

In order to achieve an optimally healed wound, appropriate aftercare should be provided and the patient needs to be warned of potential complications so that these can be recognized and treated early. In general, the wound should be elevated to minimize swelling. In the upper limb this requires a broad arm or high arm sling, in the lower limb advice to elevate the limb at home. Particularly with hand wounds, early movement should be encouraged unless an underlying nerve or tendon injury requires splintage. Advice or prescriptions for analgesic medication should also be provided.

Wounds closed by adhesive tapes should be kept dry and managed similarly to sutured wounds, with arrangements for follow-up and removal of the tapes. Following the use of tissue adhesives, any moisture will weaken and separate the adhesive leading to dehiscence. Eventually the glue will form into something similar to a scab and will separate when the underlying wound has healed.

If a dressing has been applied the patient needs to be advised when this can be removed or when it requires changing. Generally, the patient should be advised to return to the department if they are concerned about their progress.

SPECIFIC TYPES OF WOUND

PRETIBIAL LACERATIONS

Lacerations to the pretibial area are common and tend to occur predominantly in elderly people with relatively trivial injury. They are also commonly seen in patients on long-term steroid medication. The pretibial skin is fragile and because of its poor vascular supply heals poorly. The wounds often result in large flaps of poorly vascularized skin. Attempts to suture the flap back in place often result in varying degrees of skin necrosis

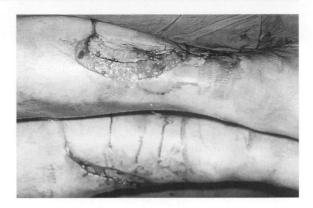

Figure 5.3: Pretibial lacerations.

from the wound edges back to the base of the flap, and secondary infection.

As in any wound, the object should be to aim for primary wound healing in as short a time as possible with the minimal inconvenience to the patient. As a result a large number of methods of treating pretibial lacerations have been described. The most aggressive approach is to excise the flap surgically and replace it with a split skin graft. This has the disadvantage of requiring an operation, although it can often be done under a local anaesthetic so that the patient can be rapidly mobilized. More commonly the flap is cleaned, with any underlying haematoma being removed, and the skin is replaced and held with adhesive wound tapes. In the latter case the skin is essentially being used as a split skin graft back on to its own donor site (Fig. 5.3).

If the skin flap is ragged, cannot be apposed and is obviously non-viable, the best option is to refer at initial presentation for the wound to be excised and grafted by a plastic surgeon before infection complicates treatment. If the skin is potentially viable, careful cleaning and apposition of the flap with wound tapes or tissue adhesive is tried. The patient can then be reviewed 3–5 days later and the viability of the skin flap reassessed. Suturing these wounds is contraindicated as the skin is often so friable that the stitches cut out or, if retained, increase the amount of skin necrosis at the edges of the flap.

HUMAN BITES

As with any animal bite wound, human bite wounds are liable to infection. However, whereas most patients will readily admit to having been bitten by a dog or a cat, the circumstances in which human bite wounds occur may leave the patient preferring to offer an alternative explanation.

Typically, the patient presents with a wound dorsal to the little finger metacarpophalangeal joint as a result of injury against their opponent's teeth. The wound commonly penetrates to the joint, disrupting the extensor tendon and the joint capsule. Fractures of the little finger metacarpal neck and retained foreign bodies in the form of fragments of the other person's teeth are also common. Untreated, the potential complications include soft tissue infection, septic arthritis of the metacarpophalangeal joint and osteomyelitis.

It is important to maintain a high index of suspicion that any wound dorsal to the knuckle joints might be caused by a human bite whatever the patient's explanation. An X-ray is valuable to rule out an underlying fracture or retained foreign body (tooth). Above all the wound must be thoroughly cleaned and debrided and then left open. Prophylactic antibiotics, usually co-amoxiclav, should be provided. The hand must be elevated in a sling and the patient brought back for review at approximately 2 days. If the patient presents late with established infection, admission for formal surgical debridement and a period of intravenous antibiotics should be arranged.

Other human bite wounds may occur. The pinna is a common target in rugby scrums. These should be treated as any contaminated wound, with thorough toilet and the use of prophylactic antibiotics followed by reassessment at approximately 2 days. Involvement of cartilage is an indication for specialist referral. With any human bite wound there is a small risk of the transmission of viral diseases such as hepatitis B and HIV. The advice of an expert on these diseases should be sought regarding prophylaxis.

ANIMAL BITES

Wounds from animal bites are common, and although dogs are the commonest source, may occur from a wide variety of animals. Similarly to the human bite, the predominant factor determining management is the risk of infection, particularly from atypical organisms such as *Pasteurella multocida*. Again, adequate wound debridement

and toilet is vital and the wounds should not be closed primarily, though delayed primary closure may be considered. The only exceptions to this rule are significant bite wounds to the face. In such cases it would be unreasonable for the wound to be left unrepaired, and therefore formal surgical excision under a general anaesthetic followed by wound closure is acceptable.

Antibiotic prophylaxis, usually with co-amoxiclav, will help reduce the rate of wound infection. It is not, however, needed in every case but must be used with wounds to the hand and where the wound has penetrated the dermis to the subcutaneous fat.

FACIAL LACERATIONS

Repair of facial lacerations requires meticulous technique to produce a scar that is cosmetically acceptable. Always be aware of the potential for injury to the major nerves of the face, such as the facial nerve, and other structures such as the parotid and lacrimal ducts. Lacerations involving the vermilion border of the lip, the nostril, the pinna or the eyelid need particularly accurate repair and should only be tackled by doctors with appropriate training. Fine synthetic non-absorbable sutures are used with care to restore tissues accurately in correct apposition. Wound healing is usually rapid and sutures can be removed early (5 days in an adult, 4 days in a child) to minimize scarring. In children with significant facial lacerations a general anaesthetic is often necessary for accurate wound closure.

HAND WOUNDS

A more detailed description of hand injuries is given elsewhere (see Chapter 27). The principal pitfalls with hand wounds are a failure to recognize a significant underlying nerve or tendon injury. Also infections, particularly from bite wounds, can enter spaces such as the tendon sheaths and produce damage that permanently restricts hand function. All hand wounds must be treated with care, with a low threshold for referral for exploration of wounds that may involve the tendons, nerves or vessels. If possible, the hand should be remobilized early, and if splintage is necessary it should be in the position of function of the hand

SCALP WOUNDS

The scalp is highly vascular and bleeds profusely when injured. Because of its good blood supply it heals well, with a low risk of infection. In assessing a scalp wound, the base of the wound should be gently palpated with a sterile gloved finger. On occasions a skull fracture will be discovered. If the laceration has penetrated the galea aponeurotica, this should be repaired separately with interrupted absorbable sutures. The scalp itself is best closed with an absorbable suture such as vicryl, as scalp sutures are notoriously difficult to find in hair when the time comes for removal.

PUNCTURE WOUNDS OF THE FOOT

Patients who have sustained injury by standing upon something often have painful injuries which appear on initial inspection to be trivial. It is important to recognize that a nail which has penetrated a foot through a patient's boot will inoculate into the soft tissues of the foot micro-organisms from the boot, sock and skin, in addition to what was present on its surface to start with. The nail may also carry with it foreign material from the boot and sock, and leave it within the foot. Puncture wounds are difficult to assess and without wide surgical exposure cannot be fully debrided. It is wise to prescribe a prophylactic antibiotic such as flucloxacillin, to check tetanus status and to arrange for review if the wound fails to settle. Extra care should be exercised when the foot is neuropathic.

NEEDLESTICK INJURY

These wounds rarely require specific treatment but there may be concern over the potential transmission of viral diseases to the injured person. Hepatitis B immunization is now provided to all health staff; however, it is increasingly common for an adult or a child to receive a needlestick injury from a needle disposed of in the community, usually by intravenous drug abusers. In these cases the source of the needle and therefore the hepatitis B and HIV status of its previous user are unknown. The risk of infection is low; however, active hepatitis B immunization on an accelerated schedule is usually provided following consultation with local public health specialists.

In the case of health staff, locally stipulated procedures for protection against hepatitis B and HIV should be followed. There is now good evidence that the low rate of infection with HIV from needlestick injury can be further lowered by providing combination antiviral therapy to those at risk. However, this is time dependent and therapy must be started with some urgency, though only when the injury has come from a known HIV-positive source. The therapy is potentially toxic and should only be started following consultation with local experts.

FURTHER READING

Simon, B. (1998) Principles of wound management. In *Emergency Medicine Concepts and Clinical Practice*, 4th edn (eds R. Barkin, P. Rosen, R. Hockberger *et al.*). Mosby, St Louis, pp. 382–96.

CHAPTER SIX

DEALING WITH CHILDREN

- Introduction
- History
- Examination
- Special tests
- Radiographs

- Analgesia
- Sedation
- Consent
- Further reading

INTRODUCTION

One-quarter of patients presenting to emergency departments are under 16 years old (Fig. 6.1). An average emergency senior house officer (SHO) will see more children in 1 week than an average paediatric senior house officer. However, most emergency department SHOs have no postgraduate training in paediatrics. Nationally, there are a number of dedicated paediatric emergency departments, which have a number of advantages over general emergency departments (Table 6.1).

There are also a number of disadvantages to dedicated paediatric emergency departments (Table 6.2).

The majority of children seen in British emergency departments are seen in general departments. However, general departments should ensure that child care is given a high priority (Table 6.3).

The purpose of this chapter is to outline an approach to children for staff who have no

Table 6.1: Advantages of dedicated paediatric departments

Staff become more familiar with the management of childhood emergencies.
Education and training of staff is focused on children.
Staff who are interested in children will gravitate to these departments, improving the quality of care.
The physical environment is designed to cope with children.
The resuscitation room is designed for children.
Children are protected from violent and abusive adult patients, who can often be found at general emergency departments.
Research is aimed at children's problems.

Table 6.2: Disadvantages of dedicated paediatric departments

Injured family members are separated for treatment.
It costs more money to maintain two emergency departments.
The local population must be aware of the distinction between the two departments.
Paediatric emergency departments are confined to areas with sufficiently high population densities to make their function viable.

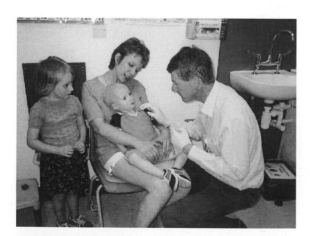

Figure 6.1: Dealing with a child in an emergency department.

Table 6.3: Facilities for children in a general emergency department

A separate area in the waiting room where children can play.
Senior medical and nursing staff with additional training and responsibility for children.
A separate resuscitation area, with appropriate equipment.
A dedicated social worker or health visitor to help with suspected non-accidental injury.

Table 6.4: Developmental milestones

90 % of children should be able to:	
Gross motor:	Lift head at 2 months
	Roll over at 4 months
	Walk well at 14 months
Fine motor:	Grasp a toy at 4 months
	Pincer grip a small object at 16 months
Language:	Say 'Dada' or 'Mama' at 12 months
Social:	Smile spontaneously at 5 months
	Indicate wants at 14 months

postgraduate training in paediatrics. Staff will find dealing with children easier if they have children of their own, or play with well children. The system of assessing children is exactly the same as for adults, namely history, examination, and special tests. However, the details do differ.

Table 6.5: Vaccination schedule for children in Britain (Department of Health (1992) Immunization Against Infectious Disease. HMSO)

3 days
BCG (if TB in family in last 6 months)
2 months
Diphtheria, pertussis and tetanus (DPT), *Haemophilus influenzae* type B (HIB) and oral polio
Meningitis C
3 months
DPT, HIB and oral polio
Meningitis C
4 months
DPT, HIB and oral polio
Meningitis C
12 months
Measles/mumps/rubella for both sexes
4–5 years
Diphtheria, tetanus and polio
10–14 years
BCG
15–18 years
Tetanus and polio boosters

HISTORY

Children under 5 years old are unlikely to give much meaningful history. The accompanying adult will usually provide the majority of the history. The relationship of the accompanying adult to the child must be ascertained and recorded in the notes. It may seem unimportant at the time, but becomes very important if child abuse is later suspected. Older children may give the best histories, as they do not interpret and distort their symptoms. Parents may interpret their children's symptoms and it is important to bear this in mind when taking the history. A common example is limping that the adult assumes must be due to trauma.

Feeding is a good indicator of a well child. It is important to ask how much the child has eaten: a hungry child who can describe all his favourite foods is probably well. As a rough guide an infant requires $150\,\mathrm{ml\,kg^{-1}\,day^{-1}}$ of milk. The parents will be surprisingly accurate about intake. If vomiting and diarrhoea are present ask exactly what the parents mean. Similarly, it is useful to ask what colour the vomit is: bile is only ever green. An enquiry about soiling and wetting of nappies is essential. More than four wet nappies in the preceding 24 h usually implies a well-hydrated baby, the exception being diabetic ketoacidosis. Unwell children are not interested in play and lack the energy to indulge in their normal activities.

Children experiencing pain and fear regress. A developmental assessment performed on an acutely ill or distressed child usually indicates greater developmental delay than is actually present. It is useful to ask the child's mother about developmental milestones (Table 6.4). The need for this is greater the younger the child is, and will depend on the presenting complaint. For instance, a developmental history is important in a 1-year-old with fits, but less important in a 5-year-old child with diarrhoea.

Immunizations should be recorded (Table 6.5). The diseases vaccinated against are now rare.

However, an incomplete vaccination record may suggest a degree of neglect. The reasons for incomplete vaccination should be recorded. A programme is currently under way to offer meningitis vaccine to all children.

All vaccines should be avoided if there is an acute febrile illness or primary immunodeficiency, or if the child is taking more than $2\,\mathrm{mg\,kg^{-1}}$ of prednisolone. Expert advice should be sought if the patient is receiving chemotherapy.

The past medical history should include questions about the delivery and the immediate postnatal period. Again, the younger the child, the more important this aspect is. Also, the relevance to the presenting complaint will vary. A prolonged stay in neonatal intensive care is extremely relevant in a breathless 1-year-old child.

Drugs and allergies should be enquired about. It is important to document what is meant by 'allergy', as the term has very different meanings for doctors and many patients. A social history should always be taken. It is essential to find out who is living at home and whether there are any siblings.

EXAMINATION

The examination of children should aim to answer similar questions to the examination of adults, although the method is very different. Observation and inspection of injured parts is much more fruitful than moving and feeling. Observation should begin after introducing yourself to the patient. Children should not be asked for their permission, as their natural response is to refuse. A firm, friendly approach with an explanation is usually appropriate. It is best to be at eye-level with children as this is less frightening (Fig. 6.2). The examination needs to be opportunistic. If you undress a baby, the parents will appreciate it if you dress or offer to dress them after the examination. A suggested method for examination is shown below: this will vary with the nature of the presenting complaint. A feverish child will need a full examination; a twisted ankle will not.

GENERAL

The first priority is to assess the general appearance of the child. Is it alert, interactive, interested,

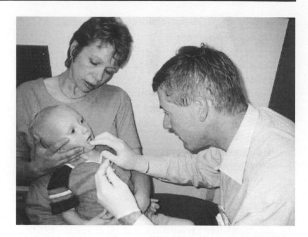

Figure 6.2: Examining a child.

happy and smiling? Or is it drowsy, lethargic, irritable and uninterested?

SKIN

Acute rashes are a source of great alarm to many parents because of the fear of meningococcal disease. It is therefore important to look at the distribution and see if the rash blanches on pressure, bearing in mind that the classic purpuric rash of meningococcal septicaemia is a late sign, and that early rashes may even look urticarial and may blanch.

HEAD

The anterior fontanelle should be assessed if present. The fontanelle becomes tense with crying, and with raised intracranial pressure. Raised intracranial pressure is usually due to head injuries or meningitis. The anterior fontanelle closes at approximately 18 months of age. It is also important to look at the eyes, asking the child to pull the lower eyelid down, if they are old enough, to permit inspection of the conjunctiva. The throat and external auditory meati must be inspected. This part of the examination is invariably upsetting for children and best left until last. It is vital to explain to the child's mother what one is going to do and how she should hold the baby. (An experienced nurse may be better at this than an inexperienced or diffident mother.) The correct way to hold a child for an ear examination is shown in Figure 6.3.

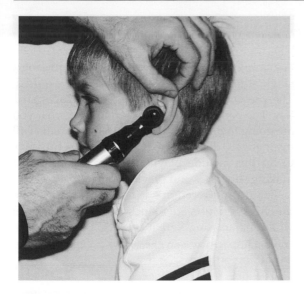

Figure 6.3: Examining a young child's ears.

Table 6.6: Normal respiratory rates for children

Age	Respiratory rate (breaths per minute)
Newborn	40–50
12 months	30–35
4 years	20–25
8 and older	12–15

NECK

The neck should always be examined for lymphadenopathy. Neck stiffness can be assessed by asking the child to kiss their knee. Kernig's sign is resistance to straightening the knee with a fully flexed hip. Brudzinski's sign is when the hips flex when the neck is flexed.

CARDIOVASCULAR SYSTEM

The capillary refill test is a useful marker of peripheral perfusion. The pulses must be examined, looking particularly for radiofemoral delay suggesting coarctation of the aorta. If cyanosis is present and does not correct with oxygen a right-to-left cardiac shunt may be present. The presence of murmurs and dyspnoea should be recorded.

CHEST

Inspection and observation are much more useful than plain auscultation. Particular attention should be paid to the upper airway. Small airways tolerate disease poorly. Stridor is an inspiratory noise caused by obstruction above the carina. If the obstruction is at or above the larynx then the noise is purely inspiratory. Below the larynx and in the trachea a soft expiratory component will be added. The respiratory rate is higher in children than in adults (Table 6.6).

Chest retraction is the indrawing of tissue beneath the costal margin, above the clavicles and between the ribs. In severe respiratory distress the sternum may be seen to bow inwards. Retraction will occur with upper and lower respiratory tract disease. Nasal flaring occurs on inspiration and indicates increased respiratory work. Expiratory grunting is produced when the glottis is partially closed, causing a delay followed by a forceful, noisy expiration. Grunting only occurs with lower respiratory tract disease.

ABDOMEN

It is most revealing to ask the child to point to tender areas and to blow his or her abdomen out and cough. If this is painless then peritonism is unlikely. Palpation should be gentle; rebound tenderness can be elicited with percussion. Herniae should be looked for, and in boys the testicles should always be inspected. A rectal examination is rarely warranted and a vaginal examination never in an emergency department.

LIMBS

Examination of the injured limb is discussed in the section on paediatric trauma and below in the section on the limping child.

SPECIAL TESTS

Blood tests are often not necessary. If they are necessary and time permits, EMLA (eutectic mixture of local anaesthetics) or amethocaine cream should be applied to anaesthetize the skin. Amethocaine has a quicker onset of action (30 min) and lasts longer (4–6 h).

RADIOGRAPHS

Children are more likely than adults to fracture bones than to have simple sprains. Guidelines such as the Ottawa ankle rules do not apply to children. A higher index of suspicion is necessary if fractures are not to be missed. Children are also harder to assess after head injuries and a more liberal approach to skull radiographs is justified. Chest radiographs are less often necessary in asthmatic children than in adults.

ANALGESIA

Children often receive suboptimal analgesia in emergency departments. This is usually due to ignorance of doses, and concern about potential overdose. Paracetamol is a very common first-line analgesic and is suitable for mild pain. A dose of $80 \, \text{mg} \, \text{kg}^{-1} \, \text{day}^{-1}$ is usually appropriate. A loading dose of $40 \, \text{mg} \, \text{kg}^{-1}$ is given.

Severe pain requires opiate analgesia. If the child can swallow, morphine solution is effective in about 20 min. Children who require fasting before an operation or who are vomiting are best treated with intravenous morphine in a dose of $0.1–0.2 \, \text{mg} \, \text{kg}^{-1}$. As with all analgesia, the end result is more important than the dose. The amount of morphine given should be titrated to the pain of the child. Intramuscular morphine has a less predictable onset of action, and should not be given to shocked children. Opiates probably cause less vomiting in children and the use of antiemetics is not routinely required. If an antiemetic is required, cyclizine is safe at a dose appropriate for the child's weight.

Local anaesthesia can also be very useful in providing analgesia. A femoral nerve block is often the best analgesia for a fractured femoral shaft. It may be less useful for knee injuries and hip injuries. Digital nerve blocks are useful for finger injuries.

SEDATION

For simple and quick procedures, such as placing a single stitch, distraction may be all that is required. The presence of the child's parents reduces anxiety. The parents should have an idea of what you are going to do before you do it. Most parents will instinctively distract upset children. Useful ways to do this include playing with a favourite toy, making silly faces and playing music.

For many procedures it is desirable to sedate the child. Sedation is a reduction in conscious level while maintaining verbal contact. Loss of verbal contact implies excessive sedation. Safety is of paramount importance.

Sedation, analgesia and anaesthesia are different states.

CHOICE OF SEDATIVE

Midazolam is a short-acting benzodiazepine which is used extensively in adults. It has variable sedative properties but is not an analgesic. There is concern that it interacts with opiates to produce hypotension. It can be given orally at a dose of $0.5–0.75 \, \text{mg} \, \text{kg}^{-1}$. It tastes bitter and needs disguising. Peak absorption occurs at 1 h and it is usually eliminated in 2 h. It does not require an intravenous cannula to be inserted, but has a number of disadvantages over intravenous midazolam:

- Gastric stasis increases the risk of aspiration.
- The pharmacodynamics are very variable.
- Onset and recovery take a long time.
- If reversal is necessary then flumazenil is unlikely to be successful because of its short half-life.
- Intranasal midazolam is another effective, noninvasive method of administering sedation; $0.5 \, \text{mg} \, \text{kg}^{-1}$ should be drawn up in a syringe and slowly squirted up the child's nose. It is important to have the child head down when this is done, otherwise the midazolam will end up on the child's clothes. The best way to do this is by lying the child head down on the parent's lap. Older children can be placed head down on a tipping trolley.

Intravenous midazolam is also used, at a dose of $0.05–0.15 \, \text{mg} \, \text{kg}^{-1}$. It is the best sedative for

Table 6.7: Side-effects of ketamine

Increased salivation can provoke laryngospasm: this can be reduced by combining the injection with atropine $0.01\,mg\,kg^{-1}$. Dysphoric reactions such as hallucinations and nightmares may occur during recovery. These are less common than in adults and can be minimized by allowing the child to wake up in a quiet, dark room. Vomiting can occur, usually during recovery, particularly if the child is disturbed. Myoclonic twitches occur at higher doses: these are benign and not related to seizure activity. It raises intracranial pressure and is contraindicated where there is a significant head injury.

older children. Flumenazil is a specific antagonist for benzodiazepines.

Intravenous sedation should only be performed by experienced staff.

Ketamine is a phencyclidine derivative. It produces a state of 'disassociative anaesthesia' by generating a functional barrier between the cortical and limbic systems. It is an extremely effective analgesic. Sedation is achieved with a dose of $2.5\,mg\,kg^{-1}$ intramuscularly and usually occurs after 10 min. It has usually worn off by 90 min. There are a number of adverse effects of ketamine (Table 6.7) and it should only be administered by experienced staff. Despite these problems, it is an extremely useful sedative and analgesic.

As with all drugs, it is important that staff become familiar with the use of sedatives. It is much better to use one preparation extensively, than to use a variety of mixtures infrequently.

CONSENT

Any procedure that has the potential for harm requires informed consent. This includes radiographs, sedation and treatment. Consent may be either implicit or explicit. The need will depend on the intended procedure. For instance, implied consent is appropriate before obtaining a radiograph. Sedating a child will require a thorough explanation and signing of a written consent form. When children are involved, the issue of who gives consent is important. Usually the parents are available to provide consent. Other adults, such as teachers, are able to provide consent by acting *in loco parentis*. The local authority provides consent for children who are in care.

Where adults are not available, an attempt should be made to contact the parents. Consent over the telephone is acceptable, provided that this is recorded in the notes. Children may consent to minor investigations and treatment, provided the doctor can satisfy him or herself that the child is competent to give consent. Usually this means that the child is over 12 years of age. Occasionally, the child's condition dictates urgent, life-saving treatment before consent can be obtained. There is no legal problem with this. Even more occasionally, parents may refuse to allow their child to be treated. A commonly quoted example is blood transfusions and Jehovah's Witnesses. In these cases, the duty consultant and the social work department should be contacted to make the child a ward of court.

If consent is refused and treatment is necessary, the child can be made a ward of court.

The issue of consent is discussed in greater detail in Chapter 9.

FURTHER READING

Morton, R. and Phillips, B. (1996) *Accidents and Emergencies in Children.* Oxford University Press, Oxford.

Strange, G., Ahrens, W., Lelyveld, R. and Schafermeyer, R. (1995) *Pediatric Emergency Medicine: A Comprehensive Study Guide.* McGraw Hill, New York.

CHAPTER SEVEN

THE ELDERLY IN THE EMERGENCY DEPARTMENT

- Introduction
- Assessment

- Specific clinical problems in the elderly
- Prior to discharge

INTRODUCTION

As the population of the UK continues to age, elderly people will represent an increasing proportion of any emergency department's workload. Not only do elderly people need emergency care more often than the younger population but the problems they present with are often more complex, with often more than one disease process present.

The functional capabilities of the patient rather than their chronological age best determine when specific age-targeted resources and approaches are required. Nevertheless, most hospitals have a rigid age limit at which a patient becomes elderly. Many elderly patients fear illness and infirmity more than death. In consequence, investigation and treatment must reflect this. Some of the problems of managing elderly patients in the emergency department include:

- Mental incapacity due to dementia may cause difficulties in obtaining an accurate medical history and informed consent. Deafness may also make communication more difficult.
- Physical incapacity resulting in poor mobility limits the activities of daily living and renders elderly people more susceptible to loss of privacy and dignity. Relatively minor injury or illness may result in a loss of ability to cope in their own home, and the doctor must have a lower threshold for seeking admission for the elderly patient.

- The presence of multiple physical and social problems is demanding of clinical and nursing time.
- Involvement of relatives, general practitioners, social services and other agencies is necessary to obtain information about the patient and to plan care.

Age alone is not a barrier to the consumption of healthcare resources.

Elderly patients with major illness may present atypical symptoms and signs. They should be managed as aggressively as younger patients. For certain conditions there is often an even greater benefit in older patients, for example in the use of thrombolysis in acute myocardial infarction.

ASSESSMENT

An accurate history is the most important component of a patient's assessment and is vital to correct diagnosis and treatment. The presence of cognitive and physical deficits makes this process more difficult; however, patience, perseverance and access to members of the family, friends and the general practitioner (GP) will often result in the required information being found. Many elderly patients are stoical and understate the severity of their symptoms.

Table 7.1: The abbreviated mental test

1. Age
2. Time to nearest hour
3. Address for recall at end of test
4. Year
5. Name of institution
6. Recognition of 2 persons
7. Date of birth (day & month)
8. Year of First World War
9. Name of present monarch
10. Count backwards from 20 to 1
    Each correct answer scores 1
    Normal = 8–10
    Moderate impairment = 4–7
    Severe impairment = 0–3

Table 7.2: Differential diagnosis of collapse in the elderly

Environmental	Poor lighting, lack of hand rails
Musculoskeletal	Arthritis, myopathy
Visual failure	Cataracts, glaucoma
Drugs	Sedatives, tricyclics, antihypertensives
Syncope	Stokes–Adams attacks, vertebro-basilar insufficiency, carotid body hypersensitivity
Cerebral	Parkinson's, cerebrovascular accident (CVA), transient ischaemic accident (TIA)
Metabolic	Electrolyte disturbance

Observations of temperature, pulse and blood pressure should be interpreted with caution. Many elderly patients with infections do not have a fever. Blood-pressure measurements regarded as normal for young adults are often abnormal for the elderly and the pulse rate may be affected by the presence of intercurrent disease or use of medication such as beta-blockers. Other physical signs such as tenderness and guarding on abdominal examination may be absent despite the presence of significant intra-abdominal pathology.

Assessment of cognitive function is essential to determine the accuracy of the history and the safety of the patient if they are to be discharged. The abbreviated mental test score is an appropriate tool (Table 7.1).

SPECIFIC CLINICAL PROBLEMS IN THE ELDERLY

'COLLAPSE ?CAUSE'

All collapses or falls must be assessed and managed appropriately. Isolated events with a clear cause, such as a trip on uneven ground, may require little medical intervention other than the treatment of resultant injury. But where the cause of the patient's collapse is not obvious, and especially if the episodes are recurrent, a full assessment is required with the aim of detecting a treatable cause (Table 7.2).

ACUTE CONFUSIONAL STATE

A breakdown in the patient's normal behaviour can be classified into three broad categories, the '3Ds':

- delirium (toxic confusional state)
- dementia (organic confusional state)
- depression (psychiatric confusional state).

Delirium (toxic confusional state)

The hallmark of toxic confusional states is the presence of a diminished or fluctuating level of consciousness. Commonly the patient's behaviour is restless and may become aggressive. Hallucinations may occur, especially at night. Again a differential diagnosis should be considered (Table 7.3) and assessment focused on detecting a treatable cause.

Fluctuating level of consciousness in a confused patient is highly suggestive of a toxic confusional state.

Treatment should be directed at the underlying cause, avoiding the use of sedation wherever possible. Reassurance and a calm, warm, quiet environment with familiar faces will often make management much easier and sedation unnecessary. Sedation when unavoidable should be titrated to response in small aliquots (e.g. 2.5 mg haloperidol intramuscularly).

Table 7.3: Differential diagnosis of toxic confusional state

Infection	Chest, urine, cellulitis
Metabolic	Hyponatraemia Dehydration Hypo- or hyperthermia Uraemia Hepatic encephalopathy
Endocrine	Hypo- or hyperglycaemia Hypo- or hyperthyroidism
Neurological	Meningitis, encephalitis, cerebral abscess Tumour Subdural haematoma Postictal
Respiratory	Infection Hypoxia Hypercapnia
Cardiac	Low-output states

Drug related	Withdrawal (alcohol,
	    benzodiazepines, opiates)
	Sedatives, diuretics,
	    antiparkinsonism

Dementia (acute organic state)

The typical findings are disorientation in time and place associated with impairment of short-term memory, cognitive function and insight. Clouding of consciousness is not a feature. If a patient with known dementia experiences an acute deterioration it is often due to a coexisting delirium state and the causes listed above should be sought.

Depression (acute psychiatric state)

There may be typical biological symptoms (poor sleep and appetite) together with hypochondriasis or social withdrawal. Some patients may appear demented ('pseudodementia') but respond well to treatment of depression, with return of normal cognitive function.

TRAUMA IN THE ELDERLY

Trauma is the fifth leading cause of death in people over 65 years of age. The elderly patient will have a reduced cardiovascular and respiratory reserve

and often has significant antecedent illness which results in a poor prognosis. For injuries of comparable severity the mortality rate in people over 75 years of age is five times that of younger people. Above 80 years of age the mortality is 25 times greater.

Injury mechanisms

The doctor should always be aware that an elderly patient's fall or road traffic accident may be the result of an underlying medical problem such as a transient dysrhythmia. Simultaneous management of both the injury and its cause may therefore be necessary.

FALLS

One in four patients over 75 years of age falls at least once each year. Of these, half fall repeatedly. Twenty-five per cent of patients who have fallen will sustain a fracture, and of these 50% will die within 12 months. Many falls are due to underlying medical problems. Thus all patients who have fallen must be thoroughly evaluated for such problems.

BURNS

The dermis of elderly patients is much thinner and thus burns tend to be deeper. The mortality rate rises sharply with age, and overall mortality in those over 60 years of age is twice that of younger patients.

NON-ACCIDENTAL INJURY

In the USA this is termed elder abuse. Patients seldom inform medical staff for fear of abandonment by their family. There is often a degree of denial or acceptance by the victim. Medical staff should have a high index of suspicion when dealing with a patient in whom there is evidence of physical neglect, unexplained medication overdoses or multiple injuries of varying ages.

Key differences

HEAD INJURY

There is an increased incidence of subdural haematoma because of increased dural vein fragility and the tendency of the brain to atrophy with age, thus allowing it greater movement within the cranium.

The overall prognosis for elderly patients with a significant head injury is poor, with over two thirds of patients over 65 years of age who present as an unconscious head injury dying.

CHEST INJURY
Advancing age reduces the compliance of the thoracic cage, and thereby reduces the ability of the thorax to withstand blunt trauma. Beyond middle age the functional residual capacity falls and the alveoli begin to collapse at the end of expiration. This phenomenon is exaggerated by recumbency. Consequently, any injury to the chest is likely to further impair an already reduced ventilatory capacity, increasing the incidence of ventilatory failure. Allied to this is the rising incidence of osteopenia with age. In consequence, even a minor fall may lead to rib fractures and even a flail chest.

Finally, because congestive cardiac failure and chronic obstructive airways disease are more common in this age group, even minor chest injuries may cause significant pulmonary compromise.

CARDIOVASCULAR RESPONSES AND INJURY
Elderly patients are less able to increase cardiac output on demand since ageing reduces the ventricular wall compliance, atrial fibrillation when present reduces cardiac output by up to 30%, and elderly patients are more likely to be taking beta-blockers, which are negatively inotropic and chronotropic.

Calcification of the aorta reduces its elasticity, increasing the risk of traumatic rupture following sudden deceleration.

ABDOMINAL INJURY
Lack of abdominal wall musculature reduces guarding and the signs of peritoneal irritation are more subtle in the elderly.

ORTHOPAEDIC INJURY
Osteopenia becomes ubiquitous with advancing age and in consequence fractures occur following relatively minor injuries (e.g. the high incidence of fractures of the femoral neck following a fall). The reduced pain perception seen in some elderly patients increases the likelihood that subtle fractures may be missed. Fractures may also be more difficult to detect radiologically, and a radioisotope bone scan should be done when clinical suspicion is high but radiographs do not show a fracture.

RESUSCITATION
To minimize mortality and morbidity resuscitation must combine vigorous treatment of haemorrhage with close monitoring to prevent fluid overload. Urinary output should be measured hourly and there should be a low threshold for measuring central venous pressures.

MYOCARDIAL INFARCTION

Atypical presentation with acute myocardial infarction becomes increasingly common with age and over the age of 85 years chest pain is not present in half of all patients. Atypical symptoms include syncope, vomiting, confusion and weakness. However, the prognosis for patients with these features is no worse than for patients presenting with the classic features of acute myocardial infarction.

INFECTIONS

Elderly people are at increased risk of developing infections, and the resultant morbidity and mortality are common. Significant infections may be present even in the absence of a pyrexia and a raised white-cell count. Pneumonia and urinary tract infections are particularly common and the doctor should have a low threshold for considering these diagnoses and treating the patient early and aggressively.

ABDOMINAL PAIN

In comparison with younger patients, abdominal pain frequently has a serious underlying cause and surgical intervention is commonly required. Again, life-threatening illness may present with non-specific symptoms and signs. Specifically, as the abdominal wall musculature atrophies patients are less likely to demonstrate important physical signs such as guarding or rebound. The omentum also shrinks with age, reducing its ability to localize disease processes such as perforation. The emergency department doctor is therefore justified in investigating elderly patients with abdominal pain and referring for a period of in-patient observation when there is any diagnostic uncertainty.

Table 7.4: Conditions inappropriately overtreated

Parkinsonism
Dependent oedema
Epilepsy
Diabetes
Hypertension

INAPPROPRIATE TREATMENT

The elderly are particularly likely victims of poly-pharmacy and the consequent problems of drug interactions and adverse effects. Certain conditions are frequently overtreated (Table 7.4).

Conversely, other conditions are undertreated, especially mental illnesses and, in particular, depression. When prescribing new medication to the elderly, particular caution should be exercised to reduce the incidence of adverse reactions and drug interactions. Overdose and other forms of suicidal behaviour are especially serious in the elderly.

PRIOR TO DISCHARGE

Before discharging any elderly patient the following must be assessed:

- Can the patient walk safely with or without an aid?
- Can the patient get home safely?
- Once home, can they cope with the activities of daily living – dressing, washing, toileting, shopping and cooking?
- Can the patient understand new or existing medication?
- Can relatives or friends continue to provide sufficient support?

If the answer to any of the above is no then either the patient will require admission or assistance must be sought from the GP, social worker and district nurse.

If a patient cannot mobilize safely they must be admitted for further investigation and rehabilitation.

CHAPTER EIGHT

ANALGESIA, SEDATION AND ANAESTHESIA

- Introduction
- Analgesia
- Local anaesthesia

- Sedation
- Emergency general anaesthesia
- Further reading

INTRODUCTION

Pain is the commonest cause of presentation to an emergency department. Effective analgesia must therefore be a high priority and a number of methods for pain relief are available to the emergency doctor. As well as oral, intramuscular and intravenous analgesia, local anaesthesia in the form of infiltration or nerve blocks is commonly used to relieve the pain of procedures such as suturing or manipulation of fractures. In addition, sedation of patients is often important to prevent distress during procedures. However, if sedation is not properly performed, this can result in uncontrolled and dangerous general anaesthesia. Finally, techniques of general anaesthesia are often required to gain definitive control of the airway and to ensure adequate ventilation. This chapter provides a description of the techniques available and appropriate for use in the emergency department.

ANALGESIA

The majority of patients attending the emergency department present with pain requiring some form of analgesia. Pain prevention and treatment must therefore form part of the management of each of these patients. It is important to evaluate each patient separately and to formulate an individual treatment plan. There are many factors that should be considered in determining the type and route of administration of analgesic drugs; these include the cause, character and severity of the pain as well as the patient's age, size, personality and any co-morbidity.

PAIN PHYSIOLOGY

Pain begins when local tissue damage occurs, resulting in the release of inflammatory mediators which in turn results in the generation of electrical impulses at the peripheral sensory nerve endings or nociceptors. These impulses are conducted to the spinal cord either by thin myelinated A fibres (sharp localized pain) or by slow unmyelinated C fibres (burning diffuse pain). Visceral pain is transmitted by vagal and sympathetic nerve fibres, is often difficult to localize, and is often referred. Further relay to the higher centres in the brain is modified within the spinal cord before the individual perceives the painful stimulus. Pain can therefore be controlled or modulated by using drugs that act at the various levels of this complex chain.

The mode of action of non-steroidal anti-inflammatory drugs (NSAIDs) is to reduce the peripheral inflammatory response by inhibiting prostaglandin synthesis. Some of the analgesic effects of aspirin and all of those of paracetamol are due to the inhibition of cyclo-oxygenase in the central nervous system. Opioid drugs modulate pain by binding to opioid receptors in the spinal cord and higher brain centres. Moreover, opioids can influence the perception of pain by binding to opioid receptors in the cerebral cortex. Local anaesthetics provide analgesia by blocking the transmission of impulses from the periphery to the central nervous system. Local anaesthetics injected into the epidural space block impulses at the spinal cord level by acting on the spinal nerve roots. Although epidural analgesia can offer excellent pain relief in other clinical settings, such as fractured ribs, it is unsuitable for emergency department use and is not discussed further in this chapter.

METHODS OF PAIN MANAGEMENT

Simple measures

Although the use of drugs is often unavoidable, the use of non-pharmacological methods of pain relief should not be ignored. Simple measures such as immobilizing a fracture, elevation of a swollen limb and the application of ice to a recent injury can be of significant benefit. The treatment of the underlying cause of the pain may also be a rapid and effective method, for example the insertion of a urinary catheter in the patient with acute retention or the reduction of a dislocated patella will produce immediate and gratifying relief. Finally, most patients in pain are anxious about the nature and severity of their condition. Anxiety heightens the perception of pain and simple reassurance may reduce the patient's distress.

Inhalational analgesia

Entonox® is a valuable adjunct in providing temporary pain relief, especially for minor procedures or during the reduction of dislocations and simple fractures. It is a 50/50 mixture of nitrous oxide and oxygen which can be safely delivered using a self-administered demand valve system. Entonox® needs to be inhaled for at least 45 s before maximum analgesia is achieved. Clear instruction to take slow, deep breaths is essential. Its effect quickly subsides once the drug is stopped, without any hangover effect. Side-effects include temporary dizziness and drowsiness. Because the drug diffuses into air spaces, its use is absolutely contraindicated

in patients with decompression sickness and undrained pneumothorax. Relative contraindications include head-injured patients owing to the risk of pneumoencephalus. In many cases it may not be sufficient to provide adequate analgesia, and therefore it may be used in combination with a regional local anaesthetic or an intravenous analgesic.

> Entonox is contraindicated in head injury, pneumothorax and decompression illness.

Enteral analgesia

Oral analgesia can be used for mild to moderate pain. The opioids and NSAIDs are the two classes of analgesics that include the majority of drugs which are commonly used in the emergency department. For mild pain paracetamol 1 g 6-hourly is often adequate. It has centrally acting analgesic and antipyretic properties and is rapidly absorbed from the gut to produce analgesia within 30 min which lasts about 4 h.

OPIOIDS

There are a variety of oral opioids of various strengths that can be used for moderate pain. These may be prescribed alone or in compound preparations with paracetamol or aspirin. Codeine is a natural alkaloid which has weak analgesic effects and produces constipation. Dihydrocodeine is a semi-synthetic derivative of codeine that has better analgesic properties than codeine but can cause confusion and disorientation in children and the elderly. Coproxamol contains paracetamol and the synthetic opioid dextropropoxyphene. It has a similar potency to codeine and is best avoided, as in overdose it may induce respiratory depression or death. Other compound analgesics include codydramol (paracetamol and dihydrocodeine) and cocodamol (codeine and paracetamol). Most departments will have a prescribing policy for compound analgesics and this should be followed. It is usually sensible practice to restrict prescribing to one of the compound analgesic drugs only. Tramadol is a new centrally acting analgesic with opioid agonist properties. It is ideal for moderate to severe pain and has fewer gastrointestinal and respiratory side-effects than morphine. Buprenorphine is associated with an unacceptably high incidence of vomiting and its use is not recommended.

NON-STEROIDAL ANTI-INFLAMMATORY DRUGS

NSAIDs have analgesic and anti-inflammatory properties and are rapidly absorbed into the systemic circulation by the oral and rectal routes. Salicylates such as aspirin are the oldest class of NSAIDs. Enteric coating of aspirin may reduce some of its gastrointestinal side-effects. The phenylacetic acids such as diclofenac are newer and can be given orally, rectally or intramuscularly. Diclofenac can also be used parenterally in the treatment of acute biliary and renal colic. Propionic acids such as ibuprofen, ketoprofen and naproxen are the best tolerated of all NSAIDs. They are particularly useful for acute soft tissue, bone and joint injuries as well as renal colic. NSAIDs can be used in conjunction with opioids such as dihydrocodeine to provide analgesia in patients presenting with chronic pain conditions such as low back pain. However, NSAIDs have their own side-effects, such as gastric irritation, nephrotoxicity, impaired haemostasis owing to decreased platelet aggregation, exacerbation of asthma and sodium retention. There is some theoretical evidence suggesting that NSAIDs may reduce bone healing in fractures, and they may be better avoided for long-term use in this group of patients. Misoprostol, a synthetic analogue of prostaglandin E_1, may be given with NSAIDs such as diclofenac to reduce some of the gastrointestinal side-effects.

> Avoid NSAIDs in patients with known peptic ulcer disease and severe asthma.

Parenteral analgesia

Parenteral analgesics are ideal for moderate to severe pain and can be broadly classified into opioid and non-opioid types. Opioid medications remain the mainstay of acute visceral pain therapy. The selection of drugs should be based on the duration of action and side-effects. The intramuscular or intravenous routes of administration are commonly used in the emergency department setting. The intravenous route is preferred as it provides a predictable and rapid onset of action. Plasma concentrations are rapidly attained, allowing easy assessment of benefit and appropriate titration of the drug. The intramuscular route has a variable absorption rate as it relies on perfusion at the site of injection and the peak plasma concentrations can be inconsistent

> Intramuscular analgesia should be avoided in patients with hypovolaemia or cardiac failure.

OPIOIDS

The most serious side-effect of opioid analgesics is respiratory depression, possibly leading to respiratory arrest (Table 8.1). Transient hypoxia with no clinical ventilatory abnormalities often occurs in the elderly and in obese patients. Careful monitoring should prevent such complications. Other side-effects include nausea and vomiting caused by stimulation of the chemoreceptor trigger zone. Centrally acting antiemetics such as cyclizine should be given, rather than metoclopramide or prochlorperazine, which are peripherally acting. Other side-effects include reduced gastric emptying, retention of urine and depression of bowel function, leading to constipation and paralytic ileus. Opioids should be carefully titrated and monitored in patients with reduced respiratory effort. They should be avoided in unventilated patients with status asthmaticus or head injuries with suspected raised intracranial pressure. Pethidine should be avoided in patient taking monamine oxidase inhibitors.

Opioid toxicity is manifested by sedation, respiratory depression and miosis and can be reversed by intravenous naloxone. Naloxone has a duration of action of 15–20 min, which is considerably shorter than that of many opioids and repeated doses may therefore be necessary. On rare occasions, establishment of a naloxone infusion may be required. In doubtful cases, a sufficient dose of naloxone should be given in order to ensure that lack of response is due to absence of opiate overdose. This is usually in the region of 2 mg.

Table 8.1: Side-effects of opioids

Respiratory depression and arrest
Hypoxia
Nausea and vomiting
Reduced gastric emptying
Retention of urine
Constipation
Paralytic ileus

- Morphine is the standard drug against which all opioids and opioid-like formulations are compared. It produces analgesia and drowsiness at higher doses. The parenteral dose is 0.1–0.2 mg kg^{-1} with a duration of action between 3 and 4 h. When administered intravenously to an adult, an initial bolus of 3–5 mg can be given followed by further 1–2 mg boluses at 5-min intervals until adequate analgesia with minimal side-effects is attained. Titration must be slow as its onset of action is slow.
- Diamorphine is a semi-synthetic opioid which is much more lipid soluble than morphine and hence faster acting. The parenteral dose is 0.05–0.15 mg kg^{-1} and it can be given intravenously, intramuscularly or subcutaneously.
- Pethidine is a synthetic drug which is commonly given either intravenously (0.5–1 mg kg^{-1}) or intramuscularly (50–100 mg adult dose). It is shorter acting than morphine (duration 2–3 h) and repeated doses may be required to maintain analgesia.
- Nalbuphine is a synthetic opioid with partial agonist effects and therefore it is associated with a ceiling to its depressant effect on respiration. It causes little cardiovascular compromise and the dosage is the same as with morphine, with an equi-analgesic effect. It is not classed as a controlled drug and is therefore commonly used by paramedics in the prehospital phase. Partial agonist effects may lessen the effectiveness of subsequent doses of opiates and make judging adequate dosage difficult. Nalbuphine is not recommended for in-hospital use.

NSAID DRUGS

Parenteral NSAIDs have an increasing role in the management of acute musculoskeletal pain as well as of biliary and renal colic. Intramuscular diclofenac has been widely used but can be painful at the injection site. Ketorolac is a newer NSAID that is also available as a parenteral preparation.

Side-effects are more common in the elderly. Patients should not be prescribed more than one NSAID at a time and the lower end of the dose range should be tried initially and titrated upwards according to response. If a patient does not tolerate one class of NSAID, a drug from another group may be tried. NSAIDs are best avoided in pregnancy. Side-effects of parenteral NSAIDs are the same as in the enteral group, as previously mentioned.

NSAIDs are best avoided in the trauma patient as they can precipitate renal impairment and deranged coagulation.

It is better to use a few drugs well rather than many badly.

LOCAL ANAESTHESIA

INTRODUCTION

Local anaesthetic agents produce a transient and reversible loss of sensation in a part of the body by blocking nerve conduction. Both sensory and motor nerves may be blocked, depending on the agent used and the anatomical level at which the agent is administered.

PHARMACOLOGY

Nerve fibres may be blocked at any level from the spinal cord to the receptor site at the periphery. Local anaesthetics block nerve conduction by interfering with the permeability of the cell membrane to sodium, thus stabilizing the membrane at the resting potential. The speed with which local anaesthetics diffuse into the cell membrane depends on the degree of myelination, the size of the nerve and the relative position of the fibre within the nerve. The smaller fibres conducting pain are more sensitive to local anaesthetic agents than the large motor fibres. Patients can therefore move their limbs during a procedure even when a local anaesthetic has been used. Similarly, a fibre may be readily blocked using a spinal anaesthetic, but the same fibre will take longer to be anaesthetized if it forms part of a larger nerve in the periphery, such as the femoral nerve.

Structurally all local anaesthetics consist of an amino group, linked through an amide or an ester to an aromatic residue. Classification is therefore based on the type of linkage:

- Ester class: cocaine is most commonly used in otolaryngology as a topical anaesthetic agent in the nose. Amethocaine and benzocaine are still used as topical agents but to a lesser extent.

Table 8.2: Summary of pharmacodynamic properties and doses of local anaesthetics

	Relative potency	Toxicity	Duration of action	Onset (min)	Maximum dose (mg kg^{-1})	Typical dose (ml) 70-kg adult
Esters:						
Procaine	1	1	Short	18	6–7	10 (of 3%)
Amethocaine	8	10	Long	15	1–1.5	6–8 (of 0.5%)
Amides:						
Lignocaine	2	2	Moderate	5	3	20 (of 1%)*
Prilocaine	2	1	Moderate	5	5	40 (of 0.5%)
Mepivacaine	2	2	Moderate	3	4	15 (of 0.2%)
Bupivacaine	8	10	Long	10	2	20–25 (of 0.5)

* 40 ml of 1% lignocaine can be used when mixed with adrenaline 1/200 000.

- Amide class: lignocaine (lidocaine) remains the standard against which the amide local anaesthetics are compared. It forms the mainstay for local anaesthetic practice. Prilocaine is considered the safest agent for intravenous blockade. Bupivacaine is a long-acting agent which is commonly used for epidural anaesthesia. The pharmacodynamic properties and doses of local anaesthetics are summarized in Table 8.2.

Adrenaline can be used as an additive in order to increase the duration of action of short- and intermediate-acting local anaesthetics by inducing local vasoconstriction. Adrenaline also allows larger doses of the local anaesthetic to be used safely by slowing absorption.

> Adrenaline should not be used in areas supplied by end-arteries, such as the toes, fingers, ears, nose and penis.

Caution should be exercised in patients with peripheral vascular disease and ischaemic heart disease.

> An easy way of converting the percentage concentration of a drug to milligrams per millilitre is by multiplying the % concentration by 10. For example, 1% lignocaine is equivalent to 10 mg ml^{-1}.

GENERAL PRINCIPLES

Local anaesthesia is cheap, simple and relatively safe to administer. It provides good and effective pain control with minimal danger to the patient

Table 8.3: Indications and contraindications for intravenous regional anaesthesia

> *Indications:*
> Any patient in whom a local anaesthetic can be used safely and effectively
> Patients with cardiorespiratory problems where general anaesthesia would be hazardous
>
> *Contraindications:*
> Patients with known allergy to local anaesthetic
> Unwilling and unco-operative patients
> Local sepsis
> Uncertain duration of surgery
> Patients with peripheral vascular disease or sickle cell disease, as there is a risk of ischaemia related to the local hypoxia
> Marked coagulation disorders
> Inexperienced user

and it is often the technique of choice in high-risk patients. Although the procedure is considered safer than general anaesthesia, deaths have been reported following equipment failure, such as cases of premature cuff deflation following Bier's block. Although patients do not need to be starved, fasting is necessary for intravenous regional anaesthesia. Many techniques can be used by the emergency doctor without the need for an anaesthetist. The indications and contraindications for using regional anaesthesia are summarized in Table 8.3.

> The maximum safe dose of lignocaine is 3 mg kg^{-1}. The maximum safe dose of lignocaine **with adrenaline** is 7 mg kg^{-1}.

PREOPERATIVE CONSIDERATIONS

Several factors should be considered before administering a local anaesthetic. These include the patient's general health, the type, site and duration of surgery, and the availability of appropriate equipment, facilities and staff. Ideally, patients should be starved because at times the regional anaesthetic may be unsuccessful or complications may arise that require general anaesthesia.

General health

A brief medical history and physical examination should be taken in all cases. Patients with ischaemic heart disease, arrhythmias, myasthenia gravis, hepatic impairment and epilepsy are at an increased risk of developing toxic reactions. Caution should be taken with debilitated frail elderly patients and with very young patients, and the dosage of the anaesthetic should be exact. A clear explanation of the procedure should be given to the patient as well as a warning that the anaesthetic will offer pain relief but pressure and pulling will be felt during the operation. It is good practice to point out the advantages associated with the chosen technique in terms of early recovery and reduced postoperative pain.

Patient monitoring

Patients undergoing i.v. regional anaesthesia to the upper and lower limbs usually require the use of large amounts of local anaesthetics. It is therefore important to ensure that resuscitation equipment is available in the department for basic life support, as well as intubation equipment and induction agents for emergency general anaesthesia. The patient should be placed on a tipping trolley and suction should be available for aspiration of any secretions or vomit. The patient should be monitored using a pulse oximeter, cardiac monitor and blood pressure. In addition to the emergency medicine specialist or surgeon a second person skilled in resuscitation, airway management and support of the circulation must be present to manage any possible adverse events. The doctor administering the i.v. regional anaesthetic should monitor the patient while a separate person performs the operative procedure.

Type, site and duration of procedure

The chosen method of local anaesthesia should provide adequate anaesthesia to the skin as well as blocking the stimuli arising from deeper structures manipulated during the procedure. The different types of regional blocks that can be used for different sites are described in detail in the next section.

The duration of anaesthesia is an important issue in deciding whether sedation or even a general anaesthetic should be offered. A mixture of a long-acting and short-acting local anaesthetic can sometimes be used to allow the procedure to be commenced a few minutes after the anaesthetic is given but at the same time allow time for a lengthy procedure to be performed. Similarly, extensive wounds which would require infiltration of doses in excess of the maximum safe dose in order to achieve effective analgesia will require some other form of anaesthetic procedure. All the drugs used should be checked before drawing up the solution. The correct dose should be carefully calculated, especially in the elderly and children. The anaesthetic should be injected slowly to minimize pain and the patient should be asked to report any symptoms of toxicity, such as tinnitus or tingling around the mouth.

Side-effects

Adverse systemic effects occur secondary to absorption of toxic amounts of local anaesthetic into the systemic circulation. Systemic toxicity is most commonly caused by accidental intravascular administration.

The most serious side-effects result from the action of the local anaesthetics on the central nervous system (CNS) and cardiovascular system. Initial symptoms of central nervous system toxicity include perioral paraesthesiae and light-headedness. With increasing concentrations of the drug the patient develops tinnitus, slurred speech, twitching of the facial muscles, irrational conversation, unconsciousness and convulsions, followed by respiratory depression, hypotension and cardiac arrest. Cardiovascular side-effects include conduction abnormalities, arrhythmias, decreased cardiac output and cardiac arrest. Severe allergic reactions are rare. Ischaemia and gangrene can occur if adrenaline is used around an end artery. Bupivacaine has the highest lipid solubility, protein

Table 8.4: Side-effects of local anaesthetics and their treatment

Treatment of toxicity:
  Stop administration of the drug
  Airway – maintenance
  Breathing – oxygen therapy
  Circulation – IV fluids
Monitor pulse, blood pressure, oxygen saturation, respiratory rate, conscious level and ECG
CNS toxicity:
  For fits – diazepam 5–10 mg IV slowly
CVS toxicity:
  Hypotension – foot elevation and intravenous fluids
  Cardiac arrhythmias – cardioversion if haemodynamically compromised
Anaphylactic reaction:
  Adrenaline, hydrocortisone, nebulized salbutamol
Methaemoglobinaemia:
  Methylene blue

binding and cardiotoxicity. Methaemoglobinaemia may result when prilocaine is used in excess of $7\,mg\,kg^{-1}$. Haematoma and bruising around the injection site are minor complications. Table 8.4 summarizes the drugs and management of the different side-effects caused by local anaesthetics.

TYPES OF REGIONAL ANAESTHESIA

Local infiltration and field block

Theses are the commonest techniques used in the emergency department. The anaesthetic is injected locally in the subcutaneous tissues in order to block sensory nerve endings. In the case of field block a wider area of anaesthesia is established by blocking the branches of nerve endings around the area to be treated. These techniques are normally used for suturing of lacerations, cleaning and debriding of wounds, minor surgical procedures and to supplement a nerve block.

Technique

Lignocaine ($3\,mg\,kg^{-1}$ max. dose) is slowly infiltrated into the wound edges, skin or tissues using a fine needle. The onset of action is about 2 min with a duration of action up to 45 min depending on whether adrenaline has been used. Excessive infiltration around the wound with local anaesthetic may distort the normal anatomy and make the operative procedure more difficult.

Upper limb blocks

Virtually all operations on the upper limb may be performed under local anaesthesia, bearing in mind the limitations and extent of anaesthesia produced by the different techniques. A regional block to the upper limb may be unsuitable for a trauma patient if the procedure is likely to be very long and when other injuries are present requiring general anaesthesia. Local infiltration or sedation may be used to supplement the block. The choice of regional anaesthesia for upper limb injuries will depend on the advantages and disadvantages of each technique, as well as the experience of the clinician with the particular block.

The following techniques are discussed below:

- Bier's block
- axillary block
- median nerve block at the wrist
- ulnar nerve block at the wrist
- radial nerve block at the wrist
- haematoma block at the wrist
- digital nerve block.

INTRAVENOUS REGIONAL ANAESTHESIA (BIER'S BLOCK)

This is commonly used in the emergency department in order to provide regional anaesthesia below the elbow. It works by diffusion of the anaesthetic out of the vascular system to act on the peripheral nerves. It is a superior technique to infiltration of the fracture site for reduction of Colles' fracture. Plain prilocaine 0.5% is the drug of choice with an onset of action between 2 and 5 min and duration of anaesthesia of up to 80 min following release of the tourniquet. Time limitation is usually due to tourniquet discomfort, which cannot be easily avoided even if a double-cuff system is used.

Contraindications These include patients with sickle cell disease, Raynaud's disease, severe hypertension and obesity, and children under 7 years old.

Precautions Although it is a simple and reliable technique there is a potential risk of toxic reactions, therefore:

- The procedure should be performed on a tipping trolley.

- Two doctors, including one experienced in the technique and another who will carry out the procedure, and a trained nurse must be present during the procedure to monitor the patient.
- Venous access should be established on both arms.
- Resuscitation equipment and drugs should be readily available.
- The tourniquet should be checked for leaks before it is applied.

Technique The arm is fully exposed and the pneumatic tourniquet is applied high on the arm. Venous access is established using a small cannula on the dorsum of each hand. The arm is elevated with brachial artery digital occlusion and exsanguinated by applying an Esmarch bandage. The cuff is then inflated to 50 mmHg above the systolic blood pressure. The prilocaine is injected slowly over 2 min (40 ml of 0.5% for a 70-kg adult; the dose is reduced in the elderly and children and may be increased to 50 ml in a large adult male). The cuff should be monitored throughout the procedure and should not be released for at least 20 min after the injection. The cannula on the anaesthetized side should be removed before the manipulation is carried out. A double-cuff system is sometimes used: the proximal cuff is initially inflated and the lower cuff subsequently inflated once the underlying skin is considered to be anaesthetic. The upper cuff can then be deflated. This system is designed to reduce patient discomfort but can result in potentially catastrophic errors if the wrong cuff is deflated. The patient should be observed for at least 1 h after the procedure.

AXILLARY BLOCK (FIG. 8.1)

This approach carries the lowest risk of life-threatening complications but produces inconsistent anaesthesia above the elbow and inadequate blockade for procedures performed in the shoulder and upper arm.

Technique The patient is positioned supine or semi-sitting with the arm abducted to 90° and the elbow flexed. A dose of 30–40 ml of 1% lignocaine with adrenaline can be used. The axillary artery is palpated as high as possible in the axilla. A short bevelled needle is inserted superior to the artery or as close to it as possible at an angle of 30–40° with the skin. A 'pop' may be felt as the needle enters the neural sheath and the patient may experience

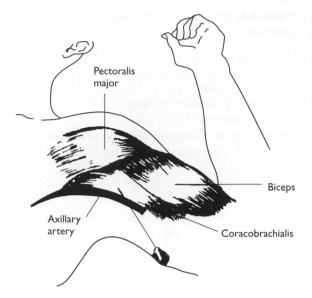

Figure 8.1: Axillary block.

paraesthesiae. If aspiration shows that the needle has entered the axillary artery the needle is advanced through the artery by piercing its posterior wall to enter the posterior part of the brachial plexus sheath. If any resistance is felt while the anaesthetic is injected the needle should be slightly withdrawn as it may be lying within the nerve. In order to encourage proximal spread of the anaesthetic the inner arm is squeezed firmly, distal to the point of injection, whilst the anaesthetic is infiltrated. The block may take 30–45 min to work fully.

MEDIAN NERVE BLOCK AT THE WRIST (FIG. 8.2)

The median nerve can be blocked at the level of the proximal skin crease as it passes just under and on the radial side of the palmaris longus tendon. It is indicated for procedures on the volar aspect of the hand in the median nerve distribution. A history of carpal tunnel syndrome should preclude this block.

Technique The hand is placed in the supine position with the wrist slightly flexed against resistance. A fine needle is inserted between the tendons of the flexor carpi radialis and palmaris longus and advanced to a depth of 1 cm. Five millilitres of 1% lignocaine are infiltrated, withdrawing the needle if paraesthesiae occur. For onset of anaesthesia, 5–10 min should be allowed.

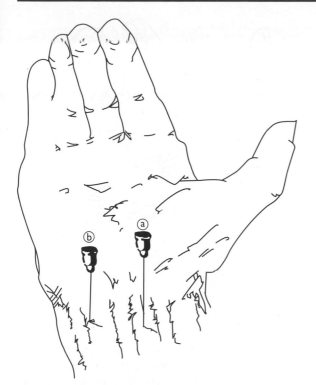

Figure 8.2: Median nerve block at the wrist.

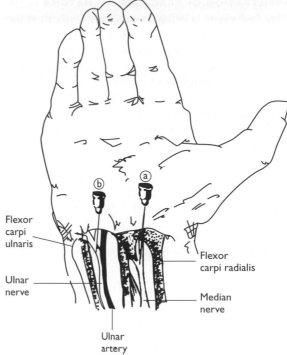

Flexor carpi ulnaris
Ulnar nerve
Flexor carpi radialis
Median nerve
Ulnar artery

Figure 8.3: Ulnar nerve block at the wrist.

ULNAR NERVE BLOCK AT THE WRIST (FIG. 8.3)

The ulnar nerve innervates the ulnar aspect of the hand by dividing into two cutaneous branches 5 cm proximal to the wrist. The dorsal branch passes under the flexor carpi ulnaris tendon and the palmar branch lies between the ulnar artery and the flexor carpi ulnaris tendon. Indications for ulnar nerve block include procedures on the ulnar aspect of the hand and reduction of fractures to the little finger and little finger metacarpal.

Technique With the hand supinated the wrist is slightly flexed against resistance in order to identify the flexor carpi ulnaris tendon. A fine needle is introduced at right-angles to the skin between the ulnar artery and flexor carpi ulnaris. If paraesthesiae are reported the needle is withdrawn slightly and, following negative aspiration for blood, 5 ml of 1% lignocaine are injected whilst the needle is slowly withdrawn. The dorsal branch is blocked by subcutaneous infiltration of 5 ml of local anaesthetic around the ulnar styloid. Before the anaesthetic is given the radial artery should be palpated to ensure that a collateral blood supply to the hand is present. Adrenaline is best avoided.

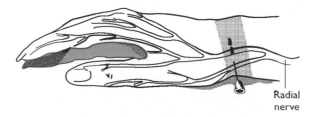

Radial nerve

Figure 8.4: Radial nerve block at the wrist.

RADIAL NERVE BLOCK AT THE WRIST

The superficial branch of the radial nerve passes under the brachioradialis tendon 8 cm proximal to the wrist to lie subcutaneously on the extensor aspect of the wrist. It then divides into several terminal branches to supply the dorsum of the hand. Radial nerve block is indicated for procedures to areas of the hand innervated by the superficial radial nerve.

Technique With the hand pronated, 5 ml of 1% lignocaine are injected subcutaneously at the level of the anatomical snuffbox around the radial border of the wrist, from the skin overlying the radial artery around to the level of the extensor carpi radialis tendon. Care must be taken to avoid intravenous injection of anaesthetic (Fig. 8.4).

INFILTRATION OF FRACTURE HAEMATOMA

This technique is being used increasingly in emergency departments for the reduction of some wrist fractures. It can easily be used by accident and emergency personnel with or without intravenous sedation, although some critics of the technique believe that the analgesia produced is less effective than regional anaesthesia (Bier's block).

Technique This technique works by blocking the nerves supplying the periosteum, bone and surrounding soft tissues at the fracture site. Using a full aseptic technique, a needle is inserted into the haematoma and fracture site and 10–15 ml of 1% lignocaine slowly injected. The fracture can be manipulated 10 min following the injection. The block lasts for approximately 1 h and remanipulation of the fracture maybe possible during this period.

Haematoma blocks should not be used for fractures sustained over 24 h ago and where there is infection of the skin overlying the fracture. Careful aseptic technique should be used as this method essentially converts a closed into an open fracture. Rapid absorption of the local anaesthetic from the haematoma can cause toxicity, and therefore the patient should be monitored and closely observed during as well as 1 h after the procedure.

DIGITAL NERVE BLOCK (RING BLOCK)

Digital nerve block is commonly used in the emergency department for simple operations on the distal two-thirds of the fingers or toes and for reductions of phalangeal fractures and interphalangeal joint dislocations. Using the dorsal approach a fine needle is introduced at the base of the radial side of the digit and 2 ml of plain lignocaine are injected while the needle is slowly withdrawn. The same procedure is repeated for the ulnar aspect. The maximum dose of anaesthetic is 5 ml. Adrenaline should never be used (Fig. 8.5). A tourniquet formed from the finger of a rubber glove can be applied to the base of the finger.

Blocks for lower limb injuries

FEMORAL NERVE BLOCK

The femoral nerve lies just lateral to the femoral artery and can be easily blocked at the level where it passes under the inguinal ligament. The femoral nerve is derived from the anterior divisions of the

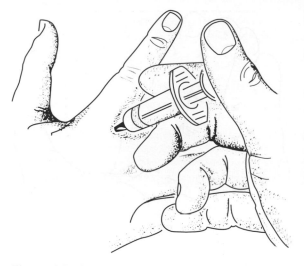

Figure 8.5: Digital nerve block.

lumbar plexus (L2–4) and supplies the anterior aspect of the thigh and the extensors of the knee. It also has a sensory distribution along the path of the long saphenous vein. In trauma patients the femoral nerve block can be used to provide analgesia for a fractured shaft of femur and fractured patella.

Technique The patient is positioned supine with the leg flat and slightly abducted. The femoral artery is identified midway along a line drawn from the anterior superior iliac spine to the symphysis pubis. A needle is inserted perpendicular to the skin just lateral to the artery as it passes below the inguinal ligament. The needle is advanced 1–4 cm deep and a palpable 'give' may be felt as the needle passes through the fascia, or the patient may complain of paraesthesiae or pain due to the needle penetrating the nerve. If this happens, the needle should be immediately withdrawn before injection of anaesthetic. Following negative aspiration for blood, 10 ml of 1% lignocaine is slowly injected. The onset of action is between 5 and 15 min, with duration of up to 1.5 h (Fig. 8.6).

COMPLICATIONS

These include puncture of the femoral artery and haematoma formation. The bleeding usually stops spontaneously with pressure. This technique can be used for all ages but it is vitally important to administer the correct dose, especially in children. There is a theoretical risk of the block masking the symptoms of a compartment syndrome, although

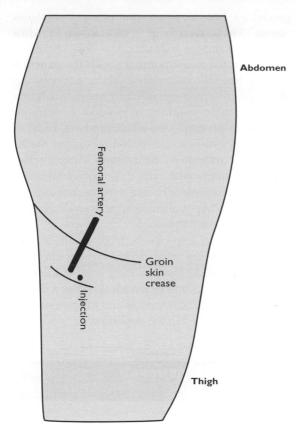

Figure 8.6: Femoral nerve block (remember **N**erve–**A**rtery–**V**ein–**Y** Fronts: **NAVY**).

this is unlikely to be clinically relevant especially if a short-acting local anaesthetic is used.

Intercostal block

This is a useful and versatile block, which can be used to provide analgesia following rib fractures. Operative procedures such as chest drain insertion are made more tolerable by performing an intercostal block. The intercostal nerves are the anterior primary rami of the thoracic nerves, which run in the subcostal groove along with the intercostal blood vessels. Lateral and anterior cutaneous branches are given to supply the intercostal muscles and the skin over the front of the thorax. The lower six intercostal also supply the anterior abdominal wall.

CONTRAINDICATIONS

These relate to the problems of causing a pneumothorax. Obese patients can be technically difficult.

Patients with chronic airway disease and emphysema may be technically easy but if a puncture occurs it can be associated with prolonged air leaks. Because of the risks of pneumothorax, bilateral intercostal blocks are rarely indicated.

Technique The patient is informed that there will be several injections. As a general rule the number of nerves to be blocked is determined by blocking one level higher and one lower than the specific area. The patient is positioned prone or on their side with the side to be blocked uppermost. The intercostal nerve can be blocked at the posterior costal angle or just posterior to the mid-axillary line to ensure blocking of the lateral cutaneous branch. A fine needle is introduced at 90° to the skin and advanced until the needle touches the bone. The needle is slightly withdrawn and redirected to pass just below the inferior border of the rib to a further depth of just 3–4 mm. Following negative aspiration for blood 5 ml of 1% lignocaine with adrenaline or 0.25% bupivacaine are injected at each intercostal level. Because of the rapid absorption of the local anaesthetic into the circulation the toxic dose should not be exceeded. The duration of action can last 4–6 h with lignocaine and adrenaline and 10–16 h when bupivacaine is used.

TOPICAL ANAESTHESIA

Topical skin anaesthesia is particularly important for children attending the emergency department. It can be used to provide skin anaesthesia prior to intravenous cannulation or injection. A thick layer of EMLA (eutactic mixture of local anaesthetic) cream 5% is applied on the skin and covered with an occlusive dressing for at least 30 min. Each gram of EMLA cream contains 25 mg of lignocaine and 25 mg of prilocaine in an oil–water mixture. It is not licensed for use on wounds or mucous membranes.

The cornea and conjunctiva can also be anaesthetized prior to removal of foreign bodies. One to two drops of a local anaesthetic such as lignocaine or amethocaine are instilled on to the eye with the patient looking up whilst pulling the lower eyelid down. The initial instillation is often associated with a stinging sensation that lasts about 30 s. The onset of action is within 30 s, with a duration of action of 15 min.

SEDATION

Both light and deep sedation are frequently required in paediatric and adult emergency practice. During light sedation the patient is drowsy or lightly asleep, with tempered response to minimally painful stimuli. Light sedation can be used during infiltration of local anaesthetics, insertion of chest drains, lumbar puncture or foreign body removal. It is normally given by the oral or intramuscular route. Deep sedation is present when the patient has a decreased level of consciousness with slurring of the speech, although still able to open the eyes to voice and spontaneously ventilate and protect their airway. Deep sedation is usually achieved by the intravenous route. Indications include procedures inflicting moderate to severe pain, such as the reduction of fractures and dislocations, incision and drainage of abscesses.

PATIENT MONITORING

The patient should be sedated for as brief a period as possible and therefore short-acting agents (midazolam) may be more useful than long-acting ones (diazepam). Resuscitation equipment must be readily available in the department and monitoring should be consistent with the depth of sedation and the degree of risk involved. For light sedation pulse oximetry and an experienced nurse may be adequate. For deep sedation, the patient should be monitored using a pulse oximeter and cardiac monitor and regular blood pressure measurements should be taken before, during and after the procedure. An experienced nurse and a skilled doctor should be present throughout the procedure and the patient must be monitored even after the procedure is finished.

> Supplemental oxygen must be administered to all deeply sedated patients.

DRUGS

Benzodiazepines such as midazolam or diazepam are commonly used intravenously to produce sedation, anxiolysis, amnesia and muscle relaxation. They produce amnesia if given before the procedure but they are not primary analgesic agents. There is a large variation in the dose required to induce sedation. The dose should be slowly titrated to the point at which the patient is drowsy but still responsive. Many patients will also have received opiates to provide analgesia, and particular caution is needed in titrating dosages to prevent side-effects and the onset of general anaesthesia. Contraindications to benzodiazepines include patients with chronic chest disease, patients who have taken other sedatives or alcohol, patients who are very aggressive, and patients with hypovolaemia which can decompensate following sedation.

Flumazenil is a specific benzodiazepine antagonist which can be used to reverse the effects of midazolam and diazepam if there is any evidence of respiratory depression or overdose. It has a shorter half-life than benzodiazepines and the patient must be safely monitored in the department.

EMERGENCY GENERAL ANAESTHESIA

General anaesthesia is a reversible drug-induced state of unresponsiveness to outside stimuli, characterized by non-awareness, analgesia and skeletal muscle relaxation. General anaesthesia can be administered in the emergency department either as part of the resuscitation of the seriously ill patient with respiratory failure or overdose, or in major trauma such as head injuries. General anaesthesia in the emergency department for minor procedures such as drainage of abscesses and manipulation of fractures has many drawbacks.

Standards for anaesthesia in any hospital location require a trained anaesthetic assistant and full monitoring, including end-tidal carbon dioxide and gas-monitoring equipment. For this reason there is a tendency to perform all emergency surgery in main theatres. Emergency general anaesthesia can be more difficult than expected and often associated with complications related to the initial problem or co-morbid conditions. For example, injured patients have a significant risk of regurgitation and aspiration of gastric contents during the induction of anaesthesia. Preoperative history may not be available and the fluid resuscitation may be underestimated, leading to unexpected complications following general anaesthesia. Emergency anaesthesia is often performed in the evening or during the night when senior help may not be readily available. In an emergency, middle-grade emergency medicine specialists may have the knowledge and experience to provide general anaesthesia in the department; however, this should primarily be the role of the on-call anaesthetist.

Before the patient is anaesthetized it is important to ensure that they are adequately resuscitated and a preoperative history is taken and the patient examined. The type of procedure, the timing of surgery, the choice of anaesthetic, as well as the availability and adequacy of anaesthetic equipment in the department, should be taken into consideration by the anaesthetist.

It is not our intention to give an in-depth description of the physiology and pharmacology of general anaesthesia as there are dedicated books for this purpose. However, a brief mention of the phases of anaesthesia (induction, maintenance and reversal) will be useful to any emergency medicine specialist as it gives an understanding of the processes involved whilst a patient is anaesthetized.

INDUCTION OF ANAESTHESIA (TABLE 8.5)

Hypnotics

An intravenous induction agent works via a still unknown mechanism to cause unconsciousness as long as it is present in the brain at sufficient levels. The brain receives a high concentration of the initial dose of the agent owing to its very high blood flow. As the drug redistributes into other tissues such as skeletal muscle the concentration of the drug in the brain is reduced to a subanaesthetic level and the patient wakes up. Hence intravenous induction agents are short acting and provide a smooth entry into general anaesthesia, after which a maintenance technique is required.

- *Thiopentone* is a short-acting barbiturate which produces sleep in 30–60 s. It depresses the myocardium and is associated with a 20% drop of the mean arterial blood pressure and a compensatory tachycardia upon induction of anaesthesia. It is therefore used with caution in hypovolaemic patients.
- *Propofol* has very short half-life and is also associated with profound hypotension and inhibits the compensatory increase in heart rate. The induction dose should be reduced to $1\,mg\,kg^{-1}$ in the elderly and in shocked patients. As it has a rapid elimination half-life it is often given as a continuous infusion to maintain anaesthesia.
- *Etomidate* is a longer-acting induction agent that is associated with a higher incidence of postoperative nausea and vomiting. It is only used for induction of anaesthesia as it depresses adrenocortical function. However, it is more potent than barbiturates and is the ideal agent for patients with poor cardiac reserve, as it tends to maintain cardiac output.
- *Ketamine*, which can be given by the intravenous or the intramuscular route, can be used in lower doses as an analgesic or in higher doses as a dissociative anaesthetic. Ketamine raises the pulse rate and blood pressure and has less hypotensive effect on induction than other agents although, paradoxically, it can produce hypotension in shocked patients. Ketamine is contraindicated in hypertensive patients, and concerns have been raised over its use in head-injured patients. The use of ketamine is associated with better airway protection than other agents. Ketamine is most commonly used in the prehospital environment for the release of entrapments and other short procedures, although it is becoming increasingly common in emergency departments as a means of sedating children, with associated amnesia. Atropine should be given to counter ketamine-induced hypersalivation. During ketamine anaesthesia, looking around with the eyes open and phonating may

Table 8.5: Dosage, distribution and elimination half-life of the most commonly used induction agents

Drug	Intravenous dose (mg kg^{-1})	Distribution half-life (min)	Elimination half-life (h)
Thiopentone	3–5	3–14	5–17
Propofol	1–3	2–4	4–5
Etomidate	0.3	2–6	1–5

occur. Nystagmus is typical, and on occasion the limbs may be placed in a position that is self-maintaining. Ketamine may be used for analgesia but its use is not recommended in the emergency department. Ketamine is probably better avoided in children under 1 year of age or those with a history of airway instability or active pulmonary infection or disease. A full stomach, significant head injury and poorly controlled epilepsy are also contraindications. For intramuscular use, $4\,mg\,kg^{-1}$ are used with $0.01\,mg\,kg^{-1}$ atropine (minimum 0.1 mg, maximum 0.5 mg) in the same syringe. If required, $2\text{--}4\,mg\,kg^{-1}$ additional doses without atropine may be given. By the intravenous route, $1\text{--}1.5\,mg\,kg^{-1}$ are administered slowly over 1–2 min. Additional doses of $0.5\,mg\,kg^{-1}$ may be given. Atropine can be given intravenously just before the ketamine dose.

Muscle relaxants

Muscle relaxants are used to facilitate intubation and to allow ventilation. They work by blocking the neuromuscular junction by either binding to the nicotinic receptors and producing depolarization or by binding to the receptors in a competitive non-depolarizing manner.

- *Suxamethonium* is a depolarizing relaxant which has the most rapid onset of all relaxants and is used primarily in predicted difficult intubations and rapid sequence induction of anaesthesia. It is given intravenously at a dose of $1.5\,mg\,kg^{-1}$ to produce fasciculations followed by paralysis within 30 s, with a duration of action between 5 and 10 min. Side-effects include bradycardia, generalized somatic pain, hyperkalaemia and histamine release, resulting in an erythematous rash and only occasionally bronchospasm. Very rarely, it causes persistent neuromuscular blockade owing to deficiency of plasma cholinesterase.
- *Atracurium* and *vecuronium* are examples of non-depolarizing muscle relaxants which are commonly used at induction and have a more delayed onset and prolonged effect (30–40 min). Atracurium is broken down in the plasma by spontaneous hydrolysis and its reversal is easy and complete. Vecuronium does not induce histamine release, thus reducing the

risk of histamine-induced hypotension and bronchospasm.

Rapid sequence induction of anaesthesia

Rapid sequence induction is mandatory in all non-fasted patients, any emergency trauma patient (trauma slows stomach emptying), intestinal obstruction or stasis, pregnancy, or in any patients with visceral pain and intra-abdominal pathology. The patient is pre-oxygenated and intubated whilst cricoid pressure is applied to prevent regurgitation and aspiration of stomach contents.

Initially the patient is given $1.5\,mg\,kg^{-1}$ of suxamethonium, immediately after the induction agent without waiting to observe its effect. A skilled assistant applies pressure on the cricoid cartilage as soon as the patient begins to feel drowsy, compressing the oesophagus between the cricoid ring and the vertebral column. The trachea can be intubated with a cuffed tube as soon as fasciculations have occurred. Cricoid pressure is released after the tube is confirmed to be in place with the cuff inflated.

Rapid sequence induction of anaesthesia should only be performed by those skilled and experienced in its use.

Maintenance and reversal of anaesthesia

Hypnosis during anaesthesia is usually maintained with volatile agents such as isoflurane, enflurane or an infusion of propofol. Relaxation during anaesthesia is maintained by the use of non-depolarizing muscle relaxants such as pancuronium, atracurium or vecuronium. Finally, analgesia is provided partly by the analgesic properties of the nitrous oxide (usually 70% NO with 30% O_2), as well as from parenteral administration of opioids such as fentanyl, alfentanyl (short-acting) or morphine. Modern non-steroidal anti-inflammatory agents such as voltarol and ketorolac are increasingly used for postoperative analgesia.

Reversal of anaesthesia is accomplished by switching off the maintenance (inhaled or infusion) whilst giving 100% oxygen and allowing the drugs to redistribute until the concentration in the brain falls. If non-depolarizing muscle relaxants are used their effect can be reversed by neostigmine, which is an acetylcholinesterase inhibitor. It works by opposing the effects of non-depolarizing neuromuscular blockers. An antimuscarinic agent such as atropine or glycopyrrolate must be given simultaneously to prevent bradycardia, profuse sweating and gut overactivity.

Any technique or procedure that is performed in the emergency department should be done safely by an experienced doctor. The emergency medicine specialists, surgeons and anaesthetists should work together in a multidisciplinary team in order to provide the best quality care for the patient concerned. At a time when clinical governance plays a pivotal role in the NHS, all procedures, ranging from a simple regional anaesthetic to emergency general anaesthesia, as well as the usage of analgesic and sedative drugs, should be routinely audited to improve the quality of healthcare provision.

FURTHER READING

Illingworth, K.A. and Simpson, K.H. (Eds) (1994) *Anaesthesia and Analgesia in Emergency Medicine*. Oxford University Press, Oxford.

Wildsmith, J.A.W. and Armitage, E.N. (Eds) (1993) *Principles and Practice of Regional Anaesthesia*, 2nd edn. Churchill Livingstone, London.

CHAPTER NINE

LEGAL ASPECTS OF EMERGENCY MEDICINE

- Introduction
- Principles of good practice
- The medical defence agencies
- Consent
- The law and mental health problems
- Child abuse
- Religious aspects of emergency medicine
- Dealing with the police
- Controlled drugs

- Requests for information
- Preservation of evidence
- Dealing with the coroner
- Giving evidence
- Negligence
- Medical protection societies
- Seeking appropriate advice
- Managing complaints
- Further reading

INTRODUCTION

It is often stated that it is only a matter of time before any doctor working in an emergency department, however competent he or she may be, is faced with dealing with either a formal complaint or legal action, usually implying negligence. It is sadly true that in this increasingly litigation-orientated age, the legal aspects of our practice have become more and more relevant, and have undoubtedly resulted in a change in the way we practise that cannot be considered entirely in the patient's best interest. Nevertheless, the majority of emergency doctors – especially those in short-term senior house officer posts – will spare themselves a great deal of potential heartache simply by attention to detail, following a few simple rules, and being aware of a small number of legal principles rather than by the practice of overtly defensive medicine.

PRINCIPLES OF GOOD PRACTICE

NOTE TAKING

Accurate, concise and legible records are an essential component of good practice in all areas of medicine. In emergency medicine good notes are vital, as statements may subsequently be required in connection with a variety of potential legal proceedings. The elements outlined in Table 9.1 should be included in the documentation of every attendance. Documentation is dealt with in more detail elsewhere (Chapter 1).

> If it's not written down, it wasn't done.

ADVICE AND REFERRALS

All emergency departments have 24-h a day consultant cover. Increasing numbers have resident middle-grade staff for the greater proportion of each day. Senior advice should always be requested if one is unsure of the most appropriate direction in which to proceed. When advice has been received, it should be clearly recorded in the case notes, together with its source. The full name of any source of advice should always be given as it may prove impossible to identify 'ortho reg' after the passage of time. If you are unhappy with any advice you receive, discuss the situation with the senior emergency doctor available: do not 'shop around' for opinions, as this will only cause irritation.

Table 9.1: Elements of note taking

Date and time
History
Examination
Investigations
Diagnosis (or differential diagnosis)
Treatment
Disposal

When making referrals, always record the name, specialty and grade of the doctor as well as the time of referral (this is also useful for audit purposes). If you wish a specialty doctor to see and assess the patient, insist that they do so and do not accept advice over the phone if you do not feel that it is appropriate. Always clearly record telephone advice.

Never be afraid to ask advice!

DEALING WITH DIFFICULT PATIENTS

A small minority of emergency department patients appear to have a genuine talent for annoying medical and nursing staff, which they are only too keen to exercise. Similarly, many patients are under the influence of alcohol or drugs rendering them uncooperative, abusive or violent. Unfortunately, these patients tend not only to be repeat offenders, but to appear when the department is at its busiest and morale is at its lowest. It is therefore all too easy to provide these patients with inadequate care and to deal with them in an inappropriate, if not hostile, manner. Every attempt should be made to deal with these patients in a normal way, for their protection (they are at risk of injury and chronic ill health) and yours. Manipulative patients are more likely to make troublesome complaints which are difficult to defend if the management is poor.

If a patient is being violent, aggressive or confrontational, it is important to attempt to avoid physical harm by unnecessarily provocative behaviour, although the patient should be informed that their behaviour is unacceptable. If physical violence appears inevitable, the patient should be restrained where possible by security services or the police. The occurrence of both physical and verbal aggression should be clearly recorded in the notes and the record countersigned by a witness.

THE MEDICAL DEFENCE AGENCIES

With the introduction of Crown Indemnity, doctors are no longer responsible for providing their own professional indemnity for matters arising from practice within the NHS. As a consequence, subscriptions to these societies have fallen dramatically. Nevertheless, all doctors working in emergency medicine are strongly advised to be a member of a medical defence agency as the cost is reasonable. These agencies provide 24-h a day telephone legal advice as well as continuing to provide indemnity for work undertaken outside the NHS, including attendance at accidents and sporting events as well as the provision of medical advice and legal reports.

CONSENT

ADULTS

For the purposes of consent, an adult is considered to be someone aged 16 years or over. Adults who are conscious and of sound mind are considered to be capable of giving or refusing consent. If, following appropriate explanation, such adults choose to withhold consent, however unwise, irrational or foolish this may appear, these wishes must be respected. Should such a refusal be made, this should be stated clearly in the notes, ideally with a written description of potential hazards as explained to the patient. Such a record should, wherever possible, be countersigned by a witness, and if they are willing to do so, by the patient.

The only exception to this occurs when the patient appears to have been brought under undue pressure by other persons to act against their best interests, and when the consequences of so doing might be serious or life threatening. In this extremely rare situation an application to court can be made regarding the lawfulness of the treatment. Such an application is made by the hospital solicitor following discussion between senior medical staff and senior hospital management.

> For the purposes of consent an adult is effectively someone aged 16 years or over.

Some adults are considered incapable of giving informed consent to a treatment or procedure. This might be because of unconsciousness or acute or chronic mental illness. In such cases it is acceptable to proceed with treatment without consent if the treatment is urgently required to save life or prevent significant deterioration. If the inability to give consent is believed to be temporary, treatment should if possible be kept to a minimum pending recovery, when a patient will be able to give their own consent to further therapy. Wherever time permits, and consent is not going to be available from the patient, the situation and the options available should be discussed with the patient's next of kin, carers or guardian.

Extreme care should be exercised when considering the necessity for consent to treat patients from mental hospitals, especially those admitted voluntarily. In such cases, a judgement must be made as to the patient's ability to give valid informed consent. Patients suffering significant mental disturbance may still be capable of understanding the medical options open to them and giving consent appropriately. Where such consent is not possible, treatment usually follows discussion among medical and nursing staff as well as relatives or guardians. If problems arise, application to the court may be necessary.

> Patients detained under the Mental Health Act should not be assumed to be incapable of giving consent.

Although many patients detained under the Mental Health Act are incapable of giving consent, and certain clauses of the Act specifically allow for certain treatments to be carried out without consent (for example electroconvulsive therapy), wherever possible informed consent should be sought from the patient. If such consent cannot be obtained, decisions regarding treatment rest with senior medical staff following discussion with relatives. In this situation, relatives cannot give or withhold consent on the patient's behalf.

Technical aspects of the Mental Health Act are discussed below.

CHILDREN

The ability of children to give consent should be based on an assessment of their ability to understand the situation which has arisen rather than on their chronological age. Any person of 16 years or over who is of sound mind is considered able to give or refuse consent to treatment on their own behalf. The Gillick Case (1985) also established that certain children under the age of 16 years are also able to give or withhold consent on their own behalf if it can be demonstrated that they are capable of understanding the consequences of their decision (so-called *Gillick competence*).

Parents or guardians are not able to overrule the wishes of a minor aged over 16 years or under 16 years who is Gillick competent. Clearly, however, the degree of understanding required will be proportional to the complexity or seriousness of the situation facing the child. The court has the power to overrule the refusal of any minor to give consent, and if the consequences of such a refusal are likely to be fatal or serious, an appropriate application should be made.

> Some children under the age of 16 years are considered legally capable of giving or refusing consent on their own behalf.

Consent to treat a child who is under 16 years and *Gillick incompetent* should be obtained from a parent or an adult with official parental responsibility. Consent from an accompanying adult or elder brother or sister without such responsibility is not adequate. If such consent cannot be obtained in time, and the proposed treatment is necessary to save life or prevent significant deterioration, the treatment can proceed without consent. If the parents refuse consent for treatment following full discussion, and this appears to be against the child's best interest, an application can be made to the court for permission to proceed without such consent. The consequences of such a refusal should be sufficiently serious to warrant this step being taken, and it should ideally only be taken after a second opinion from a senior doctor in the specialty. Such an application is made by the hospital solicitor on instruction from the duty hospital manager.

If the patient is a child of unsound mind, wherever possible consent should be sought from someone with parental (or equivalent) responsibility.

THE LAW AND MENTAL HEALTH PROBLEMS

The legislation regarding the compulsory admission to hospital of patients with mental illness is found in the Mental Health Act of 1983.

SECTION 2: ADMISSION FOR ASSESSMENT

Section 2 of the Mental Health Act 1983 allows admission to hospital for assessment, for a period of up to 28 days, either in the interests of the patient's health or for the protection of others. The admission is made on the recommendation of two doctors, one of whom must be 'approved' under the Act. The initial application is made either by the patient's nearest relative or by an approved social worker. At the end of 28 days, if not before, the patient must be discharged or detained in hospital under a different section of the Act. The patient can be discharged by the medical staff, hospital manager or nearest relative, although this course of action by relatives can be prevented by hospital authorities if clinically necessary.

SECTION 3: ADMISSION FOR TREATMENT

Patients are admitted to hospital under Section 3 for treatment of a mental disorder. The initial duration of admission is 6 months, but the doctor responsible for the patient's on-going care can extend this. As with Section 2, admission is made after two doctors have examined the patient, one of whom must be approved. The nearest relative or an approved social worker makes the initial application. Similar rules to those concerning patients detained under Section 2 apply regarding discharge. The detention of patients under Section 3 for more than 6 months is subject to regular review by a Mental Health Tribunal.

SECTION 4: ADMISSION IN AN EMERGENCY

Section 4 allows the urgent admission of a patient on the application of the nearest relative or a social worker for a period of 72 h only. The patient only needs to have been examined by one doctor, but this must have been within the 24 h preceding the admission. This doctor does not have to be approved under the Act. At or before the end of 72 h, the patient must be discharged or an application made under one of the other sections.

SECTION 5: PREVENTION OF DISCHARGE

Both medical and nursing staff have certain rights under Section 5 of the Mental Health Act which allow them to prevent the discharge of a patient who has already been admitted to hospital. In the case of nursing staff, they may restrain a patient for up to 6 h whilst awaiting medical opinion. Powers under Section 5 are not applicable to patients in an emergency department.

SECTION 135: REMOVAL TO A PLACE OF SAFETY

Under certain circumstances, a police officer accompanied by a doctor and an approved social worker may, under a warrant issued by a magistrate following an application by the social worker, remove a patient to a place of safety. Reasons for such a removal include mental illness, inability to look after oneself and ill treatment or neglect. If the patient is in a public place removal may occur without a warrant. In both cases, the patient may be detained for 72 h pending a further application. Accepted places of safety under the Act include police stations, NHS hospitals and social services residential accommodation.

SUICIDAL INTENT

Patients threatening one form or another of self-harm are unfortunately common in busy emergency departments, and it is usually clear that the behaviour concerned is attention-seeking rather than representing any genuine risk to the patient's life or health. However, great care should be exercised as a small number of patients will be genuinely at risk, and a proportion of these will be patients who have presented repeatedly with relatively trivial self-inflicted problems.

The majority of patients who present following one episode of self-harm, or threatening to carry out another, will willingly consent to treatment. Occasionally such a patient will refuse all offers of assistance. Although the patient may be threatening to commit significant self-harm, or to take their own life, unless they have been detained subject to the Mental Health Act the normal rules of consent apply. Furthermore, suicidal intent does not constitute mental illness and is not itself grounds for 'sectioning' a patient. Such a patient can only be warned of the consequences of their action and offered appropriate treatment and support. If the patient is of unsound mind, and has been sectioned under Section 2 or Section 3 of the Mental Health Act, then treatment can take place without their consent for conditions resulting from the mental illness. If the patient is rendered incapable of making an appropriate judgement of the situation by drink or drugs, treatment intended to save life or prevent serious harm can proceed without consent, pending the patient's recovery from the effects of the substances concerned.

CHILD ABUSE

The clinical features of child abuse are discussed in Chapter 39 and summarized in Tables 9.2, 9.3 and 9.4. The legal implications are discussed below.

Medical staff working in emergency departments have a clear responsibility to protect children who they believe have suffered or are at risk of suffering from abuse, whether it be physical or sexual. The consequences, to the staff as well as to the child, are only too clear from recent public enquiries. Nevertheless, it is important not to be over-zealous as the consequences of incorrect suspicions of abuse can be devastating. Every parent will know how common minor injuries are among intrepid toddlers and children, and how often the perfectly genuine explanation sounds unconvincing even to those who know it to be true.

When it is clear, or beyond reasonable doubt, that abuse has taken place, the correct action required is clear. The child should be admitted immediately under the care of the paediatrician on call. The case should be referred to a senior

Table 9.2: Characteristic injuries in child abuse

Multiple skin bruises and abrasions, including bite marks, often of different ages
Multiple fractures (check old casualty cards: some fractures may only become evident on subsequent skeletal survey)
Facial injuries, including injuries to the inside of the mouth
Signs suggestive of sexual abuse
Burns, especially from cigarettes or with an unusual history
Head injuries
Abdominal injuries

Table 9.3: Presentation of child abuse

Child usually under 3 years
Delay before presentation
Inadequate or conflicting explanation of injuries
More common in girls than boys

Table 9.4: The social background to child abuse

Young parents
Low social class
The mother's partner is often not the biological parent of the child
Large family with several small children
Social isolation
Father with a history of violent behaviour or a criminal record
Parents themselves abused, or the victims of inadequate parenting

paediatrician and discussed in detail, making any concerns clear and recording them in the notes. Where the injuries themselves require admission, there is usually no problem; however, if it is the cause of the injury that prompts admission, the situation requires considerable tact. Where possible it is better not to mention the suspicion of child abuse until the child has been admitted and appropriate arrangements for care are in place. The emergency department is not the place to make a definitive diagnosis of child abuse.

The emergency department is not the place to make a definitive diagnosis of child abuse.

If abuse or suspected abuse means that a child requires admission and the parents refuse consent, a *Place of Safety Order* lasting up to 8 days is obtained from a magistrate. Following the initial period, a *Care Order* is sought, transferring the care of the child to the local authority if it is believed they cannot safely return to the care of their parents.

Should parents attempt to remove a child who is considered to be at risk from an emergency department, they can be prevented from doing so by a police officer. If this is not possible, the social services should be contacted and the child taken into care from home under a Place of Safety Order. If the danger is considered sufficiently acute, the police are allowed to act without such an order in the first instance.

Unfortunately, the situation is often less clear. The history may be suspicious or the presentation late and the family dynamics often abnormal, but there may be no clear evidence of anything more sinister than poor parenting. In these cases, there has to be a degree of personal assessment of the possible risks to the child. It is often helpful to seek the opinion of nursing staff who have been involved in the care of the family. If there is any doubt, the child should be admitted. Most departments now have attached paediatric social workers and health visitors who will arrange to follow up families and children and offer support to parents, and referral should be made if the social circumstances of a child are a matter of concern. Couples whose parenting skills are poor, often because of their own parents' poor parenting of them, require support rather than condemnation and open suspicion, in an attempt to achieve the best for their children.

Disclosure of medical information about children to the child protection agencies is covered by the same rules of confidentiality as with all other patients. However, it is accepted that appropriate disclosures may be made if they are genuinely in the best interests of the child.

RELIGIOUS ASPECTS OF EMERGENCY MEDICINE

DEALING WITH JEHOVAH'S WITNESSES

Jehovah's Witnesses believe that it is wrong to receive blood from another person or to undergo some forms of organ transplant. However, very recently the rules regarding the prohibition of blood transfusion have been significantly relaxed. Any Jehovah's Witness over the age of 16 years is entitled to refuse such treatment, however unreasonable this attitude may seem to others. Nothing can legally be done to change their mind unless there are strong grounds for suspecting that they are not acting of their own free will, having been put under unreasonable pressure by others. If the patient is a child, however, and consent from a parent cannot be obtained in a situation in which the life or health of the child is at risk, then an application can be made to the courts to proceed with treatment without such consent. If there is no time available to obtain such permission, medical staff should carry out the necessary treatment, as it is extremely unlikely that legal action against medical staff in these circumstances would ever be successful. Gillick competence applies in these cases.

If it can be clearly and unequivocally established that a patient who is for whatever reason unable to give consent is genuinely a Jehovah's Witness, this information must be respected and the relevant treatments avoided. However, such information must be clear, and a simple statement to the effect that a friend 'thinks that the patient is a Jehovah's Witness' is not adequate.

DEALING WITH THE POLICE

Given all the problems all staff in emergency departments have to face, particularly on Friday and Saturday nights, it does no harm at all to remain on friendly terms with local police officers. Unnecessarily confrontational attitudes are therefore inappropriate. Staff are not employed to be the patient's advocate in legal matters. Nevertheless, they do have a responsibility to ensure, firstly that the patient's treatment and recovery are not compromised, and secondly that no breach of medical confidence occurs.

ACCESS TO MEDICAL INFORMATION

Police officers do not have an automatic right to see confidential medical records or to remove them from the department. Any statement containing such confidential material should only be given with the patient's written consent. If such consent is refused or cannot be obtained, the doctor may be summoned to court, where any refusal may be considered to be contempt of court. In practice, this is rarely necessary. Very rarely, an emergency may arise when withholding information might jeopardize the progress of a case where a rapid solution is clearly in the public interest. In such cases, the details should be discussed with the senior clinician involved in the case and with a medical defence organization before information is released: subsequent legal action would be very unlikely. Requests for information are usually best dealt with by a senior member of staff.

The police are not entitled to be told the time of a patient's arrival in, or departure from, the department.

Under the Road Traffic Accident Act of 1988 doctors are obliged to release the identity of patients treated as a result of a road traffic accident. In Northern Ireland, the Emergency Powers and Prevention of Terrorism Act obliges doctors to release information about injuries which may be connected with terrorist activity.

MOTORING OFFENCES

The commonest request from the police when dealing with victims of a road traffic accident is for a breath alcohol sample. Samples of breath, blood or urine can only be taken with the consent of the patient and the doctor looking after the patient, who may refuse if the patient's care would be adversely affected by the taking of such samples. Patients cannot be arrested for drunken driving whilst they remain in hospital. If a blood sample is required specifically for an alcohol level (a forensic rather than clinical test) it should be taken by a police surgeon who should be called in to carry out this task. Pressure by the police to take the sample 'in order to save time' should be firmly resisted. Diagnostic specimens cannot be used by the police without the consent of the doctor in charge of the case or the patient. Patients who refuse to give a blood or urine sample without an adequate reason are committing an offence; intoxication is not an

Do not take blood for forensic purposes – that is what a police surgeon is for!

excuse. Forensic samples may not be taken from unconscious patients.

Patients who are unfit to drive for medical reasons have a duty to inform the Drive and Vehicle Licensing Authority (DVLA) of this fact. Causes include visual disturbances, conditions associated with loss of consciousness and chronic alcohol abuse. If this situation arises, *having warned the patient of the intention to do so*, doctors have a responsibility to inform the DVLC themselves of their concern. In the acute situation, patients who clearly intend to drive whilst drunk should be warned that they will be reported, and the police informed.

THE ROLE OF THE POLICE SURGEON

The police surgeon is employed to provide medical and forensic services to the police force. The majority of such doctors are also local general practitioners. Police surgeons are trained in the medico-legal aspects of practice, and assist in taking forensic samples, examination of the victims of assault and sexual assault and assessing fitness to be detained.

CONTROLLED DRUGS

Patients with drugs in their possession are increasingly common in emergency departments, and the correct handling of such substances causes concern among medical and nursing staff. In fact, the correct response to such a situation is clearly prescribed by the law.

Once drugs, by whatever means, have come into the possession of medical or nursing staff, they must *never* be returned to the patient or a relative or friend. This could, strictly, be considered 'supplying'. The only acceptable solution is to destroy them in front of witnesses or to hand them over to the police. Unless the police are known to be involved in the case, suspecting the patient of a drugs offence, staff need not report the matter to the police as long as the drugs are destroyed. If the police are involved, destruction of the drugs is prohibited as they may be required in evidence. Medical staff may not disclose any confidential details to the police.

Controlled drugs which are legally possessed (e.g. methadone if properly prescribed to a registered addict), should be kept safe with other hospital-controlled drugs and returned to the patient on discharge.

PRESCRIPTION REQUESTS

Requests by addicts for a repeat prescription are common, usually when it can be argued that the normal legitimate source of supply is unavailable. The story is usually enhanced by much heart-rending detail regarding the consequences of a failure to prescribe. However, adequate facilities for obtaining legal supplies are now available, and the possibility that the patient may be attempting to obtain supplies for sale should be considered. If the patient does bring a prescription, ensure that it has not been altered in any way. Wherever possible, contact the doctor legally responsible for prescribing for the patient. Remember that only a doctor licensed by the Home Office can legally prescribe morphine and related drugs to an addict.

Emergency departments are not appropriate places for the uncontrolled supply of drugs to addicts, and departments that readily do so will rapidly develop a reputation they do not need and a clientele they do not want. Unless there is an overwhelming need to do so, *never* give prescriptions for controlled drugs under these circumstances.

REQUESTS FOR INFORMATION

Requests from relatives and others regarding information about a patient's condition are naturally extremely common, very often taking the form of telephone enquiries. A sensible approach should be taken, always remembering that medical information of any kind is confidential. When the relatives, or friends, accompany the patient to the department, the patient will either give consent for the disclosure of information or circumstances will render it appropriate for some details to be given. Clearly, potentially embarrassing information should not be disclosed without the patient's consent.

Care should be taken over telephone enquiries, as there is always the possibility that the caller is not who they claim to be. There are occasions when members of the press have impersonated relatives in order to gain confidential information. In general, relatives and friends should be given broad, non-specific details sufficient to allow them to do what is necessary for the patient ('they are stable'; 'they are poorly and we think you should come to the hospital'). Unless it cannot be avoided, information should not be given over the telephone that can be given better in person.

Employers are best advised that no information can be given over the telephone, although depending on the circumstances the release of broad details as above may be appropriate. Specific clinical details should not be given. It is as well to bear in mind that an accident at work may result in legal action by the patient against their employer (or vice versa).

PRESERVATION OF EVIDENCE

Many of the patients attending an emergency department have been involved in road traffic accidents or assaults, and will eventually be involved in legal action of one kind or another. Any property that may be evidence in legal action should be listed, bagged, labelled and retained.

DEALING WITH THE CORONER

All deaths occurring in an emergency department must be reported to the coroner as soon as possible. Ideally the report should be made immediately, or first thing the following morning if the death has occurred after the close of the previous working day. It is important therefore to arrange for a colleague to contact the coroner if a shift ends before the office opens. The usual point of contact is with the coroner's officer, who is a police officer and not medically trained. It is important to keep the details of the patient accurate, concise and free from unnecessary technical jargon. Until the coroner is satisfied, a death certificate cannot be issued and there will be inevitable delays in completing the formalities associated with a death. Once a death has been reported, the coroner's officer may contact the patient's general practitioner, who in cases of death due to apparent natural causes may be prepared to issue a death certificate based on their previous knowledge of the patient's medical history.

GIVING EVIDENCE

There are two types of medical evidence:

- evidence of fact
- expert opinion.

Evidence of fact, the kind of evidence junior doctors are usually called upon to give, describes what actually happened as far as the facts are known to the witness. Opinion evidence is usually, but not always, given by consultants and is intended to help the court ascertain the significance of information put before it. Experts also give evidence of fact. Junior doctors should be careful in both written and oral evidence to restrict themselves to details of which they have personal knowledge and not be tempted to offer opinions which their experience is unable to justify.

WRITING LEGAL REPORTS

All doctors working in an emergency department will sooner or later be required to complete a statement for the police on a patient they have treated. Ideally, each department will be able to provide a sample statement demonstrating correct practice. Failing this, it is advisable for new doctors to seek the advice of a senior doctor before submitting statements. A sample statement is given in Figure 9.1.

The statement should begin with the time of attendance of the patient at the department and the time they were seen by a doctor. The grade of the doctor should be recorded.

'John Smith attended the Accident and Emergency Department at Blankshire Royal Infirmary at 21.00 on Wednesday the 24th October 1997 and was seen by me, James Smith MBBS, as casualty officer at 23.15...'

The statement should included details of the medical history and of any injury received. It is acceptable, for example, to state that the patient attended as the result of an alleged assault, but details of any incident obtained from the patient are not evidence when repeated by a doctor and should be included in the form 'the patient stated that…'.

A precise description of the nature and location of all injuries should be given, together with their dimensions. Clearly labelled diagrams are acceptable, although ideally injuries should be carefully described and their relation to anatomical features given. A clear distinction should be made between the information gathered by the writer and information acquired from the notes. It is not the role of the junior doctor to offer any opinion regarding the causation and timing of the injuries.

GOING TO COURT

Although medical staff are frequently warned that they may be required to give evidence in court, in most cases they will not actually be asked to attend. If attendance at court is likely, it is essential that the original notes and X-rays are obtained and that you are familiar with them. It is usually helpful to discuss the case with a senior member of the department's medical staff. The majority of times a senior house officer or registrar is called to court it will be as a witness of fact, and it is important not to be tempted to give evidence beyond the facts as available. Expert witnesses will be called (and paid!) to give expert opinion.

NEGLIGENCE

In order for a complaint of negligence to succeed, three criteria have to be met: there must be a duty of care, there must be a failure to fulfil this duty of care and, finally, harm must have arisen as a result of this failure of care. A doctor who commences the treatment of a patient has a duty of care to that patient. A hospital doctor does not have a duty of care to a patient who collapses in the street, and is not negligent if they fail to offer assistance in this situation, although a general practitioner does have a duty of care to such patients within their own practice area. Once any doctor commences the treatment of such a patient, a duty of care exists.

The expected standard of care from any medical practitioner will depend upon their seniority and

Witness Statement

(CJ Act 1967, s.9 MC Act 1980, ss. 5A (3a) and 5B MC Rules 1981, r.70)

Statement of _____ Dr David Jones

Age if under 18 __Over 18__ (if over 18 insert 'over 18'). Occupation __Medical Practitioner__

This statement (consisting of ____1____ pages each signed by me) is true to the best of my knowledge and belief and I make it knowing that, if it is tendered in evidence, I shall be liable to prosecution if I have wilfully stated anything which I know to be false or do not believe to be true.

Dated the __21st__ day of __June__ __18 2001__

Signature _____ David Jones

I, David Jones, am a medical practitioner currently employed as a Senior House Officer in the Accident and Emergency Department of St. Elsewhere's Hospital, Anytown.

I was on duty in the department on the 5th of May 2001 when I examined Peter Smith (Date of birth 20.1.81) of 63 Riverside, Anytown at 2004 hours.

He told me that he had been punched in the face that afternoon. On examination I found a 4 centimetre laceration to the right eyebrow region. No other injury was found. The wound was closed by the insertion of 5 sutures under local anaesthetic. He was advised to have the sutures removed in 5 days. He was then discharged.

Signature _____ David Jones _____ Signature witnessed by _____ Sue Martin

P.T.O.

Figure 9.1: A sample police statement.

experience, although any doctor will be expected to confine their activities to those at which they are competent.

Failure of that duty of care is usually determined by the Bolam test. The Bolam test implies that a doctor is not negligent as long as there is a body of expert medical opinion in agreement with the treatment given, even if a substantial body of medical opinion believes it to be incorrect. In the Bolam case, the judge stated:

'A doctor is not guilty of negligence if he has acted in accordance with the practice accepted as proper by a responsible body of medical men skilled in that particular art'.

Thus the level of performance required to avoid a complaint of negligence will effectively be determined by peer review. This is likely to be particularly contentious in matters of clinical judgement where no obvious error or malpractice is evident. The burden of proof of negligence usually lies with the patient unless the medical error is apparently so obvious that the doctor is called to refute the allegation.

Common measures of damage caused by or attributed to medical negligence include pain, suffering, loss of function, disfigurement and death (or reduced life expectancy). In addition, the patient may allege that loss of employment or financial hardship has arisen as a consequence of a doctor's actions.

If it is likely that an incident has occurred that might subsequently result in a claim of negligence, it is essential firstly that exhaustive and accurate notes are made and secondly that a consultant is informed. Once litigation has been initiated, the involvement of one of the medical defence agencies is vital and membership of one of these organizations should be taken out by all doctors working in emergency medicine. As a consequence of *Crown Indemnity*, introduced as a result of the rising costs of private medical defence cover, the employing NHS Trust is responsible for the negligent acts of its employees. This responsibility, however, only extends to work done under contract, and acts such as stopping at the scene of an accident or crowd cover at sporting events are specifically excluded.

It might be said that the commonest cause of patients resorting to the formal complaint and redress procedure is not that mistakes have been made, but rather that the relationship between the doctor and patient has failed. Sometimes the attitude of the patient may make this inevitable, but in general an honest and open explanation with obvious concern and regret will go a long way to achieving a more amicable solution to the situation. Admission that a mistake has been made will not prejudice any future legal action. Where there is any doubt, expert legal advice should be sought.

MEDICAL PROTECTION SOCIETIES

In defending a case of negligence, hospitals and health agencies will be motivated not only by attempts to preserve their reputation, but also by attempts to save unnecessary expense. This latter concern is all the more important now that damage payments can be in excess of £1 000 000, and Trusts do not have unlimited funds out of which they can be paid. It is possible therefore that the specific concerns of individual doctors can be lost in what appear to be more important problems. Membership of a defence organization allows the provision of individual expert advice to each doctor and is essential in this increasingly litigious environment. In addition, these organizations are able to provide legal advice concerning a broad range of subjects, such as consent, contracts, fitness to practice and dealing with the police. Doctors taking part in regular medical cover for events outside their normal employment should also ensure that they have adequate cover as such events are not covered by Crown Indemnity (see above).

SEEKING APPROPRIATE ADVICE

Emergency medicine is a challenging specialty with an inexhaustible range of potential patients, illnesses and injuries. No single doctor can ever have seen or read about every condition that they might confront. It is essential therefore, that appropriate help and advice is sought where necessary. Alternatively, where the problem is unusual or the cause is not immediately obvious, it may be necessary to seek the advice of an emergency medicine consultant or registrar with more general experience of emergency medicine. Never be afraid to ask for advice. Junior staff must not take decisions which are beyond their experience. Emergency medicine is not about making 'courageous' decisions, often under pressure from other specialties who are reluctant to see or admit a patient, it is about making safe decisions in the best interests of the patient, and ultimately of the doctor. Where departmental or national guidelines are available, they should be followed.

MANAGING COMPLAINTS

The majority of doctors will, usually through no fault of their own, receive a complaint whilst working in emergency medicine. Some actions can be taken which will aid in the management of such complaints, at the time the patient seen. Always keep accurate, legible and thorough notes. However great the provocation, always try to maintain a civil relationship with the patient. Patients are more likely to sue doctors whom they perceive to be unpleasant than those they perceive to be incompetent. If a patient is aggressive, abusive, drunk or unco-operative, record it on the casualty card and have the statement witnessed.

Complaints are usually sent either to the department manager or senior consultant or direct to the Trust. All Trusts now have a complaints and litigation department. When asked for a statement following a complaint provide a clear statement based on the available records. Ensure that information is gathered from other members of staff who were present. Discuss the case with the consultant. If there is any possibility of legal action being taken, contact the medical defence agency and keep them informed.

FURTHER READING

Knight, B. (1991) *Simpson's Forensic Medicine*, 10th edn. Edward Arnold, London.

Knight, B. (1992) *Legal Aspects of Medical Practice*, 5th edn. Churchill Livingstone, Edinburgh.

Montague, A. (1996) *Legal Problems in Emergency Medicine*. Oxford Handbooks in Emergency Medicine, Oxford University Press, Oxford.

MEDICAL AND SURGICAL EMERGENCIES

CARDIAC ARREST

INTRODUCTION

Optimal outcome for a patient suffering cardiopulmonary arrest (CPA) is dependent on a number of time-critical links in the 'chain of survival'. Essential amongst these is rapid recognition of the emergency, access to early basic and advanced life-support skills, rapid transfer to definitive care and treatment of an underlying cause.

The objectives of this chapter are to describe discrete subsets of patients brought to the emergency department in CPA and their varying outcomes. The personnel, relevant equipment and most up-to-date Resuscitation Council (UK) guidelines on resuscitation of adults and children in CPA are included. The importance of post-resuscitation care in patients successfully resuscitated is highlighted, as well as guidance on when it is appropriate to stop resuscitation. Important additional principles in resuscitating patients in certain 'special circumstances' are also covered.

HETEROGENEITY OF CARDIAC ARREST IN THE EMERGENCY DEPARTMENT

Patients suffering CPA who present to the emergency department are a diverse group. Ischaemic heart disease is the commonest cause of cardiac arrest in adults. In practice, however, outcome can be disappointingly poor despite the patient being given the best possible treatment. It is important to anticipate this at an early stage in the resuscitation, thus allowing relevant information to be rapidly collated during an intense period in which there are many different facets to concentrate on. Patients fall into a number of broad groups with differing chances of survival (Table 10.1).

Often patients arrive in the emergency department having suffered a prehospital cardiac arrest and having been resuscitated by paramedic staff with advanced life-support skills for at least 20 min or more following collapse. If CPA persists on arrival in the resuscitation room, the outcome is extremely poor (less than 5% survival) irrespective of the type of initial rhythm.

> Patients arriving at hospital in cardiac arrest despite full resuscitation procedures by paramedics are very unlikely to survive.

Table 10.1: Categories of cardiac arrest patients seen in emergency departments

Prehospital cardiac arrest without return of circulation on arrival in resuscitation room
Prehospital cardiac arrest with return of circulation
Cardiac arrest during transport to hospital
Cardiac arrest in the department
Paediatric cardiac arrest

The patient may have suffered a cardiac arrest in the prehospital phase and have been successfully resuscitated by paramedics. These patients will often have had a witnessed arrest where the primary rhythm was ventricular fibrillation (VF) and have been successfully treated by early defibrillation. They will arrive in the department having had basic post-resuscitation care only and may still be in an unstable condition.

However, if the cardiac arrest occurred in the presence of paramedic staff or just prior to arrival in the resuscitation room and the initial rhythm is VF, the expected outcome should be a discharge rate from hospital of 30–50%. Non-VF cardiac arrest rhythms will still have a poor outcome (less than 10% survival) even in the best system.

A patient who has a cardiac arrest in the emergency department with a primarily cardiac aetiology and with VF as the first rhythm should have a successful outcome, with survival rates exceeding 50%.

Studies in children suffering a prehospital cardiac arrest have shown a uniformly dismal outcome, with a rate of survival to hospital discharge of less than 5% irrespective of the initial rhythm. The majority of survivors leave hospital with significant neurological disability. Those emergency medical service (EMS) systems with well-developed prehospital paediatric advanced life-support skills have results which are only slightly better (less than 10% survival rates).

In order to deal with such variation and the time-critical nature of the event, appropriate organization is a crucial factor. Effective management of a cardiac arrest requires a methodical approach, consistent adherence to resuscitation guidelines and joint multidisciplinary management for those patients who achieve a stable cardiac output in the resuscitation room. This also prevents an inordinately prolonged resuscitation attempt in a hope-less situation.

In addition, it is important to appreciate that neurological outcome cannot be reliably forecast in this acute state until a period of 12–24 h of controlled ventilation, cardiovascular and cerebral support has been completed. Early input from intensive care unit staff is therefore essential. Organization and appropriate use of personnel and equipment are described below.

> The quantity and quality of survival cannot be predicted early after resuscitation from cardiac arrest.

PERSONNEL

Expertise in resuscitating patients from cardiac arrest comes through training and clearly defined roles for team members. Such members should be familiar with each of the responsibilities outlined in Table 10.2.

The team leader is pivotal in running a well-organized resuscitation and must be authoritative but responsive to useful suggestions from other

Table 10.2: Roles of the cardiac arrest team

Person A (airway): Prepare airway equipment Support airway and ventilation at 12 ventilations per minute
Person B (cardiac compression): Institute CPR Maintain compressions at 100 per minute Count aloud when CPR is not in progress (one off, two off, etc.) Inform team leader at 10 off Inform team leader when tiring
Person C (defibrillation): Place gel pads on chest Read rhythm via paddles If VF or possibly VF, defibrillate; if not, then place ECG leads on chest
Person D (vascular): Gain vascular access Give intravenous drugs with chaser fluids Take blood samples and arterial blood gases as asked to do so by team leader
Person E (documentation/drugs): Prepare drugs for administration Document the rhythm, time and intervention performed
Person F (relatives/runner): Take relatives to quiet room or stay with them if they wish to stay in the resuscitation room Gain a history from relative and inform team leader if appropriate (e.g. anaphylaxis, overdose)
Person G (team leader): Prepare team Delegate tasks clearly Confirm cardiopulmonary arrest, check airway and endotracheal tube position **Co-ordinate resuscitation** Organize post-resuscitation care if appropriate Organize debrief if appropriate

members of the team. Instructions should be given clearly, though in a polite manner. The team leader must be supportive towards other members of the team during and after the event. Above all the leadership role is accomplished in a 'hands off' manner unless an essential practical procedure has not been adequately performed by the team member (failure to intubate the trachea).

It is important that the team leader also gains information from paramedics at an early stage regarding the time of arrest, interventions performed, the presence of bystander cardiopulmonary resuscitation (CPR) and any intervening return of circulation. The prehospital times and events should be taken into account when deciding on how long to persist with efforts at resuscitation and the team leader should discuss termination of resuscitation, if appropriate, with the other members of the team so that the decision to stop treatment is shared and agreed by the whole team.

> Termination of the resuscitation should be a team decision.

EQUIPMENT

All resuscitation equipment should be checked on a daily basis and, if time allows, prior to the arrival of a patient in the resuscitation room. The team leader should ensure that team members are all confident in the use of the equipment, especially the defibrillator (Table 10.3).

In the future a technique of hands-free defibrillation may become increasingly commonplace allowing for safer practice.

AIRWAY AND VENTILATION IN CARDIAC ARREST

Endotracheal intubation is the gold standard method for controlling the airway and oxygenating the patient. However, this manoeuvre requires skilled personnel and appropriate equipment. In the meantime, a number of basic airway interventions should suffice to maintain some level of ventilation. These include mouth-to-mouth ventilation with simple airway manoeuvres (jaw thrust or

Table 10.3: Defibrillation

> Do not allow anyone to use a defibrillator who has not been trained to do so.
> Apply gel pads to the patient's chest and select the energy required.
> Paddles should be charged either whilst in the defibrillator or once on the patient's chest (preferably the latter). Paddles should be held either on the chest or in the locating slots – never in mid-air.
> Apply paddles firmly over the apex of the heart and to the right of the upper sternum.
> Visually and vocally (loudly) ensure there is no physical contact by team members with the patient or the trolley.
> Deliver the shock and check for a change in the rhythm. If there is no change in the rhythm, do not delay defibrillation to check the pulse during a cycle of three defibrillatory shocks.

chin lift), oropharyngeal (Guedel) airway and bag/valve/mask ventilation. The laryngeal mask airway is achieving increasing popularity as a means of securing the airway in order to ventilate a patient in CPA. A number of studies have suggested that this device is a rapid and easier alternative to endotracheal intubation in patients with cardiac arrest, especially when staff do not regularly intubate.

> High inspired concentrations of oxygen must always be provided.

VASCULAR ACCESS

The most commonly used technique is to insert a cannula in an antecubital vein. However, during cardiac arrest it is essential to have a neutral chaser fluid running to ensure entry of drugs to the central circulation. This is usually accomplished by infusing crystalloid through the cannula after drug administration. Cannulation of the external jugular veins is also popular as the veins are distended in cardiac arrest and this route, though not strictly central venous access, offers rapid access to the central circulation and heart.

Alternative techniques include cannulation of an internal jugular, subclavian or femoral vein, although these will be dependent on the expertise of the operator. Intraosseous line insertion in children is a safe, reliable and efficacious route of drug administration. However, it is more difficult to insert in children over 6 years of age owing to the increase in bone density.

RESUSCITATION ALGORITHMS

The basic and advanced algorithms for adults and children in cardiac arrest are shown below. They are the result of collaboration between the American Heart Association, the European Resuscitation Council and other international resuscitation councils. The Guidelines 2000 for CPR and Emergency Cardiovascular Care are a comprehensive evidence-based resource and have now been adopted by the Resuscitation Council (UK).

BASIC LIFE SUPPORT IN ADULTS (FIG. 10.1)

Basic life support (BLS) is an essential prerequisite for a patient in cardiac arrest until advanced life-support (ALS) measures are available. The presence of bystander BLS is a major factor in a successful outcome, especially for patients suffering a prehospital cardiac arrest. However, even when performed optimally it provides only 20–30% of a patient's normal cardiac output.

It is important to consider a number of specific issues related to this algorithm. BLS is only a 'holding measure' and experienced help with ALS skills and equipment is essential to achieve a successful outcome. Therefore if there is a single rescuer, they must decide when to leave the patient to summon assistance (dependent upon location). The Resuscitation Council (UK) recommends that if the likely cause of unconsciousness is trauma, drowning,

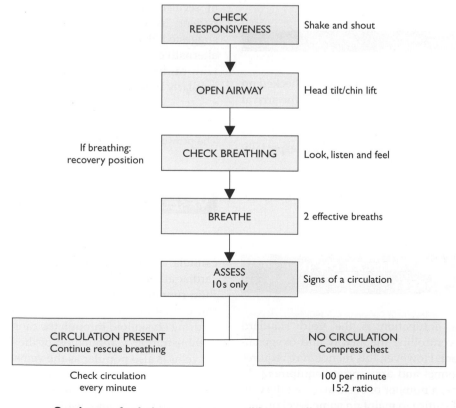

Figure 10.1: Adult basic life support.

or if the victim is an infant or child, the rescuer should perform resuscitation for about 1 min before going for help. This is based on the assumption that respiratory support is more likely to have an impact on these types of patients.

However, if the victim is an adult and the cause of unconsciousness is not trauma or drowning, the rescuer should assume that the patient has a heart problem and therefore seek help immediately after it has been established that the victim is not breathing. In these patients ALS intervention, particularly a defibrillator, is essential.

BLS should not be interrupted whilst waiting for ALS manoeuvres unless the patient makes a movement or takes a spontaneous breath, in which case their carotid pulse should be checked for up to 10 s.

ADVANCED LIFE SUPPORT IN ADULTS (FIG. 10.2)

The European Resuscitation Council 2000 Advanced Life Support (ALS) recommendations have been combined into a single algorithm as shown. One of the major recent changes is the recommendation that following tracheal intubation, cardiac massage should be performed continuously at a rate of 100 per minute without interruption for the 12 ventilations per minute. This maintains a higher coronary perfusion pressure.

The main points to consider are that the doctor must interpret the ECG rhythm in the clinical context and treat the patient not the monitor. VF or pulseless ventricular tachycardia (VT) are the most

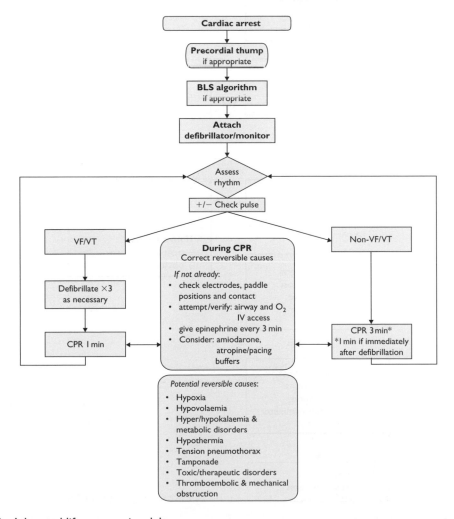

Figure 10.2: Advanced life support in adults.

redeemable rhythms but defibrillation must occur with minimal delay in order to achieve success. If the rhythm is not VF or VT it is essential to positively exclude pathologies (Fig. 10.2) which are potentially reversible causes of asystole or electromechanical dissociation. Epinephrine remains the drug of choice in resuscitation although evidence as to its exact efficacy remains limited. Amiodarone has now gained acceptance as the drug of choice in patients with resistant ventricular fibrillation and tachycardia.

PAEDIATRIC BASIC LIFE SUPPORT

The principles of paediatric BLS (Fig. 10.3) are similar. An infant is defined as being under the age of 1 year and a child between 1 and 8 years of age. Over the age of 8 years treatment algorithms are the same as for an adult, although different techniques to attain adequate chest compression may be required.

The commonest cause of childhood cardiac arrest is hypoxia and up to five rescue breaths

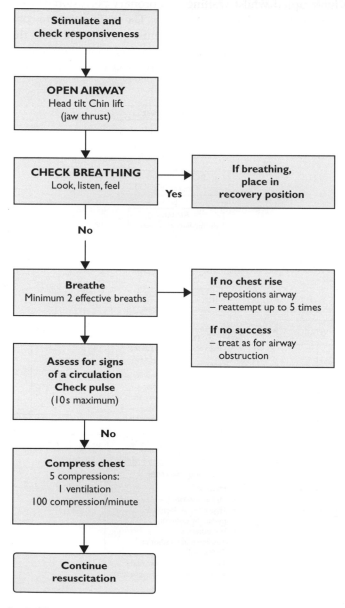

Figure 10.3: Paediatric basic life support.

should therefore be given initially, each of which should make the chest rise and fall. A minimum of two effective rescue breaths must be given. Check the pulse by feeling for a carotid pulse in the child or a brachial pulse on the inner aspect of the upper arm in an infant. If there is no pulse, or if in infants the rate is less than 60 beats per minute, start chest compression in combination with rescue breathing. In a child the required hand position is with the heel of one hand over the lower half of the sternum. In an infant the tips of two fingers are placed one finger breadth below an imaginary line joining the infant's nipples. Resuscitation should

be performed for 1 min before going for assistance, and then the rescuer should consider taking the infant or child with them.

PAEDIATRIC ADVANCED LIFE SUPPORT (FIG. 10.4)

The algorithm is similar to that for adults. However, a much greater proportion of children will have asystole or electromechanical dissociation (EMD) as the presenting rhythm with their

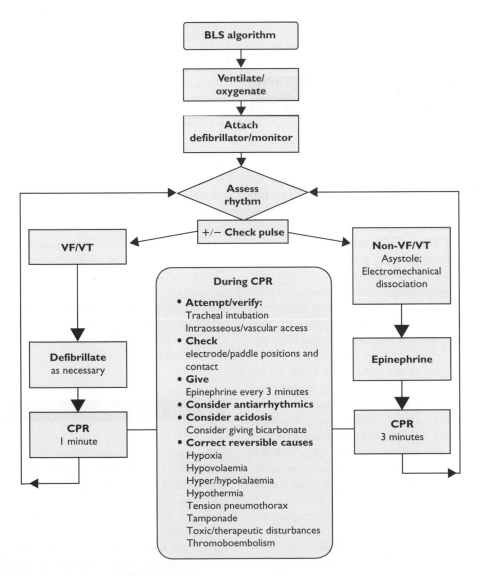

Figure 10.4: Paediatric advanced life support.

cardiac arrest. The prognosis is poor. Epinephrine is the main resuscitation drug. The first dose is $10 \mu g\,kg^{-1}$ ($0.1\,ml\,kg^{-1}$ of 1 in 10000 solution) intravenously. The second and subsequent doses are $100 \mu g\,kg^{-1}$ (1 ml of 1 in 10000 solution or 0.1 ml of 1 in 1000 solution). A dose of $100 \mu g\,kg^{-1}$ can be given by the endotracheal route if vascular access has not been attained. The intraosseous route is a safe, reliable and relatively rapid vascular access technique, especially in children under the age of 6 years. Alternatives include cannulation of the femoral vein, venous cutdown or cannulation of a central vein, depending on the level of expertise of the operator. A fluid bolus of $20\,ml\,kg^{-1}$ (repeated if necessary) should be given if there is any suggestion of hypovolaemia or any other reversible cause of shock.

CO-ORDINATING A RESUSCITATION EVENT

Proper preparation and co-ordination will lead to an orderly sequence of events in the acute resuscitation period. The resuscitation can be divided into three stages. In emergency practice there is often advanced warning from the ambulance service that a patient in cardiac arrest is about to arrive. This allows time for preparation, with the team leader allocating the team their roles. It is important also to check the relevant equipment. In some departments there are facilities to video the resuscitation for education purposes, or a senior colleague may be asked to view the resuscitation and provide constructive criticism at the end.

After the arrival of the patient the team leader must co-ordinate a rapid and safe transfer from the ambulance stretcher. It is then necessary to confirm the absence of a pulse and to attach a cardiac monitor to assess the first rhythm. Instruct rapid defibrillation if the patient is in VF or VT. If the initial rhythm is asystole or EMD the team commences basic life support. The leader must ensure staff are performing roles effectively and establish the initial resuscitation algorithm and request the interventions required.

Following the initial assessment and commencement of resuscitation the team leader is responsible for obtaining relevant information from

Table 10.4: Information from the paramedics required by hospital cardiac arrest team

Was the cardiac arrest witnessed? If so, at what time did cardiac arrest occur?
Was bystander CPR performed?
At what time were the ambulance service called?
What treatment has been administered?
Have there been any periods of return of spontaneous circulation?
What is the patient's past medical and drug history?
Are any relatives present? What do they know of the patient's condition?

the paramedic staff. The information required is shown in Table 10.4.

Throughout the resuscitation the team leader must ensure compliance with the resuscitation algorithm and monitor the effectiveness of the treatment being provided. Particular attention should be paid to supporting and replacing tiring team members. Clinical information should be used to positively exclude reversible pathology and attempt to identify underlying causes (Fig. 10.2). A team member may be asked to obtain any relevant history from relatives, if present. If successful, post-resuscitation care should be provided prior to transfer to a ward or intensive care unit. If the resuscitation attempt is unsuccessful the team leader should inform relatives as soon as possible. The team leader also has the responsibility to debrief the team. Particular attention should be paid to areas in which the team performed well, whilst also attempting to highlight areas where a change in practice or extra training might improve performance in the future.

WHEN TO STOP

There are a number of common features which are associated with a poor outcome in cardiac arrest (Table 10.5). The presence of any one or more of these factors will influence the team leader in deciding what further resuscitation efforts are appropriate. In the presence of asystole persisting for longer than 20 min or EMD with no treatable cause, prolongation of the resuscitation attempt is generally futile. In younger patients, hypothermic

Table 10.5: Factors associated with poor outcome in cardiac arrest

Unwitnessed cardiac arrest
No bystander CPR
Asystole or EMD as presenting rhythm
Prolonged cardiac arrest without return of
    circulation
Co-morbid processes

Table 10.6: Post-resuscitation investigations

12-lead ECG
Chest X-ray
Arterial blood gases
Full blood count
Urea and electrolytes
Blood sugar
Serum calcium
Cardiac enzymes

patients and those following poisoning or near-drowning, prolonged attempts may on occasions produce a neurologically intact survivor.

POST-RESUSCITATION CARE

Most patients will require a period of intensive post-resuscitation care depending upon the degree of cardiovascular and cerebral compromise they have suffered. The place of their definitive care may be an intensive care unit or a coronary care unit. However, it is essential that prior to leaving the resuscitation room the patient's condition is optimized and they are prepared for a safe transfer.

Prior to transfer out of the emergency department the airway must be reassessed. It should be secured by endotracheal (ET) intubation if unprotected. If the patient is already intubated, check the position of the ET tube and make sure it is well secured. The work of breathing is assessed if the patient is not anaesthetized. Consider the possibility of pneumothorax or aspiration of gastric contents as potential complications. Assessment of the circulation includes the pulse rate, rhythm and the blood pressure. Cerebral function examination must include recording the Glasgow Coma Scale (GCS) and pupillary reaction.

Ensure normothermia by keeping the patient covered and continue monitoring with non-invasive blood pressure, ECG monitoring, pulse oximetry and end-tidal CO_2 if the patient is intubated. Essential post-resuscitation investigations (Table 10.6) include a bedside blood sugar, full blood count, urea and electrolytes, serum calcium, cardiac enzymes, arterial blood gases, ECG and a chest X-ray. If the ECG demonstrates features of acute myocardial infarction, thrombolysis should be considered. Prior to transfer to intensive care or

a ward, confirm that adequate amounts of oxygen, resuscitation equipment and drugs are taken for the transfer.

Following successful treatment of cardiac arrest, patients will broadly fall into three categories. Those with a patent (self-protected) airway can be transferred to the coronary care unit for monitoring. In patients with a significantly depressed conscious level (GCS less than 12) a period of 12–24 h controlled ventilation, cardiovascular support and manoeuvres to optimize cerebral oxygenation is recommended in the European Resuscitation Council guidelines. After this time formal re-evaluation of any cerebral hypoxic injury can be made. A small group of patients will be those found to have a history of terminal malignancy or long-standing severe incapacity. These patients must be carefully discussed with senior staff from the admitting medical team, intensivists and, most importantly, the relatives. A clear and joint decision on the appropriate level of care to be given can then be made. This must be documented carefully in the notes.

BREAKING BAD NEWS

Breaking bad news to relatives must be done by experienced medical and nursing staff. They must prepare themselves both physically and emotionally before meeting the relatives. It is essential to introduce yourself and confirm exactly who you are speaking to. The bad news should be provided early and in unequivocal terms. Always give the impression that you have time to talk and listen. Information must be given in language that is simple, considerate and honest. Be prepared to reiterate the main points. Give the relatives the opportunity to ask questions and see the body once it has been cleaned and prepared by staff. Such an approach will go some way towards helping them to cope with an extremely traumatic and sudden event.

Debriefing with the team is almost as important, especially where a young patient died or the resuscitation attempt was perceived not to run smoothly. The timing and framework of such meetings must be carefully planned and chaired.

CARDIAC ARREST IN SPECIAL CIRCUMSTANCES

In certain specific situations of CPA it will be necessary to modify the standard ALS algorithms. These conditions may occur in isolation or be coexistent.

POISONING (SEE CHAPTER 15)

Either at the onset or during the resuscitation phase it may become obvious from history given by relatives or the paramedics that the cardiac arrest is due to poisoning of some kind. A number of specific drug therapies may help to produce a stable cardiac output (Table 10.7).

Management

Once a stable cardiac output has been attained, look for possible signs of drug administration (needle marks, blistering in the mouth) and perform a gastric lavage with charcoal therapy unless specifically contraindicated. A standard series of tests should be carried out as outlined above in the section on post-resuscitation care. Serum paracetamol and salicylate levels should be measured.

NEAR-DROWNING

This results from asphyxiation in water. In most cases it is associated with aspiration of fluid (90%). As a result pulmonary vasoconstriction occurs, leading to pulmonary hypertension. This leads to disruption of the pulmonary microstructure. In the remaining 10% the dry drowning phenomenon

Table 10.7: Antidotes for poisoning

Naloxone for opiate toxicity
Glucagon for beta-blocker poisoning
Sodium bicarbonate for tricyclic antidepressant toxicity
Atropine for organophosphate poisoning
Oxygen for carbon monoxide poisoning

results from intense glottic closure leading to profound hypoxia.

In treating the near-drowning patient cardiopulmonary resuscitation should be commenced as soon as possible; however, specific attempts to empty the lungs of water are unnecessary. There may be associated pathology which has resulted in the patient's immersion and this may require specific treatment (epilepsy, alcohol or drugs). Hypothermia may occur during immersion in cold water. Neurologically intact survival has been reported despite immersion times up to 1 h and resuscitation should be prolonged. Children have a greater likelihood of survival in such circumstances and attempts should be made to regain a core temperature of at least 33–35°C.

It is important to recognize the possibility of neck injury in patients removed from a swimming pool or shallow water, especially if there is any history suggestive of a diving injury. If the patient is successfully resuscitated there is a strong likelihood of adult respiratory distress syndrome, and close monitoring of respiratory function on an intensive care unit is indicated.

HYPOTHERMIA

Mild hypothermia is defined as a core temperature between 33 and 35°C. Moderate or severe hypothermia supervenes at a temperature less than 33°C. It may manifest in healthy individuals either as a result of the environment or be triggered by alcohol, drugs or a variety of coexisting medical conditions. Principles of initiating and terminating resuscitation should be modified in such circumstances, as profound hypothermia can both mimic cardiorespiratory arrest as well as having a protective effect on vital organs.

It is essential to exclude a very slow arterial pulse in hypothermic patients prior to starting closed chest compression, as physical movement can trigger the onset of ventricular fibrillation. The history from the paramedics or family will often be helpful. A low-reading thermometer should be used to record a core (rectal) temperature. If the diagnosis of hypothermia is confirmed active and passive rewarming methods must be employed whilst CPR is ongoing. These include warmed humidified oxygen, warm blankets for body and head, irrigation of stomach and bladder with warmed fluids, and possibly also the peritoneal cavity. In centres where it is available, cardiopulmonary bypass apparatus produces rapid rewarming and has resulted in a number of neurologically intact survivors.

If the patient is in VF and severely hypothermic (less than 30°C), the rhythm is unlikely to convert with defibrillation until the core temperature has been raised to at least 30°C. Defibrillation can then be repeated. There is no evidence that anti-arrhythmics have any role in such patients. Once the hypothermia has been corrected to between 33 and 35°C decisions can be made on how long to continue resuscitating the patient, taking into account the circumstances of the incident. In those patients successfully resuscitated the underlying cause or associated pathologies must be identified and treatment instituted. This will be a major factor affecting eventual outcome. Children have a much greater likelihood of survival and good neurological function than adults; however, such survivors have usually suffered severe hypothermia.

PREGNANCY

This is an extremely unusual circumstance of cardiac arrest where two lives are at risk. The causes include trauma, pulmonary embolism, amniotic fluid embolism, eclampsia and placental abruption. In established cardiac arrest standard CPR should be instituted. In addition, however, the following principles must be followed. It is essential to relieve the pressure on the inferior vena cava from the uterus either by a purpose-made wedge under the right side of the casualty or by manually moving the uterus to the left. A senior obstetrician and paediatrician must be called immediately, and if resuscitation has been unsuccessful for 5 min, emergency caesarean section to try and save the life of a third-trimester fetus may be appropriate. O-negative blood should be given as soon as possible in cases where haemorrhage from trauma or abruption is thought to be the likely cause.

FURTHER READING

Resuscitation Guidelines (2000) Resuscitation Council, UK.

CARDIAC EMERGENCIES

INTRODUCTION

The treatment of cardiac emergencies mandates critical decisions early in a patient's management. Time should not be wasted on exhaustive history taking. Appropriate questions will focus on:

- making a diagnosis
- identifying confounding chronic medical conditions, in particular pathology that might be aggravated by the presenting problem or influence the emergency department management (e.g. diabetes mellitus)
- accurately recording medication to ensure that avoidable drug interactions do not occur.

Identifying risk factors for ischaemic heart disease is only appropriate for the emergency physician if the diagnosis is in doubt or discharge is planned.

SYMPTOMS OF CARDIAC DISEASE

CHEST PAIN

Every patient who presents with chest pain should have a working diagnosis at the time of discharge or admission. The pain may not have a cardiac cause (Table 11.1).

Table 11.1: Non-cardiac causes of central chest pain

Aortic dissection
Oesophageal reflux, hiatus hernia, and oesophageal spasm (which is relieved by nitrates)
Costochondritis (Tietze's syndrome)
Massive pulmonary embolus (a dull, aching pain)
Psychological causes, including hyperventilation

Chronic stable angina

Narrowing of the lumen of a coronary artery by an atheromatous plaque may restrict the blood flow to the myocardium to such an extent that an increase in the oxygen demand of that tissue cannot be met. This occurs in chronic stable angina. Symptoms are provoked by an increase in myocardial work that generates an oxygen demand in excess of that which can be supplied by narrowed coronary arteries. Transient ischaemia in the downstream myocardium gives rise to angina.

The pain of angina is heterogeneous, although it is often described as a 'heavy feeling', tightness or retrosternal pressure. Radiation occurs commonly to the left or both arms. Patients sometimes complain of pain restricted to the left arm, shoulder or hand. Pain may be felt in the jaw, or give rise to symptoms similar to indigestion. Some people complain of dyspnoea rather than chest pain. Trigger factors are often identified by the patient, such as cold weather, large meals or stressful situations.

Table 11.2: Canadian Cardiovascular Society classification of stable angina

Class I	Angina on strenuous activity only
Class II	Minor restriction of normal activity
Class III	Marked restriction of normal activity
Class IV	Any physical exertion without angina is impossible. There may be pain at rest

Chronic stable angina has been classified by the Canadian Cardiovascular Society (Table 11.2).

Particular attention should be paid to the efficacy of any self-administered short-acting nitrate preparations (e.g. sublingual glyceryl trinitrate). A simple episode of chronic stable angina is, by definition, relieved within a few minutes. An episode of angina lasting longer than 15 min should raise the possibility of acute myocardial infarction (AMI).

Unstable angina

The term *unstable angina* encompasses more than one pathophysiological situation. The common feature is an acute deterioration in coronary blood supply, resulting in either new symptoms or a significant worsening of previously stable angina. Three groups of patients can be identified:

1   Anginal chest pain now occurs at rest.
2   A sudden deterioration in the exercise capacity of a patient with chronic angina.
3   New onset of angina at low levels of physical activity.

Admission is essential so that symptoms can be controlled and appropriate investigations undertaken. The aim of subsequent interventions is to prevent myocardial infarction.

Prinzmetal (variant) angina is often unprovoked. It is the result of coronary vasospasm, which gives rise to transient ST segment elevation on the electrocardiogram without the development of Q waves (which would indicate AMI). Only two-thirds of such patients have angiographic evidence of coronary artery disease. Although it may not be possible to identify trigger factors there is a tendency for pain to recur at the same time of day.

Myocardial infarction

The classic description of the pain of AMI is that it is central, severe, crushing, radiating to one or

Table 11.3: Aetiology of pericarditis

Idiopathic
Viral (Coxsackie B, echovirus, HIV)
Post-myocardial infarction
Bacterial (staphylococcus, streptococcus, meningococcus, tuberculosis)
Malignant
Connective tissue diseases
Uraemia

both arms, and prolonged. There is associated sweating (diaphoresis) and nausea. Unfortunately the history of AMI may be even more heterogeneous than that of angina and patients, particularly the elderly and diabetics, may present with atypical chest pain, syncope or sudden death.

Presentation of acute myocardial infarction is frequently atypical.

Aortic dissection

The pain of a dissection of the thoracic aorta may mimic AMI. If the dissection involves a coronary artery the ECG demonstrates an injury pattern, further exacerbating any diagnostic dilemma.

Aortic dissection more commonly causes severe interscapular back pain, which patients describe as 'tearing'. Corroborating evidence in the form of a relatively normal electrocardiogram, a normal or high blood pressure despite the patient appearing shocked, and a blood pressure differential between the two arms supports the diagnosis of aortic dissection.

Pericarditis

There are many causes of pericarditis (Table 11.3). The pain of pericarditis is typically central, sharp and constant. It may be aggravated by movement, inspiration and swallowing. Relief may be obtained by sitting forward.

With the accumulation of a pericardial effusion, the intensity of the pain is reduced.

BREATHLESSNESS

Most patients presenting to an emergency department with breathlessness secondary to cardiac

Table 11.4: New York Heart Association classification of heart failure

Class I	No limitation of ordinary activity
Class II	Mild restriction of ordinary activity
Class III	Marked restriction of ordinary activity
Class IV	Physical activity impossible without symptoms; may have dyspnoea at rest

disease have suffered an acute deterioration in left ventricular function leading to pulmonary oedema. Pulmonary oedema is defined as an increase in pulmonary extravascular water owing to transudation, or exudation in excess of the capacity of pulmonary lymphatic drainage. Cardiogenic pulmonary oedema is a transudate resulting from an elevated pulmonary venous pressure.

Pulmonary venous hypertension may develop gradually. Lying flat increases systemic venous return, which in turn elevates pulmonary venous and capillary pressure. Transudation of fluid (pulmonary oedema) is the result of the failure of the left side of the heart to respond to the increase in left atrial pressure. The resulting breathlessness on lying down is termed *orthopnoea*. Paroxysmal nocturnal dyspnoea is a distressing symptom which often wakes patients from sleep. There is a terrifying feeling of breathlessness (sometimes described as 'drowning') which is only relieved if the patient sits upright. Wheeziness is a frequent symptom of patients in acute pulmonary oedema. Bronchospasm is believed to be the cause.

Patients may complain of a deterioration in exercise tolerance. It is useful to be aware of the New York Heart Association classification of heart failure (Table 11.4).

Patients who are breathless should have respiratory pathology excluded, although it is common to find elements of pulmonary infection, heart failure and chronic obstructive pulmonary disease in the same patient.

SYNCOPE

Syncope is a transient loss of consciousness. It is often possible to exclude a seizure on the basis of the history, witness accounts and examination findings that do not suggest a postictal state. A blood glucose estimation is mandatory. Acute hypoperfusion is the commonest cause of cerebral anoxia. An ECG is indicated for all patients who have sustained an episode of syncope.

Simple faints

Simple faints occur at any age. Patients often provide a history of a precipitating situation, for example the soldier on parade, standing in a hot room, or exposure to noxious or shocking visual stimuli. There is an unpleasant constellation of presyncope symptoms (nausea, sweating, a 'sinking' feeling in the epigastrium and dimming of vision) as the systemic vascular resistance falls. There may be an associated bradycardia. The subsequent reduction in cerebral perfusion causes the victim to lose consciousness. The simple faint is characteristically aborted by lying the victim flat and elevating the legs. If the victim remains upright cerebral hypoperfusion will persist. Patients frequently vomit immediately after a simple faint.

Only diagnose fainting after excluding serious causes of syncope.

Micturition syncope may occur when an elderly male gets out of bed to pass urine. The mechanism of the fall in systemic blood pressure is a combination of a change in posture and reflex vasodilatation after elimination of the efferent vagal stimulus from the distended bladder.

Cardiac syncope (Stokes–Adams attack)

A sudden loss of consciousness occurs without warning. Recovery in less than 30s is usual. The underlying cause is an arrhythmia leading to a temporary reduction in cardiac output. Transient sinus node arrest and complete heart block are common precipitating arrhythmias. Characteristically there is no 'postictal' state. Observers often remark that the victim was pale but became flushed during the early recovery phase.

Exertional syncope

This is a sinister symptom that may affect patients who have an obstruction to their left ventricular outflow tract. Aortic stenosis and hypertrophic obstructive cardiomyopathy prevent the left ventricle from increasing the cardiac output in the face of an increase in tissue oxygen demand and reduced afterload. These patients are also prone to serious arrhythmia.

Postural hypotension

Postural hypotension is defined as a fall in the systolic blood pressure of at least 25 mmHg, or to a systolic pressure below 90 mmHg on assuming an upright posture. The victim may feel 'light-headed' or lose consciousness. The mechanism is frequently relative hypovolaemia, or a loss of vasomotor compensation for the gravitational reduction in venous return to the heart (Table 11.5).

The patient must remain supine for at least 5 min before having the blood pressure measured sitting, on standing, and then again after a further 2 min standing for the examination to be maximally sensitive.

Carotid sinus hypersensitivity

Increasingly recognized as a cause for syncope in the elderly, the carotid sinus may become sensitive to very light external pressure (e.g. a tight collar, head turning and shaving). Sinus node arrest, sinus bradycardia or a high degree of atrioventricular block may be induced. Properly performed *unilateral* carotid massage (for at least 6 s) provokes an episode of sinus node arrest of at least 3 s in susceptible individuals. Carotid sinus massage is contraindicated if there is a carotid bruit, and this finding is only significant if the presenting symptoms are provoked. Such patients should be referred for a specialist cardiology opinion and permanent pacemaker insertion may be required.

Table 11.5: Causes of postural hypotension

Dehydration
Drug induced: antihypertensives, drugs commonly prescribed in the elderly, such as diuretics, vasodilators, anti-parkinsonian medication
Autonomic dysfunction: the elderly, diabetic neuropathy
Endocrine causes: Addison's disease
Malignant vasovagal syndrome

PALPITATION

This is an awareness of the beating of the heart. The context in which this symptom occurs is critical. Palpitations may be the result of anxiety, or simple premature atrial or ventricular ectopic beats in an otherwise fit individual. Alternatively, they may be a symptom of an arrhythmia associated with chest pain, hypotension or near syncope. Rapid assessment of the haemodynamic status is followed by evaluation of a 12-lead electrocardiogram, with an extended rhythm strip if required.

MYOCARDIAL INFARCTION AND UNSTABLE ANGINA

The incidence of acute myocardial infarction and unstable angina is approximately 2 per 1000 population per year, divided equally between the two.

PATHOPHYSIOLOGY

A detailed description of the pathogenesis of an atheromatous plaque is beyond the scope of this text. However, it is appropriate to consider the acute events that affect a plaque, leading to a presentation in the emergency department.

Three pathological processes are considered when one attempts to rationalize medical therapy for patients with unstable angina: severe coronary atheroma, thrombus formation and vasoconstriction. Pure vasospasm is rare. Progression of an atheromatous plaque narrows the lumen of the affected artery, restricting the flow of blood to the downstream segment of myocardium. Symptoms are dictated by the oxygen demand of that particular area of myocardium, and the degree to which the stenosis limits blood flow to that area. As the disease progresses there is such a limitation of flow through the diseased artery that angina occurs at very low levels of physical activity, and ultimately at rest. Characteristically, patients give a history of worsening of previously stable symptoms and an increasing requirement for short-acting nitrate preparations. The logical treatment for these patients is the early use of beta-blocking agents to reduce heart rate and myocardial oxygen consumption (although many of these patients will already be 'beta-blocked').

The severity of the stenotic lesions, multiple vessel involvement and left main stem coronary artery involvement often necessitate surgical management for many of these patients.

The role of thrombus in the progression of a stenosis without infarction has yet to be fully elucidated. Pre-existing collateral branches may protect some areas of myocardium from infarction, even after total occlusion of an artery. Plaque rupture of a low-grade lesion may give rise to thrombus formation without complete occlusion of the artery. However, coronary flow reserve is severely restricted. A combination of aspirin and heparin is currently the best medical therapy for this group of patients. If rapid stabilization is not achieved percutaneous transluminal angioplasty (PTCA) offers an effective treatment for discrete lesions.

Coronary vasoconstriction may narrow the luminal diameter by up to 30% (within the physiological range). This is an inappropriate response if the artery is diseased, and is thought to result from the loss of functioning endothelium and a reduction in the synthesis of nitric oxide (a potent vasodilator). Nitrates provide exogenous nitric oxide and may dilate constricted arteries. Nitrates also reduce cardiac work by a reduction of preload and afterload.

Variant angina has been discussed. A good response is usually observed to parenteral nitrate preparations if an acute episode has not been aborted at home.

Targeting pharmacotherapy to specific pathological processes is seldom possible in the acute situation and aggressive, empirical treatment is indicated.

EMERGENCY MANAGEMENT

Ideally, patients presenting to an emergency department with chest pain will have an ECG performed before they are seen by a doctor. This minimizes any delay to thrombolysis for suitable patients.

Patients with evidence of infarction or ischaemia on their initial ECG, or unrelieved chest pain, should have intravenous access established immediately. Blood should be drawn for a full blood count, urea and electrolytes, random glucose and lipid profile. The timing of the chest pain and local policy will dictate the need for cardiac enzyme estimation, the results of which are unlikely to alter the initial management. The electrocardiogram may demonstrate ST segment depression, T-wave inversion, evidence of previous infarction (Q waves), or may be within normal limits.

> Thrombolysis is a time-critical intervention.

A chest radiograph may be obtained but must not delay treatment, particularly thrombolysis. Alternative causes for the chest pain, such as aortic dissection, are sought, as is radiological evidence of left ventricular failure.

UNSTABLE ANGINA

Patients suffering from unstable angina require urgent hospitalization. It is a condition with an untreated mortality approaching 20% 3 months after onset. This can be reduced with intensive medical therapy (Table 11.6).

Thrombolysis has no proven benefit in unstable angina. Urgent angiography might be considered by the in-patient team for selected high-risk patients and those who do not respond to medical therapy.

ACUTE MYOCARDIAL INFARCTION (AMI)

In the UK more than 250 000 people die each year as a result of AMI. Thirty per cent of deaths occur in the first 2 h after infarction. The in-hospital mortality is between 10 and 20%.

PATHOPHYSIOLOGY

The majority of AMIs are the consequence of occlusion of a coronary artery at the site of an

Table 11.6: Emergency department management of unstable angina

Oxygen
Aspirin – 300 mg chewed
Nitroglycerine (buccal or intravenous)
Heparinization – subcutaneous enoxaparin 100 U kg^{-1} every 12 h
Diamorphine (intravenous) – titrated to response
Consider short-acting beta-blocker (intravenous metoprolol – 5 mg repeated twice if required) if pain persists or recurs

atheromatous plaque. Two processes may lead to thrombus formation:

- Plaque rupture with subsequent thrombus formation beneath the plaque and on the surface: this commonly results in fatal AMI.
- Plaque erosion.

Plaque erosion is believed to be the precipitating event in most cases of non-fatal AMI, and is thought to be unrelated to the degree of stenosis. Platelets adhere to the exposed subendothelial matrix, forming microthrombi and stimulating smooth muscle proliferation and vasoconstriction. An erosion with a large surface area may result in the formation of an occlusive thrombus.

Some patients have a more 'stuttering' course suggesting intermittent occlusion, with spontaneous recanalization. The dynamic nature of coronary arterial occlusion is only now being fully appreciated. A quarter of patients may give a history of unstable angina in the weeks leading up to AMI. The window for intervention with reperfusion strategies may be broad in this group of patients.

Complications arise after AMI because of changes in electrical depolarization and contractility. The evolution of an AMI in a segment of myocardium takes several hours. Regions of relatively uninjured tissue surround areas of irreversibly damaged myocardium. Some of this is potentially salvageable. The interface between infarcted and relatively unaffected myocardium is electrically unstable and may be the ectopic focus of an arrhythmia.

The result of impaired contractility is pump failure, which is dependent on the mass of infarcted myocardium. Heart failure is observed after infarction of more than 25% of the left ventricle. Loss of more than 40% of the left ventricle almost invariable results in cardiogenic shock.

The surrounding viable myocardium adapts to neighbouring myocardial death by hypertrophy and enlargement of the cardiac chambers. This process is known as remodelling and is thought to be detrimental to cardiac function. Autolysis of infarcted myocardium results in structural weakness, which may result in ventricular free wall rupture, acute mitral incompetence due to rupture of the papillary muscles, or an acute defect of the ventricular septum. Thrombus can form in the left ventricle after substantial anterior infarction, which may be the source of systemic emboli.

CLINICAL FEATURES

Chest pain has been discussed. It is important to note that AMI is not always associated with chest pain, and up to one quarter of events may go unrecognized by the victim. 'Silent MI' is thought to be more common in diabetics than in the general population.

A severe episode of angina, lasting longer than 15 min with or without nausea, vomiting and sweating should be regarded as an AMI until proved otherwise. The clinical features are otherwise the result of complications:

- abnormalities of heart rhythm
- left ventricular failure leading to pulmonary oedema
- cardiogenic shock
- acute ventricular septal defect, or mitral insufficiency causing acute pulmonary oedema.

ELECTROCARDIOGRAPHY IN ACUTE MYOCARDIAL INFARCTION

A variety of ECG appearances (including normal) are consistent with a diagnosis of AMI. More than 1 mm of ST segment elevation in at least two contiguous chest or limb leads is highly suggestive of AMI.

> Always interpret ECGs carefully – do not rely on computer-generated diagnoses.

ST segment elevation (Fig. 11.1)

ST elevation can occur without myocardial infarction (variant angina). However, ST elevation is the most specific ECG indication of full-thickness AMI. A convex upward pattern develops in the leads facing the infarcted ventricle, often with ST depression in the leads opposite the infarcted tissue. The diastolic isoelectric line may be depressed, accentuating the ST elevation. ST elevation may resolve completely after thrombolytic therapy, or it may take several days to resolve. Persistent elevation suggests a left ventricular aneurysm or a large akinetic myocardial segment.

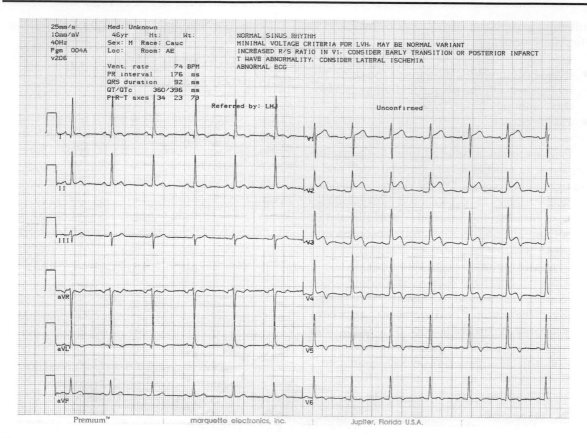

Figure 11.1: Acute anterior myocardial infarction. Note the presence of the changes described in the text.

T-wave changes

The earliest ECG indication of AMI is often confined to the T waves. The T waves become prominent and peaked before elevation of the ST segments. The T waves invert within hours of a full-thickness AMI. Symmetrical T-wave inversion may be the only change seen in patients with limited (non-Q-wave) infarction. This group of patients does not benefit from thrombolysis, but has a high probability (40–60%) of progressing to full-thickness infarction. T-wave changes in isolation are non-specific and may be present for many years. The history and appropriate use of biochemical markers is crucial for the effective management of these patients.

Q waves

Q waves are the ultimate and permanent ECG evidence of full-thickness infarction. Pathological

Q waves are at least 25% of the height of the subsequent R wave (or more than 3 mV), and more than 40 ms (one small square) in duration. There is an association with a reduction in the height of the R wave in the same lead (loss of R-wave height may be the only indication of AMI).

Left bundle branch block

New left bundle branch block (LBBB) is an important finding. Thrombolysis is indicated, and in most institutions is given if there is only a suspicion that LBBB is new with a good history. Unfortunately, access to the patient's previous ECGs is often delayed.

Localization of AMI

Anterior infarction implies involvement of the left anterior descending coronary artery, and is

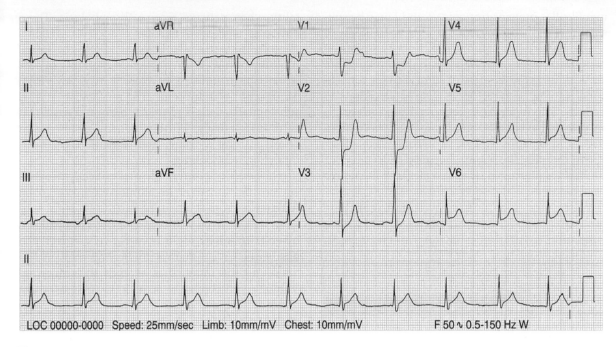

Figure 11.2: True posterior myocardial infarction.

diagnosed from ECG changes in the precordial leads (V2–V6). Lateral extension is observed in leads I, aVL and II. ST depression may occur in leads III and aVF. Changes in II, III and aVF indicate inferior wall infarction, which is usually the result of occlusion of the right coronary artery or its posterior descending branch. There may be changes in the lateral limb leads and the anterior chest leads. True posterior infarction (Fig. 11.2) is the result of circumflex artery occlusion and is diagnosed by a dominant R wave in V1, and ST depression in V2 and V3.

BIOCHEMICAL MARKERS

Biochemical markers have a limited role in identifying patients suitable for thrombolytic therapy, as by definition these individuals must have unequivocal ECG changes. Although required by convention to confirm the diagnosis after admission, biochemical markers continue to have a role in identifying subendocardial AMI in patients with equivocal ECGs. Until recently, the only strategy for the definitive exclusion of AMI was to admit patients for 3 days and document three

consecutive sets of normal cardiac enzymes (usually creatine kinase and lactate dehydrogenase). This is still practice in many parts of the UK, and is not within the remit of the emergency department. Alternative markers of myocardial injury have been identified with high sensitivity, high specificity and an early peak concentration, which makes their use in the emergency department a viable proposition. Early, safe discharge of patients with chest pain has significant resource-saving implications.

The cardiac-specific isoenzyme creatine kinase (CK-MB) has been in use for several years. Even this isoenzyme is not entirely specific for myocardial injury, and transient elevations are observed after intramuscular injections, heavy physical exercise and trauma. A rise in CK-MB is usually seen between 3 and 8 h post infarction. However, with a peak value up to 30 h post event, CK-MB in isolation is not a satisfactory test to allow discharge from the emergency department.

Some emergency departments in the UK are taking on the role of excluding AMI in patients with chest pain but an inconclusive ECG, using short-stay observation and chest pain assessment units. Recently evaluated biochemical markers such as the myofibrillar proteins troponins T and I may be suitable for this purpose. Troponin T has a sensitivity of nearly 100% when estimated at least 12 h after an episode of chest pain and some departments are already using this in place of admission for conventional cardiac enzyme series. Lesser elevations in troponin T concentration (between 0.1 and 0.2 μg l^{-1}) are detected in unstable angina, and have poor prognostic implications for cardiac events in the subsequent months. Troponin T remains elevated for 10–15 days after AMI. It is also elevated in chronic renal failure.

Other strategies under investigation include continuous ST segment monitoring, CK-MB mass estimation, myoglobin estimation, and using combinations of markers.

MANAGEMENT OF AMI

The diagnosis of AMI is initially made on the basis of the history, physical examination and the electrocardiogram. Biochemical markers are used to confirm the diagnosis or exclude AMI when the ECG is inconclusive. However, there should be no delay in instituting therapy whilst awaiting laboratory confirmation.

- *Oxygen*. Oxygen should be routinely administered in high concentration.
- *Analgesia*. Patients may receive *Entonox* (a 50% mixture of oxygen and nitrous oxide), a synthetic opiate agent or sublingual glyceryl trinitrate in the prehospital environment. On arrival, intravenous access should be established and adequate opiate analgesia administered via this route. Diamorphine or morphine sulphate should be titrated until the patient is pain free. The provision of intravenous antiemetics is recommended at the same time. If the pain recurs, a nitrate infusion may be started or the opiate dosage repeated.

THROMBOLYSIS

Thrombolysis has revolutionized the early management of AMI. A meta-analysis performed by the Fibrinolytic Therapy Trialists (FTT) Collaborative Group of nine randomized controlled trails calculated an 18% proportional reduction in mortality when patients receive thrombolysis. These data also suggested that for every 1000 patients treated, 18 deaths would be avoided. The ISIS 2 trial demonstrated a reduction in mortality of 53% when aspirin and streptokinase were given within 4 h of onset of symptoms. The mechanism of this substantial benefit is primarily early and sustained coronary patency. Further benefit is the result of myocardial salvage, and alterations in post-infarction remodelling.

The benefit of thrombolysis is critically dependent on the timing of its administration. If given within 6 h of onset of symptoms the evidence suggests that 30 lives will be saved per 1000 patients treated. This falls to 20 lives between 6 and 12 h post onset. Unless there is doubt concerning symptoms and the infarct has evolved in 'stuttering' fashion (with persistent acute ECG changes) there is no indication for thrombolysing patients who present more than 12 h after the onset of chest pain.

Who is eligible to receive thrombolytic therapy?

- Onset of symptoms less than or equal to 12 h prior to presentation.
- One of the following ECG criteria:
  - at least 1 mm ST segment elevation in at least two contiguous limb leads
  - at least 2 mm of ST segment elevation in at least two contiguous chest leads
  - new left bundle branch block, or left bundle branch block of unknown vintage with a convincing history
  - dominant R wave in V1 with ST depression in the right chest leads (true posterior infarction).
- No contraindications to thrombolytic therapy (Table 11.7).

It is strongly recommended that the emergency physician should not breach the relative contraindications to thrombolysis without the opinion of a senior member of the in-patient team who will be taking over the patient's subsequent management.

Which is the most appropriate agent?

Thrombus is broken down by the action of plasmin on fibrin. Plasmin is formed from plasminogen by the cleavage of a single peptide bond. All the

Table 11.7: Contraindications to thrombolytic therapy

> *Absolute contraindications:*
> Active internal bleeding
> Altered conscious level
> Cerebral infarct within the last 6 months, or *any* history of cerebral haemorrhage
> Known bleeding diathesis
> Persistent severe hypertension
>   (diastolic > 120 mmHg, systolic > 200 mmHg)
> Pregnancy
> Trauma or surgery in the previous 2 weeks, which might result in inaccessible haemorrhage
> Significant head trauma in the previous month
> Possible aortic dissection, or pericarditis
>
> *Relative contraindications:*
> Active peptic ulcer
> Prolonged cardiopulmonary resuscitation
> Current warfarin therapy
> Haemorrhagic conditions of the retina
> Ischaemic or embolic stroke within 6 months
> Trauma or surgery between 2 weeks and 2 months prior to presentation
> Chronic uncontrolled hypertension
>   (diastolic > 100 mmHg)

currently available thrombolytics activate plasminogen. The agents differ in several respects: half-life, 'fibrin specificity' (whether clot-bound fibrin or circulating fibrinogen), side-effect profile, rates of coronary recanalization, and cost. In the UK at the present time the two agents most commonly used are streptokinase and recombinent tissue plasminogen activator (rt-PA). Reperfusion arrhythmias occur with both agents.

STREPTOKINASE

Streptokinase forms a complex with plasminogen, which acts on another plasminogen molecule to form plasmin. This action is not specifically directed at plasminogen bound to the occlusive thrombus. Streptokinase induces neutralizing antibodies, which are effective from approximately 4 days post administration. A second administration of streptokinase is therefore not indicated after this time. Hypotension is a common side-effect which usually responds to stopping the infusion for a few minutes. Raising the patient's legs will often normalize the blood pressure, as will the judicious use of volume expanders if there is no evidence of

pulmonary oedema. The infusion can be restarted at the same, or if necessary at half the rate. Severe anaphylactic reactions are fortunately rare. Streptokinase is less expensive than rt-PA and remains the agent of choice for most patients.

> *Streptokinase* – 1.5 million units in 100 ml of normal saline over 1 h.

RT-PA

Recombinant tissue plasminogen activator binds to fibrin, specifically activating plasminogen at the site of the thrombus (it is fibrin specific). Experimental recanalization rates are therefore higher than with streptokinase. It is a recombinant molecule which should not induce allergic reactions, and remains effective after repeated administration. Subgroup analysis of the *GUSTO* trial (global utilization of streptokinase and tissue plasminogen activator for occluded coronary arteries) identified a group of patients who are most likely to gain a good result from the considerably more expensive agent. The following criteria should be satisfied before rt-PA is administered to patients who have not previously received streptokinase:

- anterior myocardial infarction
- less than 4 h since symptoms started
- age less than 75 years (local hospital policy may differ).

rt-PA is less likely to exacerbate hypotension and is the agent of choice for patients with persistent hypotension (some authors would recommend urgent angioplasty in patients with cardiogenic shock if the local facilities are available).

Intravenous heparinization is commenced at the time of rt-PA administration and is continued for 24 h. The rationale behind this is to prevent early reocclusion owing to the short half-life of rt-PA.

> *Alteplase (rt-PA)* – intravenous 15 mg bolus, followed by 50 mg infusion over 30 min, followed by 35 mg over 60 min. Simultaneous 5000 U bolus of intravenous heparin followed by an infusion starting at 1000 U h^{-1}.

Thrombolytic agents related to rt-PA with single bolus administration regimens (e.g. tenecteplase) are being introduced. These will enable further reductions in door-to-needle times and replace rt-PA.

Intravenous beta-blockers

The ISIS 1 (International Studies of Infarct Survival) trial demonstrated a statistically significant survival benefit for patients who received an intravenous beta-blocker after infarction. This was most marked in the first 48 h after AMI, owing to a reduction in deaths from cardiac rupture and ventricular fibrillation. Intravenous atenolol and metoprolol have been recommended, and are likely to be of most benefit in the following patients:

- elderly patients (>65 years) with a large anterior infarction, a resting sinus tachycardia, and/ or persistent hypertension
- thrombolysis, or PTCA contraindicated or not feasible
- extensive AMI in whom thrombolysis has been delayed.

Beta-blockers should be withheld if there is any evidence of heart failure, hypotension or atrioventricular block. These patients should be discussed with the in-patient team prior to administration.

Aspirin

ISIS 2 confirmed the additional survival benefit of aspirin. It should be given within the first 24 h after AMI, at a dose of at least 150 mg if not contraindicated. It is then continued indefinitely. It is now common practice for paramedics to administer aspirin to patients with cardiac chest pain.

PERCUTANEOUS TRANSLUMINAL CORONARY ANGIOPLASTY

Despite proven efficacy, availability and ease of administration, currently available thrombolytics have limitations. Only 50% of patients achieve normal flow through the affected artery, and a further 50% of this group develop recurrent ischaemia. PTCA has been advocated for patients who fail to achieve reperfusion after thrombolytic therapy. It is recommended that patients who have received timely thrombolysis and are still suffering severe chest pain, associated with persistent ECG changes, with or without shock, should be discussed with a cardiologist with a view to consideration of PTCA.

COMPLICATIONS OF AMI

POST-INFARCTION ARRHYTHMIAS

The recognition and early treatment of arrhythmias has been instrumental in reducing the mortality of AMI over the last three decades. The commonest arrhythmias observed are sinus tachycardia, premature atrial contractions and premature ventricular contractions (80–100% of patients). Primary ventricular fibrillation (VF) occurs in between 5 and 10% of patients with AMI. Immediate defibrillation is an extremely effective therapy, and monitoring is therefore of paramount importance.

TACHYCARDIAS

Most tachycardias respond to simple treatment strategies, and it is not the role of the emergency physician to create a toxic pharmacological 'soup' before finally resorting to a specialist opinion. Life-threatening haemodynamic compromise mandates synchronized direct current (DC) cardioversion (preferably with anaesthetic assistance) or defibrillation. Most other arrhythmias respond to the correction of electrolyte abnormalities and the use of a single agent. Lignocaine and amiodarone are the most effective agents and the emergency physician should be familiar with their use.

Sinus tachycardia

The significance of a persistent sinus tachycardia (after the provision of adequate analgesia) has been mentioned, and although never the *primary* cause of haemodynamic compromise it indicates that a large area of myocardium has been infarcted, and an adverse prognosis. The use of intravenous beta-blockers has been discussed, but it must be first established that the tachycardia is not a secondary response to ventricular failure.

Atrial fibrillation (Fig. 11.3)

Atrial fibrillation (AF) complicates approximately 10% of AMIs and is indicative of extensive infarction. Chaotic atrial activity is conducted intermittently to the ventricles. The loss of the atrial

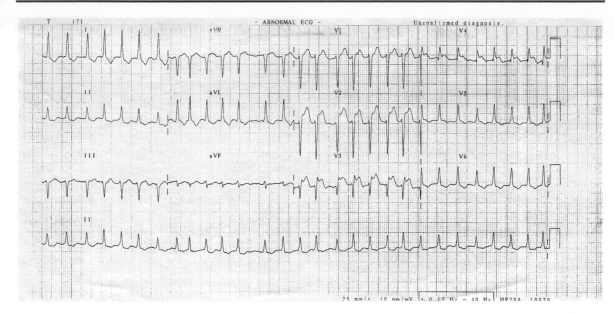

Figure 11.3: Atrial fibrillation.

contribution to ventricular filling, as well as the coexisting ventricular damage, often results in haemodynamic compromise. The ECG diagnosis is seldom problematic: an irregular narrow complex tachycardia, with no recognizable P waves. The management depends on the condition of the patient, the duration of the arrhythmia and the ventricular rate:

■ Patients with a very fast ventricular rate who are shocked should be cardioverted with a synchronized direct current shock (an anaesthetist should be called to perform a rapid sequence induction of anaesthesia).

■ Self-limiting episodes which are *not* associated with a significant fall in mean arterial pressure, with a ventricular response <110 beats per minute, are common, and require no treatment unless they persist after the acute phase.

■ Episodes which persist for longer than 30 min, with a ventricular rate of more than 110 beats per min, should be treated with intravenous amiodarone.

Amiodarone is safe and well tolerated in the short term. Unlike digoxin, amiodarone offers a good chance of cardioversion (75%). Although the ideal route of administration is via a central line, a large peripheral vein can be used if the infusion is for 24 h only, and the dilution is less than $2\,mg\,ml^{-1}$.

Atrial flutter and supraventricular tachycardia

These narrow complex tachycardias (Figs 11.4 and 11.5) are seen less frequently after AMI than is AF. Adenosine will cardiovert supraventricular tachycardias and will make flutter waves more obvious by reducing the ventricular response in atrial flutter. It is a naturally occurring purine nucleotide which blocks atrioventricular nodal conduction, with a half-life of less than 15 s. The 'sawtooth' atrial activity of atrial flutter with two-to-one block is not always obvious, but this tachycardia should always be considered in patients with a constant heart rate between 145 and 155 beats per minute. Atrial flutter requires the same treatment as AF.

> *Adenosine* – 3 mg rapid intravenous bolus into a large vein followed by 6 mg, then 12 mg if there is no response. All boluses are followed by a rapid 10 ml saline flush. Contraindicated in asthma.

Ventricular tachycardia (Fig. 11.6)

The documented incidence of this broad complex tachycardia after AMI is approximately 10%. Occasionally, a supraventricular tachycardia is

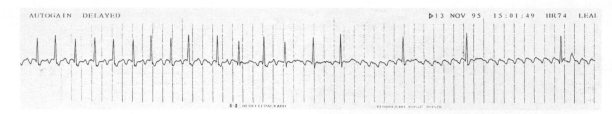

Figure 11.4: Atrial flutter.

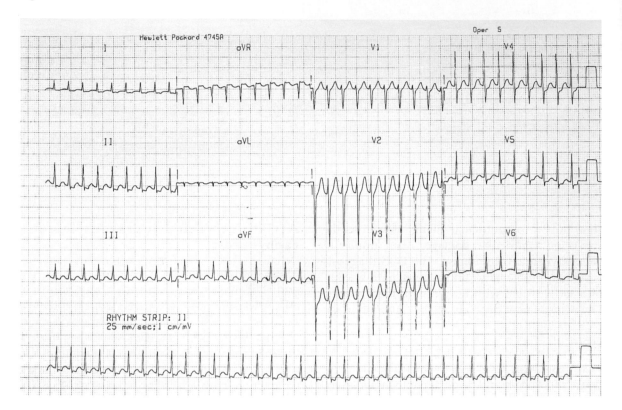

Figure 11.5: Supraventricular tachycardia.

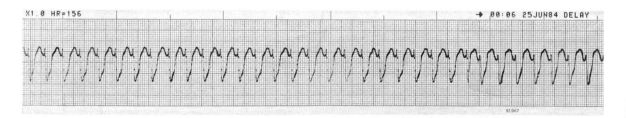

Figure 11.6: Ventricular tachycardia.

conducted with a bundle branch block, giving it a broad complex morphology. It is always safest to assume a tachycardia is ventricular in origin. Certain features of the ECG strongly support a diagnosis of VT:

- QRS duration >0.14 s
- right bundle branch block morphology
- extreme axis deviation
- chest lead concordance (the dominant QRS deflections are in the same direction)

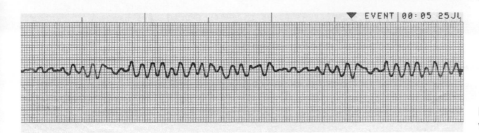

▼ EVENT | 00:05 25JL

Figure 11.7:
Ventricular fibrillation.

- fusion or capture beats (occasional narrow morphology QRS, as a P wave is conducted normally)
- dissociated P-wave activity.

Non-sustained episodes of VT and runs of premature ventricular contractions are very common (a lot more than 10%). The occurrence of frequent episodes of non-sustained VT, which do not settle after the acute phase, is a poor prognostic indicator of outcome in the after AMI (15% mortality in the first year). This is not improved by prophylactic antiarrhythmic therapy.

The haemodynamic state of the patient is the critical factor in the treatment of sustained VT. Patients who are pulseless should be defibrillated immediately and receive cardiopulmonary resuscitation (see Chapter 10). Patients who are conscious but hypotensive should be anaesthetized and cardioverted with a synchronized DC shock. The European Resuscitation Council peri-arrest guidelines also include chest pain, heart failure and a rate more than 150 beats per minute as indicators for early electrical cardioversion.

If the systolic blood pressure is more than 90 mmHg, intravenous lignocaine is recommended, initially as a bolus. This is followed by a continuous infusion and is effective in a fifth of cases. Serum potassium should be maintained between 4.0 and 5.0 mmol l^{-1}, and if the patient has been on long-term diuretics, consideration should be given to administering intravenous magnesium.

Lignocaine – 100 mg bolus (50 mg in small patients) followed by an infusion of 4 mg min^{-1} for 30 min, 2 mg min^{-1} for 2 h, and then 1 mg min^{-1}. The initial bolus may be repeated once if an infusion is not rapidly available. Lignocaine is also available as a 1 mg or 2 mg ml^{-1} solution in 5% dextrose.

If lignocaine is not effective, amiodarone is the favoured second-line agent in those who are haemodynamically stable. The same applies for patients who suffer recurrent episodes of VT despite a continuous lignocaine infusion. The lignocaine infusion must be discontinued first. Expert advice should always be sought. Some authors recommend synchronized DC cardioversion if lignocaine alone is ineffective in cardioverting sustained VT.

Ventricular fibrillation (Fig. 11.7)

Primary ventricular fibrillation (VF) has an incidence of between 5 and 10% after AMI. Episodes occurring within the first 4 h after AMI have a good long-term prognosis after successful defibrillation. VF affecting patients who are already haemodynamically compromised (secondary VF) has a much worse prognosis.

Chaotic electrical activity results in no co-ordinated ventricular contraction. Consciousness is lost almost immediately. However, it is not uncommon for there to be some respiratory effort for several seconds, which might delay defibrillation if this fact is not appreciated by the observer. Early defibrillation is an effective treatment and is covered in the advanced life-support algorithms (Chapter 10). Following a cardiac arrest it is important to relieve pain, correct electrolyte abnormalities and treat the underlying AMI (with thrombolysis if appropriate). Intravenous lignocaine or amiodarone may be indicated for recurrent episodes.

Idioventricular rhythm (Fig. 11.8)

A broad complex, regular rhythm, without P waves, at a rate between 60 and 90 beats per minute, is seen in 8–23% of patients. It is usually well tolerated and may be a sign of coronary reperfusion after thrombolysis. Specific therapy is not indicated.

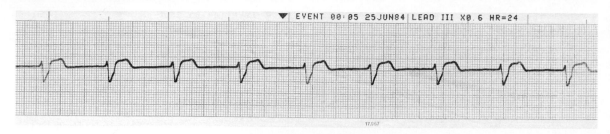

Figure 11.8: Idioventricular rhythm.

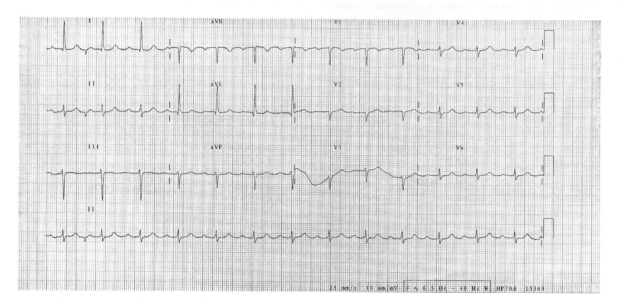

Figure 11.9: First-degree heart block.

BRADYCARDIA

Sinus bradycardia

Sinus bradycardia is observed in approximately 40% of patients with AMI. It is commonly seen in the first hour after an inferior MI, with reperfusion of the right coronary artery as a result of increased vagal tone. Ischaemia of the sinus node is an alternative mechanism. Specific treatment is seldom indicated. Prolonged sinus node arrest (more than 3 s) and hypotension require urgent therapy in the form of an intravenous bolus of atropine. Atropine reverses parasympathetically mediated bradycardia and reduced systemic vascular resistance. Small boluses of atropine should be used (0.5 mg) as increased vagal tone affords some protection against the induction of VF and infarct extension.

Doses of atropine below 0.5 mg may paradoxically induce a further reduction in heart rate. Persistent bradycardia may necessitate the insertion of a temporary pacing wire.

> Bradycardia should only be treated if causing haemodynamic compromise.

Heart block

Atrioventricular block is a poor prognostic indicator. The extent of the myocardial damage, rather than bradycardia itself, determines the ultimate prognosis. Temporary pacemakers have not been conclusively demonstrated to reduce mortality in heart block after AMI.

An increase in the PR interval (first-degree heart block, Fig. 11.9) is most often seen acutely

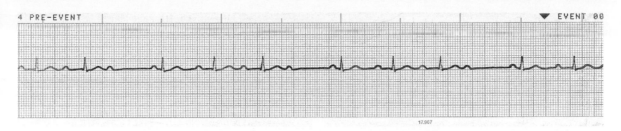

Figure 11.10: Mobitz type I second-degree heart block (Wenckebach phenomenon).

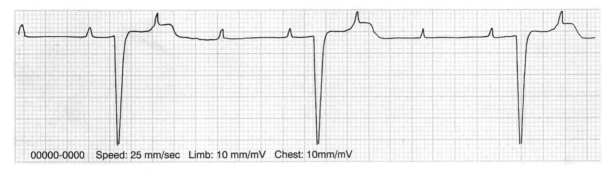

Figure 11.11: Mobitz type II second-degree heart block.

after inferior MI, and in isolation requires no therapy. A progressive lengthening of the PR interval merits increased vigilance, as it may be a sign of impending higher degrees of block.

Second-degree heart block has been classified into Mobitz types I and II:

- Mobitz type I second-degree heart block (the Wenckebach phenomenon – Fig. 11.10) complicates around 15% of inferior MIs. There is a progressive lengthening of the PR interval and then failure to conduct a P wave. Compete heart block seldom follows and asymptomatic patients do not require treatment.
- Mobitz type II (Fig. 11.11) is diagnosed by the sudden failure to conduct a P wave without a proceeding lengthening of the PR interval. This most often complicates an acute anterior MI, when there has been massive myocardial damage (in particular the septum and bundle of His). The prognosis is bad and a poorly tolerated broad complex third-degree heart block often follows. A temporary pacing wire is indicated. Atropine and emergency transcutaneous (external) pacing may be required as a temporizing measure.

Third-degree (complete) atrioventricular block (Fig. 11.12) complicates 10% of inferior MIs. The ventricular escape rhythm is a narrow complex bradycardia arising within the atrioventricular node, with a rate generally exceeding 40 beats per minute. Treatment is indicated if the patient is symptomatic or there are episodes of asystole longer than 3 s. Small doses of atropine are effective in some of these cases. If third-degree heart block recurs, or persists in spite of drug treatment, a pacing wire is indicated.

The mortality of third-degree heart block following anterior AMI is approximately 80%. A pacing wire is indicated in all cases. The escape rhythm is a broad complex, profound bradycardia, which is often associated with cardiogenic shock, which may not significantly improve when pacing is achieved.

The insertion of transvenous pacing wires is beyond the scope of this text and of most emergency departments. Improvements in transcutaneous pacing technology (Fig. 11.13) have meant that an increasing number of high-risk patients can be monitored via pacing electrodes, and externally paced on demand whilst in the resuscitation room. It is essential that emergency physicians are familiar with the system that is available within their departments.

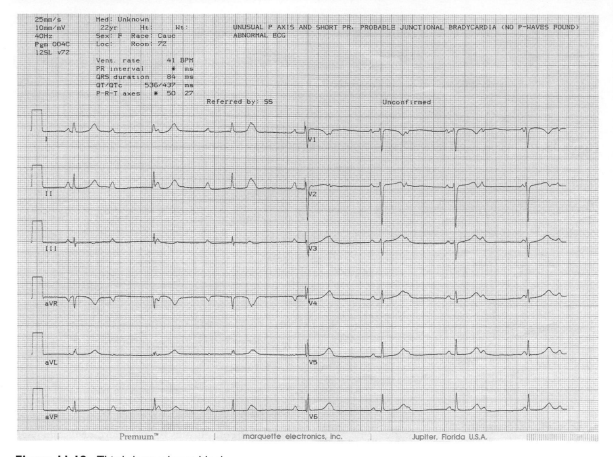

Figure 11.12: Third-degree heart block.

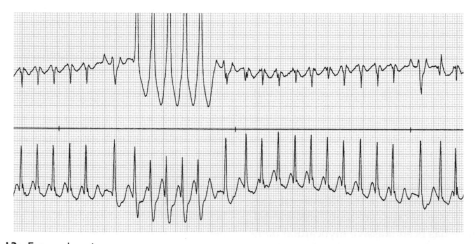

Figure 11.13: External pacing.

LEFT VENTRICULAR DYSFUNCTION

Cardiogenic pulmonary oedema is a common complication of AMI. It may be a direct consequence of extensive left ventricular damage or the result of an arrhythmia. Potentially reversible pathology must be considered at an early stage. As well as the appropriate management of arrhythmia, this might include reperfusion strategies (thrombolysis, PTCA) or urgent echocardiography if an acute mechanical defect is suspected.

Patients in acute left ventricular failure are usually extremely anxious. The following physical signs support the diagnosis:

- tachypnoea
- pallor
- cyanosis
- sweating
- tachycardia
- basal crepitations
- elevated jugular venous pressure
- third heart sound and 'gallop rhythm'.

Pulmonary oedema requires rapid and aggressive treatment (Table 11.8).

Hypotension and poor peripheral perfusion are signs of cardiogenic shock. Heart failure as a consequence of massive myocardial damage carries a poor prognosis. A new pansystolic murmur should be sought in every case, and if present raises the potential diagnosis of an acquired ventricular septal defect or acute mitral insufficiency. However, it is more common for these complications to arise later within the first week after AMI. A 12-lead ECG excludes correctable rhythm disturbances.

A chest radiograph (Fig. 11.14) confirms the diagnosis of pulmonary oedema but should not delay treatment. If the clinical state of the patient does not improve rapidly arterial blood gases should be obtained. Hypoxaemia may already be evident from pulse oximetry readings. A metabolic acidosis indicates reduced oxygen delivery and lactic acid production. Carbon dioxide retention is a preterminal sign of alveolar hypoventilation and mandates an immediate anaesthetic opinion.

Patients suffering from acute pulmonary oedema (Fig 11.14) who do not respond to initial treatment measures are likely to benefit from respiratory support. Hypoxaemia is the result of venous admixture or the shunting of blood through flooded alveoli. The application of positive end-expiratory pressure (PEEP) is believed to be effective by forcing fluid down the bronchial tree and recruiting previously unventilated alveoli. There is no evidence (as was previously believed) that fluid is forced back into the circulation. However, the

Table 11.8: Management of acute cardiogenic pulmonary oedema

1. Sit patient up and administer high-flow oxygen
2. Intravenous loop diuretic (frusemide)
3. Parenteral nitrate: buccal initially, intravenous if required to maintain systolic blood pressure between 100 and 120 mmHg
4. Small aliquots of diamorphine to reduce anxiety, with some associated haemodynamic benefit
5. Consider inotropic agents
6. Early respiratory support (IPPV, CPAP) for patients who remain hypoxic and/or hypercarbic after initial therapy

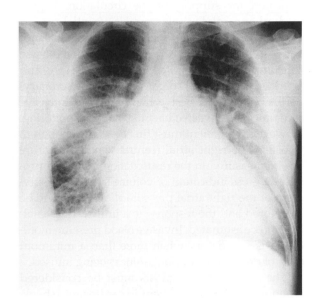

Figure 11.14: Acute pulmonary oedema.

subsequent increase in total lung volume increases the capacity of the interstitium to hold liquid.

Glyceryl trinitrate (Nitronal, Tridil, Nitrocine) – 0.6–12 mg h^{-1}.
Isosorbide dinitrate (Isoket) – 2.0–10 mg h^{-1}. Up to 20 mg h^{-1} may be required.

Continuous positive airway pressure (CPAP) supplies PEEP via a tight-fitting face-mask in spontaneously breathing patients who are able to tolerate it. At the present time this facility is seldom available in the resuscitation room, and most patients in acute respiratory failure secondary to pulmonary oedema who are not stabilized rapidly by medical therapy require endotracheal intubation and intermittent partial pressure ventilation (IPPV). PEEP should be titrated against the cardiac output, which may be impaired if it is set too high.

Patients who present to emergency departments in cardiogenic shock have an extremely poor prognosis. A mortality of at least 80% has been estimated. However, recent studies using aggressive strategies aimed at early reperfusion have yielded more encouraging data (survival rates between 20 and 70%).

Patients who present with a systolic blood pressure less than 90 mmHg should have central venous access established as soon as possible. Inotropes are indicated for support of the circulation. Urgent medical or cardiological referral is essential.

The optimal use of inotropes requires a balance between increases in heart rate, myocardial oxygen consumption, systemic vascular resistance (pre- and afterload) and vital organ (including coronary) perfusion. This is best achieved in the intensive care unit with invasive haemodynamic monitoring. However, the patient must first be stable enough to transfer. The right atrial (central venous) pressure can be measured in the resuscitation room and provides a gross indication of volume status. Measurement of the right atrial pressure allows trends to be monitored and the response to a limited fluid challenge to be estimated. Invasive blood pressure monitoring is mandatory when more than a minimum dose of dopamine or dobutamine is being infused.

The long-term prognosis must be considered when resuscitating a patient in cardiogenic shock, rather than solely the short-term normalization of haemodynamic parameters. The following must be considered early for the patient's management:

- Are attempts at coronary reperfusion appropriate? Specifically, thrombolysis with rt-PA, PTCA or coronary artery bypass grafting.
- Would the patient benefit from temporary mechanical support of the circulation (intra-aortic balloon counterpulsation)?
- Have mechanical causes of deterioration been excluded? Urgent echocardiography to exclude cardiac tamponade, post-infarction ventricular septal defect (VSD) or acute mitral regurgitation.

An aggressive approach is recommended with an early cardiology opinion in all but the very elderly or those with severe coexisting pathology.

CARDIOGENIC SHOCK DUE TO RIGHT VENTRICULAR INFARCTION

Acute right ventricular failure may be seen following an infero-posterior AMI. Agents which reduce preload (nitrates and diuretics), loss of atrial systolic contraction (AF) and concomitant left ventricular dysfunction result in a markedly reduced cardiac output. The mortality of cardiogenic shock due to right ventricular infarction is around 20%. It should be suspected in patients with the following features:

- hypotension after inferior AMI
- raised jugular venous pressure
- clear lung fields
- ST elevation in a chest lead on the right side of the chest in a 'mirror image' position of the V4 lead (V4R).

These patients require a high right-sided filling pressure, and may also require inotropic support of the right ventricle. In the resuscitation room the response to a fluid challenge should be observed (200 ml of colloid or crystalloid initially) and inotropes started empirically if there is no increase in mean arterial pressure. Nitrates and diuretics should be avoided and arrhythmia treated promptly. Atrioventricular dissociation mandates the urgent insertion of a sequential atrioventricular (dual chamber) pacemaker.

MECHANICAL COMPLICATIONS OF MYOCARDIAL INFARCTION

Mechanical complications of AMI will rarely be observed in the emergency department as their peak incidence is between 3 and 5 days after AMI. Therefore most patients will already be in hospital.

Ventricular septal defect

Ruptures of the ventricular septum characteristically occur 4–5 days after anterior AMI. If a patient has received thrombolysis, this complication is sometimes seen earlier. Patients present with severe left ventricular dysfunction. Ninety per cent of patients have a new systolic murmur. Urgent referral is essential. The diagnosis is made by echocardiography or cardiac catheterization. A mortality of

90% is observed with medical therapy, which may be reduced by 50% by urgent surgical correction.

Papillary muscle rupture

Acute mitral insufficiency due to papillary muscle rupture also occurs in the first week after AMI. Severe pulmonary oedema and, in some cases, cardiogenic shock develop rapidly. A new systolic murmur is identified in 50% of cases. Echocardiography will identify the flail leaflet. Early referral and surgery is indicated but the mortality remains high.

Left ventricular free wall rupture

Cardiac rupture is the cause of 10–20% of in-hospital deaths. It is commonest in hypertensive men who have suffered an anterior AMI. The incidence is reduced by the early administration of beta-blockers. Survival is extremely rare. A few patients have a more subacute presentation with a more gradual accumulation of a pericardial effusion. The management is volume replacement, pericardiocentesis and immediate surgical repair.

> Mechanical complications of myocardial infarction require early surgery.

POST-INFARCTION PERICARDITIS

Patients may develop pericarditis in the first week after AMI. The symptoms are of a characteristic,

well-localized pericarditic pain. A friction rub is often heard and there is an association with extensive infarction and a poor prognosis. A haemodynamically significant effusion is very uncommon. The post-myocardial infarction (Dressler's) syndrome is now rare. An autoimmune reaction to antigens exposed by myocardial necrosis results in delayed symptoms of chest pain, fever, pleuropericarditis and pleural effusion. A good response is seen to anti-inflammatory agents or steroids.

CARDIAC FAILURE

The management of acute heart failure has been discussed in the context of acute coronary syndromes.

Chronic heart failure affects 1–2% of the general population and has a complex aetiology (Table 11.9). Asymptomatic left ventricular dysfunction is believed to have at least twice the prevalence of symptomatic cardiac failure. The most common presentation in the emergency department is of an acute decompensation of chronic heart failure. Nearly half of all the patients who suffer from chronic heart failure require an admission to hospital each year.

The management of acute-on-chronic left ventricular failure is almost identical to the treatment of cardiogenic pulmonary oedema in the setting of an acute coronary syndrome. Intravenous loop diuretics and parenteral nitrate preparations are the mainstay of acute therapy. Reversible causes of an acute deterioration in cardiac function are

Table 11.9: Aetiology of cardiac failure

Myocardial pathology	Ischaemic heart disease	
	Hypertension (including pulmonary)	
	Dilated cardiomyopathy	
	Restrictive cardiomyopathy	
	Infiltrations (amyloid)	
Valvular pathology	Ventricular hypertrophy and overload (most lesions)	
	Increased left atrial pressure but ventricular function normal (mitral stenosis)	
Pericardial pathology		
Non-cardiac causes	High-output failure	Anaemia
		Thyrotoxicosis
		Paget's disease of bone
		Septicaemia
		Arteriovenous fistulae

actively sought and treated where possible (AMI, arrhythmia, pulmonary infection, hypoxaemia).

Progressive right-sided cardiac failure with dependent oedema and an elevated jugular venous pressure (progressing to hepatomegaly, ascites, pleural effusions and cachexia) is most commonly secondary to chronic left ventricular dysfunction and may require admission for intensive diuretic therapy, optimization of vasodilators, control of AF and attention to nutrition. Heart failure secondary to non-cardiac disease mandates aggressive treatment of the underlying cause.

ARRHYTHMIAS

Arrhythmias following AMI have been discussed. The management principles remain the same for patients whose primary problem is an abnormality of cardiac rhythm:

- Patients should be treated according to symptoms and haemodynamic status.
- Electrolyte abnormalities should be corrected.
- Pharmacotherapy should be limited to a small number of drugs with which the emergency physician is familiar.
- DC cardioversion is the treatment for tachycardia if the patient is shocked.
- Compromising bradycardia that does not respond rapidly to medication requires emergency transcutaneous pacing.

ATRIAL FIBRILLATION (AF)

Approximately 1% of the population over the age of 70 years is in AF, and more than 5% of those over 80 years. It is the most common sustained arrhythmia detected in the emergency department.

Causes of AF include:

- atrial distention due to mitral valve disease
- hypertensive heart disease
- impaired left ventricular function of any aetiology
- pulmonary embolus
- metabolic abnormalities (such as thyrotoxicosis)
- pericardial disease
- cardiac trauma.

AF is chaotic atrial depolarization with no co-ordinated atrial contraction. There are no P waves on the ECG and the baseline is irregular. The ventricular response is limited by the refractory period of the atrioventricular node and is also irregular. Unless there is a bundle branch block or an accessory pathway, the QRS complexes are narrow.

AF has been categorized according to the duration of symptoms. This has some weight in predicting whether a return to sinus rhythm is feasible, as well giving an indication of the risk of thromboembolus. Many patients are asymptomatic and AF is an incidental finding. The clinical features of AF are the consequence of:

- patient awareness of the fast irregular heart beat
- a reduction in cardiac output (due to reduced diastolic filing time and the loss of atrial systole)
- the increased myocardial oxygen demand in patients with coronary artery disease (angina)
- emboli originating from left atrial thrombus.

A return to sinus rhythm is the aim for all patients other than the very old or infirm, in whom AF is suspected to be long-standing. In this group of patients attempts at cardioversion are likely to be unsuccessful. Even with adequate control of the ventricular rate there is a significant risk of embolism in patients with a structurally abnormal heart, hypertension, previous stroke or diabetes. Approximately 15% of patients in chronic AF have an episode of embolization each year.

Episodes of paroxysmal AF revert to sinus rhythm spontaneously, usually within 24 h of onset. Some patients require emergency treatment for symptomatic relief. Historical features may help to identify precipitating factors such as alcohol excess or non-compliance with medication. It is not always clear how long the patient has been in AF, and treating the patient according to haemodynamic status is of paramount importance. Persistent AF may be defined as an episode lasting between 24 and 48 h.

Shocked patients should receive synchronized DC cardioversion after general anaesthesia (initial energy 100 J). Relatively asymptomatic patients can be observed. Some authorities recommend intravenous amiodarone as the first-line agent to restore sinus rhythm for patients who do not spontaneously revert to sinus rhythm within 24 h. Rapid control of the ventricular rate, good tolerance even in ventricular impairment, and efficacy in restoring sinus rhythm are significant advantages of this drug. The requirement for immediate anticoagulation (heparinization initially) remains the subject of debate.

Episodes of AF that last less than 48 h are unlikely to result in significant atrial thrombus formation. Cardioversion of these patients is believed to be safe without prophylactic anticoagulation. Synchronized DC cardioversion is an effective therapy if chemical cardioversion is unsuccessful.

If there is a possibility that the patient has been in AF for longer than 48 h, this should be assumed to be the case. If ventricular rate control is required, digoxin is the most suitable agent. Patients are loaded orally or intravenously depending on the urgency of the situation. Consideration may be given to elective cardioversion after a minimum of 3 weeks' anticoagulation. Ventricular rate control can also be achieved with beta-blockers (metoprolol) or calcium-channel blockers (diltiazem or verapamil), although digoxin is the first-line treatment in the UK.

All patients in chronic AF should be considered for indefinite anticoagulation. After successful elective cardioversion anticoagulation should be continued for a further 4 weeks.

RE-ENTRANT TACHYCARDIAS

Paroxysmal regular narrow complex tachycardias (supraventricular tachycardias) most commonly arise from electrical circuits in the region of the atrioventricular node. A re-entrant tachycardia is the result of repeated circulation of an impulse between the atria and the ventricles. In order for this to occur there must be at least two conducting pathways. The additional pathway may be within the atrioventricular node or anatomically distinct (an accessory pathway or bypass tract).

Supraventricular tachycardia

The commonest form of paroxysmal supraventricular tachycardia is atrioventricular nodal re-entry tachycardia (AVNRT) (Fig. 11.15). If an ectopic impulse generated in the atrium reaches the abnormal conducting pathway during its prolonged refractory period, anterograde conduction can only take place down the normal pathway. A subsequent retrograde impulse generated in the ventricle may then reactivate the atria via the abnormal pathway, which rapidly becomes excitable. This cycle of mutual activation and reactivation results in a narrow complex tachycardia between 150 and 250 beats per minute. P waves are superimposed on the QRS complexes because atrial and ventricular activation are simultaneous. If P waves are identified an alternative diagnosis should be considered.

AVNRT is most common in females between the ages of 10 and 50 years and is usually well tolerated. Vagal manoeuvres such as Valsalva, splashing cold water on the face, and carotid sinus massage are sometimes effective, and the arrhythmia is reliably terminated by intravenous adenosine. Verapamil is an effective second-line therapy. Occasionally, patients require synchronized DC cardioversion. Long-term therapy includes prophylactic antiarrhythmics (e.g. a beta-blocker), and radiofrequency ablation of the abnormal pathway following electrophysiological evaluation.

Atrioventricular reciprocating tachycardia (Wolf–Parkinson–White syndrome)

Wolf–Parkinson–White (WPW) is a pre-excitation syndrome. Pre-excitation is a phenomenon whereby the ventricles are activated earlier than via normal atrioventricular nodal conduction. Therefore, there is a short PR interval and slurring of the initial component of the QRS complex (Fig. 11.16). Recurrent tachycardia in conjunction with these ECG features characterizes WPW.

In the general population pre-excitation is found in fewer than 3 in 1000 people, and unlike AVNRT there is a male preponderance. Most patients with WPW syndrome have their first episode of tachycardia before the age of 40 years, and approximately 50% have an episode before they are 20 years old.

Patients with WPW may develop AF. Patients may be severely compromised, as the ventricular response may be extremely fast. AF with a rapid ventricular rate is associated with an increased risk of developing VF, owing to rapid conduction down the accessory pathway.

Hypotensive patients with a narrow or broad complex tachycardia should be immediately cardioverted with a synchronized DC shock. Adenosine

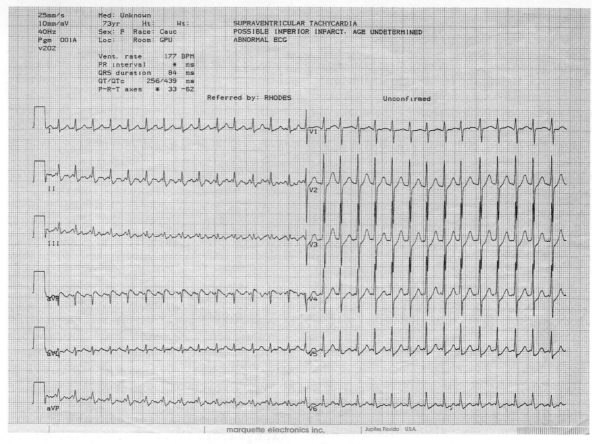

25mm/s
10mm/mV
40Hz
Pgm 001A
v202

Med: Unknown
73yr   Ht: Wt:
Sex: F Race: Cauc
Loc: Room: GPU

SUPRAVENTRICULAR TACHYCARDIA
POSSIBLE INFERIOR INFARCT, AGE UNDETERMINED
ABNORMAL ECG

Vent. rate   177 BPM
PR interval   * ms
QRS duration   84 ms
QT/QTc   256/439 ms
P-R-T axes * 33 -62

Referred by: RHODES   Unconfirmed

marquette electronics inc.   Jupiter, Florida U.S.A.

Figure 11.15: AVNRT – supraventricular tachycardia.

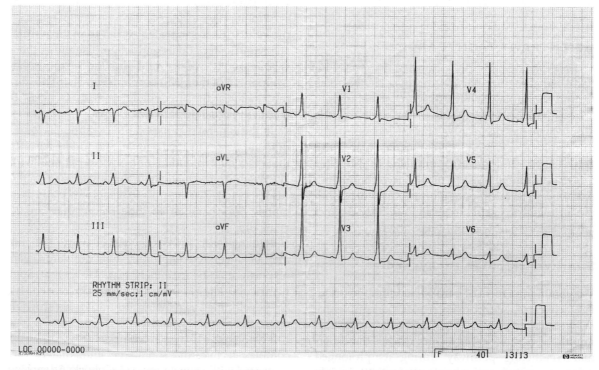

RHYTHM STRIP: II
25 mm/sec; 1 cm/mV

LOC 00000-0000

F   40   13113

Figure 11.16: Wolf–Parkinson–White syndrome.

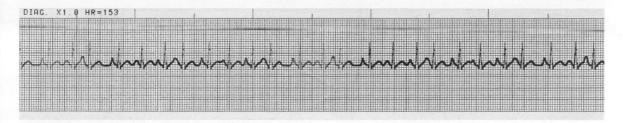

Figure 11.17: Atrial tachycardia.

cardioverts most patients from AVNRT. Care must be taken to not treat pre-excited AF with adenosine, digoxin or verapamil, as blockade of the AV node may lead to one-to-one conduction of the chaotic atrial activity down the accessory pathway, and hence VF. It is recommended that a specialist opinion is obtained before administering a second agent if there is no response of an AVRT to adenosine.

Atrial tachycardia (Fig. 11.17)

Between 5 and 10% of patients who present with a paroxysmal supraventricular tachycardia have an ectopic focus in the left or right atrium. Unifocal atrial tachycardia has rate that is usually less than 250 beats per minute, with morphologically abnormal P waves preceding each QRS complex. Atrioventricular nodal blocking agents are ineffective. Adenosine or vagal manoeuvres may be required to demonstrate that the atrioventricular node is not required to maintain the tachycardia. Continued rapid atrial activity with AV block is seen but the tachycardia is not terminated. Unifocal atrial tachycardia with variable block may be caused by digoxin toxicity.

The therapy for unifocal atrial tachycardia should address the underlying cause. Patients who are stable although clinically toxic to digoxin should have their electrolytes corrected and further doses withheld. A serum potassium of more than $8 \, mmol \, l^{-1}$ or haemodynamic compromise have been regarded as indications for the administration of digoxin-specific antibody fragments (*Digibind*). A short-acting beta-blocker may be used to control the ventricular rate.

Atrial flutter (Fig. 11.18)

Atrial flutter is less common than AF and almost never occurs without serious underlying cardiac pathology, in particular mitral valve disease and ischaemia. The mechanism of this arrhythmia is a re-entry circuit involving the right atrium and the interventricular septum. The rate of atrial depolarization is 300 per minute. The AV node will not allow conduction at this rate, and typically a two-to-one block results in a constant ventricular rate very close to 150 beats per minute. Flutter waves may not be visible on the ECG unless the degree of AV block is increased (adenosine or vagal manoeuvres). At higher degrees of AV block the 'sawtoothed' pattern of atrial depolarization is readily appreciated.

The degree of symptoms is variable. Palpitations are common. Hypotension is treated by sychronized DC cardioversion. Amiodarone, digoxin and beta-blockers have all been used to good effect. However, amiodarone combines ventricular rate control with a high probability of a return to sinus rhythm. Semi-elective DC cardioversion is an extremely effective treatment for drug-resistant cases. Consideration should be given to anticoagulation, although the risk of embolization is less than with AF.

VENTRICULAR TACHYCARDIA (FIG. 11.19)

Ventricular tachycardia (VT) is the most common broad complex tachycardia (QRS duration more than 120 ms). Alternative causes of a broad complex tachycardia such as SVT with aberration, are diagnoses of exclusion. Certain ECG features which may help in the differentiation of VT from a broad complex SVT have been discussed above.

VT is defined as the occurrence of three or more consecutive ventricular beats at a rate of more than 100 per minute. It can be further classified into sustained or non-sustained VT, depending on whether an episode is respectively more or less than 30 s.

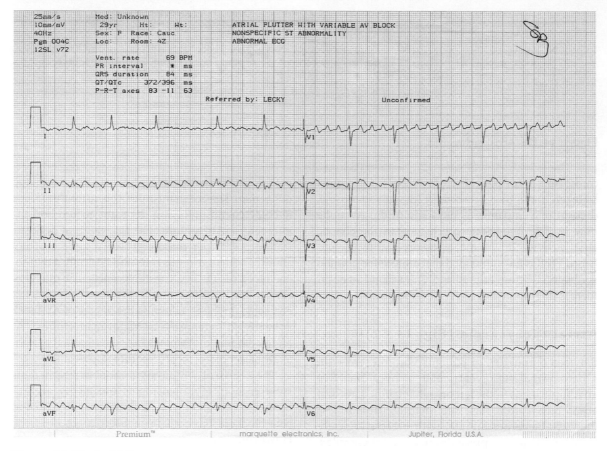

Figure 11.18: Atrial flutter.

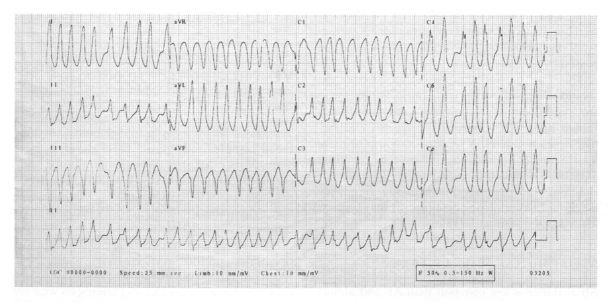

Figure 11.19: Ventricular tachycardia.

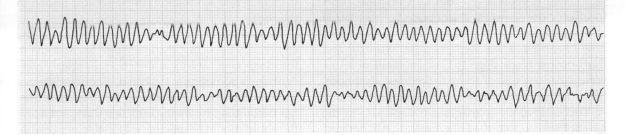

Figure 11.20: Torsade de Pointes.

VT is frequently observed in the early phase after AMI. It may also arise from re-entry circuits at the margins of an old infarct. VT is a recognized feature of most disorders that affect heart muscle (including toxins), and may occasionally be seen in young people with structurally normal hearts. It is recommended that all broad complex tachycardias are assumed to be ventricular in origin until proved otherwise.

Haemodynamically stable patients with sustained VT or recurrent symptomatic non-sustained VT should be treated with intravenous lignocaine or amiodarone. Hypotensive patients require synchronized DC cardioversion. Patients who do not have a pulse should be immediately defibrillated in accordance with the Advanced Life Support Algorithm.

Torsade de Pointes

Torsade de Pointes is a form of polymorphic VT (Fig. 11.20). There is an association with sudden death and a different management strategy is indicated.

Most antiarrhythmic agents are either ineffective or make the situation worse (including lignocaine). Intravenous magnesium sulphate is effective in most patients. DC cardioversion is an effective therapy for resistant or compromised cases.

Expert advice should be obtained, unless haemodynamic compromise mandates immediate cardioversion.

BRADYCARDIA

A secondary sinus bradycardia is a common observation in many disorders whose primary pathology is non-cardiac:

- pre-terminal event as a consequence of hypoxia
- hypothermia

- increased vagal tone
- metabolic disturbances such as hypothyroidism
- electrolyte disturbances – hyperkalaemia
- acutely raised intracranial pressure.

The two most common cardiac lesions that result in a pathological slowing of the ventricular rate are atrioventricular block and sinus node disease.

ATRIOVENTRICULAR BLOCK

Myocardial infarction has been discussed as a cause of atrioventricular block. Other causes include:

- idiopathic fibrosis
- aortic valve disease
- congenital AV block
- anatomical congenital heart disease.

First-degree heart block (Fig. 11.9) is diagnosed by a PR interval of more than 0.21 s. The PR interval is measured from the onset of the P wave to the onset of the QRS complex. First-degree heart block does not cause symptoms but may herald higher degrees of block, depending on the clinical context. First-degree heart block is sometimes seen in athletes with high vagal tone. No action is required.

Second-degree heart block is classified into type I (Fig. 11.10) and type II (the Mobitz classification). High vagal tone has been implicated in the aetiology of some cases of type I second-degree block, which is diagnosed by an increasing PR interval prior to a non-conducted P wave. In these cases the prognosis is good. However, in the absence of increased vagal tone type I block may be as dangerous as type II.

Mobitz type II atrioventricular block (Fig. 11.11) does not exhibit a progressive lengthening of the PR interval before a failure of conduction. A common pattern is a ratio of two P waves to one ventricular response (2:1 block). Complete heart block exhibits complete dissociation between atrial and ventricular activity. First-degree and Mobitz type I heart block are asymptomatic. Mobitz II and third-degree block (Fig. 11.12) may result in a low ventricular response leading to tiredness, dyspnoea, heart failure and syncope (a Stokes–Adams attack).

The emergency management depends on the haemodynamic state of the patient. All patients other than those with first-degree heart block require admission. Atropine, isoprenaline infusion or transcutaneous pacing may be required as holding strategies until arrangements are made for the insertion of a temporary transvenous pacing wire.

SICK SINUS SYNDROME

The sick sinus syndrome is caused by idiopathic fibrosis of the sinus node. It most commonly affects the elderly. The presenting symptoms are usually syncope and dizziness. There is impairment of sinus node activity or of conduction of impulses from the sinus node to the atria. The clinical features are a consequence of profound sinus bradycardia, sino-atrial block or sinus arrest. Some individuals also experience episodes of supraventricular tachycardia (the tachy/brady syndrome). Sino-atrial block is diagnosed by intermittently dropped P waves resulting in a pause that is a multiple of the normal P to P interval.

Symptomatic patients and those with pauses of longer than 3 s should be paced. Twenty-four-hour ambulatory ECG monitoring may be required to establish the diagnosis.

COMPLICATIONS OF PERMANENT PACEMAKER SYSTEMS

It is now possible to pace the atrium, the ventricle or both chambers in physiological sequence. The mode of pacing is conventionally described as a three-letter code:

- The first letter indicates the chamber that is paced (A, V, or D for dual).
- The second letter refers to the chamber which is sensed.
- The third letter refers to the type of sensing (inhibition (I), triggered (T), dual type (D)).

If there is rate modulation the letter R is added to the code.

Immediate complications may present to the emergency department and include haematoma of the chest wall and local infection. Surgical intervention is sometimes indicated. Pneumothoraces as a consequence of subclavian venepuncture may not become symptomatic for a few days and a low threshold should be maintained for obtaining radiographs of the chest. Displacement of a pacemaker lead occurs in less than 1% of patients and may be evident as a return of the original bradycardia, failure to capture (a pacing spike seen on the ECG but no subsequent native electrical depolarization), or a failure to sense appropriately.

Long-term complications occur with a breakdown of the insulation of the lead. Patients may complain of muscle twitching, and over-sensing can result in inappropriate variations in the heart rate. Fracture of the pacemaker lead may follow trauma. Patients with unichamber ventricular devices may complain of tiredness, dyspnoea and lethargy as a result of the loss of atrial transport (the pacemaker syndrome).

Defibrillation can be achieved safely in the presence of a permanent pacemaker if the paddles are placed at least 12 cm from the device. The pacemaker should be checked as soon as possible after defibrillation.

VALVULAR EMERGENCIES

Patients who have lesions of the heart valves occasionally present to the emergency department. Most require conventional management of heart failure or other medical problems. A detailed description of each lesion is beyond the scope of this text. It is more appropriate to focus on situations that require specific emergency department management.

The majority of people who have a heart murmur will already have been investigated and the diagnosis may be obtained from scrutinizing hospital records, echocardiography reports, or even asking the patient. The incidental finding of a cardiac murmur does not automatically indicate that admission is required. Patients who are symptomatically well may be referred for out-patient investigation. Advice to avoid strenuous activity should be given, and the possible requirement for antibiotic prophylaxis for certain procedures should be discussed.

THE MITRAL VALVE

The commonest cause of mitral stenosis remains rheumatic heart disease. Patients may present to the emergency department for several reasons:

- worsening dyspnoea, including paroxysmal nocturnal dyspnoea (PND) and pulmonary oedema
- haemoptysis, due to pulmonary congestion
- palpitations
- systemic embolization, most commonly seen in the presence of atrial fibrillation.

The characteristic murmur of mitral stenosis is a mid-diastolic 'rumble' with presystolic accentuation (this is lost in atrial fibrillation). There is a loud first heart sound and an opening snap, which precedes the murmur.

Acute post-infarction papillary muscle dysfunction leading to mitral regurgitation has been discussed. Chronic mitral insufficiency may be tolerated for many years. The onset of atrial fibrillation may cause a patient to become symptomatic for the first time. Breathlessness on exertion is a common symptom. Otherwise, the presentation is similar to mitral stenosis. Relatively asymptomatic individuals can be followed up as out-patients. Heart failure is treated in the conventional manner, and previously undocumented atrial fibrillation mandates admission. The risk of embolization is sufficient that patients should be considered for immediate and indefinite anticoagulation. Some invasive procedures require prophylactic antibiotic coverage.

THE AORTIC VALVE

The incidence of sudden death in patients with aortic stenosis is approximately 25%. Syncope induced by exertion is a particularly sinister historical feature. Symptoms tend to appear late in the course of the disease, so it is vital that the diagnosis is not missed when patients are examined. It is worth revising the physical signs:

- slow-rising poor-volume pulse, best felt in the carotid
- systolic thrill in the carotid pulse or over the aortic area

- ejection systolic murmur, loudest in the aortic area
- normal or low blood pressure with a narrow pulse pressure
- third and fourth heart sounds
- forceful apex beat (heart not enlarged).

The ECG may show one or more of the following: left ventricular hypertrophy, left ventricular strain, left bundle branch block, left axis deviation and P mitrale.

Afterload reduction is poorly tolerated by patients with severe aortic stenosis because of the limitation of stroke volume. Vasodilators should be avoided. A new diagnosis of symptomatic aortic stenosis (especially if there has been exertional syncope) mandates an urgent cardiology opinion, echocardiogram and admission. Urgent valve replacement may be indicated.

The two commonest causes of acute aortic insufficiency are infective endocarditis and dissection of the aortic root. Acute cases comprise 20% of the total, and acute left ventricular failure is the usual presentation.

RIGHT-SIDED HEART LESIONS

Acute valvular lesions of the right side of the heart are much less common than those affecting the left side. *Staphylococcus aureus* endocarditis of the tricuspid valve is seen in intravenous drug users. These patients are acutely ill and septic. With destruction of the valve clinical signs become more obvious: elevated jugular venous pressure, pulsatile hepatomegaly, peripheral oedema and ascites. A blowing pansystolic murmur is heard at the lower left sternal edge. Pulmonary incompetence is most often secondary to chronic pulmonary arterial hypertension.

INFECTIVE ENDOCARDITIS

Infective endocarditis is an uncommon condition. It is a multisystem disease caused by infection of the heart valves and adjacent endocardium. There are 1500 cases per year in the UK, with a mortality of approximately 15%. Although infective endocarditis may arise in a previously healthy valve, pre-existing anatomical derangement provides the optimal conditions for bacterial colonization. A 'jet' lesion chronically damages the endocardial impact site, with the formation of a sterile platelet–fibrin thrombus. This area is susceptible to transient bacteraemia. A generalized reduction in host immunity (e.g. alcoholism and renal failure) may predispose the 'normal' heart valve to infection.

Prosthetic heart valves and defective native valves are at risk from recognized sources of bacteraemia:

- dental procedures
- urogenital procedures
- intravenous drug abuse
- endoscopy (or contrast studies), particularly of the lower gastrointestinal tract
- intravenous cannulation (should be restricted to patients in whom it is essential).

The disease may be acute and rapidly overwhelming, or run a more chronic course.

Clinical features

The clinical features of infective endocarditis are a manifestation of its multisystem involvement:

- *Infection* fever, weight loss, cachexia, splenomegaly, arthralgia
- *Cardiac* a new or changing cardiac murmur, arrhythmia, conduction disturbances, heart failure
- *Embolic* stroke, mesenteric infarction, renal, recurrent pneumonitis
- *Immunological* glomerulonephritis, splinter haemorrhages, mucosal petechiae, Osler's nodes, Janeway lesions, Roth spots.

Investigations

At least two sets of blood cultures should be taken from different sites before the administration of empirical antibiotic therapy to patients who are severely ill. A full blood count may reveal anaemia and a neutrophilia. The erythrocyte sedimentation rate and C-reactive protein are often high. Urinalysis should be performed to exclude glomerulonephritis, and an ECG, although non-specific, may demonstrate conduction disturbances (suggesting abscess formation). The valvular vegetations may be visualized by echocardiography.

Antibiotic therapy

Once a diagnosis of infective endocarditis is strongly suspected empirical anitibiotics should be administered. A combination of intravenous benzylpenicillin and intravenous gentamicin is a suitable empirical choice unless the history is suggestive of a staphylococcal aetiology, in which case flucloxacillin should also be given. An early microbiological opinion should be obtained, usually at the time that the first sets of cultures are taken.

Current recommendations for antibiotic prophylaxis for patients at risk of endocarditis undergoing medical or dental procedures can be found in the *British National Formulary*.

DISEASE OF HEART MUSCLE

CARDIOMYOPATHIES

The cardiomyopathies have been classified according to clinical, echocardiographic, pathophysiological and morphological findings on biopsy and post mortem:

- dilated cardiomyopathy
- hypertrophic cardiomyopathy
- restrictive cardiomyopathy.

Dilatation and hypokinesis of the left ventricle, which is not associated with valvular disease, ischaemia, hypertension or systemic disease, is classified as dilated cardiomyopathy. The presenting features are those of left ventricular dysfunction and embolization. Specific emergency management is not required other than the treatment of complications.

Hypertrophic cardiomyopathy (HCM) is defined as hypertrophy of an undilated left ventricle that cannot be explained by pressure or volume overload. It has a prevalence of approximately 1 in 5000. Autosomal dominant inheritance has been described (possibly as many as 50% of cases), as well as sporadic mutations. Cardiac function is affected by a progressive impairment of diastolic filling of the left, and sometimes the right ventricle. Atrial fibrillation and ventricular arrhythmias are common.

At the most severe end of the spectrum of HCM, sudden deaths of apparently fit young individuals receive widespread publicity. A more benign course is observed in some individuals, usually those who have survived to middle or later life. Patients with a family history of sudden cardiac death at a young age are at the highest risk of sudden death themselves. Some patients are entirely symptom free. Exertional breathlessness, angina and syncope are frequent historical features.

Syncope on exertion is a highly sinister symptom.

Examination reveals a systolic murmur through the narrowed left ventricular outflow tract, and a murmur of secondary mitral insufficiency may also be heard. ECG findings are non-specific. Left ventricular hypertrophy by voltage criteria with no other discernible cause should raise the index of suspicion, but may be a normal finding in the athletic heart. Young patients with exertional symptoms, especially syncope, require echocardiography.

Restrictive cardiomyopathy is a disease of unknown aetiology, which is sometimes familial. There is stiffness of the left ventricle and impaired diastolic function, leading to an excessive rise in diastolic pressure with small increases in volume. The course of this illness is chronic and progressive, with the development of congestive cardiac failure.

MYOCARDITIS

Viral infections are the most common cause of myocarditis. Although most cases are subclinical, the diagnosis should be suspected in anyone who presents with a 'flu-like' illness with myalgia as a prominent symptom. Most patients make a complete recovery. In some patients a severe dilated cardiomyopathy develops.

The cause of the myocardial damage is either a direct effect of toxins or secondary immune-mediated necrosis.

The prodromal illness may be non-specific (fever, myalgia, sore throat, headache, diarrhoea). The cardiac manifestations include heart failure, syncope, heart block, chest pain and sudden death. A tachycardia out of proportion to the systemic illness may be observed. A third heart sound is a frequent finding. The ECG may reveal arrhythmia,

ST segment and T-wave changes, or poor R-wave progression.

The management is supportive. Patients without haemodynamic compromise are admitted for bed rest, cardiac rhythm monitoring and confirmation of the diagnosis (usually to exclude ischaemia). Although most patients recover completely, approximately 15% suffer progressive ventricular dysfunction. Aggressive inotropic support and mechanical support of the circulation is indicated for those with severe ventricular impairment.

PERICARDITIS

Inflammation of the pericardium is frequently asymptomatic. It may be a feature of a severe systemic disorder, or a self-limiting condition in an otherwise fit individual.

CLINICAL FEATURES

Patients frequently complain of a prodromal flu-like illness before the development of the characteristic chest pain. The pain is typically sharp and varies with respiration. It is exacerbated by lying down and swallowing, and relieved by sitting forward. Occasionally, patients present with isolated shoulder pain. The associated friction rub has been compared to the sound of 'Velcro', and is best heard using the diaphragm of the stethoscope at the lower left sternal edge with the patient holding their breath.

INVESTIGATION

Electrocardiography (Fig. 11.21)

ECG changes appear from hours to days after the onset of symptoms of pericarditis. Concave ST elevation is characteristically seen in most leads except aVL and V1. Unlike in AMI the T waves remain upright, and PR segment depression occurs in 80% of patients (best seen in lead II). Serial ECGs may be required to exclude AMI. It should also be noted that the ECG may be normal in acute pericarditis.

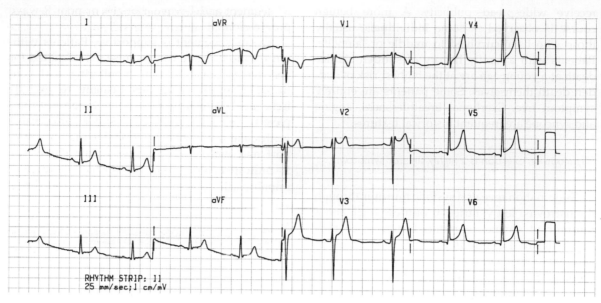

Figure 11.21: The ECG in pericarditis.

Chest radiograph

The chest radiograph is usually unremarkable in acute pericarditis.

Echocardiography

Small pericardial effusions are identifiable by echocardiography (as little as 15 ml). Thickening of the pericardium may be visualized in constrictive pericarditis.

Laboratory tests

The exclusion of ischaemia is paramount. Rigorous exclusion of an underlying systemic disorder may be required in atypical cases.

MANAGEMENT

Most patients are haemodynamically stable. Arrhythmias should be treated aggressively if there is haemodynamic compromise. Cardiac tamponade is diagnosed clinically by the following signs:

- low cardiac output state
- muffled heart sounds
- distended neck veins

- Kussmaul's sign (paradoxical elevation of jugular venous pressure on inspiration).

Urgent pericardiocentesis is indicated for these patients, preferably under ultrasound guidance if time allows. 'Blind' pericardiocentesis is indicated for impending cardiac arrest (Fig. 11.22).

Most patients suffering from acute postviral pericarditis require only symptomatic treatment with a non-steroidal anti-inflammatory agent. Some patients may be discharged from the emergency department. However, appropriate investigation must have been completed and a senior medical opinion obtained.

HYPERTENSIVE EMERGENCIES

AETIOLOGY AND CLINICAL FEATURES

Between 1 and 2% of patients who have essential hypertension develop a hypertensive emergency (Table 11.10). The untreated mortality of hypertensive crises approaches 90% at 1 year. With currently available therapy the 5-year survival rate is nearly 75%. Hypertensive emergencies are more common in males and people of African or Afro-Caribbean descent. Hypertension may be a secondary phenomenon to many conditions.

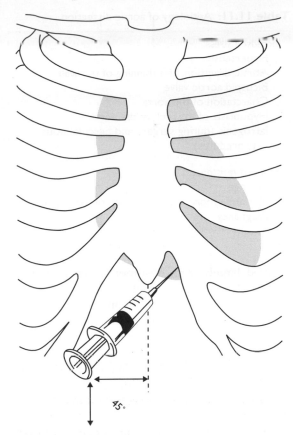

Figure 11.22: Pericardiocentesis. The patient is positioned semi-upright and a 16–18 gauge intravenous cannula is advanced in the angle between the xiphisternum and the left costal margin towards the left shoulder, 45° to the skin.

Table 11.10: Hypertensive emergencies

Hypertensive left ventricular failure
Hypertensive encephalopathy
Hypertension associated with AMI or unstable angina
Aortic dissection
Hypertension associated with acute renal failure
Hypertension associated with intracerebral or
    subarachnoid haemorrhage
Phaeochromocytoma
Eclampsia and pre-eclampsia

A hypertensive crisis is a situation where severe sustained hypertension results in life-threatening cardiovascular, neurological and renal damage.

True hypertensive emergencies mandate aggressive and rapid control of blood pressure. If a true emergency does not exist there are serious consequences associated with reducing the blood pressure too quickly.

Malignant hypertension presents with very high levels of blood pressure (a diastolic of more than 130 mmHg) and retinal haemorrhages. Papilloedema may be present. Headaches occur in 85% of patients and blurred vision in 60%. Chest pain and dyspnoea suggest cardiovascular involvement, which may be angina, AMI or left ventricular failure (LVF). Hypertensive encephalopathy is the result of the breakdown of cerebral autoregulation and may develop over several weeks. The clinical manifestations of hypertensive encephalopathy are heterogeneous, such as headache, vomiting, confusion, coma, focal signs and fits.

MANAGEMENT

A single diastolic blood pressure reading in an asymptomatic patient of more than 130 mmHg needs to be repeated after the patient has been sat in a quiet room for a short interval. Many patients will then prove to have a blood pressure that is low enough to allow safe discharge. Individuals who are hypertensive, with advanced retinopathy but no other evidence of end-organ dysfunction, do not require parenteral therapy. Oral agents are favoured over sublingual, which may cause a precipitous fall in the blood pressure of some patients. Many agents have been used with success. Admission is indicated for these patients. Oral therapy is likewise preferred for patients with a history suggesting subacute or chronic hypertensive encephalopathy on a background of chronic hypertension. The failure of cerebral autoregulation in hypertensive encephalopathy exposes these individuals to the risk of further neurological damage if the blood pressure is reduced by more than 25%.

Parenteral control of hypertension is indicated for certain situations. Blood pressure should be reduced by up to 25% of the peak level. The following situations demand immediate blood pressure reduction:

- AMI or angina – intravenous glyceryl trinitrate is a suitable agent. Intravenous beta-blockers, such as esmolol or metoprolol, are an alternative. Opiate analgesics are essential.

- LVF – intravenous glyceryl trinitrate.
- Aortic dissection – see below.
- Blood pressure control may be indicated if there is evidence that hypertension induced by spontaneous intracerebral or subarachnoid haemorrhage is damaging other end organs. Sodium nitroprusside or labetalol given intravenously are suitable agents.

Hypertensive encephalopathy demands a slightly less immediate reduction in blood pressure, which can also be achieved using nitroprusside or labetalol.

Pre-eclampsia should be managed with the early involvement of the obstetricians. Intravenous labetalol or hydralazine (a vasodilator) can be used to control hypertension, and magnesium sulphate is the anticonvulsant of choice.

FOLLOW-UP OF HYPERTENSIVE PATIENTS

Most patients who are hypertensive but do not reveal evidence of end-organ damage do not require admission. Appropriate follow-up is essential and can be arranged via the general practitioner or urgent specialist out-patient appointment. The British Hypertensive Society has recommended that patients with a systolic blood pressure more than 200 mmHg, or a diastolic more than 110 mmHg, should be treated if this level is sustained on three separate occasions over 1–2 weeks.

AORTIC DISSECTION

The wall of the aorta has three layers: from the lumen outwards – intima, media and adventitia. Aortic dissection is the longitudinal cleavage of the media by a dissecting column of blood. The affected aorta is not commonly aneurysmal; the term *dissecting aortic aneurysm* should be avoided.

EPIDEMIOLOGY AND PATHOGENESIS

The incidence of aortic dissection has been estimated in industrialized countries to be between 5 and 10 cases per million per year. These figures have been

Table 11.11: Aetiology of aortic dissection

Increased stress:
　Hypertension
　Aortic dilatation, and thinning of the wall
　Bicuspid aortic valve
　Coarctation of the aorta
　Hypoplasia of the arch of the aorta
　Iatrogenic (during surgery and percutaneous procedures)

Reduced resistance:
　Old age
　Marfan's syndrome, Ehlers–Danlos syndrome
　Pregnancy

derived largely from post-mortem examinations. The incidence is approximately twice that of acute rupture of an abdominal aortic aneurysm (although many fewer patients who suffer thoracic dissection reach hospital alive). It is more common in males and has a peak incidence between 50 and 70 years. A structural weakness in the wall of the thoracic aorta predisposes an individual to dissection when an initiating stress of sufficient magnitude is applied.

Medial degeneration is a process characterized by loss of smooth muscle cells and elastic tissue, with subsequent scarring and fibrosis. It is part of the ageing process to a varying degree, but may be accelerated in some individuals, particularly in the presence of arterial hypertension. The incidence of aortic dissection in a population is related to the prevalence of major risk factors, which lead to an imbalance between applied stress and aortic wall resistance (Table 11.11).

Once there has been a breach to the intima the pulsatile flow of blood is able to enter the vessel wall by separating its layers. The entry point of the dissection is variable and dependent on local factors. The ascending aorta, in particular the convexity 1–2 cm above the aortic sinuses, is the entry point of around 60% of dissections. The aortic arch is the entry point in 10%, and 30% arise just distal to the left subclavian artery.

A false lumen is formed within the wall on the aorta. Further progression of the dissection is determined by the blood pressure. Rarely, the false lumen ruptures internally into the true lumen, limiting further extension. Much more likely is a catastrophic external rupture through the adventitia.

CLINICAL FEATURES

Although patients may present with syncope (5%) or as a cardiac arrest, the commonest clinical scenario (in the patient who reaches hospital) is a sudden onset of severe chest and interscapular pain (see above), hypertension and an unremarkable electrocardiogram. The pain may migrate down the back as the dissection propagates.

Consider aortic dissection in patients with severe tearing interscapular pain.

Subsequent clinical findings are the result of complications. Heart failure may be observed if there is acute aortic insufficiency. An early diastolic murmur at the left sternal edge should be sought in all patients when aortic dissection is in the differential. Hypotension suggests cardiac tamponade from an intrapericardial rupture of a lesion of the ascending aorta, or external rupture of the dissection somewhere along its length.

Compression or occlusion of branches of the aorta may result in ischaemic complications such as focal neurological abnormalities, stroke, upper or lower limb ischaemia, renal failure, mesenteric ischaemia and myocardial infarction. Palpation of all peripheral pulses and a rapid neurological examination are mandatory in all cases of suspected aortic dissection. Proximal dissections give rise to pulse discrepancies in half of cases, most commonly because of subclavian artery obstruction. Involvement of the spinal and vertebral arteries leads to ischaemic paraparesis in approximately 4% of cases.

EARLY MANAGEMENT

Urgent specialist referral is essential for anyone suspected of having an aortic dissection. Appropriate management must be initiated before definitive investigations have been performed. Liberal doses of intravenous morphine or diamorphine are required to control the severe pain of an acute aortic dissection. Although lacking sensitivity and specificity, the chest radiograph is likely to be the first investigation performed.

Certain abnormalities on the chest radiograph are suggestive of aortic dissection (Fig. 11.23):

- widened mediastinum

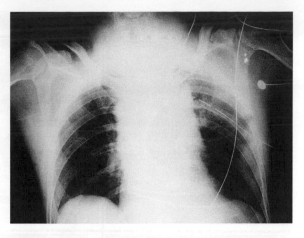

Figure 11.23: Chest X-ray of a patient with aortic dissection.

- abnormal aortic contour – localized bulges, diameter change, and obliteration of the aortic knob (differentiation from the tortuosity seen in chronic hypertension may be difficult)
- the 'calcium sign' – intimal calcification separated from the outer wall of the aorta by 5 mm or more
- double density of the aorta, suggesting a false lumen
- left-sided pleural effusion.

Control of hypertension is the critical early intervention.

Control of arterial hypertension is the critical intervention in patient management whilst advanced imaging is arranged, and different drug regimens have been used with success.

Invasive arterial monitoring is thought by many authorities to be essential once aggressive blood pressure management is commenced. This allows for 'beat-to-beat' observation of blood pressure as well as increased accuracy. A central line allows accurate fluid balance, will give an early indication of tamponade, and provides vascular access should there be a sudden deterioration.

Rapid control of hypertension is required, which can only be achieved by intravenous medication (in contrast to the management of accelerated hypertension). Therapy should be determined by a senior specialist.

The goals of therapy are to maintain a heart rate between 60 and 80, and a systolic blood pressure

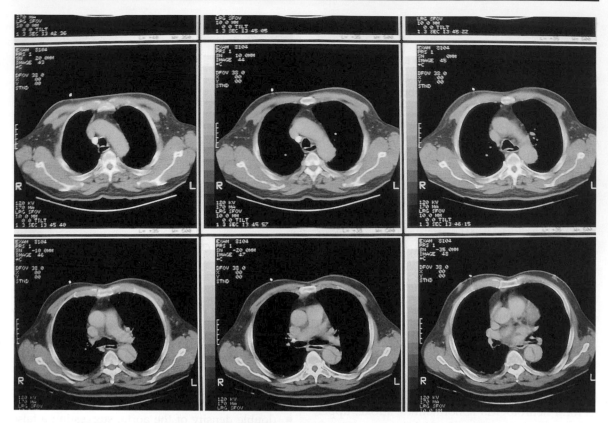

Figure 11.24: CT scan showing an aortic dissection.

between 100 and 120 mmHg. The blood pressure must be adequate to ensure renal perfusion, and the urine output should be monitored with a urinary catheter. Peripheral pulses should be observed.

INVESTIGATION

Echocardiography

Although convenient, safe and readily available, transthoracic echocardiography is limited by unacceptably low sensitivity (80%) and only slightly higher specificity (93–97%). Experience with transoesophageal echocardiography (TOE) suggests that a high degree of sensitivity (95–100%) can be obtained at the cost of the added distress for the patient of an uncomfortable and invasive procedure. It is available in a limited number of centres in the UK at present.

There may still be a role for transthoracic echocardiography, especially where TOE is unavailable, as a primary screening investigation in an unstable patient. Evaluation of myocardial performance and valvular function is reliable using transthoracic echocardiography, and pericardial effusions can be identified.

Computerized tomography (Fig. 11.24)

Where available, dynamic contrast-enhanced computerized tomography (CT) has a high sensitivity and specificity. An intramural haematoma can be identified before it ruptures either through the intima or the adventitia. CT will also visualize a thrombosed false lumen, which may have been missed by conventional aortography. Spiral CT scanners are now extremely rapid, but the scanning room remains 'out of bounds' to the unstable patient.

Aortography

Historically the standard against which new imaging modalities has been judged, aortography remains the investigation of choice in many hospitals. The entry site, aortic valve regurgitation and branch involvement can be identified, but intramural haematomas and thrombosed lumina may be missed. It is an invasive investigation that requires a catheter to be passed into a potentially abnormal aorta. It is not suitable for unstable patients for the same reasons as CT scanning.

Magnetic resonance imaging

Magnetic resonance imaging (MRI) is non-invasive, highly sensitive and specific, and does not require the injection of contrast media. As an imaging modality it has few of the disadvantages of those already discussed but is currently restricted by availability, image-acquisition time and monitoring limitations. It is only suitable for stable patients, and may have a role in follow-up.

FURTHER READING

Ahmed, J., Crossman, D., Jenkin, R. and Morris, F. (1997) *ECG Interpretation in Emergency Medicine*. Arnold, London.

RESPIRATORY EMERGENCIES

INTRODUCTION

Respiratory emergencies are common causes of emergency department attendances and of hospital admission. They range from acute severe life-threatening emergencies such as acute asthma to long-standing chronic obstructive pulmonary disease (COPD). In the former, careful application of treatment guidelines will be lifesaving; in the latter optimal management will require close co-operation with appropriate specialists, including intensivists, together with a detailed knowledge of the patient's past medical history. In conditions such as acute asthma, the dangers of inappropriate discharge have been amply demonstrated over the years. Many chest conditions are characterized by the possibility of acute catastrophic deterioration for want of timely intervention.

COMMUNITY-ACQUIRED PNEUMONIA

Community-acquired pneumonia (CAP) is a common cause of hospital admission. The incidence of CAP is approximately 2 per 1000 adults per year, and 20% of affected patients require hospitalization. The overall mortality is between 5 and 10%.

AETIOLOGY

The microbiological aetiology of CAP is diverse and in the majority of patients the responsible organism is not identified. *Streptococcus pneumoniae* is a Gram-positive encapsulated bacterium which is the most common identifiable cause of CAP. It is believed to be responsible for approximately 40% of all cases. *Haemophilus influenzae* is a Gram-negative pleomorphic rod which has both capsulated and unencapsulated forms. The type b serotype causes 95% of all human *H. influenzae* infections and is more likely to affect people with chronic debility, a compromised immune system or chronic lung disease. Data from hospitalized patients in the USA suggest that these two organisms may be responsible for only 25% of cases of CAP requiring admission. *Mycoplasma pneumoniae*, *M. legionella* and *Chlamydia pneumoniae* account for a further 15% between them. Viruses, most commonly influenza and parainfluenza, cause up to 17% of cases. Between one- and two-thirds of cases do not yield a specific microbiological diagnosis despite intensive investigation. Patients managed without hospital admission are often treated effectively using empirical therapy.

CLINICAL FEATURES AND ASSESSMENT

A 'typical' case of pneumonia presents with an abrupt onset of fever, cough, pleuritic chest pain and breathlessness. The cough may take a few days to become productive. *Streptococcus pneumoniae* (the most common), *Haemophilus influenzae*, *Legionella*, *Moraxella pneumoniae* and *Staphylococcus aureus* present in this way, although purely clinical criteria lack the specificity to reliably differentiate from 'atypical' cases. The atypical presentation is more insidious over several days, with less pyrexia, less sputum and milder respiratory impairment. *Mycoplasma pneumoniae*, *Chlamydia pneumoniae* (TWAR strain), *Moraxella catarrhalis* and *Coxiella burnetti* have a tendency to present in this manner. Mental confusion and gastrointestinal symptoms are suggestive of *Legionella* infection, which is sometimes classified as atypical.

Patients presenting to the emergency department may be in danger of suffering a catastrophic deterioration if appropriate therapy is not initiated without delay. The presence of at least two of the following three criteria is associated with a 20% mortality:

- respiratory rate more than 30 breaths per minute
- diastolic blood pressure 60 mmHg or less
- serum urea more than $7 \, \text{mmol} \, l^{-1}$.

Other features have been advocated as markers of severe CAP (Table 12.1).

Most patients are well enough to allow an appropriate history to be taken before a thorough examination is performed. Approximately 70% of

Table 12.1: Indicators of severe community acquired pneumonia

History:
  Age more than 60 years
  Chronic lung disease
  Severe concurrent illness
  Alcoholic

Clinical examination:
  Atrial fibrillation
  Confusion
  Diastolic blood pressure less than 60 mmHg
  Increased respiratory rate (more than
    30 breaths per minute)

Investigations:
  Urea more than $7 \, \text{mmol} \, l^{-1}$
  White cell count less than 4 or more than
    $20 \times 10^9 \, l^{-1}$
  PO$_2$ less than 60 mmHg
  Acidosis
  Serum albumin less than $35 \, \text{g} \, l^{-1}$
  Multilobar X-ray shadowing

Microbiological features:
  Bacteraemia
  Legionnaire's disease
  Staphylococcus or Gram-negative infection

patients who have pneumococcal pneumonia complain of pleuritic chest pain. Seventy-five per cent of patients produce rust-coloured sputum, and an association with herpes labialis is a well-recognized feature of pneumococcal pneumonia. CAP during an influenza epidemic raises the possible diagnosis of *Staphylococcus aureus* infection.

Common findings in the examination of the respiratory system include a raised respiratory rate (even if the patient appears well), reduced chest movement on the side of the pleuritic pain, and signs of consolidation. These may be difficult to elicit in a noisy department. Localized reduced air entry, crackles or bronchial breathing support a diagnosis of focal consolidation. Increased tactile and vocal fremitus may also be present. A chest radiograph is essential.

Other clinical features may give an indication of less common aetiological agents. *Mycoplasma pneumoniae* affects young people, in particular when they are living in a confined space (e.g. military camps and boarding schools). The organism lacks a cell wall (a feature that confers resistance to first-line antibiotics) and is dispersed widely throughout the community. Mycoplasma may be responsible for up to 25% of all cases of CAP. Extrapulmonary complications of mycoplasma are rare but potentially very serious:

- myocarditis and pericarditis
- erythema multiforme
- haemolytic anaemia and thrombocytopenia
- myalgia and arthralgia
- meningo-encephalitis
- gastrointestinal disturbances.

The definitive microbiological diagnosis of pneumonia is beyond the remit of the emergency physician. What is vital is the identification of those patients who require admission for investigation, and the provision of timely supportive and empirical antibiotic therapy for those in danger of a precipitous deterioration.

All patients should have appropriate investigations performed.

Chest radiograph (Fig. 12.1)

A chest radiograph allows assessment of the extent of the consolidation, the presence of a pleural effusion, cavitation and pre-existing pulmonary disease.

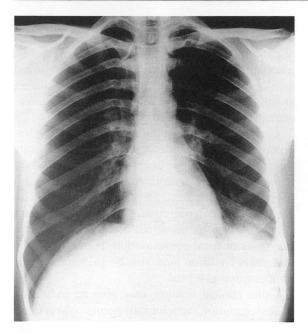

Figure 12.1: Left lower lobe community-acquired pneumonia.

Arterial blood gases

Hypoxaemia in CAP is the result of shunting of blood through alveoli filled with consolidation and venous admixture. Oxygen saturation should always be assessed by pulse oximetry. Most patients require arterial blood sampling to confirm that oxygenation and ventilation are adequate. Septic or profoundly hypoxic patients demonstrate a metabolic acidosis.

Full blood count

The white blood cell count is almost always more than $15\,000 \times 10^9$ in patients with pneumococcal pneumonia. In viral and atypical cases it is frequently normal. Evidence of haemolysis, suggesting cold agglutinin elevation, may be found in approximately 50% of cases of *Mycoplasma* pneumonia.

Biochemistry

As discussed above, the urea and albumin have prognostic importance. Hyponatraemia suggests the syndrome of inappropriate anitidiuretic hormone. Dehydration and acute renal failure are a consequence of severe CAP. Abnormal liver-function tests are detected in 30% of patients with pneumococcal pneumonia.

Microbiology

The emergency physician has a limited role in the definitive identification of the causative organism. Blood cultures should be taken, preferably before the administration of empirical antibiotics. Blood culture results are insensitive but specific. Sputum should be sent for immediate Gram stain and culture. Fifty per cent of patients with pneumococcal pneumonia will have a positive culture of their sputum. Urine examination for *Legionella* antigen allows early diagnosis for patients with a suggestive clinical picture. Baseline and convalescent sera are required to demonstrate a rising titre in specific antibodies to atypical organisms. The results of serological tests are not likely to be available in the emergency department.

ANTIBIOTIC THERAPY

The choice of antibiotics in the emergency department is largely empirical, based on the presence of clinical clues and local policy, which may have to take account of local patterns of antibiotic resistance.

CAP without markers of severity

Patients who do not have any other significant medical problems can be treated with oral amoxycillin. Amoxycillin/clavulanic acid (co-amoxiclav, Augmentin®) by mouth is an alternative for those suffering from a significant coexisting chronic illness. A macrolide antibiotic such as erythromycin or clarithromycin is an alternative if the patient is allergic to penicillin, and is the preferred first-line agent during a *Mycoplasma* epidemic.

Intravenous antibiotics are reserved for patients in whom absorption is thought to be unreliable, who are vomiting, or with severe disease.

Severe CAP

An intravenous combination of a second- or third-generation cephalosporin, such as cefotaxime or cefuroxime, with clarithromycin is suitable initial therapy. If *Staphylococcus aureus* is suspected, flucloxacillin should be added (particularly during an epidemic of influenza).

INTENSIVE THERAPY

The presence of one of the following features mandates admission to an area of high-intensity monitoring, preferably an intensive care unit:

- severe respiratory failure:
  respiratory rate > 30 breaths per minute
  mechanical respiratory support required
- haemodynamic compromise:
  shock
  inotropic support required
  persistent oliguria
- acidosis:
  pH less than 7.30
- disseminated intravascular coagulation.

These patients should be monitored invasively. They should all be assessed regarding the need for respiratory support.

COMPLICATIONS

Certain pneumococcal serotypes are associated with a severe systemic illness, haemodynamic instability and disseminated intravascular coagulation (serotype 3). Self-limiting pleural effusions commonly complicate pneumococcal pneumonia. Large and persistent effusions will require aspiration to improve respiratory function and exclude an empyema. Empyema is more likely to be due to *Staphylococcus aureus* or Gram-negative bacilli. Pericarditis as a complication of CAP is well described.

PULMONARY EMBOLUS

The incidence of pulmonary embolus (PE) in the UK is approximately 1 per 1000 per year. Most episodes occur in hospital or shortly after discharge. It has been estimated that PE is a contributory factor to up to 20% of in-hospital deaths.

AETIOLOGY

More than 70% of proven PE arise from a documented proximal deep venous thrombosis (DVT). In many cases this DVT is not evident clinically. It is widely accepted that PE is underdiagnosed. It has been shown that approximately 50% of patients with proven DVT have high-probability ventilation/perfusion scans for the presence of PE, despite an absence of respiratory symptoms. The risk of PE from an isolated calf DVT remains the subject of some controversy.

Major risk factors for PE have been identified (Table 12.2). In addition, prolonged air travel and obesity are regarded as independent risk factors.

The use of oestrogens, including the oral contraceptive pill and hormone-replacement therapy, is associated with relatively less risk when low-dose regimens are used. An underlying primary abnormality of coagulation is rare and routine screening is only justified for those aged under 50 years, with a family history, recurrent episodes and no other precipitating factor. Such abnormalities include:

- the antiphospholipid antibody syndrome
- congenital deficiencies of antithrombin III, protein C, protein S and plasminogen
- resistance to activated protein C, caused by the Leiden mutation to the factor V gene (present in 3% of the population and conferring a 10-fold increase in risk).

Table 12.2: Major risk factors for pulmonary emboli

Surgery: Major abdominal, pelvic, hip and knee surgery

Malignancy: Abdominal, pelvic and disseminated

Pregnancy

Lower limb pathology and immobility: Fractures, varicose veins, spinal cord injury and stroke

Cardiorespiratory disease: Acute myocardial infarction and severe disabling disease

Age more than 40 years

Previous episode

Trauma

Thrombotic disorders

CLINICAL FEATURES

The most common symptom experienced in acute pulmonary embolism is dyspnoea. This affects approximately 70% of individuals. Others features in descending order of frequency are:

- tachypnoea
- pleuritic chest pain
- apprehension
- tachycardia
- cough
- haemoptysis
- leg pain
- clinical DVT.

Clinical features in isolation are unreliable in either proving or disproving the diagnosis. The highly sensitive features are non-specific, and the highly specific features are insufficiently sensitive. The same applies to general investigations, which have most value in demonstrating an alternative cause for the patient's symptoms.

The clinical effects of an episode of pulmonary embolism are determined by the extent of the obstruction of the pulmonary vasculature, the release of vasoactive and brochoconstricting mediators from activated platelets, and the pre-existing health (particularly cardiac) and age of the victim. A 25% obstruction of the pulmonary arterial tree significantly increases right ventricular afterload and causes right ventricular dilatation. A previously normal right ventricle is not capable of increasing the pulmonary artery pressure above 60 mmHg. The dilated right ventricle impairs diastolic filling of the left ventricle by displacing the interventricular septum. Manoeuvres that increase venous return and hence left ventricular end-diastolic volume may improve symptoms (e.g. putting the patient 'head down' and volume loading).

Presentations of pulmonary embolism can be divided into one of three groups:

- circulatory collapse (massive PE)
- pulmonary haemorrhage
- isolated dyspnoea.

Massive PE is a recognized cause of sudden death. Lesser degrees of pulmonary arterial obstruction result in hypotension, chest pain (characteristically a dull, central 'ache') and syncope. Physical examination may, in addition, reveal jugular venous engorgement, tachycardia, tachypnoea and a third heart sound.

Pulmonary haemorrhage is typically the consequence of a peripheral embolus and accounts for 60% of episodes. Patients complain of pleuritic chest pain or haemoptysis. Because the infarcted area is potentially small the ventilation/perfusion mismatch may be insufficient to cause any abnormality of arterial blood gas tensions. There is no haemodynamic disturbance, although the respiratory rate may be elevated and a pleural friction rub heard. Tachycardia is a common feature, as is a low-grade pyrexia.

Sudden dyspnoea without any other symptoms occurs with a central occlusion. Patients are usually hypoxic.

The British Thoracic Society (BTS) guidelines for the management of pulmonary embolism identify one particular group of patients who are likely to present to the emergency department. Young patients presenting with pleuritic chest pain are a common management problem. A balance must be struck between sensitivity, in order that pulmonary embolism is not missed, and limiting unnecessary investigations and admission. Young women with no other risk factors, who are on the oral contraceptive pill and who present with pleuritic pain have a very low risk for PE if the following criteria are fulfilled:

- age less than 40 years
- respiratory rate less than 20 breaths per minute
- normal chest radiograph.

INITIAL INVESTIGATIONS

The use of pulse oximetry may give the first indication that a tachypnoeic patient is hypoxic. This should be confirmed by arterial blood sampling, which also typically reveals evidence of hyperventilation. A lactic acidosis is almost invariable in patients who have collapsed with a massive PE. It is vital to remember that with small, peripheral PE arterial gases may be normal. Conversely, high-risk patients with chronic respiratory disease may have pre-existing abnormalities of gas exchange.

The primary role of chest radiography is the exclusion of alternative diagnoses such as pneumonia, pneumothorax or pulmonary oedema. Massive or central PE often have normal radiographs.

Recognized radiological features include the following:

- dilatation of a pulmonary arterial trunk and areas of oligaemia suggest extensive obstruction
- wedge-shaped peripheral opacities suggest small infarctions
- small pleural effusions
- elevation of a hemidiaphragm.

The insensitivity of chest radiography must be emphasized. In the presence of hypoxaemia a normal radiograph provides strong supportive evidence of PE.

The lack of specificity of any of the associated electrocardiographic (ECG) abnormalities is well documented. The exclusion of significant myocardial ischaemia is the most useful function of the ECG. Sinus tachycardia, atrial fibrillation, right axis deviation, right bundle branch block and T-wave changes are consistent with the diagnosis of PE. Right heart strain is seen with massive PE.

DEFINITIVE IMAGING

In the presence of PE isotope ventilation/perfusion (V/Q) scanning demonstrates areas of normally ventilated lung which have a reduced blood supply (a V/Q mismatch). This is a widely available non-invasive investigation. However, V/Q scans can seldom be accessed through the emergency department and this is usually the task of the in-patient medical team. V/Q scans are reported as high probability, intermediate probability, low probability and normal. A scan reported as high probability (multiple large or moderate-sized V/Q defects) has a specificity for the correct diagnosis of PE of 86–92%. A normal scan correctly excludes PE in at least 96% of cases. There are some circumstances where interpretation may be imprecise:

- previous PE (unless old scans are available)
- left ventricular failure may cause regional abnormalities of perfusion
- chronic obstructive pulmonary disease (there may be local defects in perfusion because of chronic damage or hypoxic pulmonary vasoconstriction, as well as defects in ventilation)
- pulmonary fibrosis (patchy defects seen routinely)
- vascular compression by a centrally situated malignancy, resulting in a perfusion defect.

Clearly, a V/Q scan is not the appropriate investigation if the patient is unstable (Fig. 12.2). Pulmonary angiography is indicated if the victim is hypotensive, or if other investigations have not yielded a definite diagnosis. Pulmonary angiography is a safe investigation but must be performed in an environment of intensive monitoring. The fatal complication rate is between 0.5 and 1.3%, and many of these deaths are likely to be related to the underlying pathology. Low molecular weight contrast has reduced this complication rate even further (1 in 300 non-fatal complications).

The latest generation of spiral CT scanners is capable of identifying clot from the pulmonary trunks to the segmental arteries. However, small peripheral PE may be missed by CT and are better visualized using angiography. Where available, spiral CT is likely to have a role in the rapid evaluation of patients with major emboli and isolated dyspnoea.

Under certain circumstances it is appropriate to evaluate the lower limb venous system to obtain indirect evidence of thrombo-embolism. The BTS guidelines recommend lower limb imaging by compression ultrasound with colour Doppler imaging or venography:

- as the first-line investigation in patients with a clinical DVT
- in patients with chronic cardiorespiratory disease, in whom a V/Q scan would be uninterpretable
- following an intermediate probability V/Q scan.

D-Dimer is a breakdown product of fibrin and is elevated in the presence of thrombus (90% of patients with PE proven by V/Q scan). It is also elevated in other hospitalized patients and therefore has a low specificity for reliably detecting PE. Where the clinical suspicion is low, a normal D-dimer probably excludes a PE.

Transthoracic or transoesophageal echocardiography has a role in the evaluation of unstable patients. The associated findings are right ventricular dilatation, tricuspid regurgitation, abnormal septal movement and a failure of the inferior vena cava to collapse on inspiration. The actual clot is most likely to be visualized by transoesophageal echocardiography. Echocardiography will also help to exclude other causes of cardiovascular collapse, such as cardiac tamponade.

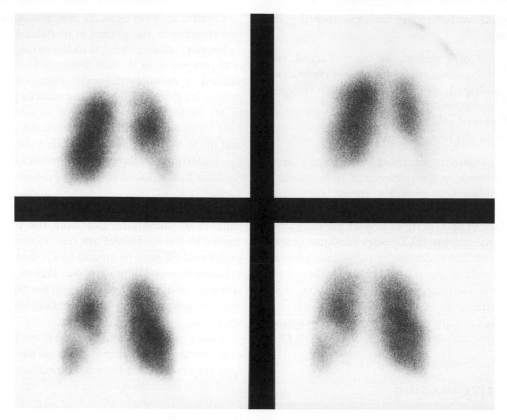

Figure 12.2: V/Q scan showing ventilation/perfusion mismatch. Top: Ventilation scan. Bottom: Perfusion scan.

INITIAL MANAGEMENT

The management of PE follows the conventional ABC lines. Stable patients should be heparinized whilst arrangements are made for further investigation. Subcutaneous low molecular weight heparin may replace intravenous unfractionated heparin in the future.

> *Intravenous heparinization* – loading dose of 5000 IU, followed by an infusion of 400–600 IU kg^{-1}day^{-1}. The activated partial thromboplastin time is measured after 6 h and maintained between 1.5 and 2.5 times the control.

Hypoxic individuals should receive high-concentration oxygen and titrated analgesia. Hypotension is initially treated with a fluid challenge. Central venous access is required, and the central venous pressure should be maintained between 15 and 20 mmHg. Inotropic support is indicated if the response to adequate filling is not maintained. Vasodilators should be avoided.

Heparin has been shown to prevent recurrent pulmonary embolism, but has no effect on the mortality of individual events. At present the two therapies available for life-threatening PE are thrombolysis and embolectomy.

Thrombolysis has been shown to result in more rapid resolution of thrombus. However, conclusive demonstration of a survival benefit in massive PE is awaited. Thrombolysis is indicated for life-threatening PE. If time and facilities allow, echocardiography or pulmonary angiography should first confirm the diagnosis.

Streptokinase and recombinant tissue plasminogen activator (rt-PA) are suitable agents and can be administered into a peripheral vein. There is a lower incidence of aggravating haemodynamic compromise with rt-PA.

> *Streptokinase* – 250 000 IU over 30 min, followed by 100 000 IU h^{-1} for the subsequent 24–72 h.
> *rt-PA* – 10 mg intravenous bolus, followed by an infusion of 90 mg over 2 h (1.5 mg kg^{-1} if patient less than 65 kg). Full intravenous heparinization commenced when the APPT ratio falls below twice the control.

Surgical embolectomy is indicated for life-threatening PE if there is a failure to respond to thrombolysis, or thrombolysis is contraindicated (see Chapter 11). An alternative strategy to open embolectomy is transcutaneous suction or fragmentation of the embolus using interventional radiology techniques. The insertion of an inferior vena cava filter should be considered if anticoagulation is contraindicated, or there is recurrent PE despite adequate anticoagulation.

SPONTANEOUS PNEUMOTHORAX (FIG. 12.3)

Pneumothorax is defined as air in the pleural space. The pressure within the pleural space is usually negative. If this negative pressure is lost the elastic recoil of the lung causes it to collapse, partially or completely, towards the hilum. The effect on ventilation is proportional to the volume of air in the pleural space, and the size of pneumothorax that a patient is able to tolerate is dependent on their premorbid respiratory and cardiac function.

A pneumothorax may be the result of trauma, or occur spontaneously. The latter is usually the result of the rupture of tiny apical bullae, which

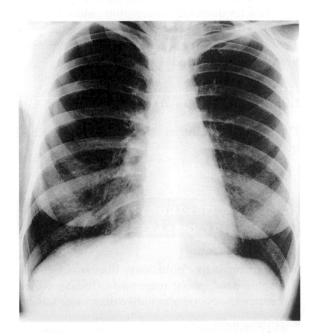

Figure 12.3: Right-sided spontaneous pneumothorax.

are believed to be congenital. Spontaneous pneumothorax commonly affects young fit males who are generally tall and thin, although patients with the following conditions also have an increased incidence:

- chronic obstructive pulmonary disease
- asthma
- cystic fibrosis
- Marfan's syndrome
- Ehlers–Danlos syndrome
- congenital cysts
- honeycomb lung.

It has been estimated that the incidence is approximately 1 per 8000 population per year in the UK.

> Remember pneumothorax as a cause of acute deterioration in asthma.

CLINICAL FEATURES

Simple spontaneous pneumothoraces present with a sudden onset of unilateral chest, shoulder or back pain. Dyspnoea is a feature of large pneumothoraces, or smaller pneumothoraces in the presence of chronic respiratory disease. Occasionally, patients are aware of the curious sensation of the collapsed lung 'flopping about' within the chest.

Specific examination findings may be subtle if the lesion is small, and an index of suspicion should be maintained in the susceptible groups of patients. Reduced breath sounds and hyper-resonance are highly suggestive of a pneumothorax in a previous healthy chest, but may also indicate a massive bulla in a patient with emphysema.

A tension pneumothorax is the result of a pleural defect acting as one-way valve, allowing air to enter the pleural space but not permitting air movement in the opposite direction. A rapid rise in the intrapleural pressure forces the mediastinum to the opposite side, impeding the ventilation of the other lung and obstructing venous return to the heart. The resulting acute pulmonary and circulatory failure has an untreated mortality of 100%. Features of a tension pneumothorax are:

- extreme respiratory distress
- hyperexpansion
- absent breath sounds
- hyper-resonance,

all on the affected side. The jugular veins may be distended. Respiratory distress is followed rapidly by respiratory failure, shock and cardiac arrest. Tension pneumothorax is one of the treatable causes of pulseless electrical activity.

MANAGEMENT

Chest radiography is contraindicated if a tension pneumothorax is suspected. Immediate needle thoracocentesis should be performed:

1 A 14-gauge intravenous cannula over needle is connected to a syringe.
2 The cannula is inserted perpendicularly through the second intercostal space in the mid-clavicular line of the affected side whilst aspirating.
3 With the free aspiration of air the stylet is removed, leaving the cannula draining the pleural space.
4 A hiss of air and an improvement in the condition of the patient confirms the diagnosis.
5 An intercostal tube should then be inserted before a check radiograph is obtained.

In recent years the management of spontaneous simple pneumothoraces has become more conservative, with the increasing use of percutaneous aspiration for symptomatic individuals, and fewer intercostal tubes are now inserted than in the past. The BTS has produced guidelines for the management of spontaneous pneumothoraces, which reflect this change in practice. These guidelines form the basis of subsequent recommendations in this section.

Patients who do not have pre-existing lung disease require treatment for either symptom relief or complete collapse of the lung. Patients with minimal symptoms should be allowed home with a clinic appointment and arrangements for a repeat radiograph in 7–10 days. If a patient is dyspnoeic or has complete collapse (*not* features of tension), simple aspiration is the first-line treatment:

1 An area is prepared over the second intercostal space in the mid-clavicular line.
2 Local anaesthetic is infiltrated down to the pleura until air is aspirated.
3 A cannula-over-needle is attached is inserted as for needle thoracocentesis.
4 A 50-ml syringe is attached to the cannula via a three-way tap.

5 Air is aspirated into the syringe and then voided to the atmosphere by turning the three-way tap to 'off to the patient'.
6 Aspiration is continued until resistance is felt, 2.5 l have been aspirated, or the patient starts to cough excessively.
7 An inspiratory check radiograph is obtained to confirm that the pneumothorax is now insignificantly small or completely resolved.

Patients may be discharged if aspiration has been radiologically proved to be successful. The follow-up is the same as for those treated conservatively. Patients are advised to return immediately if they suffer any deterioration in their symptoms, and should not fly until follow-up has been completed and all evidence of pneumothorax has resolved.

Patients with chronic respiratory disease are managed slightly differently. The size of the pneumothorax as well as the symptoms is significant. All patients with chronic lung disease should be admitted for overnight observation. A small pneumothorax has been classified by the BTS as collapse of the lung less than halfway towards the heart border. Complete collapse results in an airless lung, separate from the diaphragm. Moderate collapse is an intermediate state between the two.

Patients with chronic lung disease, a small pneumothorax and minimal symptoms should be admitted for overnight observation. Moderate and complete collapse should be treated initially by aspiration. If this is not successful an intercostal tube drain is indicated.

Intercostal tube drainage

The technique of intercostal drainage is described in Chapter 23.

CHRONIC OBSTRUCTIVE PULMONARY DISEASE

Chronic obstructive pulmonary disease (COPD) is a chronic progressive respiratory disease which encompasses several alternative diagnostic labels:

■ chronic bronchitis
■ emphysema

- chronic obstructive airways disease
- chronic airflow limitation
- some cases of chronic asthma

Airways obstruction is the defining feature of COPD, which may be partially reversible. A failure of spirometric tests, such as the forced expiratory volume in 1 s (FEV_1), to return to normal values in between exacerbations differentiates COPD from asthma. The most significant factor in the aetiology of COPD is cigarette smoking. COPD is responsible for more morbidity than asthma.

CLASSIFICATION

The BTS has recommended a classification of COPD based on steady-state symptoms and the FEV_1 (Table 12.3).

MANAGEMENT

The long-term management of COPD is beyond the scope of this text. Presentations to the emergency department are frequent although greater efforts are now being made to try and keep COPD

Table 12.3: British Thoracic Society (BTS) classification of chronic obstructive pulmonary disease (COPD)

Severity	FEV_1 (% predicted)	Symptoms and signs
Mild	60–80	No abnormal signs Cough Minimal dyspnoea
Moderate	40–59	Dyspnoea on moderate exertion Cough Persistent findings on auscultation (variable)
Severe	<40	Breathless on minimal exertion or at rest Prominent cough and wheeze Hyperinflation, cyanosis, polycythaemia and signs of cor pulmonale

patients in their own homes. In addition to initiating emergency therapy, the emergency physician has a role in identifying patients who are suitable for discharge.

Acute exacerbations of COPD are characterized by worsening of previously stable dyspnoea, increase volume of sputum and increased wheeze. Sputum may become purulent, suggesting a bacterial infection, and increasing ankle oedema is secondary to right-sided heart failure. Viral infections are common precipitating causes of acute deteriorations in patients with COPD, and influenza outbreaks continue to result in the emergency services being overwhelmed by such patients.

The decision to admit or treat at home depends on a number of factors. Does the combination of physical symptoms and social circumstances mean that an individual will receive adequate care at home? Previously good general health and function are important features in favour of out-patient treatment, as long as this management strategy is supported by objective data such as arterial blood gas measurements. Patients already receiving long-term oxygen therapy are likely to require admission. In some hospitals in the UK, out-patient therapy is supported by hospital-based teams of nurse specialists, who provide treatment at home such as regular nebulized medication.

The treatment of an acute exacerbation of COPD is summarized in Table 12.4.

In the acute situation it is often safest to prescribe oral corticosteroids (prednisolone 40 mg once daily). Before a patient is discharged on inhaled medication their inhaler technique must be assessed. 'Spacer' devices are often indicated. Follow-up arrangements at hospital or with the general practitioner must be in place.

Patients with moderate or severe exacerbations who do not respond to nebulizers should receive intravenous aminophylline and will need admission. Continuous oxygen therapy is mandatory at an inspired concentration of 24 or 28%, with arterial blood gases measured within 1 h unless a further deterioration occurs. Chronic carbon dioxide retention desensitizes the normal homoeostatic mechanisms to increases in carbon dioxide concentration. The major stimulus of ventilation under these circumstances is hypoxia. The use of high concentrations of oxygen in these patients may critically reduce minute ventilation and lead to a potentially fatal respiratory acidosis.

Table 12.4: Treatment of an acute exacerbation of COPD

Increase bronchodilators	Antibiotics	Oral corticosteroids
Worsening symptoms of COPD (nebulized salbutamol 5 mg +/− ipratropium bromide 500 μg)	2 out of 3 of: Increased breathlessness? Increased sputum volume? Purulent sputum?	Either: Already on systemic steroids Previously documented response to steroids Airway obstruction refractory to bronchodilators Or: First presentation of airway obstruction?

Aminophylline – intravenous loading dose of 250 mg over 20 min, followed by maintenance infusion of 0.5 mg kg^{-1} h^{-1}. Omit loading dose if already taking oral theophylline preparation (and check blood level).

When to administer respiratory support is a decision to be taken by the most senior medical and intensive care unit opinion that is available. A pH of 7.26 or a rising PaCO$_2$ warrant consideration for the institution of respiratory support. There are currently four options available in the UK for the management of worsening acute-on-chronic respiratory failure due to COPD:

- intubation and intermittent partial pressure ventilation (IPPV)
- non-invasive IPPV (only suitable for co-operative patients and only available at some centres in the UK)
- intravenous doxapram
- palliative care.

There is a strong case for instituting IPPV in the following circumstances:

- The patient enjoys a reasonable quality of life in between exacerbations.
- There is a clear and potentially reversible cause for the deterioration.
- It is the first presentation of respiratory failure.
- There is insufficient information concerning the individual's premorbid state on which to make a decision to limit therapy.

The use of the respiratory stimulant doxapram is being re-evaluated. It should be considered as a short-term adjunct if IPPV is contraindicated in patients with hypercapnic respiratory failure who are becoming drowsy or comatose. In some centres doxapram has been superseded by non-invasive ventilation.

Doxapram – intravenous infusion of 1.5–4 mg min^{-1} adjusted according to response.

ACUTE ASTHMA

As a result of wider usage of prophylactic medication and more timely prescription of steroids for exacerbations, the mortality from asthma has been declining. This should not encourage complacency in the management of acute episodes, which has been the subject of evidence-based guidelines produced by the BTS. In the UK asthma still accounts for between 1000 and 2000 deaths per year.

Some patients with acute pulmonary oedema due to left ventricular failure and other causes will wheeze (hence the old confusing name of cardiac asthma). This can lead to diagnostic confusion. The age of the patient and previous medical history will give important clues and, in addition, patients with left ventricular failure tend to be cold, pale, clammy and shut down. Cardiac-type chest pain is also often present. None of these features is typical of asthma.

ASSESSMENT OF SEVERITY

Patients commonly give a history of worsening symptoms of wheeze, cough (especially at night), breathlessness and, in particular, chest tightness. A failure to respond to their normal 'reliever' medication is a frequent complaint.

A mild acute exacerbation results in a peak expiratory flow rate (PEFR) of more than 75% predicted or previous best.

Moderate acute asthma is characterized by:

- PEFR between 50 and 75% of predicted (derived from widely available nomograms) or best when well
- respiratory rate less than 25 breaths per minute
- heart rate less than 110 beats per minute
- ability to talk normally or count to 10 slowly in one breath.

Any one of the following features indicates a *severe* attack:

- PEFR between 33 and 50% of predicted or best
- respiratory rate of 25 or more breaths per minute
- heart rate of 110 beats per minute or more
- unable to complete a sentence in one breath.

One of the following indicates a *life-threatening* episode:

- PEFR less than 33% of predicted or best
- silent chest, cyanosis or feeble respiratory effort
- bradycardia or hypotension
- exhaustion, confusion or coma.

Arterial blood gas sampling is mandatory if oxygen saturation is less than 92% when measured by pulse oximetry. Arterial blood gases should also be measured if there are markers of life-threatening severity, and in severe episodes unless there is an immediate response to treatment. The following arterial blood gas results indicate a severe episode and that an intensive care unit opinion is required:

- normal or elevated $PaCO_2$ (more than 40 mmHg)
- PaO_2 less than 60 mmHg irrespective of oxygen therapy
- acidosis (pH less than 7.36).

INITIAL MANAGEMENT

The initial treatment of acute asthma is summarized in Table 12.5. Patients with any of the markers for severity should receive nebulized salbutamol (5 mg) and nebulized ipratropium bromide (500 µg). Oral prednisolone should be given (30–60 mg) unless

Table 12.5: Management of acute severe asthma

Immediate:
    High flow oxygen via non-rebreathing system
    Nebulized salbutamol 5 mg
    Prednisolone 40 mg by mouth

If life-threatening features present:
    Add nebulized ipratropium bromide 500 µg
    Intravenous aminophylline or intravenous
        salbutamol
    Portable chest radiograph

the patient cannot tolerate oral medication, in which case intravenous hydrocortisone (200 mg) is the agent of choice. It should be remembered that the effects of corticosteroid are not observed for several (more than 6) hours. Wheezy patients without any markers of severity may have a trial of an inhaled beta$_2$-agonist, possibly via one of the available spacer holding chamber devices. Such a method achieves comparable drug delivery to nebulization, but precludes concurrent oxygen administration by anything other than nasal cannula.

If there are any life-threatening features, consideration should be given to intravenous hydrocortisone and intravenous bronchodilators. Intravenous aminophylline (see above) is the preferred agent unless the patient is already on an oral theophylline preparation. If this is the case aminophylline may be infused at the maintenance rate without the loading dose (also check blood level), or alternatively intravenous salbutamol may be used.

Salbutamol – slow intravenous bolus 250 µg (over 10 min). Intravenous infusion of 3–20 µg min^{-1}, adjusted to heart rate and response (start at 5 µg min^{-1}).

The evidence that either intravenous agent will have a dramatic benefit is lacking, and monitoring and repeated assessments are therefore essential. A portable chest radiograph should exclude pneumothorax, collapse and pneumonia but should not impede the initial treatment.

Patients without life-threatening features should be reassessed 20–30 min after the initial nebulized medication. If there has been little or no response, the nebulized salbutamol should be repeated and intravenous medication considered.

Severely ill patients may have nebulized salbutamol repeated every 15–30 min and ipratropium bromide repeated every 4–6 h. Continuous high-flow oxygen is mandatory at all times.

Indications for intensive care unit admission are:

- exhaustion, confusion or coma
- elevated $PaCO_2$
- hypoxia (<60 mmHg) on high-flow oxygen.

The need for IPPV should be evaluated in each case on its merits. Hypoxia despite high-flow oxygen, respiratory arrest, confusion and coma are absolute indications for IPPV. A slightly elevated $PaCO_2$ may be tolerated as long as the patient remains alert with no evidence of hypoxia.

Once a patient has been established on IPPV no attempt should be made to normalize the $PaCO_2$ at the risk of pressure-related trauma to the lungs (a strategy known as permissive hypercapnia).

COMPLICATIONS

Pneumothorax is seen in 0.5% of patients who attend hospital with acute severe asthma. IPPV is a particular risk factor. This is often difficult to detect clinically and may be life threatening. Mediastinal emphysema and segmental and lobar collapse are seldom clinically significant. Arrhythmias may be a consequence of hypoxia, acidosis, bronchodilator therapy or hypokalaemia (as a result of high-dose beta$_2$-agonists and corticosteroids). Nausea and vomiting suggest theophylline toxicity in appropriate patients.

DISCHARGE OF ASTHMATIC PATIENTS

Patients with no markers of severity after one nebulizer when reassessed 30 min later may be suitable for discharge. The PEFR should be at least 75% of predicted or best. Certain patients should have a lower threshold for admission to hospital:

- seen in the afternoon or evening

- significant worsening or recent onset of nocturnal symptoms
- previous severe episodes with rapid onset
- concern over social circumstances or the ability of patients or relatives to assess severity reliably.

Patients who have symptoms of moderate severity may have a second nebulizer and a further assessment 30 min after that. Discharge may be possible if a significant improvement has occurred. All patients with initially acute severe or life-threatening asthma should be admitted, irrespective of improvement.

If discharge is planned some attempt should be made to identify the reason for the patient's deterioration. Although viral infections are often the precipitating factor in acute episodes, evidence of a more chronic deterioration suggests under-treatment or poor compliance with medication. Exposure to tobacco smoke and to allergens should be considered.

Any patient who is discharged should have firm arrangements for follow-up with the general practitioner, a specialist liaison nurse or a hospital clinic. Patients with moderate symptoms should continue prednisolone for several days after discharge, with the recommendation that they be reassessed in the community before stopping (although a gradual reduction in the dose is not required). Inhaled medication should be optimized and inhaler technique checked. If the patient does not have one, a peak flow meter and a PEFR diary should be provided. Written communication with the general practitioner is essential.

FURTHER READING

Krome, R., Ruiz, E. and Tintinalli, J. (1995) *Emergency Medicine: A Comprehensive Study Guide*. McGraw Hill, New York.

Wetherall, D., Ledingham, J. and Warrell, D. (1995) *Oxford Textbook of Medicine*. Oxford University Press, Oxford.

CHAPTER THIRTEEN

NEUROLOGICAL EMERGENCIES

- Introduction
- Coma
- Headache
- The acutely confused patient
- Seizures

- Dizzy spells
- Syncope (collapse query cause)
- Stroke
- Further reading

INTRODUCTION

Neurological emergencies, like other life-threatening conditions, require doctors to assess, recognize and treat the underlying condition in a timely fashion. It is especially important to identify and treat reversible primary causes of cerebral injury as well as minimizing secondary damage from hypoxia, cerebral oedema and hypoglycaemia. In conditions where the diagnosis is not obvious it is essential to maintain an open mind and formulate a clear but sensible differential diagnosis based upon the available history and examination. Careful and repeated evaluation to exclude all other possibilities is necessary before judgements are made regarding functional illness.

The objective of this chapter is to describe the seven common neurological presentations to the emergency department (Table 13.1), with an overview of their initial management and differential diagnosis.

Table 13.1: Common neurological presentations to the emergency department

Coma
Headache
Confusion
Seizures
Dizzy spells
Syncope
Stroke

COMA

Coma is defined as a state of reduced level of consciousness where there is no purposeful interaction with the surroundings.

> The Glasgow Coma Score (GCS) in coma is 8 or less.

It is important to employ the dictum 'assume the worst' when assessing a comatose patient and to follow a structured approach. The initial approach to the comatose patient must include an assessment of the airway, breathing and circulation – a primary survey. Any life-threatening abnormalities that are detected must be immediately corrected. A more detailed assessment follows to document the level of consciousness and to help formulate a differential diagnosis for the cause of the coma (Table 13.2).

INITIAL ASSESSMENT AND MANAGEMENT

Airway obstruction is common in comatose patients as the protective airway reflexes are lost and the tongue may fall backwards against the posterior pharyngeal wall. There is also a high incidence of vomiting and subsequent aspiration.

Table 13.2: Differential diagnosis of coma

T	Trauma
I	Infections (CNS, extracranial sepsis)
P	Postictal (epilepsy), psychogenic
S	Syncope, subarachnoid
A	Alcohol
E	Encephalopathy (hypertensive or hepatic)
I	Insulin (hyperglycaemia or hypoglycaemia)
O	Overdose
U	Uraemia, electrolytes (high or low sodium, potassium, calcium, magnesium) or metabolic (adrenal or thyroid)

Table 13.3: Initial investigations for coma

Full blood count
Urea and electrolytes
Blood sugar
Amylase
Arterial blood gases
Chest X-ray
ECG

High-flow oxygen must be administered to all comatose patients through a well-fitting face mask with reservoir bag. If there is any suggestion of trauma from the history or examination, it is essential to suspect a cervical spine injury and immobilize the neck. Simple airway manoeuvres such as chin lift or jaw thrust are usually sufficient to correct any airway obstruction initially. Endotracheal intubation will be necessary if the patient's oxygenation remains inadequate despite optimizing the airway, or if the airway is not secure and the patient remains at risk of aspiration. Therefore an anaesthetist should be called sooner rather than later. Intubation, when required, should be carried out using a rapid-sequence induction technique.

Having opened and protected the airway, the respiratory rate and pattern should be assessed and recorded. A pulse oximeter is a vital adjunct to assess adequacy of oxygenation. Respiratory compromise is commonly a result of cerebral injury and if ventilation is inadequate or shallow, assisted ventilation must be provided. The combination of respiratory depression and constricted pupils suggests poisoning with opiates and an intravenous injection of naloxone should be administered.

Coma with respiratory depression and small pupils suggests opiate intoxication.

The circulation is assessed by examining the pulse for rate and character, and measuring the blood pressure and capillary refill time. Venous access is obtained through a peripheral vein and blood samples are taken for a standard series of tests (Table 13.3). A bedside blood glucose estimation must be performed early to rule out hypoglycaemia as a cause of the coma. If hypoglycaemia is identified, thiamine (100 mg intravenously) should be given before giving glucose if there is clinical suspicion that the patient is suffering from alcoholic liver disease. This will prevent the onset of Wernicke's encephalopathy. If there are signs of inadequate tissue perfusion a fluid challenge of 500 ml boluses (up to a maximum of 1500 ml) of an isotonic crystalloid should be given.

Next the conscious level is assessed. It is important to record the individual components (eye opening, best motor response and verbal response) of the GCS. The pupils must be examined for size and reaction and any obvious lateralizing motor signs sought. At this stage it is important to make sure that the patient is completely undressed and that a baseline core temperature is taken. Appropriate measures to maintain normothermia must be taken.

OBTAINING A HISTORY

This is essential and provides most of the information required to begin to formulate a differential diagnosis. Information should be gathered from the prehospital personnel as to the exact circumstances of the incident. Further information will also need to be obtained from the patient's family and general practitioner. A history of drug use or abuse, possible recent head trauma, notable medical history and, most importantly, events leading up to the incident must be elicited.

PHYSICAL EXAMINATION

Examination must be structured into a general assessment to exclude an extracranial cause for the coma and a detailed neurological examination. Neurological assessment in the emergency department is subdivided into that performed rapidly in the primary survey and the remaining more detailed examination in the secondary survey.

The primary survey neurological assessment consists of the GCS and the pupillary responses (size, asymmetry and response to light). These assessments must be repeated regularly to detect signs of improvement or deterioration.

> Assessment of the conscious level must be repeated regularly to detect improvement or deterioration.

The secondary survey neurological assessment is a more detailed examination that includes cranial nerve assessment and examination of the optic fundi. An assessment of the tone, power, co-ordination, sensation and reflexes in the limbs is also performed. The level of detail in the examination of such patients will depend on the conscious level, the degree of co-operation and the level of concern regarding neurological disability. Physical examination may provide enough information to suggest meningeal irritation, raised intracranial pressure (papilloedema) or lateralization suggestive of an intracranial space-occupying lesion.

Hysterical coma is a clinical diagnosis considered after detailed physical examination shows no abnormality. It is suggested by flickering of the eyelids, roving eye movements and, if necessary, an ice-water caloric response. It is, however, a diagnosis that should be considered with the greatest caution and it may still be necessary to admit the patient for observation.

FURTHER INVESTIGATION

The need for further investigations (Table 13.4) will be based on an established differential diagnosis. Failure to develop a clear differential diagnosis mandates further investigations. In a patient who has not significantly improved despite therapy and where the exact diagnosis remains uncertain, urgent CT scan is essential.

MANAGEMENT

After stabilizing the patient a clear management plan must be devised. There may be a need to

Table 13.4: Further investigations for coma

CT scan
Blood cultures
Coagulation screen
Serum calcium, magnesium and liver function tests
Paracetamol and salicylate levels
Carboxyhaemoglobin levels
Urinalysis for ketones and drug screen

institute further therapy before transfer, depending upon the individual pathology identified. More detailed discussion of these conditions is provided below.

It is essential that details of the primary and secondary surveys, investigations ordered with available results, a clear differential diagnosis limited to the three most likely causes for the coma and the further management plan are clearly documented in the notes. Involvement of a senior colleague from the medical team must occur prior to transfer from the resuscitation room. Most patients in persisting coma will require continuing management on an intensive care unit.

HEADACHE

Headache is a symptom caused by a variety of pathologies related to numerous structures of the head and neck. Patients with headaches present to the emergency department for three main reasons: first, the patient is a regular headache sufferer but on this occasion the headache is refractory to their standard medication (migraine); second, the headache is new and part of a constellation of other symptoms suggestive of a systemic illness which may in itself be serious (meningitis or cranial arteritis) or benign (influenza, sinusitis); and, finally, the headache is new and relatively sudden in onset or severe in nature. The pain is out of all proportion to anything the patient has suffered before (subarachnoid haemorrhage).

For this group of patients the goal of the emergency department doctor is to be able to categorize the headache into benign (the patient can be allowed home with appropriate advice), or likely to have serious underlying pathology (meriting admission for further investigation and urgent treatment). The important causes are outlined in Table 13.5.

Table 13.5: Differential diagnosis of headache

Benign:
   Tension headache
   Migraine
   Cluster headaches
   Drug-induced headache
   Viral illness
Serious:
   Vascular event (subarachnoid haemorrhage,
      thunderclap headache, coital cephalgia,
      hypertensive crisis)
   Temporal arteritis
   Drugs (carbon monoxide)
   Infection (meningitis, encephalitis, acute sinusitis,
      brain abscess)
   Neoplastic disease (raised intracranial pressure
      due to a tumour)
   Others (acute angle closure, glaucoma, benign
      intracranial hypertension)

The history in this situation is again the most crucial component in reaching a clear diagnosis. Clinical examination is often normal and basic investigations have no real role to play in making the decision to admit.

The clinician should aim to elicit the baseline health and chronicity of previous headache-related illnesses. It is essential to establish what made the patient decide to visit hospital on this occasion. The acuteness of onset of the headache, the associated symptoms and other factors, such as travel abroad, or factors suggesting immunocompromise, should also be elicited. Special consideration should be given to clues in the history and examination, which are more likely to be associated with serious pathology and to merit admission (Table 13.6).

Detailed examination is essential in order positively to exclude conditions outlined in Table 13.5. It is essential to look for a pyrexia and, if present, to identify a clear focus of infection. Clinical signs of meningism, raised intracranial pressure or focal neurological deficit provide obvious markers of a serious underlying pathology indicating the need for admission and further investigation.

Outlined below are four causes of headache which present to the emergency department. The first two are serious and must be identified and admitted for urgent treatment. The latter two are common and benign but may well demonstrate features of the first group and merit admission for observation.

Table 13.6: Factors suggesting serious pathology underlying headache

Sudden onset of severe headache
Pain worsens on exertion or with manoeuvres
   that raise intracranial pressure
Any associated neurological deficit
No clear trigger factor
Level of pain is out of proportion to patient's usual
   symptoms

SUBARACHNOID HAEMORRHAGE (SAH)

This condition results from the rupture of a berry aneurysm or arteriovenous malformation of one of the cerebral vessels. Patients classically describe a sudden and very severe headache that may be occipital or generalized. The onset of the pain may be likened to a blow on the back of the neck or head. Associated symptoms and signs include vomiting and meningism followed by a decreasing conscious level with neurological deficits. With this presentation there is no difficulty in diagnosis. The prognosis is worse in those patients who have had previously unrecognized warning bleeds.

Sudden onset of severe headache is a hallmark of subarachnoid haemorrhage.

However, patients are still inadvertently sent home by emergency department staff having had a subarachnoid haemorrhage. They usually fall into one of the following categories: they may be poor historians or, more often, the victim of poor history-taking by the doctor; the sudden severe headache may have improved significantly by the time they arrive in the department; or the patient may have a high pain threshold with a degree of stoicism.

Patients with an SAH can be graded on clinical grounds according to a scale developed by the World Federation of Neurological Systems (WFNS), as shown in Table 13.7. Patients with grades I to III have a much better prognosis than grades IV and V. However, a proportion of this latter group will have potentially reversible pathology (hydrocephalus or intracerebral haematoma) associated with their SAH. All such patients must therefore be discussed with the neurosurgical team.

Table 13.7: WFNS grading for subarachnoid headache (SAH)

Grade	GCS	Motor deficit
I	15	–
II	14–13	–
III	14–13	+
IV	12–7	+/–
V	6–3	+/–

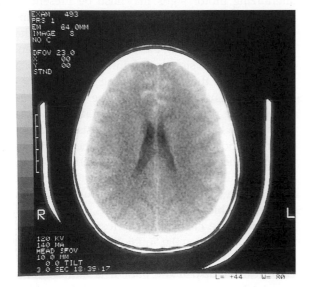

Figure 13.1: CT scan of a patient with subarachnoid haemorrhage.

CT scan (Fig. 13.1) should be performed as the first-line investigation. On occasions this may be negative or inconclusive, especially if presentation is late. In such cases admission for lumbar puncture is essential in order to look for blood or xanthochromia in the cerebrospinal fluid. A small proportion of cases will still have equivocal results despite a history strongly suggestive of SAH. These cases should also be discussed with the neurosurgical team as such 'sentinel' headaches may be the first signs of an impending major SAH.

Treatment in the resuscitation room will consist of securing a patent airway and if necessary providing controlled ventilation. Referral to the admitting medical or neurosurgical team is then appropriate. Nimodipine therapy has been shown to reduce secondary cerebral ischaemia and can be instituted if there is likely to be significant delay following consultation with the appropriate specialists.

It is essential to maintain the hydration of the patient prior to neurosurgical treatment. Failure to do so has been shown to adversely affect outcome.

CRANIAL ARTERITIS

These patients are usually elderly. The most commonly affected vessels are the superficial temporal, vertebral, ophthalmic and posterior ciliary arteries. The major symptom is usually headache but this is often associated with myalgia involving either the jaw or scapulo-humeral girdle. Malaise, anorexia and a variety of other non-specific symptoms may also be elicited.

On examination it is important to look specifically for thickening and tenderness of the scalp and temporal vessels. The erythrocyte sedimentation rate (ESR) or plasma viscosity is usually raised but these are not 100% sensitive. If cranial arteritis is clinically suspected it should be treated and the patient referred for further investigation.

Treatment consists of prednisolone, 60 mg orally, and referral for urgent bilateral temporal artery biopsy.

TENSION HEADACHES

These patients present with a plethora of vague symptoms associated with a severe vice-like headache, and which have usually been present for days or weeks. There are usually a number of stressors in the patient's background history. A detailed normal examination in conjunction with calm reassurance will often produce rapid results.

MIGRAINE

Migranous headaches have a variety of presentations. They are often lateralized, throbbing in nature, and have associated visual disturbances in the form of field defects and visual hallucinations. They are often associated with nausea and vomiting. Focal neurological deficits such as weakness or aphasia may also occur.

Patients usually have a clear history of migraine and are familiar with common trigger factors for their condition. These include specific foods, alcohol, stress, menstruation or lack of sleep.

Differentiation from subarachnoid haemorrhage may, however, be difficult. If there is any doubt (especially where there is persisting neurological deficit) the patient should be admitted for observation and urgent CT scan. Treatment consists of simple therapeutic manoeuvres such as rest in a darkened room and simple analgesics. A variety of vasoconstrictor medications (ergotamine or sumatriptan) are rapidly effective, having a high affinity for serotonin 1 receptors.

OTHER SIGNIFICANT CAUSES OF HEADACHE

A variety of other conditions may present to the emergency department with headache and other vague symptoms. Very occasionally, this will be the first presentation of serious pathology (tumours). A detailed history in conjunction with a full examination often identifies these patients.

THE ACUTELY CONFUSED PATIENT

An acute confusional state may be the initial presentation of a patient before progressing to coma. The initial management, diagnostic work-up and differential diagnosis are therefore exactly the same as for coma. Most causes of acute confusional state are the result of processes outside the central nervous system (see Chapter 7).

Amongst the most important of the potential causes and the most difficult to exclude in the confused patient is CNS infection. Three specific diagnoses are listed in Table 13.8.

BACTERIAL MENINGITIS

Infection of the leptomeninges and cerebrospinal fluid is commonly caused by one of three bacteria, *Neisseria meningitides*, *Haemophilus influenzae* or

Table 13.8: Central nervous system infections

Bacterial meningitis
Viral encephalitis
Cerebral abcess

Streptococcus pneumoniae. Spread may be local via the bloodstream from the nasopharynx, sinusitis, middle-ear infection, or from infection elsewhere (osteomyelitis, endocarditis).

The symptoms of meningeal irritation include headache, vomiting, photophobia and a variable conscious level. The clinical signs on examination are also often non-specific, with fever, neck stiffness and drowsiness progressing to coma. Specific neurological signs with cranial nerve palsies or lateralizing motor signs may also be present in more advanced cases. The presentation of symptoms and signs can be minimal or atypical in the immunocompromised, the elderly and children. Confusion, drowsiness, minimal pyrexia or a seizure may be the only presenting signs.

Management is based upon the level of certainty of the patient having bacterial meningitis. If it seems a likely or certain diagnosis (especially if pyrexia and confusion are present) then empirical antibiotic therapy must be instituted immediately. It is helpful, however, to perform a standard infection screen, including blood cultures, a clotted specimen of blood for antigen tests, clotted blood for polymerase chain reaction tests and a throat swab, prior to giving the antibiotics. Ceftriaxone (or cefotaxime) and benzyl penicillin are the standard empirical therapy. If the patient is immunocompromised and has signs of meningeal infection, the case should be discussed with a senior doctor in infectious diseases or the microbiologist. Investigations should never delay treatment if there is a high likelihood of the presence of meningitis.

If the patient has signs of raised intracranial pressure an urgent CT scan must be performed to exclude hydrocephalus or a focal mass lesion. A lumbar puncture should not be performed in such circumstances. A patient in whom there is a low risk of meningitis (unlikely but needs admission for observation) should have the above investigations performed and be admitted under the medical team for observation and lumbar puncture.

VIRAL ENCEPHALITIS

The commonest cause of viral encephalitis in the UK is herpes simplex virus (HSV). Such infections can have a similar prodrome and presentation to bacterial meningitis although patients tend to have a greater cerebral irritability and are more likely to suffer from epileptic seizures. It is an important diagnosis to consider as early empirical treatment with intravenous aciclovir can reduce the high mortality rate of 50–60%. The presentation may be one of abnormal behaviour and hallucinations progressing to coma and seizures.

Consideration should therefore be given to adding aciclovir to antibiotic therapy in the emergency department if a CNS infection is likely, the patient has marked cerebral irritability and there is no obvious diagnosis. Definitive diagnosis can often be very difficult.

CEREBRAL ABSCESS

A collection of pus within the cerebral parenchyma is due often to middle-ear or sinus infection. It may also be the result of septic emboli from an endocarditis. The presentation is again similar to that of bacterial meningitis, with meningeal irritation causing generalized symptoms of headache, vomiting and pyrexia, or specific cranial nerve palsies, visual field defects or hemiparesis. If the patient presents late, marked cerebral irritability may progress rapidly to coma.

The history from relatives and friends is essential, especially regarding any previous ENT illnesses or operations. If the diagnosis seems at all likely, a contrast-enhanced CT scan must be performed. Empirical treatment with antibiotics (benzyl penicillin, cefotaxime and metronidazole) is essential. Flucloxacillin or nafcillin may be added if staphyloccus is suspected. After confirmation by CT scan, the case should be regarded as a neurosurgical emergency. Measures to control raised intracranial pressure (dexamethasone, mannitol and hyperventilation) can be helpful until neurosurgical intervention is performed.

SEIZURES

Patients presenting to the emergency department suffering from epilepsy are usually having a generalized seizure or are in the postictal recovery stage. A number of other more unusual types of epilepsy can also present and be easily missed or misdiagnosed. The World Health Organization classification is shown in Table 13.9.

Table 13.9: WHO classification of epilepsy

Generalized seizures:
  Absence attacks (*petit mal*)
  Myoclonic seizures (myoclonic jerks, clonic seizures)
  Tonic–clonic seizures (*grand mal* or major fits)
  Tonic seizures
  Atonic seizures
Partial seizures:
  Simple, without impairment of consciousness (motor, sensory, aphasic, amnesic, olfactory) including Jacksonian, temporal lobe and psychomotor epilepsy
  Complex partial seizures with impairment of consciousness
  Partial seizures, either simple or complex, evolving into a generalized tonic–clonic seizure

The common causes for presentation to the emergency department are those patients with known epilepsy who have a further fit due to poor control, poor compliance or triggering of the seizure by other coexisting illness. A seizure may also be secondary to other serious illness, for example CNS infections, drugs overdose, (alcohol, tricyclic antidepressant overdose, amphetamines), metabolic causes (hypoglycaemia, hyponatraemia), inflammatory lesions, acute vascular events or chronic cerebrovascular disease.

A patient may attend the emergency department with a first fit, having previously been fit and healthy. The patient may be in a postictal state at presentation, in the midst of the first seizure or in status epilepticus.

Status epilepticus is present if seizures occur in succession without the patient regaining consciousness in between and lasting for longer than 20 min.

Status epilepticus is usually due to a generalized seizure, although other rarer forms, such as absence or complex status, may occasionally present, and as a result are usually misdiagnosed.

Initial management principles are similar to those outlined in the management of coma. Maintenance of a clear airway plus high-flow oxygen is essential while intravenous access is being gained. Simple manoeuvres (jaw thrust) may be necessary to keep the airway clear. Insertion of an oropharyngeal (Guedel) airway may be impossible and if the patient remains cyanosed, a nasopharyngeal airway provides a good alternative. The most popular first-line agent for drug treatment is intravenous diazemuls given in small aliquots until control is achieved; however, its action is short-lived and it can easily cause both respiratory and cardiovascular depression.

In patients who continue to fit or have been in status for 20–30 min or longer prior to arrival in the resuscitation room, diazemuls should not be used alone. A second-line agent such as intravenous phenytoin is often successful and is given as a loading dose ($18\,\text{mg}\,\text{kg}^{-1}$) over 30 min at an early stage in such patients. Other alternatives include chlormethiazole or clonazepam, although side-effects very similar to those of diazepam may occur.

If the second-line agents are not successful, anaesthetic staff must be contacted urgently for consideration of barbiturate sedation with sodium thiopentone, endotracheal intubation, and monitoring on the intensive care unit.

A bedside blood sugar estimation should always be performed in such patients. Alcoholic patients presenting with an acute seizure must be given intravenous thiamine prior to correction of hypoglycaemia.

Once acute control of the seizure has been obtained it is essential to identify a likely trigger factor. Baseline investigations and an infection screen may give some indication. A CT scan of the brain should be performed if no clear diagnosis has been made.

PATIENTS PRESENTING WITH A FIRST FIT

These patients are normally alert and orientated but there is a history that they were seen to have a 'fit'. As much information as possible should be gathered from anyone who witnessed the event. The patient should be questioned regarding prodromal symptoms and the time required to recover fully from the event. As complete a history as possible will differentiate those who have had a vasovagal event (usually postural, short lived, and with rapid and full recovery) from those with epilepsy.

Common trigger factors for an isolated fit are excess alcohol ingestion or drug abuse. A period of postictal confusion is suggestive of a fit. On examination, evidence of tongue biting, hyporeflexia and urinary incontinence may also help confirm the diagnosis.

The patient should be informed that they may suffer from epilepsy and advised not to drive or cycle until a definitive diagnosis of epilepsy has been excluded. If there is no doubt about the diagnosis, the Driver and Vehicle Licensing Authority will need to be informed and the patient should be advised to do this. Swimming is allowed if others are aware of the possible diagnosis. Any advice given must be documented in the notes.

Referral to a neurologist for assessment is indicated. Treatment is not indicated at this stage. Further investigations will include an EEG (which is not diagnostic but, if abnormal, will support the diagnosis) and CT or MRI scans to exclude a structural cause.

DIZZY SPELLS

Dizziness may be described by patients in many ways. The common causes are benign, whereas others will require follow-up and treatment. The causes are outlined in Table 13.10. In order to elicit the correct diagnosis, careful and meticulous history-taking is required. The initial categorization into vertiginous and non-vertiginous dizzy spells is dependent upon the patient being able to distinguish a sense of movement, which is often rotational, although on occasions there may be a sense of falling sideways or forwards. Specific causes as outlined in the categories in Table 13.10 can then be sought.

Most causes of dizziness do not require admission to hospital (unless they are very debilitating, e.g. acute labyrinthitis). Appropriate follow-up must be arranged if serious pathology is suspected.

SYNCOPE (COLLAPSE QUERY CAUSE)

This diagnostic challenge provides a classic opportunity for the doctor in the emergency department to miss a significant problem, with unfortunate consequences (Table 13.11). The patient is often well at presentation, wishes to go home, but has

Table 13.10: Differential diagnosis of dizziness

Vertiginous

Labyrinthine:
  Acute labyrinthitis (often viral)
  Benign positional vertigo (common after head
    trauma)
  Menière's disease
  Alcohol
  Middle ear disease

Eighth-nerve disease:
  Acoustic neuroma
  Ramsay Hunt syndrome (geniculate zoster
    infection)
  Ototoxic drug treatment

Brainstem:
  Vertebrobasilar vessel disease (TIA or stroke)
  Migraine
  Demyelinating disease
  Tumours (acoustic neuroma)

Non-vertiginous

Cardiovascular:
  Postural hypotension
  Vasovagal syncope
  Arrhythmias
  Aortic stenosis

Drugs

Ocular:
  Poor acuity
  Diplopia

Metabolic:
  Hypoglycaemia
  Hyperventilation

Table 13.11: Causes of syncope

Common and benign causes:
  Vasovagal attack
  Orthostatic hypotension
  Cough or micturition syncope
  Carotid sinus sensitivity

Infrequent but serious causes:
  Cardiac arrhythmias and mechanical obstructive
    cardiac lesions (aortic stenosis)
  Vertebrobasilar disease or carotid artery disease
  Seizures
  Metabolic causes (hypoglycaemia, Addison's
    disease)
  Autonomic dysfunction (secondary to disease
    or drugs)
  Hypovolaemia (gastrointestinal bleed, abdominal
    aortic aneurysm)

---

suffered a collapse for which there is no obvious cause. A meticulous history is again essential.

Symptoms leading up to the event will often provide clues suggesting a benign cause. Relevant past history and any persisting symptoms subsequent to the event will provide further clues: for example, drowsiness and headache are common after a seizure but are usually not present after a faint. Examination may reveal a heart murmur or carotid bruits, although these may be unrelated to the event.

Screening investigations in the emergency department are usually of little help. The decision to be made is whether admission to hospital is merited in order to observe the patient and minimize the risk of a further more serious event occurring. Patients in certain groups, for example those aged over 45 years, those with a history of heart disease or an abnormal ECG at presentation, all possess a higher risk of further events or death. The clinician should therefore have a lower threshold for admitting such patients for further observation and investigation.

STROKE

A stroke is a neurological deficit of sudden onset with symptoms lasting more than 24 h and vascular in origin. It occurs as a result of ischaemic infarction due to cerebrovascular disease or emboli, commonly from the heart or as a result of intracerebral haemorrhage. Underlying pathologies include atheromatous disease, hypertension and berry aneurysms. Rare causes include vasculitis, infection and trauma.

Clinical presentation is often with the sudden onset of signs and symptoms. In some cases there may be a step-wise progression over a number of days. Classification of these signs is based initially on whether the underlying pathology is thrombotic (90%) or haemorrhagic. Thrombotic strokes can then be further subclassified according to the area of brain affected and consequent neurological deficit.

Cerebral hemispheric infarcts (from the middle cerebral artery, 50–60% of lesions) present with contralateral hemiplegia, dysphasia (if affecting the dominant cortex), sensory loss and homonymous hemianopia. Lacunar infarcts involve smaller branches, causing infarcts around the basal ganglia, thalamus and pons. Depending upon the territory affected, the disability may be purely motor, purely sensory, cerebellar or a mixture of these components. Finally, brainstem infarction is due to basilar artery thrombosis. This results in severe disability and is associated with a high mortality rate. Clinical signs include coma, quadriplegia and cardiorespiratory dysfunction.

Management in the emergency department is aimed in the first instance at reaching a clinical diagnosis and providing supportive treatment.

Early CT scan is often indicated to confirm the nature of the lesion. Recent research has suggested a potential role for the use of thrombolytic agents in thrombotic stroke to reopen occluded cerebral vessels. As yet this is not common UK practice and only a small proportion of patients may potentially benefit from its use. Aspirin has been proven to reduce further vascular events in confirmed thrombotic stroke by 25%.

Confirmed cerebellar haematomas and large intraparenchymal cerebral haematomas, detected on CT scan, should be discussed with the neurosurgical team. Progressive deterioration in level of consciousness following stroke may be due to obstructive hydrocephalus, which is amenable to surgical treatment.

TRANSIENT ISCHAEMIC ATTACKS (TIAs)

A focal neurological deficit lasting for less than 24 h which is due to thrombotic or embolic disease is classified as a transient ischaemic attack (TIA). The symptoms or signs may affect the carotid or vertebrobasilar territory and cause motor, sensory, visual or speech deficits.

Carotid territory disease leads to a contralateral weakness and numbness. Associated dysphasia may occur and the patient may also complain of a curtain coming down to impair vision (amaurosis fugax).

Vertebrobasilar disease is more difficult to diagnose, with variable weakness, dizziness and ataxia. There may be associated dysarthria.

If the symptoms have completely resolved and baseline investigations reveal no obvious cause, the patient can be discharged. Aspirin will significantly reduce further events or progression to a stroke. Further follow-up investigation for TIAs is required. Surgical treatment is beneficial in patients with severe carotid stenosis.

FURTHER READING

Guly, U. and Richardson, D. (1996) *Acute Medical Emergencies. Oxford Handbooks in Emergency Medicine.* Oxford University Press, Oxford.

Shah, S. and Kelly, K. (1999) *Emergency Neurology.* Cambridge University Press, Cambridge.

Smith, P.E.M. (1998) *Key Topics in Neurology.* Bios Scientific Publishers, Oxford.

CHAPTER FOURTEEN

GASTROINTESTINAL EMERGENCIES

- Introduction
- Assessment of abdominal pain
- Formulating a differential diagnosis

- Investigations
- Specific conditions
- Further reading

INTRODUCTION

The abdomen more than any other body region can easily confound one's ability to reach a clear diagnosis. Recognition of gastrointestinal emergencies relies heavily on eliciting a clear and lucid history in combination with careful examination. The main aim in the emergency department is to differentiate those patients who can be safely discharged home with appropriate advice from those who need admission for a period of observation, investigation or resuscitation prior to emergency surgery.

ASSESSMENT OF ABDOMINAL PAIN

Abdominal pain is a common presentation to the emergency department. Patients may have a range of pathologies, from the acute surgical abdomen to the vague discomfort associated with a short bout of food poisoning. If on initial assessment the patient is systemically unwell, the clinician should optimize oxygenation and tissue perfusion by adherence to the principles of the ABC system prior to taking a detailed history and examination. The history more than anything else will narrow down the options in the differential diagnosis. Examination will provide further clues. Particular

points to clarify within the history are:

- the pain – its onset, character, location, radiation, and alleviating and exacerbating features
- associated symptoms – diarrhoea, vomiting, change in bowel habits, haematemesis, melaena, absolute constipation (no passage even of flatus) and genitourinary symptoms
- menstrual history in females
- notable past medical history of abdominal pain or other relevant pathology
- dietary habits, alcohol ingestion, medication history
- family history of abdominal pain (recent or long-standing)
- other symptomatology to detect extra-abdominal causes such as diabetes mellitus.

It is important on physical examination to maintain an open mind and to examine the whole patient rather than just the abdomen. The general appearance of the patient, especially whilst positioning themselves to be examined, provides useful information. Acute pain manifested in the facial expression and any signs of dehydration should be sought. Abdominal examination begins with inspection for signs of abdominal distension, scars or bruising. A differential diagnosis of distension is given in Table 14.1. Visible peristalsis, although uncommon, is strongly suggestive of small bowel obstruction.

Auscultation of the abdomen may be difficult in a noisy department. However, an attempt should

Table 14.1: Causes of abdominal distension

Fat
Flatus
Fetus
Fluid
Faeces

Table 14.2: Differential diagnosis of adult acute abdominal pain

Appendicitis
Constipation
Infection – viral or bacterial gastroenteritis
Pancreatitis
Peptic ulcer disease – haemorrhage, inflammation or perforation
Biliary tract disease – cholecystitis, ascending cholangitis
Inflammatory bowel disease – inflammation, haemorrhage or perforation
Strangulated hernias
Small bowel obstruction due to adhesions or bands
Genitourinary causes – infection, renal calculi
Gynaecological emergencies – ruptured ectopic pregnancy, pelvic inflammatory disease, torsion of ovarian cyst
Leaking abdominal aortic aneurysm
Mesenteric ischaemia
Sigmoid volvulus
Acute diverticular disease (acute inflammation, abscess, haemorrhage, perforation, large bowel obstruction)
Colorectal carcinoma (obstruction or perforation)
Testicular torsion
Non-specific abdominal pain which resolves without operation
Metabolic causes (diabetic ketoacidosis, uraemia, hypercalcaemia, porphyria)
Other medical causes (acute myocardial infarction, pneumonia)

be made to listen carefully in all quadrants of the abdomen. Abnormal bowel sounds may be high-pitched (suggesting small bowel obstruction) or low-pitched. Absence of bowel sounds can be suggestive of visceral pathology or an ileus.

Always exclude pregnancy in women of child-bearing age.

Percussion can help differentiate distension due to a gas-filled viscus from that due to fluid (shifting dullness). Pain on gentle percussion is a subtle sign of rebound tenderness and peritonism and should not be elicited more than is absolutely necessary.

Palpation of the abdomen may help to localize the pathological process. It is important to ask the patient where the pain is and to start the examination in the opposite quadrant. The examination should proceed in a circular fashion around the abdomen, first with light palpation and then deep. Tenderness, guarding and rigidity should all be sought. Careful examination should also detect abnormal masses such as an enlarged organ or the tender pulsation of an abdominal aortic aneurysm. Examination of the genitalia, hernial orifices, femoral pulses, both loins and the back is mandatory. All males should have their testes examined to exclude torsion as a cause of abdominal pain. Females should have a vaginal examination where appropriate. A rectal examination should always be performed. The assessment is completed by examination of the urine with a dipstick test.

Patients with severe abdominal pain must be given adequate intravenous opiates titrated to their pain; appropriate examination can then take place. Judicious use of opiates will not mask the signs of true peritonism.

Correct use of titrated opiate analgesia makes abdominal assessment easier.

FORMULATING A DIFFERENTIAL DIAGNOSIS

At this stage the clinician should have formulated a differential diagnosis. The commoner causes of acute abdominal pain are listed in Table 14.2. It is better to review the history with the patient than to order a further battery of tests if no clear diagnosis is forthcoming. In addition there are essential decisions to be made regarding:

- allowing the patient home with possible follow-up

Table 14.3: Differential diagnosis of abdominal pain in children

Constipation (may be related to poor diet, stress or an anal fissure)
Appendicitis (more often atypical, with few of the classic signs present)
Strangulated hernia
Torsion of the testis
Mesenteric adenitis
Small bowel abnormalities (intussusception, Meckel's diverticulum, volvulus)
Basal pneumonia

Table 14.4: Initial investigations

Full blood count
Urea and electrolytes and blood sugar
Amylase
Mid-stream urine specimen
Chest X-ray (erect)
Plain supine abdominal X-ray
ECG

Table 14.5: Further investigations

Liver function tests and calcium
Blood cultures
Coagulation profile
Ultrasound
CT abdomen with double contrast
Intravenous pyelogram

- baseline investigations
- consultation with the surgical team regarding admission.

Pathology in individual organs will commonly be due to either infection, inflammation or trauma. Uncommon causes include vascular events, complications of tumours, and medical causes.

The assessment of children with abdominal pain is more difficult. The common and important additional causes are outlined in Table 14.3.

A careful history and examination, concentrating on the general demeanour of the child as well as any abdominal signs, should raise suspicions of intra-abdominal pathology. It is vital to maintain a low threshold for asking for an experienced surgical opinion (see Chapter 40).

INVESTIGATIONS

At this stage the clinician should have narrowed the differential diagnosis down to two or three possibilities. Investigations are divided into baseline tests (Table 14.4) and a series of further investigations which are helpful in diagnosing a number of specific pathologies (Table 14.5). Routine ordering of a wide range of investigations is not good practice and only those investigations that will aid decisions regarding diagnosis and treatment should be performed.

Often a period of observation and further investigation is necessary when a definitive diagnosis is proving elusive. An ECG must be performed in any patient likely to suffer from cardiac disease.

Atypical cardiac pain can present as abdominal pathology.

SPECIFIC CONDITIONS

The following section describes a number of common and important conditions that present to an emergency department. Their clinical presentation, relevant investigations and appropriate initial management are outlined.

MANAGEMENT OF ACUTE GASTROINTESTINAL HAEMORRHAGE

The principles of managing this group of patients can be applied to any patient who presents with an acute abdominal emergency and who is systemically unwell.

The mortality and morbidity of such patients is minimized by having clear and jointly agreed management guidelines with senior physicians and surgeons. Presentation to the emergency department will commonly be with a history of haematemesis or with melaena or both. Less often the patient will also present with postural hypotension and cardiovascular collapse. In certain circumstances signs of

Table 14.6: Causes of upper gastrointestinal haemorrhage

Peptic ulceration (70–90%)
Gastric erosions and gastritis (usually due to drugs or alcohol)
Mallory–Weiss tear
Peptic oesophagitis

Less commonly:
   Oesophageal or gastric varices
   Carcinoma
   Aortoduodenal fistula (from graft or aneurysm alone)
   Small bowel causes (Meckel's diverticulum, inflammatory bowel disease, angiodysplasia)

Table 14.7: Causes of lower gastrointestinal haemorrhage

Malignant and benign colonic tumours
Diverticular disease
Inflammatory bowel disease
Angiodysplasia
Gastroenteritis
Anorectal causes (tumours, haemorrhoids, fissures)

an acute-on-chronic blood loss may manifest as angina and dyspnoea or general lethargy.

A rapid history and examination will generate a number of likely differential diagnoses. Those for upper gastrointestinal haemorrhage are shown in Table 14.6 and for lower gastrointestinal haemorrhage in Table 14.7.

Higher-risk patients can be identified in the early stages. Such patients are those aged over 60 years, with an initial systolic blood pressure less than 100 mmHg, co-morbid conditions (e.g. liver disease or myocardial ischaemia), an initial urea greater than $10 \, \text{mmol}\,l^{-1}$ and an initial haemoglobin less than $10 \, \text{g}\,\text{dl}^{-1}$. These patients need aggressive management with the early involvement of a surgeon.

Immediate management

The first priority is maintenance of an intact airway and provision of a high-inspired concentration of oxygen. The work of breathing and respiratory rate should be assessed and recorded. A high respiratory rate may be the result of hypovolaemia as well as being an indicator of primary respiratory distress. It is essential to assess the character and rate of pulse and to record a manual blood pressure reading. Two large-bore peripheral venous cannulae should be inserted and blood taken for baseline investigations. In addition, a coagulation profile, liver function tests and serum calcium should be requested. Blood should be ordered (O negative received in 5 min, group specific in 10 min, or fully cross-matched in 45 min) depending upon the urgency of the situation. If peripheral access is not possible, femoral vein cannulation, intravenous cutdown or central venous cannulation should be performed.

The circulating volume should be replenished with blood as soon as it becomes available. In the interim, warmed crystalloid should be used. The response to boluses of 1000 ml should be evaluated. The primary survey and the patient's response to therapeutic interventions should be continually reassessed. Once the patient is stable, a more detailed examination can be performed and further information sought from the paramedics or relatives. Relevant further investigations must be instituted as indicated and the appropriate specialties involved at an early stage depending upon local policy. Emergency endoscopy will assist in diagnosis as well as allowing the treatment of certain conditions.

Additional specific measures

Oesophageal varices, if present, are best treated with injection sclerotherapy and ligation. Bleeding can be controlled in up to 90% of cases.

Treatment with one of a number of newer agents, including octreotide or terlipressin, is an alternative. Given as an infusion they have been found to be safe, effective and easy to use. Vasopressin is an alternative, although it has a number of side-effects and there is some evidence in controlled studies to suggest that it is not effective.

The Sengstaken–Blakemore tube is a useful device in massive and exsanguinating haemorrhage from oesophageal varices. Various modifications exist and it is important to be familiar with the device used locally. The patient should be intubated at this stage to protect the airway. Cimetidine or omeprazole given at an early stage will contribute to minimizing bleeding from gastric erosions. Vitamin K and clotting factor replacement should be considered if there are overt or laboratory features of a coagulopathy.

Mortality in these patients is minimized by having a clearly defined early care pathway for their management. In patients with known alcoholic cirrhosis oesophageal varices must be positively excluded, although many patients will be found to be bleeding from peptic ulcer disease.

GASTROENTERITIS

This diagnosis should be made with caution as a number of potentially serious abdominal pathologies may produce diarrhoea and vomiting. These include acute appendicitis, small and large bowel obstruction and inflammatory bowel disease. Infective gastroenteritis is dealt with in Chapter 19.

CONSTIPATION

Patients, especially children and the elderly, often present to the emergency department with abdominal pain as a result of constipation. The history alone will often provide the diagnosis although physical examination may identify impacted stool. Plain radiography will confirm a loaded lower gastrointestinal tract, but the diagnosis should not be made on radiographic appearances alone.

> Serious causes of abdominal pain must be excluded before considering constipation as the diagnosis.

A clear cause for the constipation must be identified. Advice will range from simple reassurance and dietary advice to referral to the surgical team for follow-up of anal fissures, haemorrhoids, or further investigation for a possible underlying neoplasm. Occasionally, constipation may be the presentation of hypothyroidism.

Severe pain on defecation merits careful examination of the anal area. The elderly patient or one who is embarrassed or unable to communicate clearly may not complain of anorectal pain. Important pathologies include perianal abscess, perianal fistula, haemorrhoids (possibly thrombosed), an anal fissure or even an anal canal tumour.

ACUTE GASTRITIS AND OESOPHAGEAL REFLUX

Patients with acute gastritis and oesophageal reflux present with acute upper abdominal pain and often give a history of previous similar problems. The pain is worse on bending or when lying down to sleep. The examination is often normal. ECG examination and further investigation to exclude atypical cardiac pain may be appropriate, as well as a chest X-ray to exclude perforation of an intra-abdominal viscus if the pain is severe and associated with abdominal signs. Treatment with simple antacids will often resolve symptoms. Follow-up by the patient's general practitioner is important as a change in drug treatment or investigation by endoscopy might be required.

PEPTIC ULCERATION AND PERFORATION

Approximately 10% of the male population are affected by peptic ulceration, duodenal ulcers being commoner than gastric. Epigastric pain is the predominant feature and examination will usually reveal localized tenderness unless acute complications ensue. Chief amongst these is either haemorrhage or perforation.

With a perforated peptic ulcer, pain increases in severity and spreads rapidly to the rest of the abdomen owing to the peritonitis induced by the release of gastric contents. Clinical examination reveals board-like rigidity in a patient who looks markedly unwell and may have cardiovascular compromise. After a number of hours the pain may improve somewhat but signs of a rigid abdomen remain. Vomiting and abdominal distension may ensue as a result of paralytic ileus. The erect chest X-ray will show air in the subdiaphragmatic region in 75% of cases (Fig. 14.1).

Treatment in the emergency department consists of oxygenation, intravenous fluids to maintain perfusion, nasogastric aspiration of stomach contents and broad-spectrum parenteral antibiotic therapy (cefuroxime and metronidazole). Early surgical treatment will minimize mortality, although very ill or frail patients are occasionally managed non-operatively.

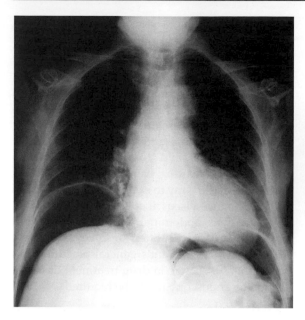

Figure 14.1: Air under the diaphragm on an erect chest X-ray in a patient with a perforated peptic ulcer.

CHOLELITHIASIS

Acute cholecystitis follows obstruction of the cystic duct by gallstones, though occasionally it may be due to a primary infective process. Obstruction results in gallbladder distension due to retained secretion and mucus and secondary infection. The patient is usually female and over 40 years. Persistent severe pain in the right upper quadrant or epigastrium is a predominant feature, although it may become intermittently worse. Other symptoms include nausea, vomiting and sometimes constipation. Examination reveals a pyrexia with associated guarding and rigidity in the right hypochondrium. Jaundice is not usually a feature and the gallbladder is rarely palpable. Pain on inspiration whilst the right subcostal region is palpated (Murphy's sign) is commonly present.

Elderly patients with cholecystitis often present with atypical symptoms and signs. In one series of over 200 such patients, only 15% presented with epigastric or right upper quadrant pain, 55% were afebrile at presentation, and nausea and vomiting were present in only 40%.

Standard acute investigations in the emergency department are usually unhelpful. Plain radiography may show gallstones (Fig. 14.2), although

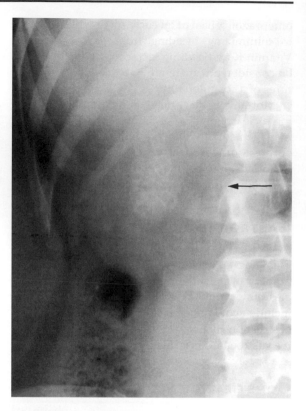

Figure 14.2: Gallstones on a plain abdominal radiograph. The gallbladder is full of faceted calcified stones. In addition, several calculi to the right of L2 lie within the common bile duct (arrow).

unfortunately 90% will be non-opaque. The serum amylase may be slightly raised. Ultrasound will confirm the diagnosis in most cases (> 90%), showing an inflamed gallbladder with stones. Failure to confirm the diagnosis on ultrasound should lead to other diagnoses being considered.

Treatment in the emergency department consists of intravenous opiates titrated to produce pain relief, intravenous fluid therapy, antibiotics and referral to the surgical team. Cholecystectomy is now commonly performed in the acute inflammatory phase during the initial admission.

In contrast to acute cholecystitis, biliary colic is the result of the passage of small calculi from the gallbladder through the cystic duct into the common bile-duct. Patients experience recurrent episodes of epigastric or right upper quadrant pain associated with nausea and vomiting. The pain often radiates to the right scapular region. Examination reveals right upper quadrant tenderness.

The main priority is pain relief. Pethidine is preferred by some as it is said to relax the sphincter of Oddi at the lower end of the common bile-duct. Parenteral non-steroidal anti-inflammatory drugs are often also effective. Patients may require admission for observation and pain relief. Investigation is by ultrasound to demonstrate the presence of calculi and definitive treatment is cholecystectomy.

PANCREATITIS

Acute inflammation of the pancreas has a multitude of triggers. The commoner causes in patients presenting to an emergency department include cholelithiasis, alcohol and blood-borne or lymphatic infections.

The presentation is varied depending on the severity of the attack. An acute attack is heralded by severe continuous epigastric pain radiating through to the back and lower chest. Nausea and vomiting may also be present.

Examination findings depend very much upon where in the spectrum of severity the patient lies. Marked epigastric tenderness may be the only sign. In severe disease the patient may be comatose, hypotensive, pyrexial, and have abdominal rigidity.

Standard investigations will reveal the diagnosis (markedly raised amylase); however, a posterior perforation of a peptic ulcer can cause moderately raised amylase levels. In addition one needs to identify a possible cause and pre-empt any possible complications of the pancreatitis. Those patients at most risk are best identified using Ranson's criteria (Table 14.8), with any three criteria being indicative of severe pancreatitis. A mortality rate of 16% is quoted for those with three or four criteria and more than 40% with five or more criteria. Hence, close biochemical monitoring of arterial blood gases, blood sugar, potassium and calcium, as well as blood cultures to exclude systemic infection, is necessary. An early contrast-enhanced CT scan will confirm the diagnosis and provide information on the degree of pancreatic necrosis.

Treatment is supportive and should be aimed at optimizing oxygenation and tissue perfusion with intravenous fluids. Pain should be treated with titrated intravenous analgesia. Nasogastric tube

Table 14.8: Ranson's criteria for severity of acute pancreatitis

On admission:
Age > 55 years
White blood count $> 16\,000\,mm^{-3}$
Glucose $> 11\,mmol\,l^{-1}$
Lactate dehydrogenase $> 350\,IU\,l^{-1}$
Aspartate aminotransaminase $> 250\,IU\,l^{-1}$
During initial 48 h:
Packed cell volume decrease $> 10\%$
Blood urea nitrogen increase $> 1.8\,mmol\,l^{-1}$
Calcium $< 2\,mmol\,l^{-1}$
Arterial oxygen concentration $< 60\,mmHg$
Base deficit $> 4\,mmol\,l^{-1}$
Fluid sequestration > 6 litres

insertion and aspiration should be instituted. Controlled studies support the use of antibiotics in acute severe pancreatitis as well as indicating possible benefits from the use of antioxidants and octreotide.

Patients with cardiovascular compromise, neurological impairment or persisting hypoxia despite high-flow oxygenation and fluid therapy should be referred to the intensive care unit for joint management by the intensivists and surgeons, as mortality is significantly higher.

INTESTINAL OBSTRUCTION

Intestinal obstruction may be due to a number of mechanical causes or to functional paralysis of the bowel wall. It may be acute or chronic. Mechanical causes can be luminal (gallstones or foreign body), mural (neoplasm) and extramural (adhesions, hernial sacs). Paralytic ileus may be due to peritonitis or trauma.

Colicky periumbilical abdominal pain with vomiting suggests small bowel obstruction. Vomiting may not be a presenting feature in large bowel obstruction, in which the pain is usually localized to the suprapubic region. Complete constipation with failure to pass flatus is highly suggestive of large bowel obstruction.

Examination in the early stages will reveal abdominal distension and an increase in bowel sounds. If strangulation supervenes, the pain becomes constant and signs of peritoneal irritation

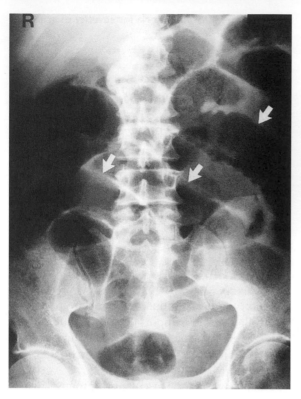

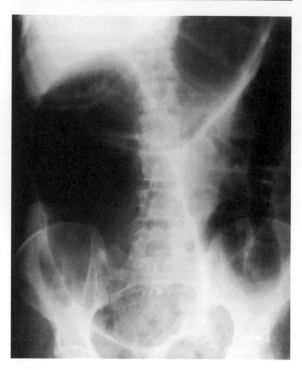

Figure 14.4: Sigmoid volvulus on a plain abdominal X-ray.

Figure 14.3: Distended loops of small bowel in a patient with small bowel obstruction.

will appear, with tachycardia. Careful examination of the hernial orifices is essential (particularly femoral and inguinal) to exclude incarceration or strangulation. Volvulus may be due to adhesions (common in small bowel obstruction) or an associated tumour (large bowel obstruction).

Plain radiology of the abdomen will reveal distended loops of small bowel and distension of the large bowel, depending on the site of the obstruction and the competency of the ileo-caecal valve (Fig. 14.3). Occasionally other diagnostic features, such as the massively distended loop of a sigmoid volvulus (Fig. 14.4) or gas in the biliary tree indicating a gallstone ileus, may be seen.

Initial management follows the basic principles of oxygenation, fluid therapy, pain relief, nasogastric aspiration and referral to the surgical team. Subsequent treatment will depend upon the clinical state of the patient and early progress with conservative therapy. Confirmed strangulation and a volvulus with signs of imminent rupture merit an urgent surgical opinion and probably early operative intervention.

APPENDICITIS

This is the commonest acute surgical presentation to the emergency department. An inflamed appendix can present in a classic manner requiring no real investigations to confirm the diagnosis, or have a delayed and atypical presentation.

Classically, initial nausea and dull central abdominal pain will move to the right lower quadrant after a number of hours. Other symptoms may include constipation, diarrhoea and frequency of micturition depending upon where the appendix lies. Examination usually reveals a pyrexia and tenderness localized to the right iliac fossa. A delayed diagnosis may result in a very ill patient with signs of generalized peritonitis secondary to a perforated appendix.

Minimal investigations are usually required to diagnose obvious appendicitis, although more difficult cases may require limited investigation to exclude other pathologies. Although the white cell count is a favourite investigation of junior surgeons, its value should not play a significant role in making decisions about patients with suspected appendicitis.

> The white cell count is of little use in diagnosing acute appendicitis.

A variety of differential diagnoses should be considered if the history or examination is atypical. Gastroenteritis, constipation, perforated peptic ulceration, cholecystitis, mesenteric adenitis, pyelonephritis and gynaecological disease may all masquerade as appendicitis.

Intravenous fluids, analgesia and broad-spectrum antibiotics, including anaerobic cover, should be instituted. Referral to the surgical team for appendectomy is required.

MESENTERIC ISCHAEMIA AND INFARCTION

This results from interruption of the blood supply to the bowel. This may be due to occlusion of a major artery by an embolus or thrombosis in an artery or vein.

Patients are usually elderly and often too ill to give a clear history. Pain associated with loose stools containing dark blood or clots is the commonest symptom. Examination usually reveals distension with progressive signs of peritonism. Bowel signs are decreased. Atrial fibrillation will suggest an embolic cause for the ischaemia.

Plain X-rays of the abdomen may show 'thumb printing', a sign of ischaemic bowel. The white blood cell count will be non-specifically and significantly raised. Treatment consists of oxygenation, fluid therapy, analgesia and urgent referral to the surgical team. The patient is often very ill with other systemic disease. A period of stabilization on the intensive care unit may be appropriate. The prognosis is poor.

DIVERTICULAR DISEASE AND DIVERTICULITIS

Inflammation of diverticulae occurs predominantly in the colon and may result in a variety of symptoms and signs. The incidence of diverticulae increases with age: 80% of people will have chronic diverticulae by the age of 80 years. However, acute diverticulitis is becoming increasingly common from the fourth decade onwards, particularly in men. Diverticular disease may be complicated by haemorrhage or perforation, resulting in peritonitis or local abscess formation. Large bowel obstruction may also occur.

Symptoms are diverse and depend upon the severity of the disease and its complications. They include lower abdominal pain, vomiting, fever, dysuria and rectal blood loss. Clinical signs may be limited to localized tenderness or progress to frank peritonitis with signs of sepsis. A lower abdominal mass may be palpable.

A standard investigation profile may reveal a high white cell count, a chronic anaemia, either large or small bowel obstruction, or free gas in the abdomen suggesting perforation. Blood and urine cultures and a coagulation screen should be carried out if there are any signs of sepsis.

Management initially consists of intravenous fluid therapy, analgesia and appropriate antibiotics (cefuroxine and metronidazole). The patient should be referred to the surgical team.

PERIANAL PROBLEMS

Although rarely life-threatening, these conditions cause considerable distress and are a common cause of presentation to the emergency department.

Abscesses

Patients present with pain, often made worse by sitting and defecation. In the case of perianal abscess, an obvious tender fluctuant mass at the anal margin will be seen. Ischio-rectal abscesses are deeper and may only be found by rectal examination. Although most are simply the result of infection of the anal glands, a number have significant underlying pathology, such as fistulae, inflammatory bowel disease, fissures and tumours. Patients should therefore be admitted and the abscess drained under a general anaesthetic following examination under anaesthetic and sigmoidoscopy.

Anal fissure

The patient complains of severe pain, most marked on defecation. The onset of symptoms is often related to the passage of a hard stool that tears the anal lining. Patients often report the presence of a small amount of blood on the toilet tissue. Pain results in spasm of the sphincters and rectal examination is often impossible. The fissure, if seen, is usually in the posterior mid-line.

Treatment is with topical and oral analgesics (constipating agents must be avoided) and the fissure will usually heal spontaneously. It is important to beware of underlying pathology such as inflammatory bowel disease and malignancies.

Haemorrhoids

Patients present to emergency departments usually as the result of one of three complications of piles.

HAEMORRHAGE

Bleeding is typically fresh and on to the surface of the stool. This usually responds to faecal softening agents but the patient may need further investigation to rule out a more sinister cause for rectal bleeding.

PROLAPSE

Patients present with pain. Reduction of the prolapsed pile may be possible after a period of application of ice with the patient resting in a head-down position. If pain is severe and the pile irreducible, early surgery may be necessary. If reduction of the pile is successful, use of faecal softeners is recommended to prevent recurrence.

THROMBOSIS

A thrombosed prolapsed haemorrhoid causes severe pain and the only treatment is surgical excision.

Perianal haematoma

This is sometimes referred to as a thrombosed external pile. It is actually a haematoma that follows rupture of a perianal vein. Relief from the acute pain can be achieved by incision to release the haematoma. Otherwise spontaneous recovery will occur.

Rectal foreign bodies

Emergency medicine folklore is full of tales of items retrieved from the rectums of the population

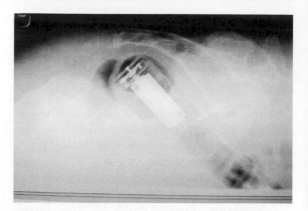

Figure 14.5: A foreign body in the rectum.

(Fig. 14.5) and imaginative explanations of how the foreign body got there. However, there are serious potential consequences, not least rectal perforation. Foreign bodies will usually require a general anaesthetic for removal.

LEAKING ABDOMINAL AORTIC ANEURYSM

This is not a gastrointestinal condition but is discussed here as it often forms part of the differential diagnosis of abdominal emergencies. This vascular emergency presents in elderly patients who collapse suddenly, having complained of abdominal pain going through to the lumbar region. The pain may mimic that of left ureteric colic, radiating to the left groin. Patients will self-select depending upon the amount of initial haemorrhage. A complete rupture into the retroperitoneum or peritoneal cavity leads to rapid death. Patients who survive to reach hospital will have had a limited haemorrhage which has temporarily tamponaded.

> Beware the elderly patient with new back pain or pain suggestive of left ureteric colic – they may have a ruptured aneurysm.

A high index of suspicion is required to positively exclude a leaking aneurysm in any patient who exhibits signs of cardiovascular collapse in association with abdominal pain. Clinical examination will often reveal a pulsatile, tender mass that may extend into the groin.

A standard blood profile should be obtained and at least 8 units of blood cross-matched. If the patient is shocked, O-negative and type-specific blood should be requested. Once the diagnosis has been made the patient should be rapidly transferred to the operating theatre for repair of the aneurysm.

If the diagnosis is less clear or the aneurysm is perceived to be a coincidental finding on clinical examination, certain investigations are essential. In particular it is important to exclude pancreatitis, myocardial infarction (ECG) and mesenteric ischaemia. An urgent ultrasound examination in the resuscitation room will often diagnose the presence of an abdominal aneurysm.

Management should be aimed mainly at obtaining immediate senior surgical help. In the mean time, high-flow oxygen should be administered, two large-bore intravenous cannulae inserted and judicious crystalloids administered to maintain the systolic blood pressure at around 90 mmHg. Intravenous opiates can be given slowly in patients with severe pain as long as the blood pressure is stable.

FURTHER READING

Moore, K. and Ramrakha, P. (1997) *Oxford Handbook of Acute Medicine*. Oxford University Press, Oxford.

CHAPTER FIFTEEN

TOXICOLOGY

- Introduction
- Poisoning in children
- Adult poisoning
- Information on poisoning
- General management principles

- Evaluation of the poisoned patient
- Treatment
- Management of specific poisonings
- Further reading

INTRODUCTION

Poisoning is a common cause of presentation to emergency departments in the UK and accounts for up to 10% of acute medical admissions. However, the mortality from acute poisoning is less than 1% and the vast majority of patients will make a rapid and complete recovery with good supportive care. The challenge is to identify those poisonings that are most likely to cause serious complications and morbidity and to institute appropriate treatment promptly.

POISONING IN CHILDREN

Accidental poisoning is the commonest form of toxic exposure in childhood. Most incidents involve inquisitive toddlers (1–5 years) sampling household chemicals and any tablets they come across. Serious morbidity is rare. Poisoning in a small number of cases in this age group can be due to non-accidental injury where a carer deliberately poisons the child, and clinicians should be vigilant for any suspicious circumstances (e.g. tablet ingestion by an infant who is not yet mobile).

Older children and adolescents may present to the emergency department after alcohol or drug experimentation or misuse, but rarely require treatment. Deliberate self-poisoning is uncommon in childhood but should be considered in children over

5 years old with normal intellectual development (often there is a family history of self-poisoning). Most of these children will need admission for psychological assessment, even if the poisoning is trivial.

ADULT POISONING

Accidental poisoning is largely due to chemical exposure at work or at home. Deliberate self-poisoning is the commonest cause of poisoning in adults. Motives for these overdoses vary from impulsive parasuicidal gestures (often younger adult females) to serious suicidal attempts.

> After deliberate self-poisoning all patients will need a psychiatric assessment.

INFORMATION ON POISONING

In the UK and many other countries a network of Poisons Information Centres provides 24-h telephone advice on the toxicity and management of poisonings (Table 15.1). An information officer or pharmacist initially answers enquiries, and medical toxicology staff are available for advice on more complex cases. In addition to a large database of information on poisonings, the Poisons Information Centres will have access to information on the

Table 15.1: Regional Poisons Information Centres

Belfast	01232 240503
Birmingham	0121 507 5588
Cardiff	01222 709901
Dublin	01837 9964 or 01837 9966
Edinburgh	0131 536 2300
London	020 7635 9191 or 020 7955 5095
Newcastle	0191 232 5131

toxicity of new products, rare ingestions or exposures, new developments and changes in existing practice.

Toxbase is an on-line computer database of poisons information run by the National Poisons Information Service centre in Edinburgh. It covers a range of drugs, household products and industrial chemicals and is used in many departments.

Unknown tablets can sometimes be identified from descriptions in the *British National Formulary* or the *MIMS Colour Index*. The Poisons Information Centres also use TICTAC, which is a computer-aided tablet and capsule identification system. For identification of plants and fungi, the CD-ROM package from the Royal Botanical Gardens, Kew, and the London Poisons Unit, Poisonous Plants in Britain and Ireland, is a valuable resource.

GENERAL MANAGEMENT PRINCIPLES

Most poisoned patients will initially present to an emergency department. Seriously poisoned patients will require admission to a medical ward or intensive care unit (ICU). In some North American centres, patients are admitted under the care of a dedicated medical toxicologist or a physician with a specific interest in toxicology. In the UK, most poisoned patients who require admission are managed by the medical team on call, though increasingly many of the less toxic poisonings are managed by emergency physicians on an observation ward. When patients present late at night or in the early hours of the morning, even if there is no risk of toxicity, admission for a short period to an observation ward can be helpful in defusing the emotional circumstances that precipitated the overdose and allowing a clearer psychological assessment later in the morning.

EVALUATION OF THE POISONED PATIENT

HISTORY

A thorough history is essential in determining management and assessing the risk posed by a particular poisoning. The important historical factors include what exactly was taken, when it was taken, how it was taken, how much was taken, why it was taken, and what else was taken (multi-drug overdoses are common, and alcohol is a frequent co-ingestant).

What was taken, when and why?

Many patients are alert and co-operative, and contrary to common opinion, most conscious patients give a fairly accurate history. Details of the time of ingestion and type of tablet are usually reasonably accurate, though actual doses ingested are less precise. Histories are less reliable in patients with a persistent high suicidal intent, patients in custody, and where illicit drugs are involved. In patients who are intoxicated or unconscious, information and corroboration are often available from friends, relatives and ambulance staff. Empty bottles or tablet packets may give a clue to possible doses ingested.

Knowledge of the patient's past medical history and any current medication is helpful, as toxicity may be potentiated in certain situations (e.g. increased toxicity of paracetamol in alcoholics). Having evaluated the medical risk, an appraisal of suicide risk must also be made. The process of evaluating the mental state and suicide risk of patients attending the emergency department after deliberate self-harm is discussed in Chapter 34.

EXAMINATION

As with any patient attending an emergency department, physical assessment of the poisoned patient starts with the ABC (airway, breathing and circulation). The patient must be capable of maintaining and protecting a patent airway. If there is any doubt, active airway management is required to protect against further compromise or aspiration. Assessment of the gag reflex is not particularly useful, as its presence does not exclude the possibility of aspiration, and testing may provoke vomiting. Evaluation of breathing involves measuring the respiratory rate and assessing the adequacy of ventilation. Observation, auscultation of the chest, and oxygen saturation will confirm adequate ventilation in most cases, though arterial blood gases should be checked if any doubt remains. Evidence of inadequate ventilation requires immediate correction. Where the cause is not readily reversible (as with naloxone in opiate overdose), assisted ventilation is necessary (intubation and mechanical ventilation). Evaluation of the circulation includes a baseline pulse rate and blood pressure (BP). Serious poisonings require continuous electrocardiograph monitoring and regular BP checks.

After assessment of ABC, a complete physical examination is undertaken to look for other signs of poisoning, injection marks, trauma (head injury or self-injury) and other disease (e.g. sepsis). In cases where unknown tablets have been taken, clues as to the type of agent taken will often arise during the course of the examination.

The neurological assessment is particularly important. An altered level of consciousness is a frequent complication of poisoning and ranges from mild drowsiness to agitation, delirium, coma and seizures. A Glasgow Coma Scale (GCS) of 8 or less strongly suggests that the patient may be unable to protect their airway and intubation is required. Pupil size and reaction are affected in many poisonings, and muscle tone, reflexes and the presence of myoclonic jerks or dystonias should also be noted.

A baseline body temperature should be recorded as many agents cause hyperthermia. Auscultation of the chest, in addition to assessing ventilation, may reveal evidence of aspiration, pulmonary oedema or bronchospasm.

A number of specific toxic syndromes may be identified on examination. The more common of these are listed in Table 15.2.

INVESTIGATIONS

The individual clinical picture dictates what diagnostic investigations (if any) are required. The

Table 15.2: Toxic syndromes

Opioid (heroin, methadone, codeine):
  CNS depression, respiratory depression, hypotension, bradycardia, miosis, hyporeflexia, rapid response to naloxone

Sympathomimetic (cocaine, amphetamine, theophylline):
  CNS excitation (agitation, paranoia, seizures), tachycardia, hypertension, hyperpyrexia, sweating, mydriasis, hyper-reflexia and tremor. Often raised glucose, low potassium and acidosis

Anticholinergic (antidepressants, antipsychotics, antihistamines):
  Delirium, hallucinations, tachycardia, dry mouth, dry skin, hyperthermia, dilated pupils, ↓ bowel sounds, urinary retention

Cholinergic (organophosphates):
  Sweating, lacrimation, diarrhoea, vomiting, urination, miosis, bradycardia, muscle cramps, fasciculations, paralysis

Serotoninergic (SSRIs):
  Mental status changes (hypomania, confusion, agitation), fever, hyper-reflexia, myoclonus, sweating, diarrhoea

---

following are needed most often:

- Blood glucose should be checked in all unconscious patients.
- Urea and electrolytes and liver function tests are usually done as baseline investigations in any ingestion with potentially significant toxicity, as well as in unconscious patients. Many poisonings cause specific electrolyte abnormalities (e.g. hyperkalaemia in acute digoxin poisoning).
- Arterial blood gases (ABGs) should be taken in patients who appear to have respiratory depression, are unconscious, or may have taken tricyclic antidepressants. ABGs are also required in suspected CO poisoning and to estimate acidosis after methanol, ethylene glycol and salicylate poisoning.
- Drug levels are useful for certain poisonings, but are not routinely required. Paracetamol and salicylate levels are most frequently done. They should not be requested on all poisoned patients, but are useful in unconscious patients and unreliable historians. Other poisonings where levels are useful include iron, lithium,

theophylline, digoxin, methanol, carbamazepine and phenytoin.

- Drug screening is available in few centres, is rarely useful, and should only be done on specialist advice.
- Electrocardiography (ECG) should be done if the patient is unconscious, has an arrhythmia, or has taken a potentially cardiotoxic overdose. A QRS complex of greater than 100 ms (2.5 small squares) in one or more limb leads can be predictive of arrhythmias and seizures after a tricyclic antidepressant overdose. Conduction blocks and QT prolongation are also seen with other pro-arrhythmic drugs.
- X-rays are usually only required for specific indications (e.g. suspicion of aspiration, iron tablet ingestion etc.).

TREATMENT

There are two main elements to managing poisoned patients. The first is the provision of good supportive care and the second is decontamination or elimination enhancement measures. Effective antidotes are only available for a small number of poisons. The most common of these are listed in Table 15.3 and their use is discussed in the text.

SUPPORTIVE CARE

Supportive care is directed at preventing or limiting the complications of a toxic exposure and is the cornerstone of good management. It is essential to ensure a patent airway, adequate ventilation and effective circulation. However, a number of specific complications are worth considering:

- Bronchospasm usually responds to standard bronchodilators.
- Hypotension can result from relative hypovolaemia, arrhythmias, decreased peripheral resistance or a direct myocardial depressant action of some toxins.
- Hypertension. The cause should be treated. Diazepam is usually sufficient after sympathomimetic overdoses. If pulmonary oedema, cardiac ischaemia or encephalopathy is present a vasodilator should be considered.

Table 15.3: Poisons and specific antidotes

Poison	Antidote
Benzodiazepines	Flumazenil (rarely needed)
Beta-blockers	Glucagon
Carbon monoxide	Oxygen
Cyanide	Dicobalt edetate, hydroxocobalamin
Digoxin	Digoxin Fab fragments
Ethylene glycol	Ethanol
Iron	Desferrioxamine
Methanol	Ethanol
Opioids	Naloxone
Organophosphates	Atropine, pralidoxime
Paracetamol	N-acetylcysteine, methionine

- Cardiac arrhythmias. Hypoxia, acidosis and electrolyte abnormalities should be corrected. Tachyarrhythmias are rarely associated with serious perfusion problems and usually require monitoring alone. Bradycardias are more sinister. Initial treatment is with atropine and any specific antagonist, depending on the cause (e.g. bicarbonate for tricyclic antidepressants, glucagon for beta-blockers and calcium for verapamil). Inotropic agents and pacing may be required.
- Cardiac arrest. The management of a cardiac arrest after poisoning follows standard advanced cardiac life support (ACLS) protocols. However, a number of important aspects are worth noting. First, poisoned patients often have a reversible cause for their arrest and are usually in good general health. Second, some antidotes given during cardiopulmonary resuscitation (CPR) prompt immediate reversal of effects, and successful resuscitation has been documented after prolonged CPR in a range of different overdoses. Hence, it is important to think of possible antidotes and be prepared to prolong resuscitative efforts when appropriate.
- Convulsions. Hypoxia and hypoglycaemia should be sought and corrected. Diazepam (usually as Diazemuls®) is the treatment of choice.
- Hyperthermia. This is treated initially with cooling. Diazepam and dantrolene may be required, and occasionally paralysis and mechanical ventilation are needed.

DECONTAMINATION AND ENHANCING ELIMINATION

Common sense suggests that when a poisonous substance has been ingested, efforts to remove it and prevent absorption should help reduce toxicity. However, most of the methods employed in the past are relatively inefficient, have been overused, and have not been shown to improve clinical outcome.

Emesis

Syrup of ipecacuanha (ipecac) has been widely used in the past to induce vomiting after toxic ingestions. It can cause drowsiness, aspiration and prolonged vomiting after use and there is no substantial evidence for any clinical benefit. As a result, it is no longer used.

> There are no current indications for the use of induced emesis.

Activated charcoal

The rationale for activated charcoal is that many drugs are carbon based and have side-chains that will adhere to charcoal. Activated charcoal has a very large surface area and adsorbs poisons in the gastrointestinal tract, preventing absorption and thereby reducing the likelihood of systemic toxicity. However, there is no strong evidence that clinical outcome after overdose is improved. The current recommendations are that a single dose of activated charcoal may be considered if a potentially toxic amount of a poison (which is known to be adsorbed to charcoal) has been ingested up to 1 h previously.

> Charcoal may be useful in some potentially toxic overdoses within an hour of ingestion.

Charcoal does not effectively bind cyanide, iron, lithium, heavy metals, alcohols, strong acids or alkali. Although charcoal is relatively safe, aspiration can occur if there is inadequate airway protection, and constipation and obstruction have been reported where repeat doses were used. A dose of $1\,g\,kg^{-1}$ is recommended for children and $50\,g$ for adults. Charcoal is unpleasant to take, but may be

Table 15.4: Gastric lavage

Ensure patient is capable of airway protection. Otherwise arrange intubation first.
Give oxygen via nasal cannulae. Lie patient head downwards in left lateral position.
Check suction.
An oral airway or mouth-guard should be placed between the teeth to prevent biting of the tube.
Lubricate and insert large-bore (36–40 French gauge) orogastric tube.
Aspirate stomach contents.
Use small cycle lavages 100–200 ml of water and then aspirate. It is not necessary to lavage until effluent is clear, and lavage is rarely indicated beyond 5 min unless tablets are still returning.
Consider leaving activated charcoal in the stomach.
On withdrawing tube, occlude it between the fingers to prevent aspiration of fluid from the tube.

more palatable if chilled or mixed with fruit juice (though this may affect efficacy). An alternative is administration via a nasogastric tube.

Repeat doses may be useful in some overdoses involving sustained-release preparations (verapamil and theophylline). Repeat doses of charcoal are thought to enhance elimination by interrupting the enterohepatic circulation of some drugs. Another possible mechanism is that the charcoal maintains a minimal drug concentration in the intestinal lumen and free drug diffuses back into the intestine down a concentration gradient, binds to charcoal and is excreted (a sort of 'gastrointestinal dialysis').

Gastric lavage

The role of gastric lavage (Table 15.4) has also been reconsidered recently. There is no evidence that it improves clinical outcome and it can cause significant morbidity. The current advice is that gastric lavage should only be considered if a patient has ingested a potentially life-threatening amount of poison and the procedure can be undertaken within 1 h of ingestion. It should also be considered in unconscious patients where the timing and type of ingestion is often unclear. Contraindications include loss of airway protective reflexes (decreased level of consciousness) and corrosive or hydrocarbon ingestion. Complications include a risk of aspiration and oesophageal rupture. Profound bradycardia leading to asystolic arrest has been recorded with gastric lavage after cardiotoxic ingestions (beta-blockers, calcium channel blockers etc.), and pretreatment with atropine to counteract any increased vagal activity in such situations is recommended. There are few indications for gastric lavage in children.

Whole bowel irrigation

Whole bowel irrigation (WBI) both decontaminates and enhances elimination by flushing the bowel of solid contents. A polyethylene glycol solution is administered orally (or via nasogastric tube) until the rectal effluent becomes clear (usually within 2–6 h). The exact role of WBI has yet to be determined, but current indications include use in 'body-packers' (drug smugglers who have ingested multiple small packets of illicit drugs), for lithium and iron poisoning (both poorly adsorbed by charcoal), and in some sustained-release preparation overdoses. If indicated, activated charcoal may be given before starting WBI. Nausea, vomiting, mild bloating and rectal irritation may occur, and antiemetics are useful.

Alkaline diuresis

Urinary alkalinization and forced diuresis was used in salicylate poisoning, on the basis that weak acids such as salicylate are more water soluble when ionized and are thus excreted in much greater concentrations when the urine has been alkalinized. Again, no clinical benefit has been demonstrated. Low-dose regimens of bicarbonate administration are sometimes still recommended for severe salicylate overdose.

Haemodialysis

Haemodialysis to increase elimination is used rarely in severe poisonings which are not otherwise easily treated by less invasive means. For haemodialysis to be effective the poison must be highly water soluble, have low molecular weight, a low volume of distribution and low protein binding. The most common indications are severe poisoning with methanol, ethylene glycol, lithium and salicylates.

Charcoal haemoperfusion

Charcoal haemoperfusion is where the patient's blood is pumped through a charcoal cartridge. For it to be effective the toxin must have a high affinity for charcoal and a low volume of distribution. Side-effects with haemoperfusion are more common than with haemodialysis and it is usually reserved for severe theophylline poisoning.

MANAGEMENT OF SPECIFIC POISONINGS

It is essential to approach the symptomatic patient methodically. The initial treatment priorities are as discussed above.

PARACETAMOL

Paracetamol is widely used as an analgesic and antipyretic agent. It is the most commonly reported cause of self-poisoning in the UK.

Toxicity

Individual susceptibility to toxicity in overdose varies, but doses of greater than $150\,mg\,kg^{-1}$ or $12\,g$ (24 tablets) can cause significant toxicity in adult patients. Doses of less than $125\,mg\,kg^{-1}$ are unlikely to cause liver damage in healthy adult patients. However, there are a number of high-risk groups of patients who are more susceptible to paracetamol hepatotoxicity (Table 15.5).

In therapeutic doses paracetamol is largely metabolized in the liver to inactive glucuronide and sulphate conjugates. A small proportion

Table 15.5: Patients at increased risk of paracetamol toxicity

Pre-existing liver disease
Malnourished/anorexic
HIV positive
Raised cytochrome P450 activity:
Drugs – anticonvulsants, rifampicin
Chronic alcoholics
Chronic paracetamol ingestion

(approximately 5%) is metabolized by the hepatic cytochrome P450 enzyme system to a toxic intermediary, *N*-acetyl-para-benzoquinoneimine (NAPBQ). This is normally rapidly detoxified by conjugation with hepatic glutathione. In overdose, there is saturation of the normal glucuronide and sulphate conjugation pathways and increased NAPBQ production. The amount of glutathione available to detoxify the increased NAPBQ is limited, and once hepatic glutathione stores are exceeded NAPBQ binds with intracellular sulphydryl groups and causes an acute hepatocellular necrosis. A small amount of paracetamol metabolism occurs in the kidneys, and saturation of renal pathways leads to acute tubular necrosis.

> Paracetamol toxicity is initially asymptomatic.

Initially, patients are usually asymptomatic despite having taken a potentially lethal overdose. Some patients have nausea, vomiting and abdominal pain. Drowsiness and metabolic acidosis have been reported after very large overdoses. Initial nausea usually settles within 24 h, and this is followed by the onset of right subcostal pain and tenderness, indicating the development of liver damage. Some may also have renal tenderness and oliguria. At 16–24 h post ingestion, prothrombin time, alanine aminotransferase (ALT), aspartatate transaminase (AST) and bilirubin levels start to rise. Nausea and vomiting reappear. Peak hepatotoxicity occurs 3–4 days after ingestion and a peak ALT or AST greater than $1000\,\mathrm{IU}\,\mathrm{l}^{-1}$ indicates significant hepatotoxicity. Jaundice can appear around this time. Patients who have taken large overdoses may develop fulminant hepatic failure with progressive encephalopathy, coagulopathy and haemorrhage, renal failure, hypoglycaemia, coma and death. Other patients with lesser degrees of hepatic failure will start to recover from the third or fourth day and complete recovery is usual.

Treatment

The treatment of patients presenting after a paracetamol overdose depends on the dose ingested, whether the patient is from a high-risk group for hepatotoxicity, and the time post ingestion.

Those patients at risk of liver damage and requiring treatment can be identified by considering the plasma paracetamol level in relation to the time of

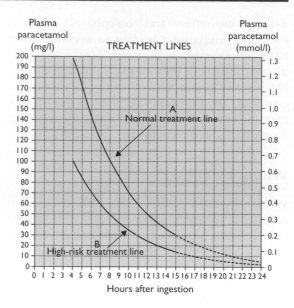

Figure 15.1: Paracetamol treatment graph.

ingestion using the paracetamol treatment graph (Fig. 15.1). This is a graph of plasma paracetamol concentrations versus time post ingestion and classically shows two suggested treatment lines. These were initially developed from observation of the natural history in untreated patients and form the basis of the guidelines on paracetamol poisoning issued by the UK National Poisons Information Service to all emergency departments. Those patients whose plasma paracetamol levels are above the appropriate treatment line at a given time require treatment. It is important that samples are not taken less than 4 h after ingestion, as early levels can be misleading.

> Where there is doubt about the timing of ingestion or the need to treat, the rule must be to treat.

N-Acetylcysteine (NAC) is the specific antidote for paracetamol poisoning and acts as a glutathione precursor preventing glutathione depletion and NAPBQ-induced hepatotoxicity. If given within 8–10 h post ingestion it affords maximum protection against hepatotoxicity. The efficacy of NAC declines thereafter, but if it is given within 16 h fulminant hepatic failure will be averted. Studies have also shown that the use of NAC up to 72 h post overdose significantly decreases both the progression to grade 3 and 4 hepatic encephalopathy and

Table 15.6: Dosage regimen for NAC

150 mg kg^{-1} NAC in 200 ml 5% dextrose infusion over 15 min
50 mg kg^{-1} NAC in 500 ml 5% dextrose infusion over next 4 h
100 mg kg^{-1} NAC in 1l 5% dextrose infusion over next 16 h

Table 15.7: Features of salicylate poisoning

Mild	Moderate	Severe
Nausea	Hyperventilation	Dehydration
Vomiting	Sweating	Confusion
Abdominal pain	Tremor	Lethargy
Tinnitus	Deafness	Convulsions
Flushing	Metabolic acidosis	Coma

death from fulminant hepatic failure. The current intravenous regimen for NAC (in adults) is given in Table 15.6.

Intravenous NAC may cause nausea, flushing, pruritus and an urticarial rash. Very occasionally, more pronounced anaphylactoid reactions occur, with angio-oedema, bronchospasm and hypotension. These reactions usually occur at the start of the infusion, or when it has been given more quickly than recommended. The infusion of NAC should be stopped and intravenous antihistamine and steroids given as required. The infusion can then be restarted at 25% of the initial rate, and increased as tolerated. Another antidote is methionine, which acts as a glutathione precursor and is given orally. However, it cannot be given to patients with nausea and vomiting and, unlike NAC, it has not been shown to be of significant benefit in patients who present after 8 h.

Fulminant hepatic failure from paracetamol poisoning has a mortality of around 50% and depends on age, use of NAC and the degree of encephalopathy on presentation. Some patients at high risk of fulminant liver failure will benefit from liver transplantation, and specialist advice should be sought early in those patients with evidence of significant toxicity. The international normalized ratio (INR) is the most specific index of liver damage and values of greater than 2 at 24 h, 4 at 48 h or 6 at 72 h indicate severe hepatic injury.

The plasma paracetamol treatment graph cannot be used to estimate risk of hepatotoxicity after a staggered overdose, and such patients should be treated with a full course of NAC and then managed according to the blood results (INR, ALT, creatinine) post infusion.

SALICYLATES

Aspirin (acetylsalicylic acid) is widely used for its analgesic, anti-inflammatory and antithrombotic actions. Understanding and management of the complexity of salicylate overdose has improved considerably over the years but fatalities, some of which should be preventable, still occur.

Pathophysiology

Salicylate overdose causes a mixture of acid–base disturbances. Initially, salicylate stimulates the respiratory centre leading to hyperventilation and a respiratory alkalosis. This is followed by a period of renal compensation with loss of bicarbonate, sodium, potassium and water in the urine (compensatory metabolic acidosis). At the same time, salicylate uncouples oxidative phosphorylation leading to reduced oxygen utilization and an increase in lactate and other organic acids. In addition, high levels of salicylate derivatives (which are weakly acidic) contribute to the metabolic acidosis. As the pH falls, there is an increase in the unionized proportion of salicylate and a greater diffusion across the blood–brain barrier, exacerbating central nervous system (CNS) toxicity.

Toxicity

The clinical features depend on age, dose ingested and stage of presentation. The elderly and the young are more susceptible to serious toxicity. A metabolic acidosis develops rapidly post ingestion in infants and small children, and a respiratory alkalosis is rarely seen under 4 years of age.

The correlation of symptoms with severity of poisoning is shown in Table 15.7. The more severe the acidosis, the more prominent the CNS effects. Electrolyte abnormalities such as hypokalaemia, hypo- or hypernatraemia, and hypo- or hyperglycaemia also present. Hypoglycaemia is commoner in children. Pulmonary oedema and renal failure are other complications.

Toxic doses and salicylate levels

Knowledge of the ingested dose helps predict which patients are at risk of significant toxicity, and serum salicylate concentrations may guide management strategies. Acute ingestions of more than $120\,mg\,kg^{-1}$ can be expected to cause some symptoms. Ingestions of more than $250\,mg\,kg^{-1}$ will cause moderate to severe toxicity, and doses more than $500\,mg\,kg^{-1}$ usually cause severe toxicity and are potentially fatal. Serum salicylate concentration should be measured at 4h post ingestion and every 2h thereafter until a peak concentration is reached. Levels of greater than $700\,mg\,l^{-1}$ ($5\,mmol\,l^{-1}$) are associated with severe toxicity and are an indication for haemodialysis. However, it is the clinical features that are more important in deciding management, as some patients who present late may have low salicylate concentrations in the presence of significant acid–base and CNS disturbances.

Treatment

Gastric lavage can be considered in adults who present within an hour of a significant overdose. Charcoal should be given to all patients and repeat doses have been recommended as they may enhance elimination. All patients with symptoms will have some degree of dehydration and should be rehydrated with intravenous fluids. Large volumes may be required. Low-dose bicarbonate will enhance elimination in patients with marked toxicity. It is essential that hypokalaemia is also corrected. Serum electrolytes, ABGs and pH and glucose should be checked regularly. Central venous access will help guide fluid replacement in moderate to severe poisoning.

Haemodialysis is the treatment of choice for severe poisoning and significantly increases elimination of salicylate. It also has the advantage of simultaneously correcting fluid and electrolyte abnormalities.

NON-STEROIDAL ANTI-INFLAMMATORY DRUGS

With the increased use and availability of non-steroidal anti-inflammatory agents (NSAIDs) intentional overdoses have increased. Significant morbidity in acute overdose is generally low. However, there are rare reports of large ingestions causing coma, metabolic acidosis, acute renal failure, seizures and death. Usually, supportive treatment is all that is required. The symptoms and signs are largely similar for all NSAIDs in overdose, with the exception of mefenamic acid, which causes convulsions much more commonly than the other agents.

Ibuprofen is the commonest NSAID encountered in overdose. The main symptoms are nausea, vomiting, abdominal pain, diarrhoea and haematemesis. Headache, tinnitus and confusion can also occur. Renal failure is most likely in patients with underlying renal disease. Ibuprofen ingestions of less than $100\,mg\,kg^{-1}$ are unlikely to cause significant symptoms and no treatment is required. For ingestions greater than this, activated charcoal may be given if the patient presents within an hour of ingestion. Adequate hydration should be maintained with intravenous fluids, and electrolyte abnormalities should be corrected. Seizures are treated with diazepam. Patients who have significant symptoms should be admitted for 24h. Patients who are asymptomatic 6h after ingestion can be considered medically fit for discharge.

XANTHINES

Theophylline and aminophylline (a theophylline derivative) are commonly used as adjuvant therapy in asthma and chronic obstructive airways disease. Theophylline has a narrow therapeutic index. Caffeine is a methylxanthine and in toxic doses shares similarities with theophylline poisoning, but serious side-effects are rare.

Toxicity

Gastrointestinal, cardiovascular and metabolic side-effects are commonest. In mild to moderate poisoning there is nausea, vomiting (often severe), haematemesis and diarrhoea. Tachycardia, agitation, dilated pupils, tremor, confusion, hypokalaemia and hyperglycaemia also occur. Severe poisoning is characterized by cardiac arrhythmias and hypotension. Seizures occur, particularly in those with a history of epilepsy, and are associated with significant morbidity. Hyperthermia, rhabdomyolysis, acute compartment syndrome and acute renal failure have all been reported.

Serum theophylline levels

In significant acute ingestions serum theophylline levels should be repeated until the concentration plateaus or starts to fall. A further sample should be drawn 4 h after the peak level to confirm a continuing decline. Serum levels of less than $20\,\text{mg}\,\text{l}^{-1}$ are unlikely to cause toxicity, while patients with levels between 20 and $60\,\text{mg}\,\text{l}^{-1}$ usually experience mild to moderate symptoms. Patients with levels greater than $60\,\text{mg}\,\text{l}^{-1}$ are at risk of severe toxicity.

Sustained-release preparations pose a particular problem as peak serum levels occur anywhere from 1 to 24 h after ingestion (mean 11 h). Peak levels in regular preparations occur 2–8 h (mean 5 h).

Treatment

Treatment is recommended for overdoses greater than 1 g of theophylline in an adult and greater than $15\,\text{mg}\,\text{kg}^{-1}$ in a child after an acute ingestion. Gastric lavage should be considered in patients presenting within an hour after a potentially significant overdose. Repeat doses of activated charcoal are recommended. Whole-bowel irrigation should be considered for significant ingestions of sustained-release preparations. Antiemetics (metoclopramide or ondansetron) should be given for nausea and vomiting and to allow the administration of repeat doses of charcoal. Hypotension usually responds to intravenous fluids or treatment of an underlying arrhythmia, but dopamine or dobutamine can be used if required. Beta-blockade with propranolol is recommended for tachyarrythmias. Lignocaine has been used for ventricular arrhythmias and adenosine can be used for supraventricular tachycardia. Correction of electrolyte abnormalities (hypokalaemia and hypomagnesaemia in particular) is important in minimizing arrhythmogenesis. Diazepam is the first-line treatment for seizures, though persistent seizures mandate intubation, paralysis and mechanical ventilation.

With severe poisoning, more aggressive means to clear serum theophylline are required. Haemoperfusion is more effective than haemodialysis and is the treatment of choice. Charcoal haemoperfusion should be considered in all patients with life-threatening toxicity (seizures and tachyarrhythmias not responding to other therapy).

BETA-BLOCKERS

Beta-blocking drugs are used mainly in the management of hypertension and ischaemic heart disease. They are also prescribed for symptomatic control in hyperthyroidism and anxiety states. They act by competitive antagonism at the beta-adrenergic receptors in the heart, peripheral vasculature, bronchi and elsewhere. There are a large number of different drugs in this class and there are considerable differences in toxicity depending on the individual pharmacological properties. The most important of these properties are lipid solubility, cardioselectivity and anti-arrhythmic activity. Propranolol has high lipid solubility and is a non-selective beta-blocker. Most experience is with propranolol, and the majority of fatalities from beta-blocker overdose have been with this drug. Atenolol and metoprolol are relatively cardioselective with low lipid solubility. Sotalol has anti-arrhythmic activity and ventricular arrhythmias (particularly torsades de pointes) may occur.

Toxicity

Most beta-blockers are rapidly absorbed and serious symptoms usually appear within 30 min to 2 h post ingestion. Symptoms may be delayed if long-acting preparations have been taken. The toxic manifestations are mainly cardiovascular and neurological. A bradycardia is usually the first sign to appear, and various degrees of heart block occur, from first-degree to complete heart block, bundle branch blocks and asystole. Hypotension occurs secondary to bradycardias and myocardial depression. Susceptible patients can develop cardiac failure and pulmonary oedema.

The more lipid-soluble agents have significant neurological manifestations. Alterations in mental status are common, ranging from drowsiness and mild confusion to convulsions and coma. Coma may also be due to cardiovascular collapse. The pupils are dilated and hallucinations have been reported.

Treatment

Gastric lavage and charcoal should be considered in patients who present within an hour of a significant ingestion. If lavage is undertaken, it is wise to premedicate with atropine. Patients who have taken significant overdoses need to be admitted to an intensive care facility. Severely ill patients will need central venous and arterial pressure monitoring to guide treatment. Atropine is given initially for bradyarrhythmias and fluid for hypotension. Glucagon is the most useful antidote and should be given early when signs of haemodynamic compromise occur. It is more effective in reversing the negative inotropic effects than the negative chronotropic effects, but should be used for both as there are few side-effects. Large doses are required.

> High-dose glucagon is a specific antidote in beta-blocker poisoning.

Second-line treatments include isoprenaline and pacing for bradyarrhythmias, and adrenaline for hypotension. Calcium has also been given for hypotension.

> Glucagon in beta-blocker overdose: adults, an initial bolus of 5–10 mg intravenously is given, followed by an infusion or further boluses.

There are successful case reports of the use of prolonged cardiopulmonary resuscitation, bypass and dialysis where other measures have failed. Seizures are treated with diazepam and hypoglycaemia with a glucose infusion.

CALCIUM-CHANNEL BLOCKERS (CCBs)

Calcium-channel blockers prevent the inward movement of calcium from the extracellular space through the slow channels of cell membranes. They have three main sites of action: the myocardial cells, cells within the specialized conducting system of the heart, and the cells of vascular smooth muscle. CCBs thus act as negative inotropes, negative chronotropes and peripheral vasodilators. Different CCBs differ in their predilection for the various sites of action. Verapamil has primarily cardiac effects, causing decreased atrioventricular node conduction and a reduction in myocardial contractility. Nifedipine acts mainly on vascular smooth muscle, leading to dilation of coronary and peripheral arteries and a reduction in blood pressure. Diltiazem has both central and peripheral circulatory actions. The majority of the newer agents (nicardipine, amlodipine, felodipine) have similar effects to nifedipine.

Toxicity

The toxicity seen in CCB overdose is an extension of the therapeutic effects. Verapamil, which is the most toxic in overdose, causes severe hypotension by a combination of heart block, myocardial depression and peripheral vasodilation. There is progressive heart block, characteristically progressing from sinus bradycardia to first-degree heart block, to junctional bradycardia to a slow idioventricular rhythm and finally to asystole. Nifedipine primarily causes hypotension due to peripheral vasodilation, and a bradycardia or reflex tachycardia may occur. Other non-specific symptoms, such as nausea, vomiting and lethargy, can occur with all types. Coma can occur secondary to hypoperfusion.

Treatment

Treatment is indicated for all but the most trivial ingestions. Even a single tablet can be fatal in toddlers. All overdoses of sustained-release preparations, even if asymptomatic, should be admitted to hospital for observation for at least 24 h. Symptomatic patients will need to be admitted to an intensive care facility with continuous ECG monitoring. Gastric lavage is indicated for patients with significant overdoses who present within an hour of ingestion. Atropine should be given prior to lavage to prevent any worsening of bradycardias from an increase in vagal tone. Activated charcoal is advised and multiple doses should be given after sustained-release preparations have been taken.

Calcium is the antidote used for bradycardia, second- and third-degree atrioventricular block and idioventricular rhythms. An initial dose of 10 ml of calcium gluconate or calcium chloride 10% is given, with subsequent doses every few minutes until the rate and blood pressure respond.

Some patients will require an infusion, and serum calcium and other electrolytes should be monitored closely. Atropine should be given in all bradyarrhythmias, but may not be effective until calcium is given. If the heart rate has failed to improve, isoprenaline can be used and ultimately transcutaneous or transvenous pacing may be required.

Hypotension is managed by treating underlying bradyarrhythmias, and with fluid replacement and inotropes. Hypotension secondary to vasodilation usually responds to fluid alone and intravenous calcium can reverse hypotension secondary to myocardial depression. Similarly, glucagon may reverse myocardial depression and hypotension, and should be tried if there is no response to ini-tial measures. All patients with haemodynamic instability need invasive haemodynamic monitoring (arterial line and central venous access).

Digoxin

Digoxin has a narrow therapeutic index and toxic side-effects are not uncommon with routine use. Digoxin binds to and inactivates the myocardial cell membrane sodium–potassium adenosine triphosphate (Na–K-ATPase) pump. This leads to a slowing of conduction through the atrioventricular node and an increased refractory period. It also causes increased intracellular calcium and increased extracellular potassium. The increased intracellular calcium is responsible for increased myocardial automaticity (and the likelihood of developing arrhythmias) and the positive inotropic action seen with digoxin.

Toxicity

The main affects are on the cardiovascular, central nervous and gastrointestinal systems. Almost any rhythm disturbance can occur with digoxin poisoning. Tachyarrhythmias are more common in older patients with chronic toxicity, whereas bradyarrhythmias are more usual in younger patients with healthy hearts. Frequent premature ventricular ectopics and accelerated junctional tachycardias with variable block are common. All grades of atrioventricular block can occur. Ventricular dysrhythmias may occur in older patients with underlying heart disease, and are often refractory.

In acute poisoning abdominal pain, nausea and vomiting (and occasionally diarrhoea) are the first signs of toxicity. Other non-specific symptoms include generalized muscle pains, headache, dizziness, drowsiness, disorientation, delirium and hallucinations. The visual symptoms of diplopia, scotomas, and yellow-green tinting of vision (xanthopsia) are well described. Hyperkalaemia is present in acute overdoses, but serum potassium is usually normal or decreased in chronic toxicity.

Serum digoxin levels are not useful in predicting severity of toxicity. Some patients with predisposing factors for digoxin poisoning and clinical toxicity will have serum levels within the therapeutic range. Conversely, others with high levels may not show any signs of toxicity, particularly if the level is taken before significant tissue distribution has occurred. None the less, the higher the serum digoxin level the greater the likelihood of toxicity.

Treatment

Activated charcoal and gastric lavage should be considered for those presenting within an hour of large deliberate overdoses. Patients may need to be premedicated with atropine prior to lavage. Symptomatic bradycardia is treated initially with atropine and then digoxin-specific antibodies (Fab fragments). In the absence of Fab fragments a pacemaker (external or transvenous) may be needed. Magnesium enhances the activity of the Na–K-ATPase pump and may be a life-saving treatment for digoxin-induced ventricular arryhthmias. Some anti-arrythmic agents (phenytoin and lignocaine) have been used in the past on the basis that they depress ventricular automaticity and increase the fibrillation threshold. However, Fab fragments, if available, are the treatment of choice for ventricular arryhthmias that do not respond immediately to conventional treatment.

Dig-Fab fragments

Dig-Fab fragments are the Fab fragment of IgG from sheep immunized with digoxin and are less immunogenic than the original digoxin-specific antibodies. Dig-Fab binds to digoxin in the vascular and interstitial spaces, creating a gradient between intravascular and extracellular areas. Treatment with Dig-Fab rapidly reverses conduction defects, ventricular dysrhythmias and hyperkalaemia. A clinical response is usually seen within 20–30 min.

Serum potassium should be corrected by conventional methods for rapid correction.

QUININE

Quinine is used for nocturnal leg cramps and in the treatment of malaria. Overdose carries a risk of significant morbidity and mortality.

Toxicity

Quinine toxicity (originally known as cinchonism) is characterized by visual deficits and blindness, tinnitus and deafness and a range of other effects. Visual effects are due to a direct toxic effect on the retina and include blurred vision, loss of peripheral vision and blindness. Pupils may be fixed and dilated. Other central nervous system symptoms include headache and dizziness, confusion, drowsiness and seizures. Nausea, vomiting, abdominal pain and diarrhoea all result from a local irritant effect of quinine. Quinine also has anti-arrhythmic activity and has cardiovascular effects similar to tricyclic antidepressant poisoning, with prolongation of the QRS and QT intervals, followed by heart block, torsade de pointes and hypotension. This is usually the cause of death in fatal overdoses. Hypoglycaemia can occur, and renal failure has been reported.

> Quinine may cause life-threatening cardiac arrythmias.

Treatment

Gastric lavage can be considered for patients who present within an hour of significant overdoses. Activated charcoal is recommended for patients who have ingested more than $20 \, mg \, kg^{-1}$. Repeat doses enhance elimination. Hypotension is treated with intravenous fluids initially. Sodium bicarbonate may attenuate QRS prolongation, and is the initial treatment for arrhythmias. Magnesium, isoprenaline and overdrive pacing have all been suggested for torsade de pointes. All patients should

be observed until the ECG changes have resolved. No treatment has been shown to have any effect on the visual symptoms and over 10% of patients can have residual visual deficits.

PHENYTOIN

Phenytoin acts by blocking voltage-gated sodium channels and thereby suppressing repetitive neuronal impulses. It also has anti-arrhythmic activity (like lignocaine). Phenytoin has a narrow therapeutic index and side-effects with regular treatment are not uncommon. It also interacts with a large number of other drugs that can either increase (amiodarone, cimetidine, sulphonamides) or decrease (alcohol, theophylline, carbamazepine) its activity. Serious morbidity after oral overdoses is rare, and the mainstay of treatment is good supportive care.

Toxicity

Symptoms occur 1–2 h post ingestion and can persist for 3–4 days after significant overdoses. Nystagmus on lateral gaze is usually the first sign of toxicity and corresponds with serum levels of more than $20 \, \mu g \, ml^{-1}$ (normal therapeutic range $10–20 \, \mu g \, ml^{-1}$). Nystagmus is followed by lethargy and increasing drowsiness, ataxia, slurred speech, confusion, coma and apnoea with large doses. Deep tendon reflexes are often brisk and the pupils are dilated and reactive. Patients are unable to walk or even stand unaided. Acute dystonias, opisthotonic posturing and involuntary movements are occasionally seen. Paradoxically, brief generalized seizures may occur at high levels, but these are rare.

Treatment

Treatment is largely supportive. Charcoal should be given to all patients and repeat doses are recommended for significant ingestions as they may enhance excretion. All patients should receive generous intravenous fluids. Seizures are treated with diazepam. Diazepam may also be needed to prevent patients from injuring themselves if they are agitated and confused. Phenytoin has a long half-life in overdose and it may take a number of days before the clinical signs resolve and the patient can be discharged home.

CARBAMAZEPINE

Carbamazepine is the treatment of choice for simple and complex partial seizures and for tonic–clonic seizures. It has chemical similarities to both phenytoin and the tricyclic antidepressants, and shares features of both in overdose.

Toxicity

Nystagmus, ataxia and drowsiness are early symptoms. Patients may hallucinate and become agitated and confused. Pupils are dilated and dystonic posturing and athetoid movements are common. Seizures and coma occur; carbamazepine also has anti-arrhythmic activity and causes hypotension, bradyarrhythmias and prolongation of the QT and QRS intervals. Respiratory depression and apnoea can occur with large overdoses. Delayed onset of symptoms can occur with the use of slow-release preparations and slow absorption from gastric concretions.

Treatment

This is symptomatic and supportive care. Gastric lavage and activated charcoal should be considered in patients who present within an hour of significant ingestions. Repeat-dose activated charcoal is recommended for significant ingestions. Hypotension should be corrected with intravenous fluids and inotropes if required. Seizures are treated with diazepam. The dystonic effects are not life threatening and no specific treatment is required. Charcoal haemoperfusion has been used effectively in a number of cases where adequate supportive care was failing.

TRICYCLIC ANTIDEPRESSANTS

Tricyclic antidepressants (TCADs) are widely prescribed for depression in the UK, though with the introduction of the safer serotonin re-uptake inhibitors they should be less commonly seen in future years. They are also used for anxiety, phobias, obsessive–compulsive disorder and nocturnal enuresis in children. TCADs are the commonest cause of drug overdose-related death from prescribed medication in the UK, North America and Australia. Over 90% of successful TCAD suicides die before reaching hospital.

Toxicity

TCADs are non-selective agents that have a number of different pharmacological actions. The antidepressant action is thought to be due to blocking of the re-uptake of the excitatory neurotransmitters noradrenaline and serotonin within the brain. They also bind to many other receptors, including histamine, alpha-adrenergic receptors, gamma-aminobutyric acid (GABA) and muscarinic cholinergic receptors. Histamine-receptor blockade causes sedation. Blockade of alpha-receptors causes vasodilation, GABA-receptor blockade predisposes to seizures and muscarinic-receptor blockade produces anticholinergic symptoms. TCADs also have a membrane-stabilizing effect on the heart and share the anti-arrhythmic and pro-arrhythmic effects of some anti-arrhythmic drugs (quinidine).

There are some differences in toxicity between the various agents, but doses of $15\,mg\,kg^{-1}$ are generally regarded as potentially fatal. Dothiepin is significantly more toxic and causes seizures more often and following smaller ingestions than other agents. Lofepramine is somewhat safer and less cardiotoxic in overdose.

The toxic effects of TCAD overdoses fit broadly into three categories: anticholinergic effects, central nervous system effects, and cardiovascular effects. Anticholinergic effects are prominent early, with tachycardia, dry mouth, dilated pupils, blurring of vision, urinary retention, agitation, hallucinations and drowsiness. In more serious ingestions there is progressive CNS depression with myoclonic jerks, seizures and coma. Hyperreflexia is present and can be a marker for increased seizure risk. Cardiovascular toxicity manifests as arryhthmias and myocardial depression. Widening of the QRS complex is the most consistent feature of TCAD cardiotoxicity and various studies have attempted to equate QRS width with risk of significant toxicity. Unfortunately it is neither specific nor sensitive. Hypotension is usually due to a combination of alpha-receptor blockade-induced vasodilation and direct myocardial depression. Intravenous fluids are often all that is required.

The three most consistent clinical features associated with significant poisoning are tachycardia, an altered level of consciousness and a widened QRS.

Treatment

The first priority is ensuring adequacy of airway, ventilation and circulation. All patients need intravenous fluids. Gastric lavage is recommended in patients who present within an hour of ingestion and in all comatose patients (after intubation to secure the airway). Activated charcoal is given after lavage. Repeat doses are generally of little benefit. Sodium bicarbonate acts as an antidote by raising serum pH and thereby increasing the plasma protein binding of the TCADs and reducing the active concentration of the drug. Bicarbonate (1–$2\,ml\,kg^{-1}$ of 8.4% $NaHCO_3$) should be given initially and subsequent doses titrated to maintain the pH in a range of 7.50–7.55. This can also be achieved by mild hyperventilation in intubated patients. Indications for sodium bicarbonate include seizures, QRS widening, arrythmias and persistent hypotension.

> Bicarbonate is effective in treating tricyclic-induced arrythmias and seizures.

Bicarbonate is the treatment of choice for arrhythmias. Other drug treatment is best avoided. If unresponsive to bicarbonate, DC shock should be considered. Magnesium can be used to treat torsade de pointes. Standard advanced cardiac life-support protocols should be followed if cardiac arrest occurs, and prolonged cardiopulmonary resuscitation has been associated with full recovery in a number of cases.

Seizures are treated with diazepam. Some severely poisoned patients may develop an anticholinergic delirium with visual and auditory hallucinations during the recovery phase of their illness, and this can last for a few days. Simple reassurance will often suffice, but diazepam and haloperidol can be used.

All patients should be observed with ECG monitoring for at least 6 h post ingestion. Patients who are asymptomatic and have a normal ECG after this time can be considered medically fit for discharge. All others require continued observation.

SELECTIVE SEROTONIN RE-UPTAKE INHIBITORS

The selective serotonin re-uptake inhibitors (SSRIs) have become the commonest prescribed antidepressant agents over the last few years. This is due in part to the low incidence of side-effects and the relative safety of these agents compared with older antidepressants. The SSRIs most commonly used in the UK are fluoxetine, paroxetine, sertraline, fluvoxamine and citalopram. They are also used for obsessive–compulsive disorder, bulimia nervosa and panic attacks.

> SSRIs are relatively non-toxic antidepressants.

Toxicity

When taken alone in overdose, the SSRIs have relatively low toxicity. However, when taken with certain other drugs they may cause the serotonin syndrome, which is potentially fatal (see below).

The commonest symptoms seen after SSRI overdose are nausea, vomiting, diarrhoea, headache, dizziness, tremor and drowsiness. Convulsions and coma may occur with large overdoses. The SSRIs have minimal cardiotoxicity, although sinus tachycardia is common.

Treatment

Care is symptomatic and supportive. Charcoal can be given to those presenting within an hour of ingesting a significant number of tablets. Patients should be observed for at least 6 h. Symptomatic patients should have ECG monitoring.

Serotonin syndrome

The serotonin syndrome is caused by the simultaneous administration of two or more agents that increase serotonin availability in the brain. It occurs from medication errors and in overdoses. It has been most commonly caused by the combination of a serotinergic agent (e.g. fluoxetine) and the monoamine oxidase inhibitors (MAOIs). The clinical picture shares similarities with the neuroleptic malignant syndrome and the heatstroke-type syndrome occasionally caused by Ecstasy

(MDMA – 3,4-methylenedioxymethamphetamine). It is characterized by changes in mental status, autonomic nervous system function and neuromuscular signs. The serotonin syndrome usually occurs within 2 h of the precipitating agent, and will resolve within 6–24 h of removal of this agent. However, severe complications can occur, and include hyperthermia, seizures, disseminated intravascular coagulation (DIC), rhabdomyolysis and death.

Treatment

Care is symptomatic and supportive. Generous hydration with intravenous fluids is important. Diazepam is used for delirium and agitation. Paracetamol and simple cooling measures are used for hyperthermia. If the core temperature is above 40°C dantrolene is given. If this fails, the patient needs to be electively paralysed (with a non-depolarizing agent) and mechanically ventilated.

NEUROLEPTICS

The neuroleptics are a diverse group of drugs used in the treatment of schizophrenia and other psychoses. The most widely used agents include chlorpromazine, thioridazine, haloperidol, droperidol, clozapine and sulpiride. The antiemetics prochlorperazine and promethazine (phenothiazine derivatives such as chlorpromazine and thioridizine) have similar effects when taken in overdose.

Neuroleptic toxicity may closely resemble that of tricyclic antidepressants.

Toxicity

The therapeutic action of the neuroleptics is blockade of dopaminergic receptors in the central nervous system. However, the neuroleptics also have activity at alpha-adrenergic, muscarinic and histamine receptors. Blockade of the alpha-receptors leads to vasodilation and hypotension, muscarinic receptor antagonism results in typical anticholinergic symptoms and histamine-receptor blockade causes sedation. Some neuroleptics also have a membrane-stabilizing action on the heart similar to some anti-arrhythmics (quinidine). Toxicity

in overdose varies, with central nervous system and cardiovascular effects being the most serious. For example, thioridazine appears to have a relatively higher incidence of arrhythmias in overdose than does chlorpromazine, which causes more sedation. Neuroleptic malignant syndrome is a tetrad of fever, rigidity, altered sensorium and autonomic instability that occurs with routine neuroleptic treatment and is not discussed further here.

Dopamine antagonism causes abnormal movement disorders such as dystonias, dyskinesia and akathisia. Tremor, hyper-reflexia, opisthotonus, oculogyric crisis and drooling all occur. These effects can be relatively mild in some overdoses, possibly due to a competing anticholinergic effect.

Anticholinergic effects are tachycardia, dry mouth, dry skin and dilated pupils. Patients with severe toxicity who are unconscious on presentation often develop an anticholinergic delirium in the recovery phase, which can persist for a number of days. Hypotension occurs secondary to alpha-receptor blockade. Cardiac toxicity is variable. Bradycardia and a wide QRS indicate severe toxicity, and the pathophysiology is similar to that seen in TCAD overdose.

With large neuroleptic ingestions there is rapid absorption of the drug leading to a decreasing level of consciousness and coma. Seizures are not uncommon and patients with seizures are often noted to have been hyper-reflexic or to have had myoclonic jerking.

Treatment

Treatment is supportive. Gastric lavage should be considered in unconscious patients (after ABC stabilization) and in alert patients who present within an hour of a significant ingestion. Charcoal is also recommended after significant ingestions. Intravenous fluids (normal saline) are given to all. Diazepam is used for seizures and for an anticholinergic delirium. Arrhythmia management follows the same principles as for TCAD overdose, with intravenous bicarbonate being first-line treatment. Other drug treatments are controversial. Magnesium is used for torsade de pointes, but its calcium-channel-blocking activity may aggravate the hypotension and heart block that can occur in neuroleptic poisoning.

Dystonic reactions are idiosyncratic reactions that occur with neuroleptic treatment and are not dose related. They can be treated with benztropine or procyclidine for adults or diphenhydramine for children.

Patients who are asymptomatic and have a normal ECG 6 h after the overdose are medically fit for discharge.

ANTIHISTAMINES

Antihistamines are widely used in the symptomatic relief of allergies and in the prevention of motion sickness and vertigo. The most commonly used preparations include chlorpheniramine, cyclizine, astemizole, cetirizine, loratidine and terfenadine. Serious toxicity after overdose is uncommon.

Toxicity

Antihistamines block H_1-receptors in the periphery and in the central nervous system. Many of the older agents also have anticholinergic activity, blocking muscarinic acetylcholine receptors.

Most symptoms are minor and are due to anticholinergic effects. Patients can be drowsy or agitated and confused, with dilated pupils, hyperreflexia and myoclonic jerks. Seizures and coma are infrequent complications. Other anticholinergic side-effects include tachycardia, dry mouth, ileus, urinary retention and hyperthermia. Hypotension can occur secondary to vasodilation. Some antihistamines, particularly terfenadine, are chemically related to the TCADs, and ECG QRS and QT prolongation and arryhthmias similar to those with TCAD poisoning have been reported. However, significant arryhthmias are uncommon. The newer non-sedating antihistamines are more selective for peripheral H_1-receptors, and usually have few CNS or anticholinergic toxic features.

Treatment

Care is symptomatic and supportive. Intravenous fluids and sedation are all that is usually required. Diazepam is used for agitation and delirium. Hallucinations may require haloperidol. The management of arryhthmias is the same as for TCAD overdose, with administration of bicarbonate to a pH of between 7.5 and 7.55. Torsade de pointes can be treated with magnesium and overdrive pacing. Patients who are asymptomatic and have a normal ECG at 6 h post ingestion can be medically discharged.

ANTICHOLINERGIC SYNDROME

Specific antimuscarinic agents (orphenadrine, benzhexol, benztropine and procyclidine) are used in the treatment of Parkinson's disease and for drug-induced extrapyramidal side-effects. They are commonly taken in overdose by patients with major psychiatric illness. In addition, a large number of other drugs have anticholinergic activity and can cause anticholinergic toxicity. These include TCADs, phenothiazines, antihistamines and antispasmodics. All these agents can cause an anticholinergic syndrome.

Toxicity

The signs and symptoms of anticholinergic toxicity are a result of blocking the central and peripheral cholinergic receptors. Depending on the drug involved, antagonism of muscarinic, nicotinic or both receptors can occur. The central effects of cholinergic blockade include agitation, confusion, disorientation, delirium, hallucinations and seizures. The peripheral effects include tachycardia, arryhthmias, hypo- or hypertension, dry mouth, dilated pupils, decreased gastrointestinal motility, urinary retention, decreased sweating, hyperthermia and vasodilation.

> The classic anticholinergic syndrome presentation is often remembered as 'Hot as Hell, blind as a bat, dry as a bone, red as a beet, mad as a hatter'.

Treatment

Treatment is supportive, with diazepam for sedation and intravenous fluids being all that is usually required. Malignant arryhthmias are managed as in TCAD poisoning. Physostigmine (a reversible acetylcholinesterase inhibitor) will reverse the anticholinergic effects but has no effect on the membrane-stabilizing (cardiac) or antihistamine effects of some of these drugs. As the anticholinergic effects are not normally life threatening and as its use has been associated with severe complications (seizures, heart block and asystole) in the past, physostigmine is not routinely recommended.

LITHIUM

Lithium salts are used in the management of mania, manic–depressive illness and recurrent depression. Lithium has a narrow therapeutic index and toxicity from long-term treatment and drug interactions is commoner than acute overdose. This is usually due to reduced renal clearance of lithium because of renal impairment or co-administration of drugs (diuretics, NSAIDs).

Toxicity

The mechanisms by which lithium toxicity occurs are poorly understood. Symptoms such as polyuria and tremor can occur within the therapeutic range. With increasing levels, further symptoms appear. These include nausea, vomiting, diarrhoea, ataxia, weakness and dysarthria, and later myoclonic jerks and confusion. In severe cases seizures, coma and acute renal failure occur. Hypotension can occur secondary to dehydration. Sinus node dysfunction and prolongation of the QT interval are often seen, but clinically significant arryhthmias are uncommon.

Serum lithium levels

The therapeutic range for lithium is $0.4–1.2\,mmol\,l^{-1}$ and concentrations of greater than $2\,mmol\,l^{-1}$ are usually associated with significant toxicity. However, in acute overdose much higher concentrations can occur without symptoms because significant tissue penetration has yet to occur.

Treatment

The mainstay of treatment is good supportive care. Gastric lavage can be considered in patients who present within an hour of a significant ingestion. Charcoal does not bind lithium and has no role. All patients require generous fluid replacement with normal saline. Haemodialysis may be indicated in severe poisonings, following expert advice.

Following an acute ingestion, if serial lithium levels taken more than 4 h apart show a decline, the asymptomatic patient can be discharged if the lithium level is less than $1.5\,mmol\,l^{-1}$ and a sustained-release preparation was not involved. All symptomatic patients require admission.

IRON POISONING

Acute iron poisoning is usually due to accidental ingestion of iron supplements or multivitamin preparations by small children who mistake them for sweets. Most ingestions are minor and patients will be asymptomatic or have minor symptoms only. Large overdoses are extremely toxic and fatalities occur.

Significant iron poisoning may follow ingestion of some multivitamin preparations.

Toxicity

Iron salts are directly caustic to the gastrointestinal mucosa, causing inflammation, ulceration, bleeding and perforation. Systemic toxicity also occurs. Under normal circumstances iron absorbed from the gastrointestinal tract is transported in the blood bound to the protein transferrin. The total amount of iron with which transferrin can bind is known as the total iron-binding capacity (TIBC). The TIBC is far greater than the total serum iron, and there is normally no 'free' iron circulating in the blood. In iron overdose the TIBC is overwhelmed and unbound iron enters the cells, interfering with mitochondrial oxidative phosphorylation and promoting the formation of free radicals, leading to lipid peroxidation and cell death. This leads to multiorgan dysfunction, particularly in the liver (where much of the iron accumulates), but also in the kidneys, heart and brain. The natural history of significant iron poisoning is often divided into four stages (Table 15.8).

Estimating toxicity

Symptoms are unlikely when a dose of less than $20\,mg\,kg^{-1}$ of elemental iron is ingested. Serious toxicity can be anticipated if a dose of more than $60\,mg\,kg^{-1}$ of elemental iron has been taken.

Table 15.8: Clinical presentation of iron poisoning

I	30–60 min post ingestion. Nausea, vomiting, haematemesis, abdominal pain, diarrhoea (often haemorrhagic), lethargy, hypotension. Metabolic acidosis, leucocytosis, hyperglycaemia.
II	Latent phase. Begins after 6–12 h and not always seen. During this stage the early gastrointestinal symptoms settle and iron is deposited systemically. This can lead to an apparent improvement of symptoms and give false reassurance.
III	Begins 12–24 h after ingestion and earlier in severe poisonings. Multi-organ failure. Cerebral dysfunction leads to increasing lethargy, convulsions and coma. Cardiovascular collapse occurs due to hypovolaemia, vasodilation and myocardial depression. Renal and hepatic failure may develop, with coagulopathy and hypoglycaemia.
IV	Occurs weeks after recovery from significant poisoning and is due to gastrointestinal scarring causing gastric outlet or small bowel obstruction.

However, accurate assessments of ingested doses are not often available. Serum iron levels usually peak 4–6 h post ingestion. Patients with levels greater than $300 \, \mu g \, dl^{-1}$ ($55 \, \mu mol \, l^{-1}$) are at risk of significant toxicity.

Abdominal X-rays may show ingested iron but up to 50% of patients who develop toxicity will have negative X-rays. The X-ray does, however, confirm a significant ingestion and indicates that continued absorption may occur.

Treatment

In significant poisonings patients are often hypotensive owing to a combination of gastrointestinal losses and peripheral vasodilation. Adequate volume resuscitation is essential. Gastric lavage can be considered in patients who present within an hour of ingestion of doses greater than $20 \, mg \, kg^{-1}$ of elemental iron. The decontamination procedure of choice is whole-bowel irrigation with polyethelyene glycol. Ileus, bowel obstruction and significant haemorrhage are contraindications to whole-bowel irrigation. Charcoal does not bind iron and has no role. Hypoglycaemia should be corrected if present.

Desferrioxamine is a potent, specific chelator of extra- and intracellular ferric iron. It combines with iron to form water-soluble ferrioxamine, which is excreted in the urine giving the urine a rose-wine colour. Desferrioxamine is given as an intravenous infusion, though rapid infusion rates can cause hypotension. This is best prevented by adequate volume resuscitation. Desferrioxamine infusion should be continued until systemic toxicity has resolved and serum iron levels are normal or low.

> Desferrioxamine is a specific antidote in severe iron poisoning.

Patients with a normal abdominal X-ray and serum iron level, who have remained asymptomatic up to 6 h post ingestion, are unlikely to develop significant toxicity and can be allowed home.

CARBON MONOXIDE POISONING

Carbon monoxide (CO) poisoning is the commonest cause of death from poisoning in the UK. In 1996 in England and Wales 887 deaths were attributed to carbon monoxide poisoning. The majority of deaths are suicides from car exhaust fumes. Carbon monoxide is a colourless, odourless, tasteless, non-irritant gas which is formed when there is incomplete combustion of carbonaceous matter. The commonest sources are car exhaust fumes, faulty domestic heaters and fire smoke.

Toxicity

CO toxicity is due to a combination of impaired oxygen delivery and utilization. Carbon monoxide rapidly diffuses across alveoli and binds with haemoglobin with an affinity of more than 200 times that of oxygen to form carboxyhaemoglobin (COHb). This leads to a reduction in the oxygen-carrying capacity of the blood and tissue hypoxia. However, it is felt that the predominant toxic effect of CO is due to the poisoning of intracellular oxygen-carrying haem proteins such as cytochrome A3 and myoglobin. This results in cellular injury, which manifests first in those tissues with the highest energy requirements (brain and heart).

The toxicity of carbon monoxide is predominantly as a cellular poison.

The presentation of CO poisoning depends on the concentration of CO and duration of exposure. The initial symptoms of CO exposure are notoriously non-specific. Frontal headache, dizziness, lethargy, nausea and vomiting are the first symptoms to appear and have frequently been misdiagnosed as 'flu' or other complaints.

Symptoms, particularly with chronic poisoning, are non-specific.

With increasing levels of COHb more marked CNS and cardiovascular symptoms appear. CNS signs include impaired cognitive function, memory deficits, gait disturbance, parkinsonism, increasing drowsiness, seizures and coma. Myocardial ischaemia occurs and patients with pre-existing ischaemic heart disease are particularly susceptible. Arrhythmias, pulmonary oedema and hypotension due to myocardial depression are other complications. ST segment depression on ECG is often seen in severe poisoning, and ST elevation can also occur (Table 15.9).

Delayed neuropsychiatric problems after CO poisoning are well recognized and occur in up to 10% of patients. Headache, memory impairment and personality changes are most frequent. These usually appear within the first few weeks.

Normal individuals have up to 5% carboxyhaemoglobin (COHb) in the blood and heavy smokers can have up to 8%. Once the patient is removed from the source of CO, blood levels start to fall. CO has a half-life of about 4 h when breathing room air, but this is reduced to around 90 min when the patient is given 100% oxygen. For this reason, COHb levels taken in hospital can only confirm the diagnosis but do not reflect severity of exposure. Recently, initial acidosis has been shown to be a good correlate with severity of poisoning. A COHb level of more than 10% is diagnostic of CO poisoning but a normal level does not exclude the diagnosis. It is important to remember that oxygen saturation measured by pulse oximetry can be misleading in CO poisoning as it does not distinguish between oxyhaemoglobin and COHb and can be falsely elevated. Likewise arterial blood gases can be misleading as they calculate the oxygen saturation on the basis of PaO_2 and pH.

Normal oximetry and PaO_2 do not exclude carbon monoxide poisoning.

A CO-oximeter uses spectophotometry to measure the different forms of haemoglobin (oxy, deoxy, meth and carboxyhaemoglobin). Hence, arterial blood gases measured by CO-oximeter are essential to give the true values for oxyhaemoglobin (oxygen saturation) and COHb.

Treatment

All patients should receive 100% oxygen to assist elimination of CO. Patients should continue with 100% oxygen for at least 6 h and until they are asymptomatic and the serum COHb is less than 5%. Hyperbaric oxygen treatment remains controversial. There are a number of reasons why hyperbaric oxygen may be useful (Table 15.10). First, hyperbaric oxygen promotes more rapid elimination of CO (the COHb half-life is reduced to 25 min with 100% oxygen at 3 bar) and increases the amount of dissolved oxygen in plasma. Second,

Table 15.9: Clinical features of carbon monoxide poisoning

Peak % COHb	Clinical features
0–10	Usually none
10–20	Headache
20–40	Severe headache, nausea, vomiting, dizziness, confusion
40–60	Syncope, seizures, coma
>60	Hypotension, respiratory failure, death

Table 15.10: Current indications for hyperbaric oxygen therapy

Loss of consciousness at any time
Any neurological sign or symptom other than headache
Cardiac arrhythmia/ischaemia
COHb greater than 20%
Pregnancy

hyperbaric oxygen has been shown to reduce the free radical concentration, and this may prevent further injury and the development of some of the delayed neurological sequelae.

CYANIDE

Cyanide poisoning usually occurs by inhalation when hydrogen cyanide is released after combustion of polyurethane, vinyl or other plastics in a house fire. Poisoning can also occur after ingestion of cyanide salts, or iatrogenically after excess use of intravenous sodium nitroprusside. Cyanide salts can also be absorbed through the skin. Some plants and fruit kernels contain significant amounts of cyanide.

Toxicity

Cyanide is a potent cellular toxin and acts by binding and inhibiting the function of important metal-containing enzymes, particularly those that contain ferric iron. This leads to disruption of mitochondrial oxidative phosphorylation by blocking the cytochrome oxidase enzyme. Cells are prevented from using oxygen, causing severe tissue hypoxia despite the presence of adequate oxygen. Anaerobic metabolism produces large amounts of lactic acid and a severe acidosis.

Absorption of cyanide following inhalational exposure is almost immediate, occurring within 10–15 min after ingestion. Initial signs and symptoms depend on the concentration of cyanide inhaled or the dose ingested. The clinical features are similar to those of hypoxia except the patient is not cyanotic (unless a respiratory arrest has occurred).

Usual initial symptoms include anxiety, dizziness, headache, palpitations, dyspnoea and lethargy. Initial cardiac effects are a sinus tachycardia, atrial dysrhythmias and ventricular ectopics. With progressive poisoning there is bradycardia, apnoea and asystolic arrest. Seizures, coma and pulmonary oedema also occur with severe poisoning. Arterial blood gases, electrolytes and a serum lactate should be taken. Significant poisoning will cause an elevated anion gap metabolic acidosis (due to raised lactate). The PaO_2 is normal, calculated O_2 saturation is normal and the oxygen saturation by CO-oximetry is normal or slightly decreased (there is a small amount of cyanide binding to haemoglobin). This is in contrast to carbon monoxide poisoning and methaemoglobinaemia, where oxygen saturation measured by CO-oximetry is significantly reduced (due to binding with haemoglobin), leading to a large 'saturation gap' between the calculated oxygen saturation and oxygen saturation measured by CO-oximetry.

Treatment

Supportive care with 100% oxygen, intravenous access and ECG monitoring is essential. Contaminated clothing must be removed and exposed skin washed (with appropriate precautions to avoid contaminating others).

In patients who are mildly symptomatic, supportive care is all that is required unless their mental status deteriorates or they become significantly acidotic.

Previously, antidote therapy was reserved for patients with moderate to severe toxicity because the specific antidotes for cyanide poisoning have significant side-effects themselves. In the UK, dicobalt edetate (Kelocyanor) was first-line treatment for severe, confirmed cyanide poisonings. More recently vitamin B_{12} in large doses has been shown to be a safer and effective alternative. Significant acidosis is treated with bicarbonate. Expert advice is essential.

CORROSIVES

Strong acids and alkalis are present in a large number of household products and are widely used in industry. Examples include sodium and potassium hydroxides (cleaning products) and sulphuric acid (battery acid, drain cleaners). Accidental exposures are common and they can cause significant local tissue destruction if splashed on the skin or ingested. Children are frequently reported to have ingested corrosive substances, but serious side-effects are rare. The extent of injury depends on the agent involved, the volume and the concentration. Hence, identification of the particular product is important.

Most acids and alkalis are irritant and the stronger agents are corrosive. Strong alkalis cause a liquefactive necrosis with saponification of fat and tissue dehydration. Strong acids cause a coagulation necrosis. The formation of a coagulum of damaged tissue tends to limit the penetrating ability of acids, whereas with liquefaction necrosis continuing penetration by alkali can produce further injury after exposure has ceased. However, deep burns still occur with concentrated acid exposures.

Ingestions

Patients who have ingested either acid or alkali can present with facial burns, drooling, oropharyngeal pain, dysphagia, vomiting, haematemesis and epigastric pain. Hoarseness and dyspnoea may indicate laryngeal oedema. Alkalis tend to cause most severe corrosive effects to the oesophagus, whereas acids usually affect the stomach more severely. Severe ingestions can result in oesophageal or gastric perforation. It is important to remember that oesophageal or gastric injury can occur in the absence of oral burns.

Acids are also well absorbed and may have systemic effects, including a metabolic acidosis, hypotension, acute renal failure and DIC. Alkaline ingestions are not usually associated with significant systemic effects.

Treatment

The majority of patients will require no treatment other than reassurance, and oral fluids can be given unless there is evidence of significant upper gastrointestinal tract injury. Patients with respiratory distress require urgent airway assessment.

Gastric lavage is contraindicated.

Neutralizing chemicals should never be given as they may exacerbate tissue damage. In large acid ingestions, nasogastric aspiration of the stomach contents can be considered. Patients with signs and symptoms of significant upper gastrointestinal tract burns should have intravenous fluids and analgesia, and endoscopy should be arranged within 12–24 h to quantify the severity of the injury. Patients with evidence of perforation or massive gastrointestinal haemorrhage will need surgery. The possibility of stricture formation and

an increased predisposition to cancer are recognized long-term complications.

For information on ocular and cutaneous chemical burns see Chapters 28 and 36.

Never give neutralizing chemicals in acid or alkali poisonings.

PESTICIDES

Organophosphates

Organophosphates are used in insecticides for agricultural and domestic use. They are also the principal toxins in nerve gases (Sarin). Poisoning with organophosphate insecticides is a significant problem in many developing countries but is fortunately rare in the UK.

Organophosphates are very toxic chemicals and act by binding to the acetylcholinesterase enzyme, leading to an increase in acetylcholine at nerve endings and the neuromuscular junction. This causes an initial stimulation of autonomic receptors (cholinergic crisis) and a depolarizing block at the neuromuscular junction and paralysis. Carbamates are the other major group of insecticides in common use and have the same mechanism of action as organophosphates, except that the carbamate–cholinesterase bond is reversible and usually reverses spontaneously within 4–8 h.

Toxicity

Organophosphates are rapidly absorbed by dermal, oral and respiratory routes. Initial presentation depends on the agent involved, concentration, and the route of exposure. After significant exposures, symptoms of toxicity will usually appear within 4 h. Nerve gases produce symptoms within minutes. The symptomatology is best understood by considering the mechanism of action. An increase in acetylcholine at the muscarinic cholinergic receptors leads to over-stimulation of the parasympathetic nervous system, with the features noted in Table 15.11.

Over-stimulation of nicotinic receptors causes tachycardia, hypertension and sweating. Accumulation of acetylcholine at the neuromuscular junction causes initial stimulation followed by depolarization

Table 15.11: DUMBELS mnemonic for signs of cholinergic excess

Diarrhoea
Urination
Miosis
Bronchospasm
Emesis
Lacrimation
Salivation

and paralysis. This appears first as fasciculations, cramps and muscle weakness. Central nervous system (CNS) effects include delirium, coma and seizures. Most deaths are due to respiratory failure. Any patient who is unable to walk unaided or has any CNS signs has had a significant toxic exposure.

Treatment

Treating staff should wear protective clothing. The patient's clothes should be removed and destroyed and the patient should be showered in a designated decontamination area. As always, maintenance of an adequate airway, ventilation and circulation takes priority. Activated charcoal should be given to all patients after oral ingestion of organophosphates. Gastric lavage can be considered in those presenting early, but antidotal therapy should be given first.

Atropine acts as an antidote by competitively blocking the action of acetylcholine at the muscarinic receptors. An initial dose of 2 mg is given, followed by repeat doses until there is evidence of adequate atropinization (pupils dilated, tachycardia and absence of oropharyngeal secretions). Large doses are often required.

The other antidote is pralidoxime, which 'reactivates' cholinesterases by binding to the organophosphates and removing them from the enzyme. It is indicated in moderate to severe poisoning but is only of use in the first 36 h (after this time the organophosphate–enzyme complex 'ages' irreversibly, destroying the cholinesterase). Diazepam is used for symptom control (anxiety, seizures) and may attenuate the toxic effects.

Plasma cholinesterase or red blood cell cholinesterase are sensitive markers of exposure but are less useful in guiding management.

PARAQUAT

Paraquat is used in weed-killers and is extremely toxic if ingested. Granular preparations for garden use contain 2.5% paraquat and severe poisoning is uncommon. However, commercial concentrated liquid preparations with 10–20% paraquat are used in agriculture and a single mouthful can be fatal.

Toxicity

Toxic exposures can be separated into three groups depending on the dose ingested. Mild poisonings can occur after ingestion of dilute solutions. Patients may be asymptomatic or have vomiting and diarrhoea, and usually make a full recovery. More severe poisonings present initially with oropharyngeal burns and gastrointestinal symptoms, as paraquat has a direct corrosive effect. This is followed by multi-organ failure and death. Significant paraquat ingestion and absorption leads to the generation of free oxygen radicals which cause lipid peroxidation, damaging cell membranes and leading to cell death. The lung is the most severely affected target organ. For this reason oxygen treatment should be avoided in the early stages. Some patients who have taken intermediate doses survive this phase but go on to develop pulmonary fibrosis and respiratory failure over the next few weeks. This is usually fatal.

Treatment

Activated charcoal should be given immediately. No specific treatment has been shown to improve outcome so care is largely symptomatic and supportive. Oxygen should be avoided in the initial stages as it may aggravate pulmonary toxicity by enhancing free-radical generation.

Paraquat absorption can be tested by a qualitative urine test. If this is negative 2–6 h post ingestion it suggests significant exposure is unlikely. Plasma concentrations can also be used to predict severity.

ALCOHOLS

Methanol

Methanol (CH_3OH), also known as methyl alcohol or wood alcohol, is used as an industrial solvent and as a component in antifreeze, copy fluids, paint removers and varnishes.

Toxicity

Methanol is metabolized by alcohol dehydrogenase to formaldehyde and then formate. Formate is the most toxic metabolite and causes a profound metabolic acidosis and ocular toxicity. The ocular toxicity is thought to be due to a direct toxic effect of formate on the optic nerve. Folate is a cofactor in the metabolism of formate, and folate-deficient patients (e.g. alcoholics) have an increased susceptibility to toxicity.

The clinical effects in the first 1–2 h post ingestion resemble mild inebriation. This is followed by a latent phase of 6–30 h, which represents the time taken for methanol to be metabolized to formaldehyde and formate (this takes longer if there is co-ingestion of ethanol). Patients then present with headache, dizziness, abdominal pain, diarrhoea, visual symptoms, drowsiness, convulsions and coma. The visual symptoms range from diplopia and blurring of vision to photophobia and blindness, and the characteristic visual complaint is of 'looking through a snowfield'. Patients may be tachypnoeic, as they attempt to compensate for the high anion gap metabolic acidosis. Pancreatitis is present in over 50% of patients. Hyperglycaemia is often present and there is an increased osmolar gap.

Treatment

Gastric lavage or aspiration should be considered if the patient presents within an hour of a significant ingestion. Charcoal does not bind to the alcohols. Sodium bicarbonate treatment is recommended if the pH is less than 7.2. Ethanol is the antidote for methanol as it has a 20-fold greater affinity for the alcohol dehydrogenase enzyme than methanol and thereby prevents the conversion of methanol to formaldehyde and formate. A loading dose should be given for all confirmed ingestions and when bloods are awaited in large ingestions and symptomatic patients. The loading dose can be given orally ($2.5 \, \text{ml} \, \text{kg}^{-1}$ 40% ethanol as whisky, gin or vodka, diluted in water) or intravenously ($7.5 \, \text{ml} \, \text{kg}^{-1}$ 10% in 5% dextrose over 30 min). Following this an ethanol infusion is commenced and maintained until methanol is no longer detected in the serum and the patient is asymptomatic. The large doses of ethanol given can cause hypoglycaemia, particularly in children, so it is important to monitor the patient's

blood sugar. Folate is a cofactor in the conversion of formate to carbon dioxide and is recommended by some to promote formate metabolism. Severely poisoned patients require haemodialysis; indications include ocular symptoms or signs, unresponsive or severe acidosis, methanol or formate levels greater than $500 \, \text{mg} \, \text{l}^{-1}$ and acute renal failure.

Patients treated early have a good prognosis, but those who present after 24 h do less well and can have residual visual and cerebral injury.

Ethylene glycol

Ethylene glycol is used mainly in antifreeze. It is odourless and has a slightly sweet taste. Like methanol its toxicity is due to its metabolites rather than the parent compound.

Toxicity

Ethylene glycol is metabolized by alcohol dehydrogenase to produce glycoaldehyde and then glycolate. Glycolate is then metabolized further by various pathways, including one to oxalate. Glycolate causes a severe metabolic acidosis and oxalate precipitates with calcium, particularly in the kidneys, leading to renal injury and symptomatic hypocalcaemia. Doses of more than 100 ml can be fatal.

Three clinical stages are seen following ingestion. The severity and progression of each stage depends on the dose ingested. Within an hour of ingestion the patient appears inebriated, with transient exhilaration, dysarthria and ataxia. Nausea and vomiting may occur. In large doses this is followed by progressive CNS depression, with drowsiness, nystagmus, myoclonic jerks, seizures and coma. A severe metabolic acidosis is present. The second (or cardiopulmonary) phase begins at around 12 h with tachycardia, mild hypertension and tachypnoea. Symptomatic hypocalcaemia may occur with tetany and cardiac arryhthmias. The ECG shows QT prolongation. Cardiac failure and circulatory collapse occur after large ingestions. The third phase is characterized by oliguria, flank pain, acute tubular necrosis and renal failure. Oxalate crystals are seen in the urine in 50% of patients at 24 h and in 75% at 36 h.

Treatment

The management of ethylene glycol poisoning is similar to that of methanol. Coma, seizures, hypotension and the presence of calcium oxalate crystals in the urine are also indications for haemodialysis. Hypocalcaemia should be corrected with intravenous calcium. Thiamine and pyridoxine are suggested in severe poisoning as they are cofactors in the further metabolism of glycolate derivatives to non-toxic metabolites. Hypomagnesaemia should also be corrected. Patients treated early have a good prognosis, but those who present after 24 h have significant morbidity and mortality.

Methylated spirits

Methylated spirits are a mixture of ethanol, methanol and water. Specific treatment is not usually required as alcohol dehydrogenase is saturated with ethanol and the methanol is cleared by the kidneys.

Ethanol

Ethanol (ethyl alcohol) is the most widely used and abused substance in our society, and is a frequent cause of attendance at emergency departments. Active treatment is most likely to be required for injuries sustained while under the influence of alcohol. Routine supportive care is all that is needed for most patients, until the effects of acute intoxication wear off. However, severe poisoning occurs when large doses of concentrated ethanol are ingested. Distilled spirits (whisky, gin, vodka etc.) typically contain around 40–50% ethanol. Ethanol is also a constituent of mouthwashes (up to 70%) and colognes (40–60%). Generally quoted fatal doses of 100% ethanol are 6–10 ml kg^{-1} for adults and 4 ml kg^{-1} for children.

Progressive CNS depression occurs leading to coma, respiratory depression, hypotension, hypothermia and a metabolic acidosis. Aspiration can occur, and hypoglycaemia is particularly common in children under 5 years and causes seizures. Treatment is supportive. It is essential to ensure adequate airway, breathing and circulation. Hypoglycaemia should be corrected.

BENZODIAZEPINES

Benzodiazepines are commonly used as anxiolytics, anticonvulsants, muscle relaxants and sedative hypnotic agents. Those encountered most frequently include diazepam, chlordiazepoxide, temazepam, nitrazepam and lorazepam. Serious morbidity and mortality are rare in pure benzodiazepine overdose. Most serious reports of benzodiazepine overdose have occurred in the setting of co-ingestion with other CNS depressants, particularly alcohol. The elderly are more susceptible to benzodiazepine-induced CNS depression. Some of the shorter-acting benzodiazepines (e.g. triazolam, midazolam) are more acutely toxic.

Toxicity

Clinical features are usually evident within 1–3 h. Generalized CNS depression occurs, beginning with drowsiness, dizziness, ataxia, slurred speech and confusion, and occasionally progresses to coma. Respiratory depression and hypotension may occur with coma. Rarely, paradoxical effects such as excitement and agitation, or delirium and hallucinations occur. This is most common in children.

Treatment

Gastric lavage and charcoal can be considered in adults who present within 1 h of having taken a potentially large overdose or who have taken other toxic substances. Most patients require only a short period of observation. They should be monitored for CNS and respiratory depression, and hypotension. Flumazenil (Anexate) is a competitive antagonist to the benzodiazepines and will reverse benzodiazepine-induced CNS and respiratory depression.

> Flumazenil should not be routinely administered to patients following benzodiazepine overdose.

However, a number of factors limit its clinical utility, and it is not licensed in the UK for use after overdose. First, the half-life of flumazenil (less than 1 h) is shorter than that of the benzodiazepines and toxicity may reoccur once its effects have worn off. More importantly, it may reverse the anticonvulsant activity of the benzodiazepines and precipitate convulsions in epileptics or in those who have co-ingested proconvulsant drugs, particularly tricyclic antidepressants. It has also been reported to precipitate arryhthmias in the presence of cardiotoxic drugs. Hence it is contraindicated in the presence of QRS widening, tachycardia, anticholinergic signs, and in mixed or unknown overdoses where the cause of coma is unclear. If alert and ambulating after 6 h of observation, patients can be medically discharged after psychiatric review if appropriate.

OPIOIDS

Opioids are drugs that interact with endogenous opioid receptors, and are used mainly for their potent analgesic effects. Morphine and codeine are naturally occurring opium alkaloids extracted from the opium poppy. Diamorphine (heroin), pethidine and methadone are synthetic and semi-synthetic derivatives of these. The less potent opioids are commonly found in popular combination analgesic preparations with paracetamol (co-dydramol contains paracetemol and dihydrocodeine, co-proxamol contains paracetamol and dextropropoxyphene).

Patients overdosing on compound analgesics must be assessed and treated for opiate and paracetamol or salicylate toxicity.

Other weak opioids are used in cough medicines (codeine linctus) and as antidiarrhoeal agents (diphenoxylate, loperamide). Because stronger opioids (heroin, morphine) can produce subjective sensations of euphoria and tranquillity, they are very addictive and widely misused. Heroin is currently the most commonly injected drug of abuse in the UK. The potency of 'street' heroin is unpredictable and accidental overdoses by intravenous drug users are a recurrent problem. Heroin smoking is also popular, but many users graduate to intravenous use. Large numbers of former heroin addicts are on methadone maintenance programmes.

Toxicity

The different opioids vary in strength and duration of action, and there is significant individual variation in sensitivity to opioids. Peak levels usually occur within 2 h of oral ingestion, an hour of intramuscular injection, and within minutes of intravenous injection. However, prolonged toxicity can be seen after ingestion of propoxyphene, sustained-release preparations of morphine and methadone (half-life 20–25 h). The CNS-depressant action of opioids can be potentiated by co-ingestion of other sedative agents (alcohol, benzodiazepines).

The classic triad of opioid poisoning is pinpoint pupils, respiratory depression and coma.

Clinical features include nausea, vomiting, constipation, urinary retention, bradycardia, hallucinations, increasing drowsiness and convulsions. Some opioids (notably pethidine) have a histamine-releasing effect which may cause flushing, an urticarial rash, pruritus and hypotension.

Respiratory depression with hypoxia and apnoea is the commonest cause of death. Non-cardiogenic pulmonary oedema occurs in some patients soon after intravenous heroin overdoses, though the mechanism for this remains unclear. Dextropropoxyphene has some membrane-stabilizing activity that may lead to arryhthmias and myocardial depression.

Treatment

The first priority is maintenance of an adequate airway, ventilation and circulation. Gastric lavage and charcoal can be considered in patients who present within an hour if sustained-release preparations or methadone have been taken orally. Hypotension is treated initially with intravenous fluids. Naloxone, an opioid receptor antagonist, is the specific antidote for opioid poisoning and is indicated for respiratory depression and coma. An initial bolus dose of 0.4 mg intravenously is repeated to a maximum bolus dose of 2 mg. Thereafter, the dose is titrated to the response. As naloxone has a relatively short half-life, re-sedation may occur and repeat doses or an infusion may be needed. In accidental and recreational overdoses it is best to use the minimum dose necessary to raise the patient's level of consciousness to a point where respiratory depression is avoided and the patient can easily be woken. Larger doses can precipitate symptoms of opioid withdrawal in addicts and they may abscond, only to collapse later when the naloxone wears off.

Naloxone has a short half-life and opiate toxicity may recur after an initial satisfactory response.

Patients with propoxyphene overdoses should have ECG monitoring until their ECGs return to normal. Propoxyphene cardiotoxicity is similar to that of the tricyclic antidepressants and alkalinization is the initial treatment. Pulmonary oedema requires maintenance of adequate oxygenation and ventilation.

It is recommended that all patients be observed for a minimum of 6 h (owing to the risk of a delayed onset of effects from long-acting opioids such as methadone). Patients who are asymptomatic, and who have not received naloxone within the previous 6 h, can be considered for discharge after appropriate counselling.

AMPHETAMINES

Amphetamine (an acronym for alpha-methylphenethylamine) is the prototype of a widely abused group of drugs. The amphetamines have structural similarities with endogenous catecholamines but have much more marked CNS stimulant effects. The effects of the amphetamines are complex, but the main features are due to indirect sympathomimetic, dopaminergic and serotoninergic actions. Different agents have differing effect profiles. Other commonly abused amphetamines are methamphetamine and the hallucinogenic amphetamine derivatives such as 3,4-methylenedioxymethamphetamine (MDMA or *Ecstasy*) and 3,4-methylenedioxyethamphetamine (MDEA or *Eve*). There are currently few licensed indications for amphetamines. Methylphenidate (Ritalin) is used in attention-deficit hyperactivity disorder and phentermine (Duromine) is used as an appetite suppressant.

Amphetamines can be taken orally, insufflated or smoked, and rank second to heroin as the most commonly injected drug of abuse in the UK. The main effects are in the CNS. Initially, there is elevation of mood and a sense of increased energy and alertness. This is followed by agitation, hyperactivity, repetitive or stereotyped behaviour, choreoathetoid movements, delirium and paranoid psychosis. Seizures may occur. Other features include flushing, tachycardia, hypertension, arrhythmias and hyperthermia.

Severe amphetamine intoxication may be complicated by myocardial infarction, cardiogenic pulmonary oedema, subarachnoid haemorrhage, intracerebral haemorrhage, acute renal failure, rhabdomyolysis, acute compartment syndrome, disseminated intravascular coagulation and adult respiratory distress syndrome.

Treatment

Treatment is symptomatic, with supportive care. Charcoal can be considered up to 1 h after ingestion. Diazepam is the drug of choice for agitation and delirium. It also helps reduce tachycardia and hypertension. Haloperidol can be considered as second-line treatment for extreme agitation and psychosis but it has the potential to lower the threshold for convulsions. Intravenous fluids are given liberally to correct volume depletion and aid thermoregulation by sweating. Hypertension (diastolic BP greater than 140) can be treated with intravenous sodium nitroprusside or nitrates. Beta-blockers can aggravate hypertension due to unopposed alpha-stimulation, though labetalol, a combined alpha- and beta-blocker, has been used. Hyperthermia is treated initially with simple cooling measures and intravenous fluids. If the patient fails to respond dantrolene (1 mg kg^{-1} intravenously over 15 min) is recommended, and if this is ineffective, the patient should be paralysed and ventilated.

MDMA (Ecstasy)

MDMA (3,4-methylenedioxymethamphetamine) is a hallucinogenic amphetamine derivative. It is widely used in the UK at dance parties and raves. It promotes a sense of euphoria, increased empathy and greater energy. The usual dose taken is 30–150 mg. Tablets or capsules sold as Ecstasy often contain caffeine, ketamine, methamphetamine, MDEA or other adulterants. Effects appear within an hour and usually last 4–6 h. Regular users become tolerant and require increased doses to achieve the same effects.

Adverse effects occur as often with 'recreational' doses as with overdoses. These include nausea, increased muscle tone, muscle pain, trismus, agitation and anxiety. These are followed by more marked hypertonia, hyper-reflexia, tachycardia, hypertension, palpitations, increased body

Table 15.12: Common street names for drugs

Amphetamines	Speed, bennies, uppers, rocks
Cannabis	Dope, ganja, grass, hash, hashish, weed, shit, pot, marijuana
Cocaine	Blow, charlie, coke, snow
Gamma-hydroxybutyric acid	GBH, GHB, liquid X
LSD	Acid, dots, purple haze
MDMA	Ecstasy, XTC, E
Opiates	Chinese crap, junk

temperature and visual hallucinations. With severe toxicity, all the same complications that occur with severe amphetamine poisoning are seen. Two other complications more specific to MDMA are hyponatraemia and hepatic injury. Hyponatraemia is partly due to users drinking excessive amounts of water in the absence of sufficient exercise to sweat off fluid. MDMA may also cause an increase in antidiuretic hormone (ADH) production. MDMA has also caused severe hepatic failure requiring liver transplant. A severe hepatitis can occur secondary to hyperthermia or due to a direct idiosyncratic drug-induced hepatotoxicity. Long-term MDMA use causes permanent serotoninergic nerve terminal destruction, and the possibility of permanent neuropsychiatric sequelae is mooted in the literature.

Management of patients who present after ingestion of MDMA is the same as for the amphetamines. Diazepam is the only treatment required in most cases. Patients should usually be observed for 6 h.

COCAINE

Cocaine is the commonest illicit drug implicated in emergency department attendances in the USA and its use is increasing in the UK. It is a naturally occurring alkaloid extracted from the leaves of the coca plant. It is sold as a powder (cocaine hydrochloride) and is usually taken intranasally ('snorted'), but can also be injected. Crack cocaine is made from cocaine hydrochloride and is a colourless crystalline substance that makes a popping or cracking sound when heated (hence the

name). Crack cocaine can be smoked, inhaled or injected.

Toxicity

Cocaine is rapidly absorbed across all mucosal surfaces. When insufflated nasally, the peak effect occurs within minutes and effects last for up to an hour. A peak effect occurs more rapidly when injected or inhaled (30 s to 2 min) and the duration of effect is 15–30 min. Cocaine is primarily metabolized by plasma cholinesterase and relative deficiency of this enzyme may predispose individuals to more significant toxicity. Recreational doses taken vary. A 'line' of coke is around 30 mg and several are usually taken. Intravenous doses are around 25–50 mg and a rock of crack cocaine is around 200 mg.

Cocaine is a potent CNS stimulant and acts by blocking presynaptic re-uptake of noradrenaline, dopamine and serotonin. This leads to sympathetic overactivity with the characteristic signs of tachycardia, hypertension, dilated pupils and sweating. It also predisposes to the development of arrythmias, seizures and hyperthermia. Users describe a sense of euphoria, increased alertness and general well-being.

Cocaine also has a membrane-stabilizing effect by causing sodium-channel blockade and may cause myocardial depression, bradycardia and hypotension.

Clinical presentation

The usual presentation is with signs of sympathetic overactivity. A life-threatening 'sympathetic storm' can occur from beta- and alpha-adrenergic stimulation.

Arrhythmias, myocardial ischaemia and infarction are well reported. Chest pain is present in up to 40% of patients who present to the emergency department after cocaine use. However, the incidence of actual infarction in these patients is around 5%. Aortic dissection has also been documented.

The more serious CNS effects are delirium, seizures, subarachnoid haemorrhage, intracerebral haemorrhage and cerebrovascular infarction. Distorted thought processes and a paranoid psychosis occur and increase the chance of accidental trauma (a significant cause of morbidity with all forms of substance misuse).

Cocaine smoking may cause a variety of respiratory symptoms including an exacerbation of asthma, thermal airway injury, pneumothorax, pneumomediastinum, pulmonary haemorrhage and pulmonary oedema. Cocaine-induced rhabdomyolysis may cause renal failure, and severe hyperthermia is another well-recognized complication.

Treatment

The mainstay of treatment is good symptomatic and supportive care. First-line treatment is benzodiazepines, which sedate and reduce central stimulation generally. Adequate sedation is essential and is best achieved with incremental doses. Intravenous fluids are given to all. Hyperthermia is treated as for amphetamines. Suspected myocardial ischaemia should be treated initially with aspirin, nitrates and morphine. The role of thrombolysis in cocaine-induced infarction has not yet been established as these patients would be at a higher risk of thrombolytic complications. In view of this, angioplasty has been recommended as a more appropriate alternative. Beta-blockers can exacerbate cocaine-induced coronary artery vasoconstriction and are best avoided. Phentolamine (an alpha-blocker) is used for severe hypertension, and may also alleviate coronary artery vasoconstriction. Sodium bicarbonate is first-line treatment for malignant arrhythmias. Lignocaine may be useful for ventricular arrhythmias after cocaine-induced myocardial infarction.

In patients who have taken 'speedballs' (a combination of heroin and cocaine, often injected) naloxone should be titrated carefully as its use has been associated with acute narcotic withdrawal, pulmonary oedema and ventricular arryhthmias, probably due to residual cocaine.

GAMMA-HYDROXYBUTYRATE

Gamma-hydroxybutyric acid (GHB) is a naturally occurring neurotransmitter. It is found in greatest concentrations in the basal ganglia and is a precursor of gamma aminobutyric acid (GABA). It has been used as an anaesthetic agent and in the treatment of narcolepsy, and by body-builders as an aid to muscle growth. More recently, it has become popular as a drug of abuse because of its euphoriant effects.

Toxicity

The neurotransmitter activities of GHB are complex and involve different receptor sites in various areas of the brain. GHB can be injected, but is usually taken orally. Absorption occurs rapidly after ingestion, and systemic effects appear within 15 min.

The clinical effects depend on the dose ingested and are often potentiated by co-ingestion of alcohol, benzodiazepines or other substances of abuse. The initial features of GHB intoxication include nausea, vomiting, urinary incontinence, dizziness, tremor, euphoric feelings, ataxia and agitation. These are followed by bradycardia, hypotension, mild hypothermia, random clonic movements of the face and extremities, myoclonic jerks, increasing drowsiness and profound coma with respiratory depression and death. A peculiar feature of the coma in GHB intoxication is that profound coma with respiratory depression leading to apnoea can be interspersed with periods of violent combativeness, usually after stimulation (attempted intubation). Most patients recover consciousness relatively quickly (2–6 h). An emergence phenomenon is sometimes seen, with myoclonic jerks, transient confusion and agitation. This is brief, and followed by full recovery of consciousness and return to normal respiratory function.

Treatment

Treatment is supportive. Particular attention to maintenance and protection of an adequate airway is essential. Some patients will require intubation and assisted ventilation for a short period. Although vomiting has been reported in up to 30% of cases in some series, aspiration appears uncommon. Fluids should be given for hypotension, and bradycardia is treated with atropine if required. Patients whose symptoms have resolved can be discharged after 6 h of observation.

VOLATILE SUBSTANCE MISUSE

Hydrocarbons present in a large number of commercial substances, such as lighter fuel, cleaning fluids, paint thinners and glue, are highly volatile and produce vapours that are inhaled by substance misusers for their intoxicating effects.

Butane, which is found in lighter fluid and many aerosols, is the commonest example. When these vapours are inhaled they produce feelings of euphoria and exhilaration. Higher concentrations lead to ataxia, slurred speech, drowsiness, and coma in extreme cases. Facial burns and excoriation of mucous membranes may occur during usage. Sudden deaths can occur from anoxia (due to direct asphyxia), respiratory depression, vagal inhibition (due to direct laryngeal stimulation, as occurs when an aerosol has been sprayed directly into the back of the oropharynx) and cardiac arrythmias (direct myocardial toxicity).

Treatment

Treatment is symptomatic and supportive care. Patients should be observed with ECG monitoring for at least 4 h and stimulants should be avoided (hydrocarbons are thought to enhance the susceptibility of the myocardium to arrythmogenesis from endogenous and exogenous catecholamines). Most patients recover quickly and if asymptomatic can be discharged home after appropriate counselling. Standard advanced life support (ALS) protocols should be followed for those requiring cardiopulmonary resuscitation.

OTHER HALLUCINOGENIC DRUGS

A wide number of drugs and plants are taken specifically for their hallucinogenic effects. Phencyclidine (PCP) and lysergic acid diethylamide (LSD) are among the most commonly encountered. Cannabis and mushrooms of the *Psilocybe* genus also have hallucinogenic effects.

PCP has a dissociative anaesthetic effect similar to ketamine. It can be smoked, injected or taken orally. It causes euphoria, dissociation, hallucinations, nystagmus and ataxia. Higher doses may cause increased agitation, delirium, muscle rigidity, seizures and coma. Hypoglycaemia may also occur. Treatment is supportive. Diazepam is the drug of first choice, with haloperidol as second-line treatment.

LSD is an extremely potent hallucinogen with psychomimetic activity in microgram doses. It is most commonly ingested from a sugar cube or blotting paper ('microdots'). Visual hallucinations, agitation, tachycardia, mild hypertension, pyrexia and dilated pupils are the commonest effects. Most patients retain insight while intoxicated. More severe sympathomimetic and CNS features such as seizures and hyperpyrexia are uncommon. The most usual adverse effects are paranoid delusions, anxiety attacks and psychoses. Diazepam is usually the only treatment required. LSD has a relatively short half-life and most recover within 4–8 h.

'Magic mushrooms' is a term used to describe mushrooms with hallucinogenic properties. In the UK the most commonly encountered are members of the *Psilocybe* genus. Psilocybin and psilocin are the active ingredients and have an LSD-like effect. The mushrooms can be eaten raw, or brewed in a tea or soup. Symptoms usually occur within 1 h and are largely similar to those of LSD, though nausea and vomiting are more common.

Cannabis (marijuana) is widely smoked in the UK and at present its use remains illegal. Tetrahydrocannabinoid is the main active ingredient. Clinical effects appear around 10 min after inhalation and 45 min after oral ingestion. The commonest effects are euphoria, relaxation and mild ataxia. Other findings include a mild tachycardia, peripheral vasodilation and conjunctival suffusion. Occasionally, patients experience panic attacks, hallucinations and paranoia, causing them to present to hospital. Treatment other than reassurance is rarely needed.

FURTHER READING

Proudfoot, A.T. (1992) *Acute Poisoning Diagnosis and Management*. Butterworth–Heinemann, Oxford.

CHAPTER SIXTEEN

HAEMATOLOGY, IMMUNOLOGY AND ALLERGY

- Haematological disorders
- Allergy and anaphylaxis
- Further reading

HAEMATOLOGICAL DISORDERS

There are three broad categories of haematological conditions that are relevant to emergency department practice:

- cellular deficiencies – anaemia, leucopenia and thrombocytopenia
- coagulation disorders
- sickle cell disease and trait.

CELLULAR DEFICIENCIES

Anaemia

Anaemia is an absolute decrease in the number of circulating red cells. Low levels of haemoglobin are tolerated especially if their onset is gradual, allowing compensatory mechanisms to function. In such cases the detection of anaemia may need no specific treatment in an emergency department, although the doctor must ensure that suitable arrangements have been made for further investigation and treatment before the patient is discharged (Table 16.1).

With rapid onset and marked reduction of haemoglobin levels, anaemia may be life threatening. In an emergency department the commonest cause of acute anaemia is blood loss, and early fluid replacement and blood transfusion may be required along with efforts to detect the source of blood loss and prevent further bleeding. The management of

Table 16.1: Differential diagnosis of anaemia

Reduced red cell production	Marrow failure or haematinic deficiency
Loss of red cells	Haemorrhage – occult or overt
Increased red cell destruction	Haemolytic anaemias

bleeding as a result of injury is dealt with in Chapter 4. Blood loss in the non-traumatized patient is most commonly into the gastrointestinal tract, although haemorrhage from a ruptured abdominal aortic aneurysm or ectopic pregnancy should also be considered in the appropriate age groups.

SYMPTOMS AND SIGNS

A general medical history may give clues to the diagnosis and a drug history must also be sought. In the absence of trauma the history should concentrate on other causes of blood loss, particularly haemorrhage from the gastrointestinal or genitourinary tracts, or from a ruptured aortic aneurysm. Acute blood loss may also manifest as thirst, confusion and reduced urinary output. If there is no haemorrhage, an underlying failure of red cell production or haemolytic process should be considered.

Bleeding from the gastrointestinal tract may be occult – always do a rectal examination.

Table 16.2: Investigations for anaemia

Full blood count
Group and cross-match
Coagulation screen
Urea and electrolytes
Glucose

The physical examination should assess the patient's response to any haemorrhage with baseline and continuing measurements of the heart rate, blood pressure, respiratory rate and conscious level. Examination of the skin may reveal pallor and sweating in the patient with haemorrhage. Haemorrhage in a non-trauma patient may be occult and a rectal examination is mandatory to detect melaena or fresh blood in the rectum.

INVESTIGATION
The investigations required in a symptomatic anaemic patient are given in Table 16.2.

Haemoglobin level may initially be normal following acute blood loss.

NON-BLEEDING CAUSES OF ANAEMIA
Decreased red cell production Examination of the red cell indices will aid in the diagnosis. A hypochromic microcytic anaemia suggests iron deficiency that may be the result of poor diet or chronic occult blood loss. Less commonly this picture is seen in thallassaemia and the anaemia of chronic disease. Macrocytic anaemia is suggestive of folate or vitamin B_{12} deficiency, and there is often a pancytopenia.

Failure of the bone marrow may occur for a number of reasons, including replacement by malignant infiltration and primary marrow aplasia. The red cells are typically normochromic and microcytic and there is often a pancytopenia.

Increased red cell destruction Increased and abnormal red cell destruction occurs in haemolytic anaemia. This may be the result of an intrinsic abnormality of the red cells, such as an enzyme deficiency (glucose 6-phosphate dehydrogenase), spherocytosis or a haemoglobin abnormality such as sickle cell disease. Alternatively, haemolysis may occur as a result of an extrinsic abnormality, such as ABO incompatibility in transfusion or an environmental cause such as drugs, toxins, infections and burns.

Table 16.3: Causes of leucopenia

Marrow	Aplastic anaemia, leukaemia, chemotherapy, idiosyncratic drug reaction
Distribution	Splenomegaly, malaria, portal hypertension
Increased utilization	Viral infection, rickettsia, autoimmune disease
Laboratory error	

TREATMENT
When the cause of anaemia is bleeding then therapy includes prevention of further loss (this often requires surgery) and restoration of sufficient circulating red cells, usually by transfusion. When the cause is other than haemorrhage, therapy is aimed at the specific underlying cause together with transfusion and the advice of a haematologist.

Leucopenia

Both leucocytosis and leucopenia are non-specific findings. The causes listed in Table 16.3 are intended to highlight this lack of specificity. Leucopenia predominantly affects one cell type, usually neutrophils. Although the patient may be highly susceptible to infection, when infection occurs it is often occult since there are insufficient cells to mount a substantial inflammatory response.

Infection in a leucopenic patient is often accompanied by few physical signs.

Thrombocytopenia

This subject is dealt with in the section on Platelet disorders (p. 195)

COAGULATION DISORDERS

Normal coagulation is dependent on the vessel wall, platelets and the coagulation cascade. Abnormalities of any of these components may lead to pathological states of reduced or excessive coagulation. As the number of patients taking anticoagulant therapy in the community increases it is also increasingly common to see patients with abnormal bleeding as a result of over-treatment.

Platelet disorders

Platelet disorders may be the result of a reduced number of platelets or failure of the platelets to function effectively. The source of bleeding is usually the capillary, and platelet disorders therefore first manifest as cutaneous and mucosal petechiae or ecchymosis. Epistaxis, menorrhagia and gastro-intestinal bleeding are the common presenting symptoms to emergency departments.

> Platelet disorders are characterized by cutaneous or mucosal haemorrhage.

Thrombocytopenia may be due to decreased production of platelets by the bone marrow (drugs, toxins or infections), increased pooling (hypersplenism), or increased destruction (drugs, idiopathic or autoimmune thrombocytopenic purpura (ITP), disseminated intravascular coagulation (DIC)). Most patients with thrombocytopenia do not manifest symptoms or signs until the platelet count falls below $50\,000\,\text{mm}^{-3}$. Spontaneous bleeding, including life-threatening central nervous system haemorrhage, may occur if the count falls below $10\,000\,\text{mm}^{-3}$.

The emergency management of thrombocytopenia is based upon the severity and the likeliest cause. Platelet transfusions will be required in patients with platelet counts of less than $50\,000\,\text{mm}^{-3}$ who are bleeding. Each unit transfused should raise the platelet count by $10\,000\,\text{mm}^{-3}$. Any patient who presents with a count of less than $10\,000\,\text{mm}^{-3}$ should receive platelets because of the risk of life-threatening spontaneous haemorrhage. Patients with ITP may not respond to platelet infusions because of circulating antiplatelet antibodies. In consequence, prednisolone 30–60 mg orally should be given to reduce this auto-immune destruction. Conditions such as DIC may be exacerbated by platelet infusions.

More rarely an adequate number of platelets are present but platelet function is abnormal. The cause is most often a drug (typically aspirin), with abnormalities of platelet aggregation and adhesion.

Coagulation factor deficiencies

The normal function of the coagulation cascade is dependent on a series of complex linked enzymatic reactions. Patients with abnormalities of coagulation typically have bleeding into the deeper tissues, specifically the joints and genitourinary tract. Diagnosis is based predominantly on interpretation of laboratory coagulation studies.

> Coagulation disorders are characterized by bleeding into joints, urinary tract or the bowel.

HAEMOPHILIA

The haemophilias are due to a deficiency of Factor VIII (classic haemophilia) or Factor IX (Christmas disease). Eighty-five per cent of patients with haemophilia have classic Factor VIII deficiency. This is an X-linked recessive disorder occurring in 1 in 10 000 live births. The disease is classified according to severity on the basis of the level of Factor VIII activity. Mild cases have more than 6% Factor VIII activity and are not at risk of excessive bleeding except after major injury or surgery. Moderate cases have 1–5% activity and severe cases have less than 1% activity and are at risk of spontaneous bleeding. Unfortunately more than 60% of haemophiliac patients fall into the severe category.

Usually haemophiliacs have no problems with minor cuts and abrasions. However, the risk in trauma is of late bleeding. As a consequence patients with a head injury should undergo CT scanning and be admitted for close observation for the development of an intracranial haematoma. Patients with haemophilia should never receive intramuscular injections, and central line placement and blood gas sampling can only be done under Factor VIII cover.

Management All patients should be discussed with an experienced haematologist. Patients with mild or moderate haemophilia may respond to treatment with desmopressin (DDAVP). In patients who respond, DDAVP can produce a three-fold increase in Factor VIII activity and a response should be seen within 1 h. DDAVP has the advantage of not being a blood product, is easily administered, and serious side-effects are uncommon.

Patients with moderate or severe haemophilia and significant bleeding will require Factor VIII concentrate. Ancillary therapies such as immobilization, analgesia and topical use of antifibrinolytic therapies such as aminocaproic acid and tranexamic acid may also be of value in the specialist setting.

Von Willebrand's disease

Von Willebrand's disease is a related disorder of a portion of the Factor VIII complex. It is caused by a deficiency or abnormality of the Von Willebrand factor (vWF) and is the most common bleeding disorder. Von Willebrand factor allows platelets to adhere to damaged endothelium and carries Factor VIII in plasma. Screening coagulation tests may be normal, although the partial thromboplastin time is usually prolonged in moderate to severe cases. The haemorrhagic tendency is highly variable. DDAVP is the mainstay of therapy for most patients, but for those with severe disease or severe bleeding, Factor VIII concentrate should be used. Bleeding from tooth sockets can often be managed with fibrinolytic inhibitor agents such as E-aminocaproic acid and tranexamic acid.

Seek advice early from a haematologist if the patient has abnormal coagulation.

Disseminated intravascular coagulation (DIC)

DIC results in the generalized activation of the haemostatic system, causing fibrin to form within vessels. This causes small vessel obstruction with tissue damage and multiple organ dysfunction. The consequent consumption of coagulation factors and platelets and secondary activation of fibrinolysis produces a generalized bleeding tendency. This may be acute and overwhelming, usually as a result of septicaemia (Fig. 16.1), acute haemolysis, shock or placental abruption. More rarely, the process may be subacute (malignancy) or chronic (liver disease, malignancy, eclampsia).

Investigations

In acute DIC a wide range of abnormalities is found on investigation. The blood count shows thrombocytopenia and examination of a blood film may demonstrate red cell fragmentation. Coagulation studies demonstrate a prolonged prothrombin time, partial thromboplastin time and thrombin clotting time. The plasma fibrinogen is low and fibrin degradation products (FDP) are raised as fibrin is formed and then broken down. In the non-acute forms there may be minimal disturbance of these markers, although the platelet count is almost always reduced.

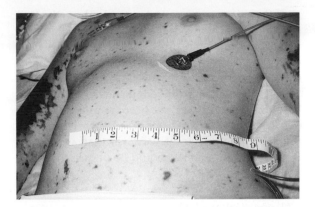

Figure 16.1: Disseminated intravascular coagulation in meningococcal septicaemia.

Management

The most important principle is to remove or treat the underlying cause. Secondary disturbances of acid–base balance and electrolytes are corrected and the advice of a haematologist should be sought on the use of fresh frozen plasma, platelets, blood and cryoprecipitate.

Over-anticoagulation

One of the commonest causes of abnormal bleeding seen in emergency departments is an acquired coagulation deficit as a result of anticoagulant therapy. Warfarin therapy requires regular monitoring to maintain therapeutic levels and prevent over anticoagulation with the attendant risk of haemorrhage. Drug interactions with warfarin are also common and may potentiate its action, resulting in a prothrombin time raised above the therapeutic range. Treatment of over-anticoagulation depends on the prothrombin time or international normalized ratio (INR), the presence of abnormal bleeding and the initial reason for anticoagulation.

The aim should be to return the INR to the therapeutic range. If bleeding is absent or minimal and the INR raised to between 4 and 6, warfarin should be withheld and subsequently reintroduced at a reduced dose. If the INR is between 6 and 8, vitamin K should be administered and the INR estimated again after 24 h. With an INR of above 8, vitamin K should be administered along with 2 units of fresh frozen plasma. The INR is checked again 6 h later and daily for 3 days. Further vitamin K may subsequently be required.

If there is severe or moderate bleeding, the INR should be normalized as rapidly as possible. The use of vitamin K and fresh frozen plasma is indicated and a haematologist should be consulted as early as possible.

Recently, genetically engineered prothrombin complex concentrate has become available. This provides a safer and more effective means of reversing the effects of warfarin than with fresh frozen plasma. Its use should be discussed with a haematologist.

Always check the INR of any patient on oral antico-agulants who presents with any abnormal bleeding.

If over-correction may cause harm, such as in the case of a patient with a prosthetic heart valve, the problem should be discussed with a haematologist and the consultant responsible for the patient's ongoing care (where possible) and consideration given to using heparin whilst antagonizing the effects of warfarin.

SICKLE CELL DISEASE

Haemoglobin S is the commonest abnormal variant of adult haemoglobin and is the result of a single amino-acid substitution on the beta-chain of haemoglobin. It is transmitted by autosomal dominant inheritance. The abnormal haemoglobin causes no significant problems when bound to oxygen but when deoxygenated it polymerizes. If significant quantities within the red blood cell polymerize, the red cell morphology is altered, forming a characteristic sickle shape. Sickling increases blood viscosity and may cause microvascular obstruction. Sickling is increased in the presence of acidosis, increased 2,3-diphosphoglycerate, vascular stasis, dehydration, infection and low oxygen tensions. Sickled red cells are rapidly haemolysed, reducing their lifespan from 120 to 10 days.

Patients with sickle cell *disease* are homozygotes for the abnormal gene and usually present following the first 6 months of life with sickle cell crises. Heterozygotes are referred to as having sickle cell *trait* and sickling usually only occurs with marked hypoxia. Patients are therefore often asymptomatic and are detected by routine screening for the abnormal haemoglobin in susceptible population groups.

Table 16.4: The sickle cell crises

Vaso-occlusive
Haematological
Infectious

Clinical features

Patients with sickle cell disease have a chronic haemolytic anaemia with a haemoglobin level in the range of $6–9\,g\,dl^{-1}$. There is often chronic hypoxia, with cardiomegaly, pulmonary hypertension and congestive cardiac failure. The splenic enlargement seen in childhood disappears in adults as a result of recurrent infarction. Renal papillary necrosis, dactylitis (hand and foot syndrome) and skin ulceration on the lower legs are further examples of tissue infarction. Patients may present to the emergency department with one or more of three types of sickle cell crisis (Table 16.4).

VASO-OCCLUSIVE CRISIS
Hypoxia, acidosis, dehydration or cold result in polymerization of the abnormal haemoglobin and a loss of elasticity with reduced ability to pass through capillary beds. Further hypoxia and acidosis are thus produced, which leads to progressive ischaemia. Symptoms vary with the organ affected, although abdominal, chest and musculoskeletal pain are uncommon. Other disease processes may be mimicked and care should be taken in assessing a patient with sickle cell disease to exclude other pathology.

HAEMATOLOGICAL
Splenic sequestration crisis occurs predominantly in children, with rapid enlargement of the spleen with sickling and infarction. The haemoglobin drops acutely and transfusion is required. With the shortened lifespan of a red cell in sickle cell disease, any impairment of bone marrow function, for example due to folate deficiency or post-infectious marrow suppression, may result in an aplastic crisis. The haemoglobin level drops even further, often to less than $2\,g\,dl^{-1}$, and the reticulocyte count is low.

INFECTIOUS
Sickle cell disease is associated with an increased susceptibility to infection. This is thought to be

a result of poor splenic function and impaired neutrophil migration. Infections with staphylococci, streptococci and *Haemophilus influenzae* are particularly common with fulminant pneumonia or meningitis. Less common, although classically associated with sickle cell disease, is *Salmonella osteomyeleitis*.

Diagnosis

The diagnosis is usually suggested by the patient, who will almost invariably know that they have sickle cell disease. The Sickledex test will confirm the presence of sickle cell disease if there is any doubt. Investigations should include a full blood count but the 'normal' white cell count is often up to $18\,000\,\mathrm{mm}^{-3}$. A fall in haemoglobin of more than $2\,\mathrm{g}\,\mathrm{dl}^{-1}$ from the patient's normal level suggests a haematological crisis. A reticulocyte count should be requested and a value of less than 5% suggests an aplastic crisis.

Additionally, urea and electrolytes are required to exclude or quantify dehydration and arterial blood gases to quantify hypoxia and acid–base disturbances. Bacteriological analyses (including urinalysis) are required to identify the source of infection.

Imaging may include a chest X-ray, although a normal film does not exclude a pulmonary crisis. Skeletal X-rays, radio-isotope scans or magnetic resonance imaging (MRI) are required if there is localized tenderness, in order to identify osteomyelitis. CT or MRI of the brain is essential in any patient with neurological abnormalities, although are unlikely to be requested by the emergency department.

Management

General measures include rehydration, which may need to be intravenously administered, and supplemental oxygen. Fluid overload should be avoided since cardiopulmonary disease is common. Patients with vaso-occlusive crises typically have severe pain and generous amounts of intravenous opiates should be given.

> Pain from vaso-occlusive crisis requires large doses of intravenous opiates.

Specific measures

Acute splenic sequestration is common in young children. The spleen enlarges rapidly and the haemoglobin falls rapidly. Pneumoccocal infection is frequently the precipitant. Treatment is with blood transfusion and antibiotics.

Any patient with sickle cell disease and a temperature higher than 38°C should be presumed to have a bacterial infection. A septic screen should be carried out with a low threshold for lumbar puncture. A broad-spectrum antibiotic such as ceftriaxone should be administered.

Parvovirus infection can cause a potentially fatal red cell aplastic crisis in which the reticulocyte count and haemoglobin level fall rapidly. The treatment is emergency blood transfusion.

If a pulmonary crisis is suspected, empirical intravenous antibiotics should be administered. If there is a significant ventilation/perfusion mismatch the patient should be anticoagulated. Cardiovascular decompensation, if severe, may indicate an exchange transfusion.

If there is any alteration of mental state or a focal neurological deficit a central nervous system crisis should be suspected. Following a CT scan a lumbar puncture should be performed to exclude meningitis and subarachnoid haemorrhage.

Localized bone pain may represent a skeletal vaso-occlusive crisis or local bone infection. Management should be discussed with an orthopaedic surgeon and antibiotics to cover *Staphylococcus aureus* and salmonella should be considered early.

> Patients with sickle cell trait have a normal red cell lifespan and are generally asymptomatic.

ALLERGY AND ANAPHYLAXIS

Hypersensitivity is an exaggerated immune response to an antigenic stimulus. Allergic reactions bridge the full spectrum of severity from minor irritations to life-threatening circulatory collapse. The skin, gastrointestinal and respiratory tracts and cardiovascular system are all commonly affected.

Table 16.5: Manifestations of anaphylaxis

Skin	Erythema, pruritus, urticaria and angioedema
Respiratory	Upper airway swelling leading to obstruction
	Acute brochospasm
Gastrointestinal tract	Nausea, vomiting, abdominal pain and diarrhoea
Cardiovascular system	Light-headedness, tachycardia, hypotension and shock. Cardiac dysrhythmias and infarction may occur

ANAPHYLAXIS

Anaphylaxis is a common medical emergency and the most severe type of allergic reaction. Symptoms may occur within minutes of exposure to the allergen. In patients who have experienced previous anaphylactic reactions there may be an aura of impending doom. Symptoms and signs are listed in Table 16.5.

Common precipitants are bee stings, nuts and parenteral antibiotics, especially penicillin. The speed of onset and severity of the reaction are related to the amount and type of allergen as well as the degree of sensitization.

An anaphylactoid reaction is clinically identical but is not triggered by IgE antibody and therefore does not require prior exposure. Radiocontrast media and non-steroidal anti-inflammatory agents are classic causal agents.

Management

Prevent further administration of the allergen.

Assessment and support of airway, breathing and circulation should be prompt and sequential. High-flow oxygen should be given via a face mask and a pulse oximeter and cardiac monitor attached. If there is laryngeal oedema or wheeze, 1 in 10 000 adrenaline should be immediately administered *intravenously* in 1-ml boluses repeated to achieve relief of life-threatening airway obstruction, bronchospam or shock. If intravenous access is not available 0.5 mg of adrenaline should be given intramuscularly every 5 min to achieve the same effect. Hydrocortisone 200 mg intravenously and 5 mg nebulized salbutamol should also be administered. Endotracheal intubation may be required but can be impossible and necessitate the formation of a surgical airway.

If the patient is shocked an intravenous infusion of 1–2 l of normal saline should be given rapidly. Further treatment may include chlorpheniramine intravenously, and patients with refractory hypotension should receive an H_2-blocker. Patients on beta-blockers may require glucagon 1 mg repeated as necessary if hypotension persists. Once the patient has responded it is important to remember that up to 20% will relapse within the next 12 h. Therefore all should be admitted and closely observed.

URTICARIA

This presents with typically itchy, oedematous transient skin swellings, often occurring in crops. There are many causes, including foodstuffs, drugs, insect stings, viral illnesses, temperature, sunlight and exercise. In chronic cases no cause is usually found.

Treatment

Most will improve with a non-sedating histamine antagonist. Refractory cases may respond to the addition of an H_2-antagonist. An attempt should be made to identify the likely cause.

ANGIO-OEDEMA

This is a well-demarcated, non-pitting oedema of deep subcutaneous tissue, predominantly involving the face and mouth. When it involves the larynx it is life threatening. Pruritus is uncommon. The causes are as for urticaria, but it appears that the angiotensin-converting enzyme (ACE) inhibitors are particularly likely to cause this condition. There is also a hereditary form related to C_1 esterase inhibitor deficiency.

Treatment

Treatment is the same as for urticaria but because of the increased risk to the airway, adrenaline should be administered early. Invasive and surgical airway techniques may be required. The use of histamine antagonists is routine. Hereditary angio-oedema responds poorly to adrenaline and requires urgent fresh frozen plasma which contains C_1 esterase inhibitor.

FURTHER READING

Wetherall, D., Ledingham, J. and Warrell, D. (1995) *Oxford Textbook of Medicine*. Oxford University Press, Oxford.

ENDOCRINE EMERGENCIES

INTRODUCTION

Disorders of glucose metabolism, specifically diabetes mellitus and its complications, are commonly seen in emergency departments. They may represent major emergencies where time-critical intervention is needed to preserve life and prevent morbidity. Thyroid, pituitary and adrenocortical disorders are less often recognized although they may be equally life threatening. Although not exclusively endocrine problems, disorders of calcium metabolism are also considered in this chapter.

HYPOGLYCAEMIA

Hypoglycaemia is one of the commonest medical emergencies seen in an emergency department. Glucose is the main energy source for the brain and prolonged hypoglycaemia can cause brain damage and death.

Hypoglycaemia is defined as a blood sugar of less than 3 mmol l^{-1}.

Most hypoglycaemic patients are diabetic and have either administered too much insulin, missed a meal or increased their activity level. Other causes include use of the biguanide hypoglycaemic drugs (metformin), malnutrition, alcohol use, liver failure, aspirin overdose, sepsis and the other endocrine emergencies of hypoadrenalism, hypopituitarism and insulinoma. The sulphonylurea hypoglycaemic drugs (glicazide) do not cause hypoglycaemia. If the patient is not a diabetic and has had proven hypoglycaemia, consideration should be given to further investigations for other rare causes, such as an insulinoma or a phaeochromocytoma.

CLINICAL PRESENTATION

Symptoms may be due to neuroglycopenia or autonomic overactivity (Table 17.1). However, in many long-standing diabetics, impairment of the adrenergic response may result in hypoglycaemia occurring without warning symptoms.

Hypoglycaemia may more rarely produce seizures or focal neurological deficits such as cranial

Table 17.1: Features of hypoglycaemia

Neuroglycopenia:
Confusion
Lethargy
Hunger
Aggression
Coma
Autonomic overactivity:
Sweating
Pallor
Tachycardia
Vomiting

nerve palsies and hemiplegia (Todd's paresis). These respond to correction of blood glucose levels although prolonged and profound hypoglycaemia may produce permanent neurological deficit.

Because of the non-specific nature of symptoms and signs hypoglycaemia may be misdiagnosed as a cerebrovascular accident, seizure disorder, migraine, Stokes–Adams attack or psychiatric illness. The value of a routine bedside blood glucose measurement for patients in emergency departments patients is obvious.

> Bedside blood glucose analysis is a vital component of early assessment in the emergency department.

TREATMENT

If the patient is conscious then glucose can be administered orally as a sweet drink or chocolate bar. If the patient is unconscious, blood should be taken and sent for laboratory blood glucose analysis and 25–50 ml of 50% glucose given intravenously as a bolus. In children 50% dextrose solutions may cause cerebral oedema and it is safer to use 10% dextrose solution in a dose of $5\,ml\,kg^{-1}$. Rapid recovery usually follows and it is often possible subsequently to discharge the patient with appropriate advice and follow-up. An insulin overdose may be deliberately self-administered by the patient as a suicidal act. In these cases further glucose may need to be administered, both as boluses and as an infusion. If severe, surgical excision of the subcutaneous area where the insulin was injected may be indicated to prevent further absorption, although this is extremely rare.

Hypertonic glucose solutions must be administered carefully as extravasation of the solution from the vein will result in necrosis of soft tissues. Following intravenous administration, local thrombophlebitis may occur if the vein is not flushed with an isotonic solution.

If intravenous access cannot be obtained, glucagon 1 mg intramuscularly may be given as a temporizing measure although this is not effective if the patient has no hepatic glycogen stores, for example in chronic alcohol abuse. When reversing hypoglycaemia in an alcoholic, thiamine should be administered concomitantly with dextrose to prevent Wernicke's encephalopathy.

If the patient fails to recover consciousness over the next few minutes, alternative diagnoses should be sought. However, permanent neurological injury may follow prolonged and severe hypoglycaemia and a head CT scan may show cerebral swelling.

HYPERGLYCAEMIA

> A random blood glucose of greater than $11\,mmol\,l^{-1}$ is diagnostic of diabetes mellitus.

Hyperglycaemia alone rarely requires urgent therapy. In the emergency department urgent correction of the cause of hyperglycaemia is only required in patients with diabetic ketoacidosis and non-ketotic hyperosmolar coma.

DIABETIC KETOACIDOSIS (DKA)

DKA occurs only in diabetics. It is characterized by hyperglycaemia and ketonaemia. Common precipitants are trauma, infection, myocardial infarction, cerebral infarction or inadequate insulin therapy. The latter is often the result of cessation of insulin in an unwell diabetic owing to loss of appetite and reduced food intake. Alternatively keto-acidosis may be the presenting illness in a previously undiagnosed diabetic.

Pathophysiology

The lack of insulin causes impaired tissue utilization of glucose with a consequent rise in blood glucose. Water is drawn osmotically out of cells, causing cellular dehydration and impaired function. The same effect in the renal tubules produces an osmotic diuresis (polyuria) with a reduction in total body water and sodium (dehydration) and thirst (polydipsia). The loss of glucose in the urine and dehydration results in weight loss.

The relative excess of glucagon (unopposed by insulin) causes the breakdown of fats and the production of ketones. These acidic molecules cause a metabolic acidosis and the consequent respiratory compensation manifests itself as Kussmaul breathing. The exhalation of ketones produces a sickly sweet smell.

Serum osmolarity (in mmol) = 2(Na + K) + urea + glucose.

The level of consciousness correlates poorly with most of the biochemical parameters. However, if a patient with DKA has a serum osmolarity of less than $340\,mmol\,kg^{-1}$ then an alternative cause of impaired consciousness should be sought (cerebrovascular accident). Nausea, vomiting and abdominal pain are common.

The diagnosis of DKA is made with a blood glucose of greater than $11\,mmol\,l^{-1}$, associated with ketonuria and a bicarbonate of less than $15\,mmol\,l^{-1}$.

Management (Table 17.2)

The first priority is to assess and ensure a patent airway. Cardiac monitoring and pulse oximetry are essential and high-flow oxygen must be administered. Venous access must be established and urgent samples sent for urea and electrolytes, blood sugar, full blood count and blood culture. Urea and electrolytes typically demonstrate hyponatraemia, hyperkalaemia and raised urea and creatinine. In DKA an arterial blood gas sample will demonstrate a metabolic acidosis with a raised anion gap. A chest X-ray, urinalysis (including ketones) and ECG should be organized. If the patient is unconscious or obtunded a nasogastric tube and catheter should be passed, as gastric stasis with vomiting and aspiration and acute retention are common. Routine catheterization is not indicated as it increases the incidence of urinary tract infections.

Correction of dehydration

In severe DKA there may be a deficit of up to 10 l of body water and 400–700 mmol of sodium. The first

Table 17.2: Management aims for diabetic ketoacidosis

Correct dehydration
Correct electrolyte disturbances
Correct insulin deficiency
Treat precipitating causes
Prevent complications

litre of intravenous fluid should be given over 30–60 min. Thereafter the rate of replacement is determined by reassessment, both clinical and biochemical. Normal saline is the most commonly used intravenous fluid but should be exchanged for dextrose when the blood sugar falls below $15\,mmol\,l^{-1}$. Furthermore, persistence of ketonaemia and ketonuria is best treated by concomitant administration of dextrose and insulin. If shock is present the circulating volume should be expanded using a colloid prior to correction of dehydration.

Correction of electrolyte and acid–base disturbance

Potassium is predominantly an intracellular ion. Total body potassium is reduced as a result of insulin deficit, acidosis, diuresis and vomiting. There is usually a 250–700 mmol deficit. Because of the acidosis and lack of insulin (both of which increase extracellular potassium levels) the extracellular potassium is often within the normal range or is raised and is therefore misleading. The aim is to maintain normal extracellular levels and replace the total body deficit over a period of days. This requires insulin to normalize function of the sodium/potassium pump and potassium supplementation. Potassium should be given at a rate of $20\,mmol\,h^{-1}$, rising to $40\,mmol\,h^{-1}$ if the level continues to fall. Serum potassium should be regularly reassessed and supplements not given if the level rises above $6\,mmol\,l^{-1}$ or if the patient is oliguric.

There is no compelling evidence that correction of acidosis in DKA with bicarbonate improves outcomes even in patients with a pH as low as 6.9. Because bicarbonate administration increases carbon dioxide levels and this diffuses into cells, there is an increase in intracellular acidosis. Moreover, once ketogenesis ceases (as a result of insulin administration) hydrogen ion production ceases and acidosis improves. Since intracardiac pH is around 6.9 it is unlikely that extracellular acidosis is negatively inotropic.

Insulin therapy

The rapid reduction of blood sugar is neither necessary nor desirable.

Low-dose insulin regimens are simple, safe and effective. Soluble insulin has a biological half-life at tissue level of 20–30 min. Five units should be given as an initial bolus followed by a sliding-scale regimen that reduces blood sugar levels at a rate of 2–4 mmol h^{-1}. Continuous insulin infusion should be continued until the ketonaemia and acidosis have resolved. The patient can then be commenced on a maintenance regimen.

Treatment of the precipitating cause

DKA does not occur in isolation and it is important to identify and treat any precipitating causes. These are infections, insufficient insulin, infarctions (myocardial or cerebral) or other intercurrent illnesses.

Complications

The major complications are hypoglycaemia, hypokalaemia and cerebral oedema. The first two can be avoided and the third minimized by regular clinical and biochemical reassessment of the patient. Early detection of cerebral oedema with the institution of hyperventilation and mannitol therapy is necessary to reduce mortality. Patients are also at risk of venous thrombosis and appropriate prophylaxis should be provided.

> Serial arterial gas sampling is not required.

Monitoring of acidaemia can be done perfectly well using venous pH measurements since mean arterial and venous pH differs by only 0.03 pH units.

> Remember identification and treatment of the precipitating cause is essential.

HYPEROSMOLAR HYPERGLYCAEMIC NON-KETOTIC COMA (HHNKC)

This is usually seen in older non-insulin dependent diabetics. There is hyperglycaemia, hyperosmolarity and dehydration but no ketoacidosis. It is much less common than DKA.

Table 17.3: Management of HHNKC

> If the serum sodium level is >150 mmol l^{-1} use 0.45% saline.
>
> Patients are usually extremely sensitive to insulin and require lower infusion rates than in DKA.
>
> Thrombotic complications are common and patients should be fully anticoagulated with a low molecular weight heparin.

The condition is usually precipitated by infection, myocardial infarction, stroke or the administration of thiazide diuretics. The mortality rate is 50%. In comparison with diabetic ketoacidosis, dehydration and hyperglycaemia are severe although there is no ketosis or acidosis. Typically, the patient presents with an altered conscious level, the greater the osmolarity the greater the neurological deficit. Focal signs, including hemiparesis, are common.

Investigations demonstrate a raised serum osmolarity. In HHNKC the serum osmolarity is usually around 380 mmol l^{-1}. Whilst there is no ketoacidosis there is often a mild metabolic acidosis secondary to dehydration and impaired tissue perfusion and a subsequent rise in lactate levels.

Management follows the same principles as for DKA with a small number of variations (Table 17.3).

THYROID EMERGENCIES

THYROID CRISIS OR 'STORM'

This is a life-threatening exacerbation of thyrotoxicosis usually occurring in an undiagnosed or poorly treated patient. There is acute decompensation of major organ systems with a significant mortality from hypovolaemia, cardiac failure and arrythmias.

History

Known precipitants of thyroid crisis include non-compliance with medication for hyperthyroidism, infection, surgery, or the recent administration of iodine, including radio-contrast media. Thyroid crisis usually occurs in known thyrotoxics but may be the first presentation of previously undiagnosed disease.

Clinical examination

High fever, warm peripheries, tachycardia and a bounding pulse are usually found and thus make the differentiation from septic shock difficult. Specific thyroid signs, such as tremor, goitre and signs of thyroid eye disease, may be found. Central nervous system effects include anxiety, proximal myopathy and coma. On occasions the presentation may be of a major mental illness.

Investigation

Baseline full blood count, electrolytes, urea and thyroid function tests should be ordered. A raised white cell count is common in thyrotoxicosis and hypercalcaemia is often found. Treatment must commence before the thyroid function test results are available. An ECG may demonstrate cardiac arrhythmia or myocardial ischaemia and the patient should be continuously monitored.

Treatment

There must be careful maintenance of fluid balance with correction of hypokalaemia. Dysrhythmias (usually atrial fibrillation) should be controlled by drug therapy, and for hyperpyrexia external cooling and chlorpromazine (50 mg IM) may be used. Specific therapies for thyrotoxicosis are shown in Table 17.4. Treatment of the precipitating cause is the main determinant of outcome.

Table 17.4: Specific emergency therapy for thyrotoxicosis

Inhibition of hormone synthesis – propylthiouracil
Inhibition of hormone release – sodium iodide
Inhibition of peripheral hormone conversion – propranolol and prednisolone
Inhibition of peripheral hormone action – propranolol

HYPOTHYROIDISM AND MYXOEDEMA COMA

Myxoedema coma is life threatening although now very rare. It represents hypothyroidism in its most severe form and is most commonly seen in elderly women with undiagnosed or undertreated hypothyroidism. Infection is again the commonest precipitant and mortality may be as high as 50%.

History

Because of the confusion or coma often seen in this condition the history may be unobtainable from the patient, and as a consequence the questioning of friends or relatives is essential. There are often pre-existing typical symptoms of hypothyroidism, including cold intolerance, lethargy, hair loss, weight gain and hoarseness. Again the presentation may be of a psychosis (myxoedema madness). There may be a history of thyroid disease or the use of drugs such as lithium or amiodarone.

Clinical signs

Confusion may progress to coma and hypothermia is common. Bradycardia is usual and a chest X-ray may demonstrate cardiomegaly and pericardial effusion. The ECG usually shows small voltage complexes and a prolonged QT interval. The other characteristics of hypothyroidism, such as periorbital oedema, macroglossia and slow-relaxing deep tendon reflexes, are often found.

Laboratory investigations

Megaloblastic anaemia is common, as is hyponatraemia as a result of inappropriate antidiuretic hormone secretion (SIADH). The patient may also present with hypoglycaemia. Thyroid function tests will show either primary (low T_4, high thyroid-stimulating hormone (TSH)), indicating thyroid failure), or secondary (low T_4, low TSH, indicating pituitary failure) hypothyroidism. The serum cortisol is often also low.

Treatment

The emergency treatment of hypothyroidism requires correction of the associated abnormalities

Table 17.5: Emergency treatment of hypothyroidism

Hyponatraemia – fluid restriction (500 ml in 24 h).
Hypoglycaemia – 50% dextrose intravenously.
Hypothermia – slow rewarming to avoid a sudden decrease in peripheral vascular resistance and vascular collapse.
Glucocorticoids – hydrocortisone until cortisol level known. Treatment of hypothyroidism secondary to pituitary failure may precipitate adrenal crisis.
Specific thyroid therapy – the choice of thyroid hormone and dose regimen is controversial and consultation with an endocrinologist is recommended.

Table 17.6: Causes of adrenocortical failure

Primary:
Idiopathic (autoimmune)
Adrenal haemorrhage (Waterhouse–Friedrichsen syndrome)
Infiltration (tumour, tuberculosis)
Drugs (ketoconazole)
Secondary:
Pituitary apoplexy (haemorrhage into a pituitary tumour)
Infarction (Sheehan's syndrome)
Tertiary:
Withdrawal of glucocorticoid therapy
Chronic adrenal insufficiency in the face of increased cortisol demands (trauma, infection)

of glucose metabolism, temperature regulation, electrolytes and glucocorticoid hormones as well as specific thyroid therapy (Table 17.5).

ADRENOCORTICAL INSUFFICIENCY (ADDISONIAN CRISIS)

Adrenal insufficiency may be acute or chronic. Each adrenal gland consists of the medulla, which secretes adrenaline and noradrenaline and is largely under neuronal control, and the cortex, which is controlled by the pituitary gland and secretes glucocorticoids, mineralocorticoids and androgens. The secretion of glucocoticoids, principally cortisol, is governed by circulating adrenocortical trophic hormone (ACTH) produced by the pituitary. The secretion of mineralocorticoids, principally aldosterone, is controlled by the renin–angiotensin system. Symptoms of adrenocortical insufficiency occur when there is a failure (relative or absolute) of glucocorticoid and mineralocorticoid secretion.

CAUSES

The causes of adrenocortical insufficiency can be classified as primary, where there is failure of the adrenal cortex, secondary where the pituitary gland fails, or tertiary (Table 17.6). The abrupt onset of symptoms often occurs in relation to a physical stressor such as injury.

CLINICAL FEATURES

The symptoms of chronic insufficiency are non-specific. They include weakness, lethargy, hyperpigmentation, anorexia and weight loss. Acutely the presentation is of shock or hypoglycaemia in a patient known to be on long-term steroids as replacement therapy or for the treatment of some other condition. Some symptoms and signs are specific to the lack of glucocorticoids (hypoglycaemia), of mineralocorticoids (hyponatraemia), or to the excess ACTH (hyperpigmentation) of secondary hypoadrenalism. Consequently, a high index of suspicion of adrenocortical insufficiency must be maintained in any hypotensive patient in whom the diagnosis is in doubt. Patients with secondary hypoadrenalism are less likely to develop shock, hyponatraemia and hyperkalaemia since the production of mineralocorticoids via the renin–angiotensin system is not pituitary dependent.

INVESTIGATION

Blood should be taken for cortisol, ACTH and aldosterone levels in addition to baseline urea and electrolytes and full blood count.

TREATMENT

Prompt correction of hypoglycaemia may initially be necessary. Urgent intravenous fluid replacement should be commenced with normal saline and 200 mg of hydrocortisone administered as an intravenous bolus. Hyperkalaemia usually improves with rehydration and the patient may require potassium supplementation later. Any precipitating cause of the crisis should be treated. Mineralocorticoid therapy in patients with primary adrenal failure is required only after the acute crisis has been corrected.

Hypopituitary crisis

It is rare to identify a patient with pituitary failure in an emergency department. Nevertheless, patients with this condition may present with an intercurrent illness or injury and management will require some knowledge of their endocrine condition. Failure of the pituitary manifests largely as failure of its principal target organs, the adrenal cortex and thyroid gland. Treatment involves replacement therapy with thyroid and glucocorticoid hormones. Additionally, if the posterior pituitary is affected lack of antidiuretic hormone results in diabetes insipidus, which requires replacement therapy with desmopressin.

Disorders of calcium metabolism

Calcium plays a vital role in many processes at the cellular and molecular level. Processes such as haemostasis, muscle contraction, immune function and the maintenance of membrane integrity therefore rely on the calcium level being tightly regulated. Ionized serum calcium is the physiologically active entity but most laboratories analyse the total serum calcium, which is often a poor indicator of ionized calcium levels.

Most serum calcium is protein bound and physiologically inactive. Fluctuations in the serum proteins therefore affect the total serum calcium level. The normal serum calcium is within a range of 2.2–$2.6 \, \text{mmol} \, \text{l}^{-1}$. When interpreting serum calcium measurements it is important to correct the reading if hypoalbuminaemia is present. To correct for protein binding 0.02 mmol should be added or subtracted to the calcium level for each gram of

Table 17.7: Causes of hypercalcaemia

Malignancy	Extensive bone metastases
	Production of parathyroid hormone-like substances
Primary hyper-parathyroidism	
Iatrogenic	Lithium
	Thiazide diuretics
	Calcium and vitamin D preparations
Granuloma	Sarcoid
	Tuberculosis
Miscellaneous	Immobilization
	Hyperthyroidism
	Paget's disease

albumin above or below $40 \, \text{g} \, \text{l}^{-1}$. Both hypercalcaemia and hypocalcaemia represent medical emergencies.

Hypercalcaemia

Causes

In emergency department practice, hypercalcaemia is most commonly a result of disseminated malignancy or the use of vitamin D preparations. A differential diagnosis of hypercalcaemia is given in Table 17.7.

Symptoms and signs

The symptoms of hypercalcaemia are typically non-specific and may be remembered using the epiphet 'bones, moans, stones and abdominal groans'. Specifically, the patient may present with a change of mental state such as drowsiness, confusion, psychosis and coma. In the renal tract, calcium impairs reabsorbtion in the renal tubules and dehydration results, with polydipsia and polyuria and ultimately renal failure. In the longer term urinary calculi develop. Gastrointestinal symptoms such as constipation and ileus are the result of reduced smooth muscle tone. Peptic ulcer disease and acute pancreatitis are also more common. Other symptoms may include pruritus. Cardiovascular effects are demonstrated on an ECG with shortening of the QT interval and widening of the QRS complexes. Profound hypercalcaemia may

Table 17.8: Treatment of the patient with hypercalcaemia

Correction of dehydration
Increase renal excretion of calcium
Reduce osteolysis
Identification and treatment of underlying cause

Table 17.9: Causes of hypocalcaemia

Vitamin D deficiency	Renal disease
	Liver disease
	Malnutrition
	Malabsorption
Parathyroid hormone deficiency	Neck surgery
	Infiltrative diseases
	Sepsis
	Pancreatitis
Calcium chelation	Fluoride poisoning
	Citrate (blood transfusion)

result in bradycardia, heart block and cardiac arrest.

Treatment

Emergency treatment should be initiated if the corrected serum calcium is greater than $3.5\,\mathrm{mmol\,l^{-1}}$ or if the patient is symptomatic. The principles of treatment are given in Table 17.8.

Expansion of the intravascular volume is the most important step in correcting hypercalcaemia. Rehydration alone decreases the serum calcium and renal calcium clearance is also increased. Up to $5\,\mathrm{l}$ a day of saline may be required and care should be taken to avoid fluid overload in patients with reduced cardiac reserve. Renal calcium excretion can also be increased by the use of frusemide, which reduces renal tubular reabsorption of calcium. Reduction of osteolysis is achieved by administration of specific drugs such as the biphosphonates (e.g. etidronidate) or steroids, which are specifically beneficial in haematological malignancies and sarcoidosis.

The measures described above will temporarily correct hypercalcaemia. Its long-term treatment and prognosis are dependent on effective treatment of the underlying cause.

HYPOCALCAEMIA

Causes

Hypocalcaemia is a relatively rare diagnosis in emergency department practice. A differential diagnosis of its causes is given in Table 17.9.

Symptoms and signs

General fatigue and irritability are common and again the presentation may be of predominantly behavioural abnormality. When the serum calcium falls below $2\,\mathrm{mmol\,l^{-1}}$ neuromuscular symptoms, including carpopedal spasm, perioral parasthesiae and seizures, may occur. Chvostek's sign (tapping over the facial nerve causes facial muscle twitching) and Trousseau's sign (spasm of the small muscles of the hand after inflation of a tourniquet to stop arterial flow) may be elicited. Calcium depletion reduces myocardial contractile strength and may therefore contribute to cardiac failure. The ECG demonstrates QT interval prolongation and dysrhythmias are common.

Treatment

Again care should be taken in confirming the diagnosis by laboratory analysis to take into account variations in serum protein levels. Hypertension, vomiting and cardiac arrythmias may occur during calcium administration and the patient must be carefully monitored. Symptomatic patients should receive 10 ml of 10% calcium gluconate i.v. over 10 min. If the serum magnesium is also low or suspected to be low, 5 mmol of magnesium sulphate should be given intravenously over 15 min.

FURTHER READING

Moore, K. and Ramrakha, P. (1997) *Oxford Handbook of Acute Medicine.* Oxford University Press, Oxford.

CHAPTER EIGHTEEN

GENITOURINARY EMERGENCIES

- Introduction
- Renal failure
- Haematuria
- Acute retention
- Acute ureteric colic
- Urinary tract infection (UTI)
- Urethritis and sexually transmitted diseases

- Prostatitis
- Scrotal pain and swelling
- Balanitis
- Phimosis and paraphimosis
- Priapism
- Penile trauma
- Further reading

INTRODUCTION

Genitourinary emergencies represent a broad range of conditions from the very common, such as urinary tract infection, to the extremely rare. A few require rapid treatment to protect life whilst others are distressing and embarrassing. An ordered assessment will allow accurate diagnosis and the initiation of effective treatment.

RENAL FAILURE

Acute renal failure can be life threatening owing to biochemical disturbances and the consequent risk of cardiac arrythmia. Patients do not, however, normally present with such a diagnosis. A range of often non-specific symptoms is much more common. In many cases, the renal failure is an incidental biochemical finding. In rare cases, however, the patient will give a clear history of monitored worsening renal function.

The distinction between acute and chronic renal failure is often dependent on test results. In the emergency department, serious and immediately treatable causes and complications should be looked for and dealt with, leaving precise diagnosis for later. Patients are unlikely to have oliguria

or anuria as primary presenting complaints unless there is a obstructive component to their renal impairment. A careful history must be taken since non-specific symptoms are common, especially nausea and vomiting. Itching, paraesthesia and tetany may all result from biochemical abnormalities. More specific symptoms may include polyuria, nocturia and oedema. It is important to ask about difficulty in voiding, poor stream and other symptoms suggesting obstruction.

In the past medical history, systemic diseases that can cause renal failure (e.g. diabetes mellitus) should be sought, as well as details of any previous renal investigations. The family history may be relevant, for example in polycystic kidney disease. Many drugs can affect renal function and a careful drug history should be obtained, especially noting drugs that the patient has recently started.

If renal failure is suspected or discovered, the causes can be categorized as follows:

- *prerenal* – hypovolaemia; decreased perfusion – for example heart failure, renal artery stenosis
- *renal* – for example glomerulonephritis, renal vein thrombosis, accelerated hypertension, connective tissue disorders
- *postrenal* – obstruction – supravesicular obstruction needs to be bilateral to produce decreased urine flow.

Table 18.1: Emergency treatment of hyperkalaemia

10% calcium gluconate slow IV injection 10 ml
10 IU soluble insulin and 50 ml of 50% dextrose given intravenously
25–50 ml 8.4% sodium bicarbonate intravenously

General examination may reveal pallor, brown or 'half-and-half' nails and scratch marks secondary to pruritis. Facial or ankle oedema and a pericardial friction rub may be present. There may be signs of systemic diseases and abdominal examination may reveal a distended bladder. Rectal examination is necessary in order to examine the prostate and check for pelvic masses.

If a patient is in or believed to be in acute or acute-on-chronic renal failure, the most important investigation is urea and electrolytes. An urgent potassium is needed to exclude life-threatening arrythmogenic hyperkalaemia. Rapid intravenous access is therefore essential. A full blood count may demonstrate anaemia and clotting studies may be deranged. Cardiac monitoring should be commenced and an ECG should be obtained. In hyperkalaemia this will show peaked T waves, broadening of the QRS complex and arrythmias, including heart block. If the serum potassium is significantly raised (greater than 6.5 mmol l^{-1}), treatment with calcium, bicarbonate or a dextrose and insulin infusion should be started immediately (Table 18.1).

> Hyperkalaemia is life threatening and must be treated immediately.

A urethral catheter should be passed where possible and any urine obtained sent for microscopy and culture. If a urethral catheter cannot be passed, a urology referral for suprapubic catheterization should be made.

The role of imaging is limited in the immediate phase though it is important to rule out a treatable obstructive uropathy early. As some contrast materials are themselves nephrotoxic, ultrasound is often requested for this purpose.

The basis of immediate treatment is to make sure that further insults to the kidneys are avoided or treated. Obstruction should be relieved, drugs such as aminoglycosides and non-steroidal anti-inflammatories (NSAIDs) should be stopped,

Table 18.2: Effects of chronic renal failure

Secondary hyperparathyroidism	Bone pain, pathological fractures and osteomalacia
Hypocalcaemia Pseudogout	Twitching, tetany
Hyperkalaemia	Arrhythmias
Hypertension	Can be severe and resistant to treatment Increased risk of encephalopathy
Poor platelet function	Bleeding, bruising
Immunosuppression	Increased risk of infection
Uraemic pericarditis	Requires dialysis
Effects of drugs	Accumulation (opiates) Exacerbate renal failure (NSAID, angiotensin-converting enzyme inhibitor (ACE-I)) Hyperkalaemia (K$^+$ sparing diuretics)

hypovolaemia and hypotension corrected and sepsis treated.

EMERGENCIES ASSOCIATED WITH CHRONIC RENAL FAILURE

Table 18.2 lists the complications of chronic renal failure that might cause a patient to present to the emergency department.

CONTINUOUS AMBULATORY PERITONEAL DIALYSIS (CAPD)

Bacterial peritonitis is a common problem for patients on CAPD. The patient presents with abdominal pain and peritonism but is often systemically well. The drained dialysate bags are cloudy and a sample should be sent to the laboratory. Staphylococci are the usual causative organisms, but a ruptured diverticulum or other surgical cause should be sought if anaerobes or Gram-negative microbes are found. Advice should always be sought from the renal unit regarding admission and current antibiotic policy. Other problems include leakage of fluid into the abdominal wall, chest or scrotum. Hernias are common.

HAEMODIALYSIS

Patients on haemodialysis may present with hyperkalaemia or pulmonary oedema, especially immediately prior to a dialysis session. Unless the condition is life threatening the arm with the arterio-venous fistula should not be used for intravenous access or bloods. Likewise, BP cuffs should never be used on this arm. Fluid overload and hyper-kalaemia require urgent dialysis, although intra-venous frusemide may buy time owing to its vasodilatory action. If the patient is in extremis and dialysis is not immediately available, venesec-tion may be lifesaving.

> Do not use a dialysis fistula for routine intravenous access.

If a dialysis patient presents with local pain, swelling and redness around the site of the arterio-venous fistula, a shunt thrombosis must be suspected. This needs rapid vascular referral.

TRANSPLANT PATIENTS

Unless the complaint is trivial, the transplant team should always be informed of the attendance of a transplant patient, even if the problem seems unre-lated. They will know the patient and advise on treatment and follow-up. Acute rejection can be mistaken for a systemic infection. There is often pain over the transplant site, decreased urine pro-duction and deranged biochemistry. Urgent refer-ral is required.

HAEMATURIA

All cases of haematuria require thorough investi-gation. Causes are shown in Table 18.3.

> Urine is discoloured by rifampicin, beetroot and myoglobin. This may simulate haematuria.

The haematuria may be painful, painless or the result of trauma; it may occur at the beginning of voiding, mid-stream or at the end. The presence of clots should be noted. An upper urinary tract source may be indicated by flank or abdominal pain,

Table 18.3: Causes of haematuria

Infection	Pyelonephritis, cystitis, parasites (schistosomiasis)
Stones	
Malignancy	Renal, ureter, bladder, prostate
Inflammation	Glomerulonephritis
Haematological	Leukaemias, platelet disorders, haemophilia, sickle cell disease
Vascular	Renal artery and vein occlusions
Congenital	Polycystic kidneys, hydronephrosis
Drugs	Warfarin and other anticoagulants, aspirin, cyclophosphamide
Others	Post severe exercise, factitious

whilst a lower source may have associated fre-quency, urgency and dysuria. A glomerular cause can present with facial or ankle swelling and arthralgia. It is important to ask about a history of preceding upper respiratory tract infection.

Pallor, purpura and oedema should be sought. A rectal examination must be performed in order to exclude a pelvic mass and to examine the prostate. Associated signs may suggest where in the urinary tract the source is. The external genitalia should be examined in order to exclude a meatal lesion.

Routine investigations as appropriate should include a mid-stream specimen of urine (MSU) for microscopy, sensitivity and culture, dipstick urine testing and full blood count, urea and electrolyte and clotting tests. If glomerulonephritis is sus-pected the laboratory should be specifically asked to look for urinary casts. If the patient shows signs of infection, blood cultures should be taken. Imaging is rarely required before referral.

All children and patients with clot retention, trauma or deranged clotting should be admitted. Urological referral and follow-up is otherwise indi-cated unless a glomerular cause is suspected, in which case medical referral is appropriate.

ACUTE RETENTION

Acute urinary retention is a common problem in men with prostatism; it is much rarer in women but can occur in atrophic urethritis or late pregnancy. Other causes include acute urethritis and urethral strictures, stones, clot retention, trauma, drugs and faecal impaction. Drugs responsible include anticholinergics, antihistamines, tricyclic antidepressants and alcohol.

It is important to distinguish between retention and true oliguria.

Examination will reveal suprapubic fullness, tenderness and dullness. A rectal examination will provide information about the prostate and exclude a pelvic mass or faecal impaction. Decreased anal tone may suggest a neurological cause.

The patient should be given every chance to pass urine on their own. Privacy and running taps may help. Otherwise urethral catheterization should be performed. If this is unsuccessful the patient should be referred for suprapubic catheterization. Once obtained, a urine sample should be sent for dipstick, microscopy and culture. Urological referral is almost invariably required.

Chronic retention can cause massive painless bladder distention. A large diuresis may follow once the obstruction has been relieved. This can produce fluid and electrolyte disturbances and it is advisable to drain the residual urine slowly.

ACUTE URETERIC COLIC

Ureteric colic is characterized by severe intermittent unilateral loin pain that waxes and wanes. Stones or blood clots may be the cause. Calcium phosphate and oxalate stones are the commonest; more rarely stones consist of magnesium ammonium phosphate, urate and cysteine. The underlying factors that lead to stone formation include infection, any cause of raised calcium in the blood or urine, hyperoxaluria and hyperuricaemia. The differential diagnosis includes pain from an aortic aneurysm or testicular or ovarian sources.

The pain may radiate anteriorly or laterally from the loin, or down to the groin and genitalia. The patient is usually sweaty and restless. Nausea and vomiting are frequent, as are dysuria, haematuria and 'gravel' in the urine. The patient will often have experienced previous episodes.

The abdominal examination is usually normal except for tenderness in the renal angle. Aortic aneurysm should be actively excluded in patients in the appropriate age group. The presence of pyrexia and rigors suggests associated infection.

The first treatment priority is analgesia. Intravenous opiates (and an antiemetic) work rapidly and are effective. Rectal and intramuscular NSAIDs can also be used and will not cause sedation or vomiting but are slower in onset of relief. There is no proven role for bolus intravenous fluids (in order to 'wash out' the stones) or for anticholinergics such as buscopan.

An urine specimen will almost invariably demonstrate microscopic haematuria; however, sieving and stone analysis are of no value in the emergency department. A full blood count, urea and electrolytes, calcium, phosphate and urate should be taken. Blood cultures are indicated if there is any sign of systemic infection. Ninety per cent of renal stones are radio-opaque and will show up on careful examination of a KUB (kidneys–ureters–bladder) film, but the incidence of both false-positive and false-negative findings with this investigation is high (Fig. 18.1). Intravenous urography (IVU), ultrasound or CT scanning may also be of value but are best performed by the specialist team.

Ninety per cent of renal stones are radio-opaque.

Patients with persistent pain after adequate analgesia, obstruction, renal impairment or evidence of infection should be admitted. Pain-free patients can be discharged home with arrangements for urological follow-up.

URINARY TRACT INFECTION (UTI)

Urinary tract infections vary in incidence and symptoms with age, although *Escherichia coli* is the most common causative organism at all ages. Young children may present with generalized abdominal pain, malaise and vomiting; the elderly are likely to present with a similar picture or be asymptomatic. Many elderly people suffer the symptoms of UTI with no infection. At all ages women are at increased risk, owing to the shorter female urethra. This risk further increases in sexually active women (so-called honeymoon cystitis).

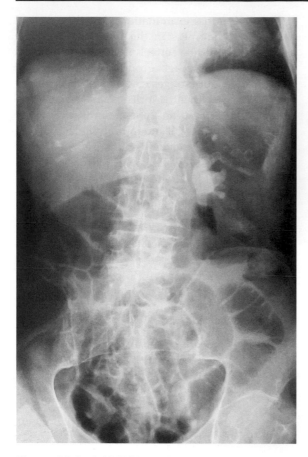

Figure 18.1: A KUB X-ray showing a renal stone.

Other predisposing factors include:

- urinary tract malformation
- vesicoureteric reflux – 40% of children with UTI
- stones
- diabetes mellitus
- immunosuppression
- incomplete bladder emptying
- bladder abnormalities: diverticulae, neuropathy, tumours.

Between the extremes of age, UTI usually presents to the emergency department in one of two forms:

- *Acute pyelonephritis (upper UTI)* – presents with loin pain, fever (with or without rigors) vomiting and dehydration. The features associated with cystitis are not prominent. Septicaemia and perirenal abscesses may, very rarely, develop.
- *Cystitis (lower UTI)* – presents with dysuria, frequency, nocturia, urgency, and smelly and cloudy urine, as well as suprapubic discomfort and sometimes haematuria.

In all cases of suspected UTI, a mid-stream specimen of urine should be analysed. Direct examination of the urine may reveal it to be cloudy and to smell offensive. Dipstick analysis will demonstrate protein, blood, leucocytes and nitrites and this information is sufficient to confirm the diagnosis and initiate treatment. Similarly, a negative dipstick examination is strongly predictive of negative microscopy and the finding of no bacterial growth on culture. Urgent microscopy if performed on an infected specimen will show leucocytes, red blood cells and bacteria (crystals, red blood cells and granular casts suggest underlying renal pathology). Culture should be performed to identify the infecting micro-organism and to confirm its sensitivity to the antibiotic used.

Patients who are:

- systemically unwell
- male
- female with recurrent infection (>3 per year)
- very young
- elderly
- pregnant
- suffering from renal impairment
- immunosuppressed

require further investigation or admission (or both) and should be referred to a urologist. Blood cultures are essential if there is a possibility of systemic infection.

Systemically unwell patients should be admitted for analgesia, intravenous antibiotics and fluids. Other patients can be discharged on oral antibiotics with advice to drink plenty of fluids. Amoxycillin (3 g) or trimethoprim (200 mg) are appropriate single-dose regimens for a woman with an uncomplicated first-time UTI. Recurrent UTIs should receive 3–5-day courses. All discharged patients should be followed up by their general practitioner or in the out-patient department.

URETHRITIS AND SEXUALLY TRANSMITTED DISEASES

Patients concerned that they have caught a sexually transmitted disease (STD) may attend the emergency department with or without symptoms. The telephone numbers of the local genitourinary medicine (GU or 'special') clinic should be prominently displayed in the waiting room. All these patients should receive a sympathetic

Table 18.4: Causes of urethral or vaginal discharge

Male	Female
Gonococcal urethritis	Normal physiological discharge
Non-gonococcal urethritis	Oral contraceptive pill – can increase normal discharge
	Atrophic vaginitis
	Gonococcus
	Candidiasis
	Chlamydia
	Trichomonas
	Gardnerella
	Retained tampon or other foreign body
	Malignancy of cervix or uterus – rare first presentation

hearing and most can then be directed to the clinic for further diagnosis, treatment and contact tracing. Even where treatment is needed or requested in the emergency department, follow-up should be arranged in the clinic.

Dysuria and discharge are the most common symptoms experienced by patients, although 5–10% with urethritis can be asymptomatic. Causes of urethral or vaginal discharge are shown in Table 18.4. Urinary frequency is also a common symptom. Urethritis is far more common as a cause of dysuria in men than other forms of UTI. Urethritis is almost always caused by an STD, although it may be a result of trauma or foreign body insertion. *Gonococcus* and *Chlamydia* are the commonest causative organisms in both sexes. Others include *Trichomonas* and *Gardnerella*.

Epididymitis (see below) is the most frequent complication of urethritis. Around 2% of patients with non-gonococcal urethritis will develop Reiter's disease. This presents with accompanying iritis and arthritis usually affecting the lower limbs. Cutaneous, cardiac and neurological manifestations are rare. Gonorrhoea can cause disseminated disease presenting with fever, arthralgia, septic arthritis and a purpuric or vesiculopapular rash.

GENITAL ULCERATION

Painful ulcers are most likely to be genital herpes. Rarer causes are Behçet's disease and chancroid. Candida or gonococcal disease may also present with multiple painful sores.

Herpetic lesions start as small vesicles which are often missed by the patient. These develop into 1–3 mm ulcers with a ring of erythema, and may coalesce. In the first episode the ulcers can be very painful with local lymphadenopathy. Patients may feel unwell, with 'flu-like' symptoms and fever. Meningitis and radiculomyelitis are rare complications.

The diagnosis is clinical but can be confirmed on viral culture of swabs. Oral aciclovir should be started if the presentation is within 6 days of the onset of the primary attack. Analgesia may be required. The patient should be referred to the GU medicine clinic for follow-up.

Painless ulcers are caused by syphilis and, less commonly, carcinoma.

GENITAL WARTS

Genital warts are usually asymptomatic unless situated at the external urinary meatus. Whatever the site, referral to the GU medicine clinic is all that is needed.

PROSTATITIS

Patients may present to the emergency department with either acute or chronic prostatitis. Causative organisms include *E. coli*, *Pseudomonas*, *Proteus*, *Klebsiella* and *Streptococcus faecalis*. Tuberculous disease is very rare.

The clinical features include urgency, frequency, hesitancy and poor stream, together with fever, rigors, dysuria, and suprapubic or groin pain. A tender, hard and irregular prostate is found on rectal examination. A prostatic abscess may develop causing severe pain. An urine specimen may show proteinuria on dipstick and the causative organism on culture. Other diagnostic tests (3 or 4 glass tests) are not the province of the emergency department. All patients should be referred to a urologist. Antibiotics must penetrate the prostatic fluid (trimethoprim) and may be required on a long-term basis.

SCROTAL PAIN AND SWELLING

The likely causes of scrotal pain and swelling vary with age (Table 18.5). It is important to remember

Table 18.5: Causes of scrotal pain by age

Neonates and infants:
   Testicular torsion
   Epididymo-orchitis
   Acute hydrocoele

Before puberty:
   Testicular torsion
   Torsion of hydatid of Morgagni
   Epididymo-orchitis
   Trauma

After puberty:
   Testicular torsion
   Epididymo-orchitis
   Torsion of hydatid of Morgagni
   Trauma
   Tumour

that inguinal hernias, abdominal aortic aneurysms and ureteric stones may be a cause of scrotal pain and also that abdominal pain may be referred from the testicles. The testicles should always be examined as part of the abdominal examination.

Always consider abdominal aortic aneurysm as a cause of scrotal pain in the elderly patient.

TESTICULAR TORSION

Testicular torsion is most frequent in neonates and around puberty. Boys with undescended testicles are at higher risk. It may present in adults but is rare after 30 years of age. Torsion presents with an acute onset of severe scrotal and lower abdominal pain. Occasionally, the lower abdominal pain may predominate. Vomiting is common. Previous short spontaneously resolving episodes may have occurred. The affected testis is red, very tender and elevated, lying horizontally. In the early stages a non-tender epididymis may be palpated anteriorly, until it is affected by oedema. The cremasteric reflex is absent.

The emergency treatment of testicular torsion is analgesia and urgent surgical referral. Failure to do this may result in loss of the testicle and reduced fertility.

Testicular torsion is a surgical emergency.

TORSION OF THE HYDATID OF MORGAGNI

The hydatid of Morgagni is a remnant of the para-mesonephric duct and is situated at the antero-superior pole of the testis. The history is very similar to testicular torsion. On examination, however, there is point tenderness at its site, where a small nodule may be felt. The rest of the testis is normal. Once again, the treatment is analgesia and surgical referral.

EPIDIDYMITIS

In young adult males epididymitis is usually secondary to urethritis, the most common causative organisms being *Chlamydia* and *Gonococcus*. In older men a UTI, with underlying urinary tract pathology, is more likely. The patient may present with dysuria, frequency, urethral discharge and a fever as well as scrotal pain. On examination there may be scrotal redness, swelling and epididymal tenderness. The testis is normal in the early stages. The urine should be dipsticked for blood and protein, and an MSU and urethral swab taken.

If it is not possible to exclude testicular torsion, urgent surgical referral is essential. If the diagnosis is clear and the patient is systemically unwell admission for intravenous antibiotics is required. Otherwise suitable oral antibiotics for the causative organism and analgesia may be given. The younger patient should be referred to the STD clinic for follow-up and contact tracing.

ORCHITIS

Bacterial epididymitis may extend and cause epididymo-orchitis. Orchitis may also be viral in origin. Mumps is the most common cause, and can produce uni- or bilateral orchitis. This typically occurs 4–5 days after the parotitis, though rarely there is no parotitis. Rare causes include TB, syphilis, leprosy and brucellosis. The most appropriate treatment is analgesia; antibiotics may be prescribed if the exact diagnosis and organism are unclear.

TRAUMA

Trauma to the scrotum can cause scrotal haematoma or testicular rupture. Both require analgesia and referral. An ultrasound scan may be needed to distinguish between the two. The former can be treated conservatively, whilst the latter requires surgical exploration and repair. Testicular haematoma may also occur following vasectomy. Scrotal wounds can be sutured unless there is complete penetration of the sac, in which case exploration to exclude damage to deeper structures will be necessary.

PAINLESS SCROTAL MASSES

Some patients may present with lumps that are pain free or only slightly tender. Minor trauma or health promotion programmes may have caused them to examine themselves for the first time. Possible causes include tumour, hydrocoele and epididymal cyst. Whilst they do not need admission, rapid out-patient follow-up should be arranged.

BALANITIS

Balanitis is a bacterial or fungal infection of the space between the foreskin and the glans. It is most common in younger boys, and can present with pain, discharge and dysuria. Appropriate investigations include a swab, MSU and dipstick urine for glucose.

The most effective treatment is amoxycillin, with referral to the general practitioner for follow-up. If the whole penis is involved, admission for intravenous antibiotics may be necessary.

PHIMOSIS AND PARAPHIMOSIS

Phimosis is constriction of the foreskin preventing retraction. If it persists after the age of 5 years, or is associated with recurrent balanitis, it requires elective surgical referral for consideration of circumcision.

Paraphimosis is an irreducible retracted foreskin. The glans distal to the foreskin can become swollen and painful, and may lead to acute urinary retention. Pressure using cold compresses should be applied for 5–10 min after which manual reduction should be attempted using lubricating gel. If this fails, urgent surgical referral is needed.

PRIAPISM

Priapism is a prolonged, often painful, erection not associated with sexual stimulation. After 12 h it may lead to intracorporeal thrombosis and long-term fibrosis and impotence. Causes include:

- iatrogenic – papaverine injection for impotence
- drugs – for example phenothiazines
- sickle cell disease
- leukaemia
- myeloma
- spinal cord trauma.

In addition, patients occasionally present with a persistent erection following the use of a constricting device (used to prolong an erection for sexual pleasure) around the base of the shaft of the penis, which they are unable to remove. A similar problem may occur when the penis is inserted into the neck of a bottle.

If the cause is unclear, a full blood count (FBC) and sickle test should be considered. If a constricting device is not the cause of a persisting erection, urgent urological referral for aspiration of the corpus cavernosum is essential.

PENILE TRAUMA

FOREIGN BODIES

Foreign bodies can be introduced into the external urinary meatus for varying reasons in adults and children. If stuck, gentle manipulation should be attempted. Lignocaine gel may be of use. Referral to the urologists may be necessary if removal is unsuccessful or there is haematuria or any possibility of urethral rupture.

ZIP ENTRAPMENT

This painful (and embarrassing) accident, affecting boys more often than men, is usually minor and easily released by the victim or parent. Severe cases will present to the emergency department. Cutting through the zip below the entrapment may allow easy removal. Where possible it is desirable to cut only the material near the zip and preserve the trouser material so that only the zip and not the trousers need replacement. In more difficult entrapments liberal application of lignocaine gel, which is then left for at least 15 min, may facilitate manipulation. Plain lignocaine may be injected but can increase soft tissue swelling, defeating the purpose. Younger boys may not tolerate the procedure well in the emergency department and may require referral for release under general anaesthesia. Circumcision is only rarely needed.

FRENULAR TEARS

The frenulum may be torn during (often vigorous) sexual intercourse. The patient complains of pain and bleeding. In most cases local pressure is all that is required. This should be followed by advice to abstain from sex for around 10 days to allow healing and prevent recurrence. If pressure does not work, referral is required.

Caution must be exercised in assessing any penile injury in a child. Consideration must be given to the possibility that the injury represents sexual abuse.

PENILE FRACTURE

The patient complains of sudden pain and loss of erection during sexual intercourse. Often this is

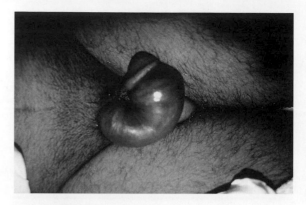

Figure 18.2: Penile fracture.

accompanied by a loud crack. On examination the fracture may be palpable, along with a visible haematoma and bend in the shaft. The appearence has been compared to that of an aubergine (Fig. 18.2). The tunica albuginea, which surrounds the corpus cavernosa, is ruptured. In up to 20% there is a urethral tear. Urgent urological referral is required for exploration and repair, otherwise the prospects for return of function are poor.

FURTHER READING

Wetherall, D., Ledingham, J. and Warrell, D. (1997) *Oxford Textbook of Medicine*. Oxford University Press, Oxford.

CHAPTER NINETEEN

INFECTIOUS DISEASES

- Introduction
- Human immunodeficiency virus (HIV)
- Travellers' illnesses
- Meningococcal septicaemia

- Gastroenteritis
- Hepatitis
- Lyme disease
- Further reading

INTRODUCTION

Infectious diseases remain the single commonest cause of illness within the community. Fortunately, most are not life threatening and are self-limiting illnesses which cause their victim no more than temporary incapacity. Many of these conditions which present to emergency departments are dealt with in specific chapters on the sick child (Chapter 40), respiratory emergencies (Chapter 12), neurological emergencies (Chapter 13), dermatology (Chapter 32) and ear, nose and throat (Chapter 37). In this chapter the remaining significant infectious diseases that present to emergency departments are covered.

HUMAN IMMUNODEFICIENCY VIRUS (HIV)

It is less than 20 years since the acquired immune deficiency syndrome (AIDS) was first recognized and its causative organism, HIV, identified. This modern epidemic has already claimed the lives of many, and millions of patients, particularly in Africa, are infected with and carrying the virus. In urban American emergency departments up to 9% of patients have been found to be carriers of HIV, although fortunately it is much less common in the UK. A number of risk factors are associated with carriage of the virus (Table 19.1).

HIV is an RNA retrovirus which may be isolated from a wide variety of body fluids. Blood, semen, vaginal fluids and transplacental spread are the established vehicles and routes for transmission of infection in humans. Following infection with the virus a patient may remain asymptomatic for many years. HIV produces AIDS by destroying cells vital to the immune response, principally the T helper cells and some monocytes and macrophages. With the progressive impairment of cellular immunity the patient develops rare opportunistic infections and tumours, which may result in their presentation to an emergency department.

CLINICAL FEATURES

The diagnosis of HIV infection is often made on the basis of the detection of antibodies to the virus during routine testing, often as the result of contact tracing. A patient may or may not be aware of their infection with the virus when they present to an emergency department with an illness related to

Table 19.1: Risk factors for HIV infection

Homosexuality or bisexuality
IV drug abuse
Multiple sexual contacts
Prostitution
Tattoos
Blood transfusion recipient
Sexual partner or child of above

Table 19.2: Markers of AIDS

Pneumocystis pneumonia
Kaposi sarcoma
Toxoplasma encephalitis
Atypical mycobacterium infections
Systemic fungal infection

HIV infection. Patients may present with symptoms of acute HIV infection after an incubation period of approximately 6 weeks. The manifestations of this (pyrexia, lethargy, myalgia) are non-specific and the significance of the illness is rarely recognized.

After a prolonged asymptomatic period of infection, immunity is sufficiently impaired to result in the development of unusual secondary infections or tumours. Certain of these illnesses are so characteristic of AIDS that their presence is almost diagnostic of the disease (Table 19.2).

The patient may also present with generalized lymphadenopathy or fever, weight loss and lethargy. Other manifestations of the disease may predominantly affect the respiratory, neurological and gastrointestinal systems as well as the skin and mucous membranes. For further details of these conditions a specific text should be consulted (see Further Reading).

INVESTIGATION AND TREATMENT

The role of the emergency department in the management of HIV-infected patients is the detection and immediate treatment of life-threatening abnormalities and referral to the appropriate specialty for definitive care. There should be a low threshold for admission for further assessment.

RISKS TO THE CARERS

The risk of acquiring HIV through occupational exposure is low; however, universal precautions should always be taken as even analysis of risk factors (Table 19.1) does not accurately predict HIV carriage. Particular care must be taken to ensure safe disposal of sharps, and all samples sent to the laboratory for analysis must be carefully labelled and the technicians warned of the potential risks.

It has now been established that following exposure to the virus, rates of seroconversion may be substantially reduced by the early (within 3 h) use of antiviral agents. Any patient or member of staff exposed to the blood of a known HIV-positive patient via parenteral inoculation or blood contact to broken or inflamed mucosa or skin must therefore be assessed rapidly. The risks and benefits of use of antiviral prophylaxis should be discussed with the patient and a specialist in HIV infection and, where appropriate, therapy commenced immediately.

> Early use of antiviral agents reduces HIV seroconversion following needlestick injury from a known HIV-positive patient.

Concerns regarding the risk of transmission of HIV to carers must not be allowed to prevent the patient from receiving optimal treatment including, where necessary, cardiopulmonary resuscitation. Above all, confidentiality must be preserved and the doctor should not reveal any details of the patient's illness without appropriate consent.

REQUESTS FOR HIV TESTING

It is not uncommon for patients to present to an emergency department requesting HIV testing. This may be the result of real and significant concerns regarding the possibility of infection. Although an emergency department is not the appropriate place to perform these tests it is important to encourage the patient to seek appropriate help, as effective prophylactic treatment is now available which reduces the risk of the development of AIDS in patients with HIV infection. The patient should be thoroughly assessed and counselled with regard to the limitations of the test and the consequences of a positive test before agreeing to the test being carried out. The most appropriate facility for this is the genitourinary medicine clinic.

> HIV testing should not be performed by the emergency department.

TRAVELLERS' ILLNESSES

Foreign travel to increasingly remote and exotic destinations is increasingly common. It is not uncommon for patients to present to emergency departments with illnesses that have developed during or following a visit to another country. The commonest presenting complaint in this group is diarrhoea, followed in order of frequency by febrile illness. Rabies is also covered here, as it remains a disease acquired only outside the UK. It is important to find out which areas the patient has visited, in what time period and what prophylactic measures (specifically antimalarial) were used and for how long. Further advice may be available from the local department of infectious diseases. Alternatively, the national centres of excellence in Liverpool or London may be contacted (Table 19.3).

DIARRHOEAL ILLNESS

Diarrhoea is a common experience for travellers to developing countries. Symptoms often develop within a few days of arrival but may be delayed or persist until the traveller returns to his or her home country. The common causal agents are shown in Table 19.4 and are predominantly bacterial.

The illnesses are typically distressing but self-limiting and not life threatening. The patient should replace fluid losses with oral fluids and a specimen should be sent for microbiological analysis. Antibiotics have a role to play in substantially reducing the length of illness. A 3-day course of a quinolone antibiotic produces rapid relief of symptoms.

Table 19.3: National contacts for tropical disease advice

School of Tropical Medicine, Liverpool	0151 708 9393
Hospital for Tropical Diseases, London	020 7387 4411

Table 19.4: Common causes of travellers' diarrhoea

Enterotoxic *Escherichia coli*
Shigella
Campylobacter
Salmonella
Rotavirus
Norwalk virus
Giardia
Cryptosporidium

THE FEBRILE TRAVELLER

The incubation period for some illnesses is prolonged (Table 19.5). The development of a febrile illness may not be connected by the patient to a recent period of travel if the onset of the illness occurs some time after return to home. It is therefore wise to enquire routinely about foreign travel when assessing a patient with a febrile illness.

The differential diagnosis is arrived at by considering the symptoms and examination findings, as well as a knowledge of the diseases a patient may have been exposed to in the area to which they travelled. Prophylactic measures used, such as antimalarial chemotherapy, should also be considered, though this does not provide complete protection.

Malaria

This must be considered and excluded in the diagnosis of any febrile illness in a patient who has travelled to a malarial area in the 3 months prior to onset. Areas of risk include India, Southeast Asia, Africa and Central or South America, although cases have also been reported in airport workers in the UK presumably bitten by mosquitoes transported to the UK on aeroplanes. The symptoms are often non-specific, with fever, lethargy and headache. The classic episodes of rigours with high fevers and vomiting may follow but often do not conform to the regular periodic pattern described elsewhere. Falciparum malaria may produce cerebral involvement, with fits and coma. Examination may reveal splenomegaly and jaundice.

A blood-film examination is essential in the investigation of a febrile patient who has visited a malarial area within 3 months.

Table 19.5: Incubation periods for travellers' diseases

Malaria	Falciparum	7–14 days
	Other	14–48 days
Paratyphoid		1–2 days
Lassa fever		4–14 days
Typhoid		7–21 days

The diagnosis is made by the finding of the malarial parasites on thin and thick blood-film microscopy. This may be initially negative, and if doubt persists regarding the diagnosis it should be repeated. Following diagnosis the patient should be transferred to the care of a specialist in infectious and tropical diseases.

Typhoid and paratyphoid

These infections, caused by *Salmonella typhi* and *S. paratyphi*, are a common cause of fever in the returning traveller. The initial symptoms are of fever, headache, myalgia and anorexia, often with abdominal bloating and discomfort. The patient may either be constipated or have diarrhoea. With progression of the illness there is alteration in level of consciousness. Typhoid is characterized by the presence of a bradycardia and rose spots (small pink macules) on the trunk. Abdominal signs may mimic a surgical emergency.

The patient should be admitted and isolated. Treatment with antibiotics leads to rapid resolution of the illness.

Viral haemorrhagic fevers

These are the most feared, although fortunately the least common, of the imported infectious diseases. The best known form is Lassa fever. The initial symptoms are non-specific and investigation should address the possibility of malaria or typhoid. If there is any possibility of the diagnosis of viral haemorrhagic fever based on the area which the patient has visited (usually west or central Africa) great caution must be exercised as blood and secretions are highly infective. Essential blood tests (to exclude malaria) should still be performed but the laboratory must be warned of the possibility of haemorrhagic fever. The patient should be discussed with a specialist in tropical and communicable disease and transferred to a unit that can provide the required degree of isolation.

RABIES

Over recent years rabies has gradually spread across Europe though it has yet to establish itself in the UK. However, it remains uncommon in Europe and is most common in the Indian subcontinent and Southeast Asia. It is acquired predominantly through animal bites, usually from dogs. Less commonly, infection may occur following contact between the infected animal's saliva and broken skin or a mucosal membrane.

The incubation period is variable but is usually between 1 and 3 months. A history of exposure may or may not be available. The initial symptoms are localized to the area of entry of the virus, with irritation or pain. A generalized illness follows, with headache and fever. Episodes of agitation occur classically characterized by hydrophobia (fear of water, with spasm of the oropharyngeal muscles). Progressive paralysis occurs and the outcome for established disease is virtually always fatal. Supportive care on an intensive care unit is required although precautions, including immunization of the carers, must be taken to prevent spread.

> Effective post-exposure prophylaxis is available for rabies.

Effective post-exposure prophylaxis is now available for patients potentially exposed to rabies. Where concern exists that a patient has been exposed to the virus, they should be urgently referred to a consultant in communicable diseases. As the incubation period for rabies is long, prophylaxis may still be beneficial some weeks after potential inoculation.

MENINGOCOCCAL SEPTICAEMIA

Infection with *Neisseria meningitidis* may result in meningitis (see Chapter 13) or a septicaemic illness, the latter often characterized by a rapid and fulminating course. It is distressing, though unfortunately not uncommon, to see a young patient rapidly deteriorate and die from this disease in a short time despite the best available therapy. It is a disease predominantly of children and young adults. Extensive public education campaigns have encouraged patients to seek help early when concerned, particularly about the appearance of a rash. Unfortunately, early symptoms are often non-specific and the nature and severity of the disease may not become apparent until too late.

In meningococcal septicaemia rash may be absent or non-purpuric.

PRESENTATION

Early symptoms of the disease may mimic upper respiratory tract infection or gastroenteritis. The rash, if present, may initially be maculo-papular, subsequently developing into the classic non-blanching purpura. Although the disease may be rapidly progressive with the rapid development of profound shock, other patients may remain deceptively well initially. The differential diagnosis of the purpuric rash includes Henoch–Schönlein purpura, toxic shock syndrome and thrombocytopenic purpura. Shock occurs as a result of intravascular fluid volume loss and myocardial suppression. Disseminated intravascular coagulation, renal failure and coma are late complications and indicators of severe disease with poor prognosis.

TREATMENT

Following recognition or even suspicion of the diagnosis high-dose parenteral antibiotics should be administered. Blood cultures should be taken to confirm the diagnosis but attempts to take blood must not delay antibiotic administration. Depending on local policy the choice of antibiotic agent may be a third-generation cephalosporin or high-dose penicillin G.

Management otherwise follows the usual emergency sequence of protecting the airway, administering a high concentration of oxygen and supporting ventilation if it is inadequate. Vascular access allows administration of intravenous fluids and invasive monitoring is required in patients with haemodynamic compromise. Patients will require to be treated in isolation, usually on a high-dependency or intensive care facility.

PROPHYLAXIS

Following the diagnosis of meningococcal infection, the emergency department should ensure that the consultant responsible for communicable

diseases is informed. It is important to provide antibiotic prophylaxis for family members and others who have been in close contact with the patient. This is not generally required for carers unless they have provided mouth-to-mouth ventilation. The usual agent used is rifampicin or ceftriaxone.

GASTROENTERITIS

Gastroenteritis as a result of food poisoning is common; however, this is a diagnosis that should only be made with caution after other significant diseases which may mimic it have been ruled out. Specifically, appendicitis, inflammatory bowel disease and large bowel malignancy may produce similar symptoms. The cardinal symptoms are diarrhoea and vomiting, although these may occur in isolation or sequentially depending on the causative organism (Table 19.6).

ASSESSMENT

The history should define the length and severity of the illness and its symptoms. A history of foreign travel and contact with others with a similar illness should also be sought. If the patient handles food, they must cease work and if a diagnosis of food poisoning is made the case must be notified to the local consultant responsible for communicable disease control. Examination and investigation should aim to exclude more serious diseases which mimic infectious gastroenteritis. An assessment of the degree of dehydration should also be made.

Table 19.6: Characteristics of types of food poisoning

	Onset	Symptoms
Rotavirus	2–5 days	Diarrhoea, vomiting, systemic illness
Staph. aureus	abrupt < 6 h	Profuse vomiting
E. coli	2 days	Diarrhoea, vomiting
Salmonella	1–2 days	Diarrhoea, vomiting
Campylobacter	< 2 days	Diarrhoea (bloody), systemic illness

Table 19.7: Clinical features of dehydration

Dry mucous membranes
Reduced skin turgor
Altered mental state (drowsy, lethargy)
Depressed fontanelle if present
Reduced and concentrated urine output
Tachycardia
Postural hypotension

Table 19.8: Oral rehydration therapy (ORT)

Fruit juices
Flat soft drinks (not diet)
Commercial oral rehydration salts – Dioralyte®,
    Rehidrat®

MANAGEMENT

These illnesses are generally self-limiting and not life threatening. Admission may be required where there is evidence of dehydration (Table 19.7), particularly in small children or the frail elderly. If the patient is fit to continue treatment as an outpatient then general advice should be provided regarding oral rehydration therapy (Table 19.8). If the patient is significantly dehydrated intravenous fluid therapy may be necessary, commencing with normal saline.

Most infective diarrhoea is caused by viral infections. Stool samples should be taken for culture and sensitivity although antibiotic treatment should be reserved for those patients with a proven diagnosis of invasive bacterial infection.

Antidiarrhoeal medication is not indicated and may be harmful. Parenteral antiemetic therapy is occasionally useful in an adult who is vomiting profusely.

HEPATITIS

This section deals with hepatitis produced by infectious agents, the hepatitis viruses (A, B and C), Epstein–Barr virus and Weil's disease as a result of infection by the spirochaete *Leptospira icterohaemorrhagiae*.

HEPATITIS A

Otherwise known as infectious hepatitis, this virus is acquired by faeco-oral transmission. Most cases are now seen in patients who have visited tropical areas. Incubation is approximately 30 days, with non-specific symptoms of nausea, lethargy and fever being followed by the development of abdominal pain, hepatosplenomegaly and jaundice. Complete spontaneous recovery usually occurs and the period of greatest infectivity has usually passed by the time the diagnosis is made.

HEPATITIS B

This is of greatest concern as a result of its high infectivity and the ability for it to be transmitted by needlestick injury. Other common forms of transmission are sexual contact and as a result of needle sharing in intravenous drug abusers. Modern techniques for screening blood donors has removed the possibility of transmission by blood products.

Protection from hepatitis B requires immunization, universal precautions against blood contamination and safe sharps disposal.

All healthcare workers should be immunized against hepatitis B and should have their antibody levels checked regularly to ensure continuing immunity. Despite this, and as a result of the potential to acquire other infections, carers should protect themselves from blood contamination by wearing gloves, eye protection and, where appropriate, protective clothing. Continuing vigilance must also occur to ensure the safe disposal of sharps.

The onset of illness follows approximately 1–2 months after infection with the virus. The illness follows a similar pattern to hepatitis A, although in some cases there is a fulminant course resulting in hepatic failure. Patients may recover completely, develop a chronic hepatitis or become asymptomatic carriers of the virus. Treatment is largely supportive and the patient should be advised to avoid other hepatotoxins (particularly alcohol).

Patients sustaining a needlestick injury from a needle contaminated by blood from a patient with hepatitis B should be managed according to local guidelines. If the patient has effective vaccination against the virus, no further action is usually required. However, consideration should also be given to the possibility that a patient carrying hepatitis B might also carry HIV (see above).

HEPATITIS C

This infection is classically associated with blood transfusion, although transmission may also occur during IV drug abuse and as a result of occupational exposure. It follows a similar course to hepatitis B though as yet no effective vaccination or prophylaxis is available.

EPSTEIN–BARR VIRUS (EBV)

Hepatitis may occur as a result of EBV infection either as an isolated illness or in association with the other features of infectious mononucleosis. Diagnosis is based on visualizing abnormal monocytes on a blood film and demonstrating a rise in antibody titres to the virus. Treatment is expectant.

LEPTOSPIROSIS

Infection occurs when there is contact between broken skin or mucosal membranes and water containing the spirochaete. *Leptospira* is carried by rats and excreted in their urine. Human infection occurs from sewers and canals, and those who work in these environments are instructed to attend emergency departments for antibiotic prophylaxis if they sustain a wound or may have had mucosal contamination. Penicillin is an appropriate antibiotic in these circumstances.

Weil's disease is characterized by a hepatitic illness with fever, vomiting, jaundice and renal failure. Treatment consists of penicillin and supportive therapy.

> Wounds potentially contaminated by water from sewers and canals should be treated with prophylactic penicillin.

LYME DISEASE

This is a tick-borne spirochaete infection. Initially an expanding red area of rash (erythema migrans) develops at the site of the tick bite, which may itself have gone unnoticed. The rash may develop a bull's-eye appearance. This is followed by a flu-like illness and subsequently there are cardiac effects including myocarditis and conduction abnormalities, peripheral nerve lesions and large joint arthropathies. A chronic arthritis may develop. Treatment with penicillin or doxycycline is thought to reduce the incidence of chronic arthropathy.

FURTHER READING

Barkin, R., Rosen, P., Hockberger, R. *et al.* (1998) *Emergency Medicine: Concepts and Clinical Practice*, 4th edn. Mosby, St Louis.

Moore, K. and Ramrakha, P. (1997) *Oxford Handbook of Acute Medicine.* Oxford University Press, Oxford.

PART THREE

TRAUMA

CHAPTER TWENTY

HEAD AND NECK TRAUMA

- Head trauma
- Neck injuries
- Further reading

HEAD TRAUMA

INTRODUCTION

Head injuries are the commonest cause of trauma deaths throughout the western world, playing a part in half of all deaths due to trauma. Each year around 5000 people die from head injuries in Britain and another 1500 are severely brain damaged. Several hundred thousand more sustain a 'minor' head injury and may present to an emergency department. Head injuries are most common in young adult males and may be due to assaults, road-traffic accidents, falls or other accidents. Head injuries due to falls are four times as likely to be lethal as those due to road-traffic accidents.

The arbitrary division of head injuries into severe, moderate and minor groups is of little clinical use, especially in the emergency department. Therefore, in this chapter head injuries will be regarded as a single entity, representing a spectrum of severity.

Severity of head injury can only be judged in retrospect.

ANATOMY

The head consists of the brain contained within a non-expansile (except in young children) box, the skull. On the front of the skull are the facial bones. Injuries to the facial bones are dealt with in Chapter 21 and are not further discussed here. The skull is covered by the scalp, which has five layers (Table 20.1).

Table 20.1: The layers of the scalp

Skin
(sub)**C**utaneous fat
Aponeurosis
Loose areolar tissue
Periosteum

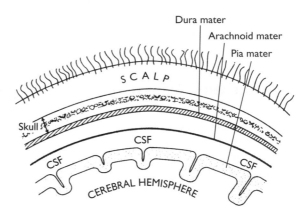

Figure 20.1: The meninges and their spaces.

The skull consists of the vault (the frontal, parietal, temporal and occipital bones) and the base, which runs obliquely along a line joining the mastoid processes with the orbits. Within the skull are three layers of meninges or brain coverings. These are, from outwards in, the tough, thick dura mater which is attached to the inner surface of the skull, the thin arachnoid mater and the pia mater, which is tightly applied to the cortex of the brain (Fig. 20.1).

These layers define the various spaces:

- The extradural space, between the dura and the inner surface of the skull. This space contains arteries grooving the skull.
- The subdural space, between the dura mater and the arachnoid mater. This space is crossed by large veins.
- The subarachnoid space, between the subarachnoid mater and the pia mater. This space contains the cerebrospinal fluid.

The brain has two cerebral hemispheres, a cerebellum and a brainstem, which is in direct continuity with the spinal cord. The brainstem consists of the mid-brain, pons and medulla. The mid-brain and pons contain the reticular activating system that is vital for consciousness. The medulla contains centres that control breathing and cardiac function. Cerebrospinal fluid is produced by choroid plexuses and leaves the ventricles of the brain to circulate in the subarachnoid space. The tentorium lies horizontally between the cerebral hemispheres and the cerebellum. The mid-brain passes through the large opening or incisura in the tentorium. The third cranial nerve (oculomotor nerve) also passes through the incisura.

INTRACRANIAL PRESSURE

Intracranial pressure (ICP) is the pressure within the skull and is normally controlled within tight limits by homoeostatic mechanisms. The cerebral perfusion pressure (CPP) is also regulated, a normal CPP being required for adequate perfusion of the brain tissue. The normal CPP is above 50 mmHg. The CPP and ICP are related to the mean arterial blood pressure in the following way:

Cerebral perfusion pressure = Mean arterial pressure − intracranial pressure.

Thus, if intracranial pressure increases, owing to bleeding within the confined skull or to cerebral oedema or swelling, the cerebral perfusion pressure will fall, compromising the blood supply to the brain and making secondary brain damage likely. This equation also explains how hypovolaemia, via a fall in mean arterial pressure, causes a reduction in cerebral perfusion.

> Falls in cerebral perfusion may result from raised intracranial pressure or reduced mean arterial blood pressure.

In addition, any increase in supratentorial pressure (e.g. cerebral swelling) can force the uncus of the temporal lobe through the incisura. This will pinch the oculomotor nerve of the same side, causing an ipsilateral fixed, dilated pupil. It also pinches the pyramidal tract on the same side, causing contralateral spastic weakness of the arm and leg. If pressure within the skull continues to rise, the Cushing response occurs, with a fall in heart rate and a rise in blood pressure. This is a preterminal event.

> Pupillary dilatation, hemiparesis, hypertension and bradycardia are late signs of raised intracranial pressure.

INITIAL ASSESSMENT OF THE HEAD-INJURED PATIENT

The Royal College of Surgeons of England produced a report in 1988 which stated that up to a third of all trauma deaths at that time were 'preventable'. Many of these deaths were in patients with head injuries who were thought to have an isolated head injury but in fact had another injury that was missed, all attention being focused on the obvious injury to the head. These complicating factors included airway problems and unidentified causes of major haemorrhage, especially abdominal injuries such as splenic lacerations. Since the Royal College of Surgeons report was published, there have been marked improvements in trauma care. A major example is the advanced trauma life support (ATLS) course that was introduced to Britain in 1988 and concentrates attention on the ABCs of resuscitation (airway, breathing and circulation, see Chapter 4). Nowhere is this approach more important than in the early management of head-injured patients, where the ABCs need to be prioritized above definitive management of the head injury itself.

> Adequate management of the airway, breathing and circulation is vital to achieving optimum outcomes in head injury.

Table 20.2: Primary and secondary brain damage

Primary	Secondary
Cerebral lacerations	Hypoxia due to airway compromise or ventilatory problems
Cerebral contusions	
Dural tears	
Diffuse axonal injury	Hypovolaemia due to blood loss
	Raised intracranial pressure due to brain swelling
	Hypoglycaemia
	Infection
	Increased or decreased temperature
	Seizures

It is important to note the distinction between primary and secondary brain injury. Primary brain injury occurs at the time of the actual insult to the head; it may be a laceration or contusion to the actual brain substance. Secondary brain damage may occur either as a secondary effect of the primary brain injury or from the effects of extracranial injuries such as hypoxia or hypovolaemia. Examples of primary and secondary brain damage are given in Table 20.2.

In general, it is fair to say that there is very little that can be done about primary brain damage after the event. There are no techniques to repair neurological tissue injured by mechanical force at the time of the trauma. Secondary damage, however, can be either prevented or treated and this is what the emergency department should be aiming to achieve. Much can be done by adhering to the ABCs of resuscitation: securing an airway, establishing good ventilation and oxygenation, and maintaining the circulation by preventing shock. In these ways, cerebral hypoxia and ischaemia can be avoided.

In the initial assessment and management of head injuries it is therefore essential to stick to the ABCs and not be immediately distracted by the head injury itself.

THE ABC OF HEAD INJURY MANAGEMENT

The airway is the first priority. If the patient is conscious and able to talk freely then his or her airway is satisfactory. If not, it will need to be secured, using the hierarchy of airway control measures (see Chapter 4). Indications for early paralysis and intubation (preferably by an anaesthetist using an induction agent and a muscle relaxant) include the following:

- Glasgow Coma Score of 8 or less
- need for surgery
- failure to maintain an adequate airway.

Throughout the management of the airway the cervical spine must be controlled, either by in-line manual immobilization or by a combination of hard collar, sandbags and tapes. However, it should be borne in mind that there is now increasing evidence that prolonged wearing of a semi-rigid cervical collar is associated with rises in intracranial pressure. This is not usually a problem during the time most patients spend in an emergency department but is relevant to intensive care management.

High-flow oxygen should be provided using a tight-fitting mask with reservoir bag. The chest must be examined thoroughly and any life-threatening problems (e.g. tension pneumothorax, massive haemothorax, open pneumothorax, flail chest), diagnosed and treated as soon as they are identified. Treatment of breathing problems is a higher priority than treatment of the head injury itself.

The state of the circulation must be assessed by measuring the pulse rate and capillary refill time, and assessing the peripheries for temperature and colour. If the patient is shocked, this should be assumed to be due to hypovolaemia from blood loss and treated as such until proven otherwise.

It is important never to presume that brain injury is the cause of shock. Other than in infants, it is not possible to lose a large enough volume of blood within the skull to cause hypotension, remembering of course that it is perfectly possible to bleed to death from scalp lacerations, although this is extremely rare.

Isolated head injuries do not cause shock.

Shock must be aggressively treated using intravenous fluids, including blood if necessary, until the patient is normotensive and has a normal pulse rate. If this cannot be achieved by fluid resuscitation, the cause of the blood loss must be found and dealt with by surgery. Again, the treatment of the circulation is a higher priority than the head injury.

Only when the patient is completely stable from the ABC point of view should attention be turned to the head injury itself. A brief history should be obtained, including a description of the mechanism of injury, the past medical history and drug history (including allergies). This information will usually have to be sought from the paramedics and relatives.

ASSESSMENT OF THE HEAD INJURY

This can be broken down into the following:

- assessment of conscious level, using the Glasgow Coma Scale
- pupillary examination
- neurological examination
- scalp and skull examination.

Assessment of conscious level

This is best achieved using the Glasgow Coma Scale (Table 20.3). This is a scoring system based on three measurements: eye-opening, verbal response and motor response. The scores for each of the three components are added together, giving a total score. It must be noted that the minimum score is 3 and the maximum is 15.

> The patient is scored using the Glasgow Coma Scale.

Painful stimuli used when measuring the Glasgow Coma Scale should be applied to the supraorbital margins; painful stimuli applied to limbs may not be perceived if there is a spinal injury.

The Glasgow Coma Scale can be used to categorize patients into the following groups:

- GCS less than 9: Patient is in coma. Severe head injury.
- GCS 9–12: Moderate head injury.
- GCS 13 or above: Mild head injury.

The main value of the Glasgow Coma Scale, however, is not in interpretation of a single reading. The scale provides an objective assessment of conscious level and by repeating the assessment trends of deterioration and improvement are detected.

Table 20. 3: The Glasgow Coma Scale

Eye-opening response (E score):	
Spontaneous	4
Eyes open to speech	3
Eyes open to pain	2
Eyes do not open	1
Verbal response (V Score):	
Oriented: knows name, age, date	5
Confused	4
Inappropriate words	3
Incomprehensible sounds	2
None	1
Best motor response (M score):	
Moves limbs to command	6
Localizes pain	5
Withdraws from painful stimulus	4
Abnormal flexion (decorticate)	3
Abnormal extension (decerebrate)	2
No movement	1

It is important to note that it is not merely the head injury that may cause changes in the level of consciousness. Hypoxia and hypovolaemia can also cause deterioration in conscious level. Any such deterioration should therefore prompt the doctor to a reassessment of the airway, breathing and circulation prior to considering the head injury itself.

> The Glasgow Coma Scale allows objective serial assessment of conscious level.

Pupillary examination

The pupils must be examined for their size and their reaction to light. A difference between the two pupils of more than 1 mm is abnormal. A fixed dilated pupil implies pressure on the ipsilateral oculomotor nerve as it passes through the tentorium until proven otherwise. A sluggish response to light may be due to head injury.

Neurological examination

A neurological examination should be carried out of the cranial and peripheral nervous systems (Table 20.4). Tone, power, co-ordination, sensation and reflexes must be examined and all results

Table 20.4: The cranial nerves

I	Olfactory	Smell
II	Ophthalmic	Visual fields in all quadrants
III	Oculomotor	Pupils, external ocular movements
IV	Trochlear	Failure of downwards outwards vision
V	Trigeminal	Teeth clench (masseter)
VI	Abducens	Lateral gaze
VII	Facial	Smile
VIII	Auditory	Hearing (both ears)
IX	Glossopharyngeal	Palate movement
X	Vagus	Parasympathetic
XI	Accessory	Shrug shoulders
XII	Hypoglossal	Tongue movement

Table 20.5: Signs of basal skull fractures

Blood or CSF leaking from the nose
Blood or CSF leaking from the ear
Battle's sign: Mastoid bruising
'Panda eyes': Bilateral periorbital bruising
Intracranial air on X-ray or CT scan
Haemotympanum

Table 20.6: Indications for skull X-ray

Loss of consciousness at any time
Amnesia at any time
Neurological symptoms or signs
CSF or blood from nose or ear
Suspected penetrating injury
Scalp bruising or swelling
Difficulty in assessing patient, e.g. very young, alcohol

Table 20.7: Indications for urgent CT scan

Skull fracture
GCS <15 after resuscitation
Penetrating injury
Fall in GCS of 2 points

Table 20.8: Indications for admission for observation

Depression of conscious level
Skull fracture (including base)
Neurological symptoms/signs
Difficulty in assessing patient
No responsible carer
Other conditions, e.g. haemophilia

Table 20.9: Indications for urgent neurosurgical consultation

GCS 8 or less after resuscitation
Deteriorating conscious level
Open brain injury
Neurological signs, e.g. pupils, lateralizing features
Abnormality on CT scan

documented. In particular, differences between the left and right sides are looked for; such differences suggest an intracranial mass lesion that may well be amenable to neurosurgery.

Examination of the scalp and skull

The scalp should be examined for lacerations, swellings and bruising. The depth of any lacerations and the presence of foreign bodies must be noted. Examination of the skull should be rigorous in the search for fractures. Vault fractures can be suspected by tenderness, swelling and bruising. The signs of basal skull fractures are summarized in Table 20.5.

Battle's sign may not be apparent until 24 h after the injury and cannot be relied on in the early assessment of head injury.

INVESTIGATION AND MANAGEMENT

Having completed the ABCs of resuscitation and assessed the head injury, critical decisions need to be made about further imaging investigation (Tables 20.6 and 20.7), whether admission to hospital is required (Table 20.8), and whether or not consultation with a neurosurgeon is required (Table 20.9).

For each of these questions, well-defined guidelines aid decision making.

Skull X-rays versus CT scans

Computerized tomography (CT) is the investigation of choice for head-injured patients. It actually gives information about the brain rather than just the box in which it is contained. Increasingly in the UK, CT scanners are available 24 h a day and easily accessed by staff working in emergency departments.

CT scans image brain injury.

The two factors that best predict the presence of intracranial haematomas are skull fractures and depressed conscious level (Table 20.10). It can be argued that any patient with either of these features should have an urgent CT scan.

It can therefore be seen that the presence of both a skull fracture and a depressed level of consciousness increases the risk of there having been an intracranial bleed by a factor of 1500. Having either puts the patient in a high-risk group and is an indication for CT scanning. Similarly, a fully alert patient with no skull fracture is at extremely low risk and can be discharged if otherwise well and in the presence of adequate supervision. It should be noted that the same relationship between skull fracture and intracranial haematoma does not apply in children.

If a skull X-ray series is performed, useful information can be gleaned from it. Skull radiographs are difficult to interpret but vault fractures can usually be diagnosed, as can penetrating injuries, the presence of intracranial air and occasionally fluid levels. However, basal fractures are not visible. When looking at skull X-rays always use all the information on the film and remember to look at the cervical spine.

Table 20.10: Risks of intracranial haematoma in an adult

Conscious level	No fracture	Skull fracture
Fully alert	1 in 6000	1 in 120
Depressed	1 in 32	1 in 4

THE SPECTRA OF HEAD INJURIES

Head injuries are notoriously difficult to classify and it is very useful to have a system to use to aid the memory and to make your findings more understandable to a neurosurgeon. Having carried out the initial assessment and resuscitation and then relevant investigations, it should be possible to describe the pattern of head injury in any given patient using the following four headings:

- fractures
- diffuse brain injury
- focal brain injury
- intracranial haemorrhage.

Each of these can be represented along a spectrum as shown in Table 20.11. The specific types of head injury are described below.

Skull fractures

Skull fractures are common but do not necessarily indicate the presence of underlying brain injury. They are, however, a useful 'flag', in that the presence of a skull fracture means that the force involved in the injury was large enough to cause bony damage. As mentioned previously, skull fracture is one of the two best predictors of intracranial bleeding (the other being reduced conscious level). For this reason all patients with skull fractures should be admitted to hospital for neurological observation and all should have a CT scan. Simple linear skull fractures (Fig. 20.2) require no specific intervention.

Depressed skull fractures (Figs 20.3 and 20.4) are difficult to diagnose but appear on skull X-ray as an area of increased opacity due to the overlying of bony fragments. Management is directed at the underlying brain injury and a CT scan is required to image the underlying brain and assess the degree of depression. To reduce the risk of convulsions, any

Table 20.11: Spectra of head injury

	Minor			Major
Fractures	Linear vault fracture		Basal fracture	Compound, depressed
Diffuse brain injury	Concussion			Diffuse axonal injury (DAI)
Focal brain injury	Contusion			Pulped brain
Haemorrhage	Extradural	Subdural	Intracerebral	Intraventricular

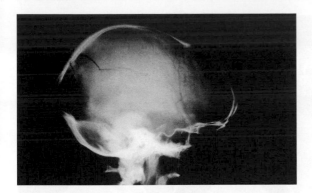

Figure 20.2: Linear vault skull fracture.

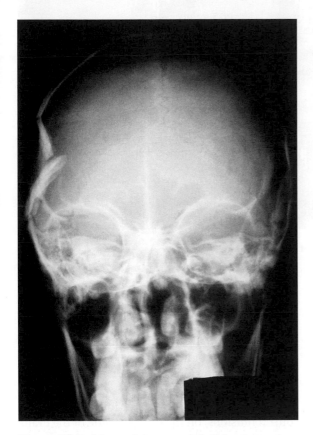

Figure 20.3: X-ray of depressed skull fracture.

fragments depressed by more than 5 mm should be elevated surgically.

Open skull vault fractures imply tearing of the dura. The brain is therefore exposed, with a high risk of infection with either meningitis or cerebral abcess. Early operation is indicated to toilet the wound, close the dura and elevate any bony fragments.

Basal skull fractures are rarely seen on skull X-rays but the presence of intracranial air or blood in the sphenoid sinus is an indirect radiological sign of this injury. The clinical features have been listed above (Table 20.5). Basal skull fractures are open fractures as a result of communication through the sinuses or the middle ear. The patient will require a CT scan to detect intracranial injury. There is no good evidence for the use of prophylactic antibiotics in patients with basal skull fractures, though the patient should be closely observed for signs of developing infection.

Diffuse brain injury

This occurs when the whole brain is subjected to shearing forces, in the form of rapid acceleration or deceleration. In concussion, the damage done is minor and temporary but in diffuse axonal injury there is permanent, structural damage as a result of shearing of the white and grey matter throughout the brain.

Concussion is defined as a brain injury with brief loss of neurological function. There may or may not be a short period of unconsciousness. Many neurological abnormalities may occur but most settle even before the patient arrives in the emergency department. For this reason, any neurological abnormalities present when the patient is seen by the doctor must not be put down to concussion. Most patients with concussion will be awake and alert when seen in the emergency department, but some confusion may persist, as may non-specific symptoms such as nausea, headache or dizziness. Neurological examination is normal. Once they are no longer confused, these patients may be allowed home with advice to return if their symptoms worsen or any new symptoms develop. Worrisome symptoms include drowsiness, vomiting, blurred vision and fits. They are usually issued with a 'head injury advice card' (Fig. 20.5) and only allowed home with a responsible carer. They should be advised to rest at home and avoid contact sports and alcohol for at least 3 weeks. Any patient who has been unconsciousness for more than 5 min should be admitted for observation.

Symptoms of concussion such as headaches, poor concentration and nausea may persist for days or weeks after a head injury, and tend to be more prolonged after occipital injuries. It is common for

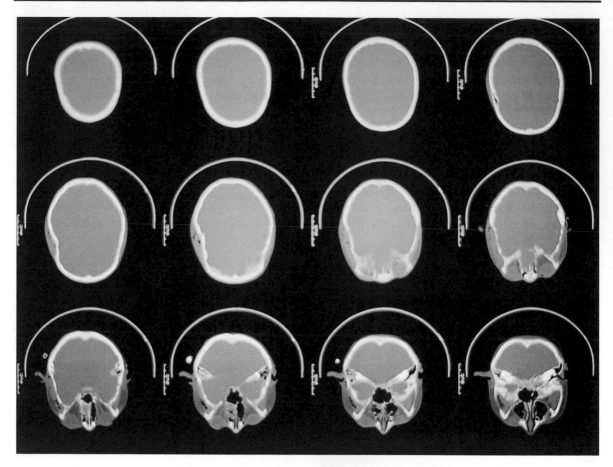

Figure 20.4: CT of depressed skull fracture (same patient as in Fig. 20.3).

patients to return to an emergency department several days after the injury as they are concerned about persistence of such symptoms. The diagnosis of post-concussional syndrome is used to describe these symptoms in the absence of significant intracranial pathology.

Diffuse axonal injury (DAI) is at the other end of the spectrum of diffuse injury from concussion and is characterized by prolonged coma, often lasting weeks. It is due to microscopic neuronal damage that is widespread throughout the brain. Surgery is of no benefit. The condition has a mortality approaching 50% and this is largely due to increased intracranial pressure from cerebral oedema. The CT scan may be normal in the early stages or show multiple punctate haemorrhages. Patients with DAI often progress into the permanent vegetative state (PVS) and will need to be cared for accordingly, with all the associated ethical problems.

Focal brain injury

In these, macroscopic damage occurs in a small area of the brain. Such injuries may need neurosurgery because of mass effects.

Cerebral contusions may be of any size and can be isolated or multiple. They may be either coup contusions, beneath the area of impact, or contracoup contusions, on the opposite side of the brain. The contusion itself may cause a focal neurological deficit if it occurs near the sensory or motor cortex, or the surrounding swelling and oedema may cause mass effects, including tentorial herniation. CT scanning will elucidate the nature of contusions.

Patients with contusions must be admitted, as delayed swelling may cause marked deterioration. Surgery is only indicated if there is significant mass effect or if bleeding occurs into the contusion. This latter eventuality is more likely in patients who abuse alcohol.

Head Injury

Children

If your child has a minor injury, we will not always X-ray it because the treatment will be just the same.

You should:

- Try to keep your child resting quietly when you get home.

- Give your child medicines, such as Calpol or Junifen, to relieve a mild headache.

Take your child to your nearest Accident & Emergency department at once if:

- They have a very bad headache that does not get better after they have taken medicine.

- They become more sleepy than usual.

- They vomit more than twice.

- You are worried about them.

Adults

For a few days you should:

- Make sure there is another adult to keep an eye on you.
- Rest quietly at home.
- Take tablets such as ibuprofen or paracetamol (both available from a chemist) to relieve a mild headache.

For a few days you should not:

- Join in any sports or strenuous activity.
- Drink alcohol or eat heavy meals.

For the attention of the person looking after you - take the patient to the nearest Accident & Emergency department at once if they:

- Become more sleepy than usual.
- Have a fit.
- Develop any unusual symptoms.

Please retain this card for future reference

Figure 20.5: Typical head injury advice card.

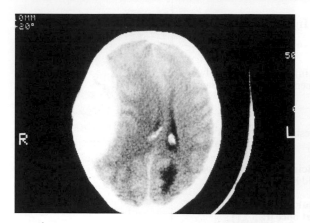

Figure 20.6: CT scan of an extradural haematoma.

Intracranial haemorrhage

Extradural (often referred to as epidural in American literature) haemorrhage or haematoma occurs as a result of a tear in a dural artery, usually the middle meningeal. The arterial tears are commonly associated with a linear skull fracture of the temporo-parietal area that crosses the skull grooves of the artery. Extradural bleeds are rare but must always be considered as they can be rapidly fatal. The typical history of an extradural haemorrhage is a lucid period followed by increasing headache, vomiting and deteriorating level of consciousness. CT scans of extradural haematomas show a typical lentiform or biconvex high-density lesion just within the skull (Fig. 20.6). Acute extradural haemorrhage requires urgent surgery to evacuate the blood and prevent the development of secondary brain injury. If treated rapidly the prognosis in terms of both morbidity and mortality is excellent. The reason for this is that the cause of the symptoms and signs is injury to and bleeding from an artery, causing a rapidly expanding mass lesion. There is usually little or no associated primary brain injury. Once the bleeding has been stopped and the clot evacuated there is no residual brain damage. For this reason, the mortality for patients who are alert before surgery is virtually zero, rising to 10–20% for those in coma.

Acute subdural haemorrhage is more common and more life threatening than extradural haemorrhage and there is frequently an associated primary brain injury. The blood usually comes from bridging veins between the cerebral cortex and dura but may come from brain lacerations or

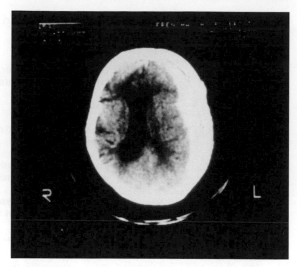

Figure 20.7: Acute subdural haematoma.

cortical vessels. As well as the problems caused by the subdural blood there is often severe primary brain injury; hence the mortality is approximately 60%. Outcome can be improved by early evacuation of the haematoma. The CT scan appearance of a subdural haematoma is typically that of a 'rind' of blood just within the skull which 'peels away' the cortex of the brain from the skull (Fig. 20.7).

Subarachnoid haemorrhage causes blood in the CSF and meningeal irritation, characterized by headache and photophobia. The haemorrhage itself is not life threatening but traumatic subarachnoid haemorrhage implies major injury to the surrounding brain tissue. Calcium antagonists such as nimodipine can be used in traumatic subarachnoid haemorrhage to cause cerebral vasodilatation and limit ischaemic brain damage.

Intracerebral and intraventricular haemorrhages (Fig. 20.8) have a high mortality rate and are usually associated with substantial brain injury. The neurological deficit depends on the anatomical situation. Neurosurgery is rarely of value in the treatment of intracerebral haemorrhage.

REFERRING HEAD-INJURED PATIENTS TO NEUROSURGEONS

The indications for neurosurgical referral have already been listed in Table 20.9. When speaking to a neurosurgeon it is useful to have a system for describing your findings (Table 20.12).

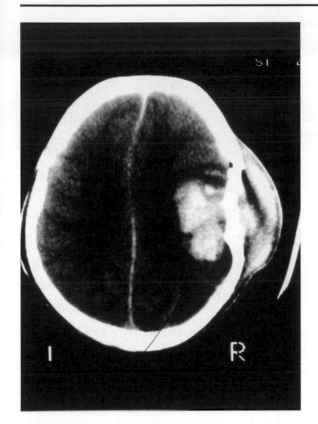

Figure 20.8: Intracerebral haematoma.

Table 20.12: Important information for neurosurgical referral

Name, age, sex
Referring hospital and consultant
Time of injury
Type of injury
Past medical history
Pulse, BP, respiratory rate
Extracranial injuries
Plain radiology findings
GCS score (E, M, V)
Pupillary size and reaction
Neurological findings
CT findings
Investigations and interventions

SPECIFIC TREATMENTS IN HEAD INJURY

These will usually only be given after discussion with the neurosurgeon who will be responsible for definitive care of the patient.

Mannitol

This is an osmotic diuretic and can be used to reduce intracranial pressure. It is important to appreciate that it is only a holding measure and that intracranial pressure will rise again unless the underlying cause is remedied. It is frequently used in the acute situation, after discussion with the receiving neurosurgeons, to keep the intracranial pressure down during transfer to definitive care. The usual dose is $1\,\mathrm{g\,kg^{-1}}$.

Controlled ventilation

Arterial carbon dioxide tension affects cerebral circulation and should be controlled to maintain it at the lower end of the normal range (4.0–6.5 kPa) as measured by blood gas analysis. This is best achieved by endotracheal intubation, paralysis and controlled ventilation. Hyperventilation to produce hypocapnia is probably not beneficial as this causes cerebral vasoconstriction. Blood gases should be measured frequently.

Fluid restriction

IV fluids should be given only sparingly in order to prevent overhydration and cerebral oedema, leading to raised intracranial pressure. This is possible only after blood loss in the chest, abdomen and pelvis has been excluded or treated. Remember that the treatment of shock takes priority over the treatment of the head injury itself.

Steroids

There is currently no conclusive evidence for the use of steroids in the early treatment of head injury. A randomized controlled trial is taking place to try and clarify this issue.

Burr holes

These may need to be considered in cases of dire emergency if neurosurgical facilities are not immediately available. The commonest situation where they may be lifesaving is in the management of extradural haemorrhage, where the patient, after a lucid interval, is suddenly deteriorating, with

Table 20.13: Checklist of equipment for neurosurgical transfer

Airway and anaesthetist. Make sure the airway is secure and that equipment is available to cope with emergencies en route (ET tubes, laryngoscope). An experienced anaesthetist should travel with the patient.

Breathing and oxygen. Ensure that the oxygen supply is adequate for the journey. Use of a gas-powered ventilator will rapidly drain the supply.

Circulation. Ensure that there are two intravenous cannulae in place and working. Exclude bleeding from the chest, abdomen and pelvis before transfer. If found it requires treatment before transfer.

Drugs and documentation. All necessary drugs (anaesthetic drugs) must be taken, as must all notes, X-rays and scans.

Equipment. If in doubt, take it. If it might go wrong, take two.

Fluids. IV fluids and blood.

reducing conscious level, a fixed dilated pupil and evolving hemiplegia. In these cases, burr holes may be placed in the temporal region of the skull, preferably by a surgeon who has experience in performing them. The best place for an exploratory burr hole is immediately above the zygomatic arch mid-way between the posterior orbital margin and the external auditory meatus. The site of the burr hole should be on the side of the suspected haematoma. This may be known from a CT scan, but if not, valuable guidelines are to explore the side of the dilated pupil (or the first to dilate) or the side of any skull fracture or external injury.

TRANSFERRING PATIENTS TO NEUROSURGICAL CENTRES

The head-injured patient will frequently need to be transferred, either within the hospital to a CT scanner or to another hospital for neurosurgical care. In either case it is essential that the patient be adequately resuscitated and stabilized before transfer and that all necessary personnel and equipment accompany the patient during the transfer.

Before transfer, the emergency department doctor must speak with the neurosurgeon who will receive the patient and communicate the information previously discussed. The neurosurgeon may clarify treatment which he or she wishes instituted before the patient is transferred (endotracheal intubation, mannitol). For the transfer itself the items in the checklist in Table 20.13 should be considered.

PITFALLS IN HEAD INJURY MANAGEMENT

Patients under the influence of alcohol or drugs

These are a common problem in emergency departments. One must never assume that drugs or alcohol are the cause of depressed conscious level in these patients who have had a head injury. They should be aggressively investigated and managed assuming that the head injury is the cause of their clinical state. There should be a very low threshold for admitting these patients for observation.

Always assume that reduced conscious level in an intoxicated head injured patient is due to the injury.

Reattenders after head injury

Frequently patients attending an emergency department following a head injury are allowed home after assessment and then reattend because of new or persistent symptoms. Studies have shown that these patients have a high incidence of intracranial lesions. There should be a low threshold for performing CT scans in this group.

Scalp lacerations

It is possible to bleed to death from a scalp wound as the scalp is an extremely vascular structure.

Bleeding from scalp wounds should be initially controlled by pressure. The skin should be infiltrated with local anaesthetic (1% lignocaine with adrenaline) and the wound thoroughly explored. Any foreign material must be removed and debris scrubbed away. It is often possible to visualize the outer table of the skull and confirm or exclude skull fracture by gentle palpation. Closure of the scalp must take account of the fact that the scalp has five layers; it is vital to close the aponeurosis as well as the skin or haemostasis will not be achieved. This can be done by either performing a two-layer closure or by taking large 'bites' of skin with the suture material to ensure that the aponeurotic layer is picked up.

Seizures

Seizures after head injury may be either generalized or focal. Both are common at the time of injury or very shortly thereafter and are not a reliable predictor of long-term epilepsy. If short, they require no treatment. If prolonged or repetitive, they may be a sign of intracranial bleeding and may cause cerebral hypoxia, brain swelling and raised intracranial pressure. They should be treated with intravenous diazepam 10 mg, repeated after 5 min if necessary. If this is unsuccessful, phenytoin should be administered as an intravenous loading dose.

Restlessness

This may be due to an expanding intracranial mass or haematoma. It may also be due to hypoxia, pain from injuries, a full bladder or painful bandages or plaster casts. Any identifiable cause of restlessness must be treated (ventilation for hypoxia, analgesics for pain). Sedatives should be withheld until neurosurgical advice has been sought. Chlorpromazine given intravenously is of value in cases of severe agitation.

Hyperthermia

Elevations in body temperature increase brain metabolism and carbon dioxide levels. Temperature should be monitored and any hyperthermia should be treated by passive cooling and inhibition of shivering using chlorpromazine.

NECK INJURIES

This section deals with injuries to the upper airway and penetrating neck wounds and their management. Injury to the cervical spine is covered in Chapter 22.

INJURIES TO THE LARYNX AND TRACHEA

Fractures of the larynx are unusual and are usually due to direct blows. There is a classic triad of hoarseness, surgical emphysema and palpable crepitus over the larynx. The diagnosis, if suspected, should be confirmed by CT scan or laryngoscopy and the patient referred to the ear, nose and throat (ENT) team.

If the airway is not compromised, management of laryngeal fractures can be conservative with in-patient observation. If the airway is partially or totally obstructed, intubation should be attempted. If this is not possible, emergency tracheostomy is indicated, followed by surgical repair of the fracture.

Trauma to the trachea may be blunt or penetrating. If penetrating, the injury requires immediate surgery and primary repair of the trachea. Blunt injuries are more difficult to diagnose and require a high index of suspicion. As with laryngeal injuries, CT scanning and endoscopy are important diagnostic adjuncts. Treatment is conservative if there is no airway compromise. If the airway is at risk, surgery is often required.

NECK WOUNDS

The most important anatomical consideration in the assessment of neck wounds is whether or not the platysma muscle is breached. Platysma is the muscle immediately deep to the skin and if it is not breached the wound may be closed in the emergency department in the normal way. If, however, platysma has been breached there is a high likelihood of damage to vital deep structures (arteries, veins, nerves, lymph ducts, larynx, trachea, oesophagus) and the wound must be formally explored in the operating theatre, where injured structures can also be repaired.

The management of patients with neck injuries follows the normal 'ABC' approach, with early initial aggressive assessment and resuscitation of the airway, breathing and circulation, whilst of course immobilizing the cervical spine. Other than stopping obvious external haemorrhage from neck wounds, the definitive management of neck injuries takes place only when the patient is stable.

FURTHER READING

Currie, D (2000) *The Management of Head Injuries. A practical Guide for the Emergency Room*. Oxford University Press, Oxford.

MAXILLOFACIAL INJURY

INTRODUCTION

Injuries to the face and mouth are assessed during the secondary survey and are not usually life threatening. However, some facial trauma may compromise the airway or cause profuse haemorrhage, and in these circumstances must be managed in the primary survey. Haemorrhage from the maxillofacial region may be so severe as both to result in hypovolaemic shock and be responsible for airway obstruction. In addition, maxillofacial trauma may be associated with concomitant cervical spine injury (in 2% of cases) and the neck must be protected in the initial management of the patient.

AIRWAY MANAGEMENT

The patient should be examined in a good light, with an assistant suctioning away blood and debris from the mouth. A wide-bore (Yankhauer) sucker is essential to help clear the airway. In some cases immediate intubation or the formation of a surgical airway will be necessary (see Chapter 4).

REMOVAL OF FOREIGN BODIES

Loose fragments of teeth and bone should be removed. Broken dentures should be taken out but intact, well-fitting dentures can be left *in situ*.

HAEMORRHAGE

The soft tissues of the mouth can bleed profusely. Intra-oral bleeding can be controlled by placing a rolled-up piece of gauze over the bleeding point and asking the patient to bite firmly down on to it. This is clearly contraindicated in an unconscious or semi-conscious patient. Alternatively, firm pressure can be maintained by an assistant. If the bleeding is sufficient to compromise the airway, the airway should be secured by anaesthesia and intubation or the formation of a surgical airway.

LOSS OF TONGUE CONTROL IN A FRACTURED MANDIBLE

Fractures of the mandible are not usually life threatening in those patients who can maintain their own airway. However, in patients with a head injury or who are intoxicated the airway may be compromised. Severe comminution of the mandible or bilateral fractures are of particular concern. The muscles of the tongue are attached to the genial tubercles in the mid-line of the mandible on the lingual aspect. Mandibular fractures that leave this segment mobile may allow the tongue to fall backwards against the posterior wall of the pharynx causing respiratory obstruction. This segment must be pulled forward and held in this position to prevent further obstruction. The tongue can be held forwards by passing a large suture (0 gauge black silk) transversely through the dorsum of the tongue and then pulling the tongue out of the mouth. The suture should be held or taped to the side of the face.

POSTERIOR IMPACTION OF THE FRACTURED MAXILLA

The maxilla articulates with the base of the skull along an inclined plane downwards and backwards. Trauma to the face sufficient to cause a fracture at any of the Le Fort levels may move the maxilla backwards down along this inclined plane. This may result in obstruction as the soft palate impinges on the posterior wall of the pharynx. Immediate management of this potentially life-threatening problem involves inserting the index and middle fingers into the mouth and hooking them behind the soft palate. The maxilla is then pulled forwards to relieve the obstruction.

DIRECT LARYNGEAL TRAUMA

This is discussed in Chapter 37

CONTROL OF SEVERE HAEMORRHAGE

Profuse haemorrhage can result from a fractured maxilla. This is best managed by a maxillofacial surgeon. Nasal Epistats® (Fig. 21.1) are inserted into each nostril and inflated using saline. Two balloons are inflated, one anteriorly and one posteriorly to exert a compressive force sufficient to stop the bleeding. Ideally, they are used in conjunction with dental props placed between the posterior teeth on both sides. Use of the Epistats® alone may cause bony separation of a fracture and make the

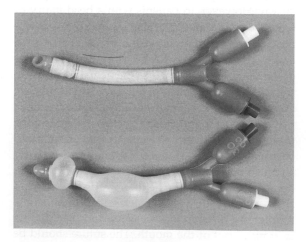

Figure 21.1: Nasal Epistats®.

bleeding worse. In severe haemorrhage from facial trauma, the priority is achieving a patent protected airway by whatever means necessary: intubation will almost always be required and experienced anaesthetic assistance should be called.

INTRA-ORAL SWELLING

Oral tissues may swell following trauma and this may cause airway obstruction some hours after the initial injury. Continued close observation of an initially patent airway is therefore necessary.

EPISTAXIS

Nasal bleeding following trauma often occurs from Little's area, which is a rich plexus of vessels on the anterior part of the septum. This can usually be controlled by direct digital pressure on the lower nose. Alternatively, bleeding can be controlled with expanding sponge packs inserted into the nostrils (see Chapter 37). If these simple measures fail to stop the bleeding the nose should be packed.

Bleeding from vessels in the posterior part of the nose may require insertion of a Foley catheter (size 12/14G) until the tip is seen just behind the palate. The balloon is then inflated with saline and the catheter pulled forwards to produce tamponade. An anterior pack can then be inserted as described.

SEPTAL HAEMATOMA

Trauma to the nose may produce haemorrhage into the subchondrial space, resulting in a septal haematoma (Fig. 21.2). This occurs commonly in children as the mucoperichondrium is loosely adherent to the underlying cartilage. The patient may complain of nasal obstruction but pain is only a feature if the haematoma becomes infected. On examination the septum appears swollen.

If an abscess occurs, cartilage necrosis will follow, causing nasal collapse and deformity. Treatment consists of draining the haematoma using a needle or through an incision if blood clot has formed. Nasal packing will prevent recurrence and antibiotics are necessary.

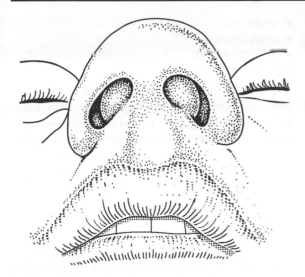

Figure 21.2: Septal haematoma.

In nasal trauma always check for the presence of septal haematoma.

CLASSIFICATION OF MAXILLOFACIAL INJURIES

Injuries can be divided into those involving the soft tissues and those affecting the hard tissues (see Chapter 38 for dental trauma).

SOFT-TISSUE INJURY

The face and scalp are well perfused and profuse bleeding can occur after trauma. Injuries include superficial cuts and abrasions, lacerations and penetrating wounds. (Intra-oral lacerations are discussed in Chapter 38.) During the secondary survey a detailed examination of the face and scalp should include assessment of motor and sensory nerve function. A deep laceration over the cheek may injure the branches of the facial nerve and movement of the face must be noted. The parotid duct may also be damaged in a deep cheek laceration, and if this is suspected (saliva may be seen extruding from the wound) the patient should be admitted for formal exploration and repair.

Foreign bodies penetrating the face or mouth should be left *in situ* and removed under general

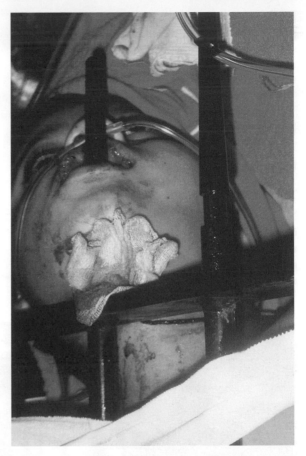

Figure 21.3: Foreign body penetrating the face/mouth.

anaesthetic unless they are causing airway obstruction (Fig. 21.3).

Wounds of the neck may involve some of the deep structures and should not be explored in the emergency department if they penetrate platysma. Penetrating neck wounds should be explored under general anaesthetic, and preoperative arteriography may be needed.

Soft-tissue wounds can be simply covered during the primary survey using gauze. During the secondary survey they should be cleaned and covered with a gauze dressing. Definitive treatment should be carried out under sterile conditions, with either local or general anaesthetic as appropriate. The wounds should be closed in layers using reabsorbable material (3/0 Vicryl or cat gut) for the deep layers and a non-reabsorbable material (5/0 or 6/0 Prolene or nylon) for the skin. Sutures on the face are normally removed at 5 days. A course of antibiotics should be prescribed and a broad-spectrum penicillin is usually given. If there is a penetrating wound into the mouth, metronidazole should be included. Where there is a possibility of significant cosmetic deficit following wound repair referral to a plastic surgeon for expert reconstruction is indicated.

BONY INJURY

Mandibular fractures

These may be unilateral or bilateral and they are classified as follows:

- dentoalveolar
- condylar
- angle
- body
- coronoid
- symphysis
- parasymphysis
- ramus.

Fractures of the mandible occur in patterns depending on the direction of the traumatic force. For example, an injury to the left side of the face may produce a fracture of the left angle and right condylar neck. A blow to the chin may result in a mid-line mandibular and bilateral condylar fractures (the guardsman's fracture, so called because it typically results from a fall forwards onto the chin – Fig. 21.4).

A patient with a fractured mandible may complain of pain and swelling over the site of the injury and be unable to open their mouth fully. They may say that the teeth do not meet together properly (Fig. 21.5). Possible associated physical

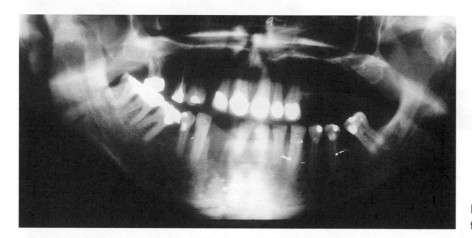

Figure 21.4: Mandibular fractures.

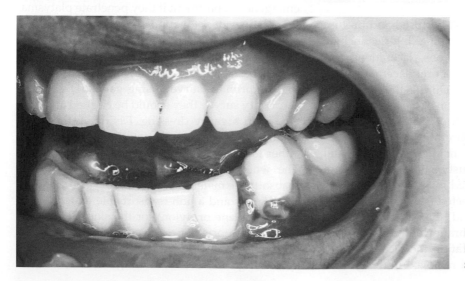

Figure 21.5: Malocclusion as a result of a mandibular fracture.

signs include:

- swelling over the mandible
- step deformity of the lower border of the mandible
- numbness over the chin (injury to the inferior alveolar nerve)
- laceration of the gingiva
- mobile teeth
- teeth not meeting properly (malocclusion)
- mobile fragments of mandible
- sublingual haematoma adjacent to fracture.

Dislocation of the jaw

Dislocation of the condylar head from the fossa may occur following trauma or after simply opening the mouth too wide, as in yawning. The patient may present with their mouth open wide and will often drool saliva. They may be unable to speak and in considerable pain. A history should indicate whether this has happened before and for how long the jaw has been dislocated.

Reduction of the dislocation depends on how relaxed the patient can be made and it may be necessary to administer an intravenous benzodiazepine prior to attempted reduction. The patient is seated in a low chair with the clinician standing in front. Both thumbs are placed on the lower teeth (or bony ridges in an edentulous patient) and sustained pressure applied in a downward and backward direction. The clinician should wrap gauze around the thumbs for comfort. Successful reduction can be felt by the clinician as the jaw goes back into place, producing instant relief for the patient. Repeated attempts at reduction should be avoided as the patient usually becomes distressed; in these circumstances it is better to manage the dislocation under general anaesthetic.

MAXILLARY FRACTURES

These may be unilateral or bilateral and may be a combination of different types, as classified below (Fig. 21.6):

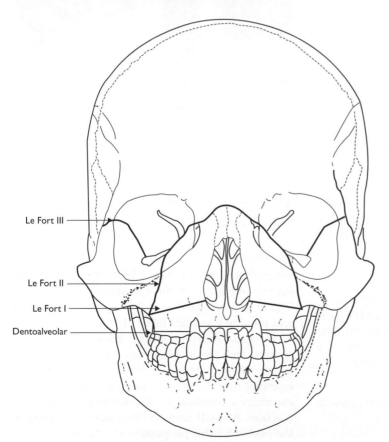

Figure 21.6: Maxillary fractures.

- dentoalveolar
- Le Fort I (low level)
- Le Fort II (pyramidal)
- Le Fort III (high level).

Plain radiographs are often difficult to interpret and may reveal different fracture levels on each side of the maxilla.

The physical signs of maxillary fracture include:

- bilateral facial swelling
- mobility of maxilla
- 'dish-face' deformity
- mouth gagged open on posterior teeth
- teeth not meeting properly (malocclusion)
- bilateral periorbital bruising and oedema.

NASAL COMPLEX

Fractures to the nose may occur following trauma from the front and from the side. The resultant nasal deformity reflects the direction of impact (Fig. 21.7).

The majority of patients with nasal trauma present with discomfort, soft-tissue swelling around the nose and possible epistaxis. Septal deviation and haematoma are sought on examination; both are rare. Patients with a septal haematoma should be referred immediately to ENT for drainage; patients with obvious septal deviation may be referred to the next convenient ENT clinic and advised to take pre-injury photographs of their face with them. Other patients may safely be reassured that in the majority of cases the swelling will settle down and their appearance will return to normal. In the event of this failing to happen, patients may require manipulation of the nose. Depending on local policy, these patients should be reviewed after approximately 1 week either in the emergency department or a specialist clinic. Radiographs are not indicated in the immediate management of simple nasal fractures.

Nasal bleeding and septal haematoma have been covered above. Severe nasal injury may disrupt the thin ethmoidal bones, and the physical signs of a naso-ethmoidal fracture are given below (Fig. 21.8):

- flattening of the bridge of the nose
- widening of the intercanthal distance (greater than 35 mm)
- nasal obstruction.

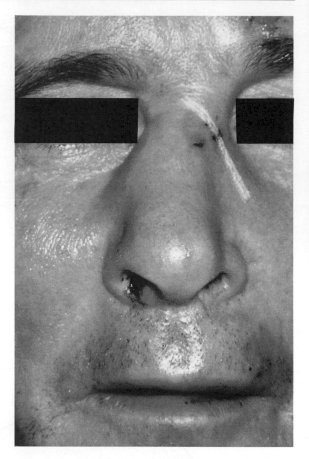

Figure 21.7: Nasal fracture.

Urgent referral to a maxillofacial, plastic or ENT surgeon is appropriate.

ZYGOMATICO-ORBITAL COMPLEX FRACTURES

Fractures in this region of the face are of particular concern because of the possibility of damage to the eye. Examination of the eye should proceed in a logical fashion, starting with the periorbital tissues and moving inwards (Table 21.1).

Marked swelling often accompanies facial trauma and the eyelids may be closed, making examination of the eye difficult. However, it is essential that the eye is examined even if only to ascertain a baseline visual acuity and pupillary reaction. A small Snellen chart may be carried in the pocket for this purpose.

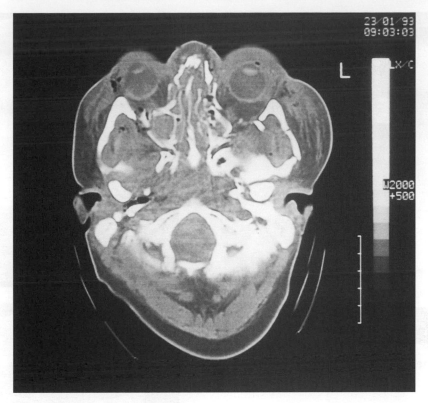

Figure 21.8: CT scan of a naso-ethmoidal fracture.

Table 21.1: Examination of the eye (summary)

Visual acuity testing
Inspection of cornea and conjunctival sac, including eversion of the upper lid
Staining with fluorescein and inspection with blue light
Pupil reactions
Assessment of anterior chamber – use a slit lamp if available
Ophthalmoscopy
Visual fields if indicated
Eye movements if indicated

In a patient with swollen eyelids, gentle pressure applied to both upper and lower eyelids for 2 min will disperse the fluid and allow the eye to be examined. An assistant can help to assess the eye as the eyelids are compressed. Eye observations should be noted on a chart and continued regularly.

Physical signs of a zygomatico-orbital complex fracture are given below:

- bruising and oedema around the eye
- subconjunctival haemorrhage
- paraesthesia of the cheek (injury to infra-orbital nerve)
- step deformity of the inferior orbital margin (Fig. 21.9)
- flattening of the cheek
- diplopia
- traumatic mydriasis
- restricted jaw opening.

Figure 21.10 is a plain radiograph of a fractured right zygomatic arch. This fracture may produce a slight concavity of the cheek if the patient is examined soon after the injury. Otherwise, there will be a swelling over the fracture for a few days. In uncomplicated zygomatic fractures, the complex of ophthalmic signs will be absent. The patient may have restricted mouth movements due to the bony fragments impinging on the temporalis muscle running beneath the arch.

A patient may give a history of injury to the orbital region (e.g. having been hit by a squash ball). There may be only slight bruising or diplopia.

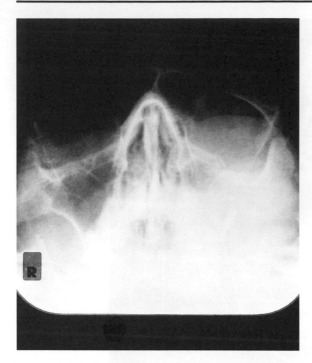

Figure 21.9: Step deformity of the inferior orbital margin.

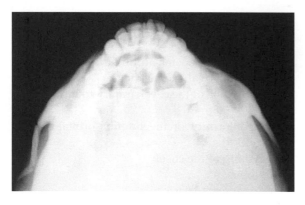

Figure 21.10: A simple zygomatic fracture.

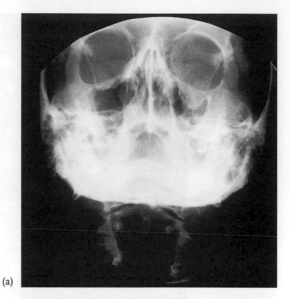

(a)

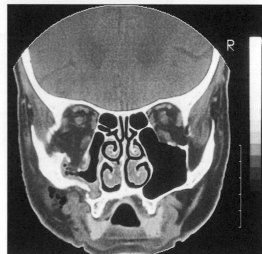

(b)

Figure 21.11: Orbital floor fracture. (a) Plain X-ray. (b) CT scan.

In these circumstances a blowout fracture of the orbital floor should be suspected and plain radiographs obtained. A blowout occurs when the thin floor of the orbit is fractured and there is herniation of the periorbital fat into the maxillary sinus. Figure 21.11(a) illustrates a left orbital floor blowout fracture and the 'tear drop' sign, which may not always be apparent.

A subsequent coronal CT scan of the orbits will demonstrate whether there is herniation of the ocular muscles as has previously been described (Fig. 21.11(b)). Examination of the eye movements may reveal some restriction of upward gaze due to trapping of the muscles in the breach in the orbital floor.

Patients with significant trauma to the eye or orbit should be referred to the ophthalmologist on call.

FRONTAL BONE FRACTURES

These may occur in isolation or in association with other facial fractures. Plain radiographs are essential and a CT scan may be required to determine the extent of the injury (Fig. 21.12).

FURTHER READING

Hawkesford, J. and Banks, J. (1994) *Maxillofacial and Dental Emergencies.* Oxford University Press, Oxford.

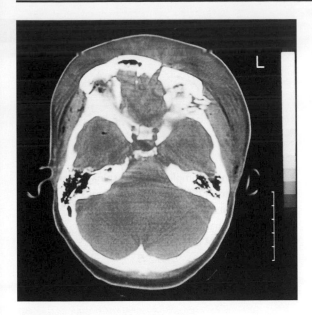

Figure 21.12: A frontal fracture.

SPINAL INJURY

INTRODUCTION

Injuries to the spine are common. Each year in the UK several hundred patients are permanently paralysed as a result of a spinal injury. In addition to these, many thousands suffer prolonged symptoms of pain and stiffness following a more minor injury to the soft tissues surrounding the spinal cord. The most common cause of spinal injuries in the western world is road traffic accidents; these can cause a range of injuries, from fractures or dislocations of any part of the spinal column to the so-called 'whiplash' injury due to sudden flexion–extension of the cervical spine. Most 'whiplash' injuries occur in drivers and front-seat passengers of cars.

The most dangerous form of transport for serious injuries is the motorcycle. Spinal injuries can also occur from falls and during sporting activities. Any patient who has fallen a distance greater than their own body height or who has been involved in a road traffic accident should be assumed to have a spinal injury until proven otherwise.

> Assume a spinal injury has occurred and immobilize the spine till proven otherwise.

The concern in all patients with spinal injury is that the spinal cord itself may have been injured. It is important to remember that the vertebrae act as a protective box for the spinal cord. Thus it is perfectly possible to injure the spinal cord without radiological evidence of vertebral injury. This is commonly the case in children and is known as 'SCIWORA' (spinal cord injury without radiological abnormality). The spinal cord, if transected, will not recover; any damage and consequent paralysis is, therefore, permanent. Patterns of paralysis include quadriplegia (where all four limbs are paralysed), paraplegia (where the lower limbs are paralysed) and hemiplegia (where both limbs on one side are affected). The suffix -paresis indicates that motor function has been disturbed in the distribution referred to (e.g. hemiparesis means loss of motor function down one side of the body).

CLASSIFICATION OF SPINAL INJURIES

Frankel's classification is probably the most useful way of describing the types of neurological deficits, rather than the distribution of the deficits. It is summarized in Table 22.1.

ASSESSMENT

As stated above, spinal injury should be assumed until proven otherwise. The most common parts of

Table 22.1: Frankel's classification of spinal injuries

Frankel A: Complete sensorimotor deficit
Frankel B: Complete motor paralysis. Sensory normal
Frankel C: Useless motor capacity. Sensory normal
Frankel D: Useful motor capacity. Sensory normal
Frankel E: Normal neurological function

Table 22.2: Patients with potential cervical spine injury

Any patient with an injury above the clavicle
Any victim of major trauma
Any trauma victim who is unconscious
Any patient who has fallen
Any patient involved in a road traffic accident (RTA)

the spine to be injured are the cervical and thoracolumbar areas; these are the most flexible parts of the spinal column. The most common sites of injury, in adults, are where these flexible parts of the spine are fixed to the more rigid thoracic spine, that is, at the lower end of the cervical spine and the upper end of the lumbar spine. In children, the upper region of the cervical spine is more commonly the site of injury.

It should be assumed that there is a risk of spinal injury in all the situations listed in Table 22.2.

In any of these patient groups the cervical spine must be immediately immobilized during the 'A' section of the primary survey, 'A' standing for 'Airway with cervical spine control'. Complete immobilization of the cervical spine is achieved only by the application of a hard ('semi-rigid') cervical collar, sandbags either side of the neck and strong tapes securing the head of the patient to the trolley (Fig. 22.1). The only alternatives to these three components of cervical spine immobilization are either the correct application of a long spinal board together with head blocks and a hard collar (Fig. 22.2), or 'in-line manual immobilization' of the spine, where the head is supported by both hands of the doctor or nurse (Fig. 22.3) and neck movements prohibited.

In some patients who are combative, full three-component immobilization of the cervical spine may not be possible and a commonsense compromise may have to be struck, with the application of a hard collar alone. It must be stressed that this

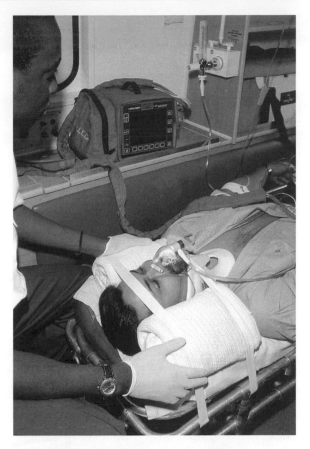

Figure 22.1: Full cervical spine immobilization with collar, sandbags and tape.

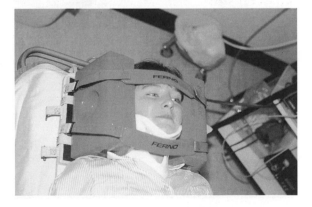

Figure 22.2: Immobilization using collar, spinal board and head blocks.

does not provide proper cervical spinal immobilization.

Immobilization of the thoracic and lumbar spine is more difficult but can be achieved by the

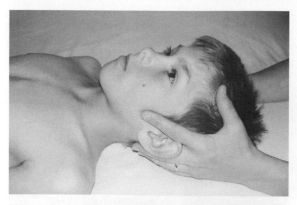

Figure 22.3: Manual in-line immobilization of the cervical spine.

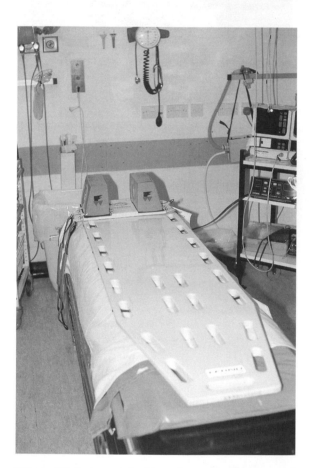

Figure 22.4: Long spinal board.

use of a long spinal board (Fig. 22.4). The complications of such boards, including pressure sores, especially of the sacrum, scapulae and heels, must be borne in mind and the patient removed from the device as soon as possible.

Once the airway has been cleared and the cervical spine has been immobilized, the rest of the primary survey can be dealt with. Spinal injury may affect the breathing component as high cord injury results in denervation of the muscles of respiration and ventilatory inadequacy. Similarly, during the assessment of the circulation, spinal injury can cause shock; this is known as neurogenic shock, and results from loss of sympathetic innervation to the cardiovascular system causing loss of venous tone. It must also be remembered that the presence of spinal injury may mask signs of abdominal injury, making the latter extremely difficult or even impossible to diagnose clinically. During the 'circulation' phase of the primary survey, any shock must be assumed to be due to hypovolaemia and treated accordingly until proven otherwise.

Definitive care of spinal injury should occur in specialist centres and transfer to another hospital may be necessary. For the emergency department clinician the maxim is 'do no further harm': further movement of an injured spine may produce further spinal or spinal cord injury. The medicolegal implications of such iatrogenic injury do not need to be stated, as injuries due to inadvertent or unnecessary mishandling constitute negligence.

Assessment of the spine is by clinical examination and imaging. Clinical examination must include inspection and palpation of the entire spine, searching in particular for areas of tenderness, steps, deformity and the presence of haematomas. As a consequence, the patient will require logrolling in order to access the whole of the spine. Log-rolling requires five people (Fig. 22.5).

The person controlling the head is in charge and responsible for ensuring the safety of the patient by checking that the rest of the team know their roles. The leader co-ordinates the role in each direction and ensures that the head remains in line with the rest of the spine whilst explaining the procedure to the patient. A second member of staff places their hands over the chest and pelvis, controlling the arm. The third person places a hand over the pelvis and under the opposite thigh. The fourth member of the team controls the opposite leg by placing two hands under the calf and ankle ('three hands over, three hands under'). The final member of the team is responsible for examining the patient's spine, the back of the head and torso. A rectal examination should also be performed. The team leader must give clear instructions ('When we

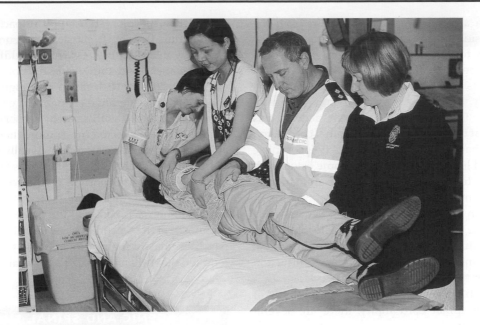

Figure 22.5: Log-rolling a patient.

Table 22.3: Clearing the cervical spine by clinical examination alone

Sober and alert patient
No painful distracting injuries
Neurologically intact
No spinous process tenderness
No neck pain
Pain-free neck movement

Table 22.4: Clinical findings suggestive of cervical spinal cord injury

Flaccidity and loss of reflexes
Diaphragmatic breathing
Flexion but not extension at the elbow
Response to pain above but not below the clavicle
Hypotension with bradycardia
Priapism
Loss of anal sphincter tone

start, I will say "1, 2, 3, roll", at the end, "1, 2, 3, down" ').

Log-rolling is followed by a full neurological examination, which must include assessment of tone, power, co-ordination, sensation and tendon reflexes. Radiological examination is initially by plain radiographs (see below), and suspected abnormalities are further investigated by computerized tomography (CT) or magnetic resonance imaging (MRI).

Cervical spinal injury can only be excluded clinically if the conditions in Table 22.3 are met.

EXAMINATION FINDINGS IN SPINAL INJURY

A patient who is conscious is often able to identify pain and tenderness at the site of spinal injury because there is loss of sensation below this level. In conscious, co-operative patients, spinal levels can often be accurately mapped out and numbness below a particular level gives valuable information about the location of a traumatic spinal cord lesion.

If the patient is unconscious and the mechanism of the injury is either a fall or a road traffic accident there is a 5% risk of a cervical spine injury. Clinical findings that suggest a cervical spinal cord injury are shown in Table 22.4.

As stated earlier the patient must be fully examined for motor strength, sensory disturbance, reflexes, and also autonomic problems such as lack of bladder or bowel control (indicated by loss of anal tone) and priapism (a sustained penile erection).

There are many tracts in the spinal cord but only three can be easily clinically examined. The first of these are the spino-thalamic tracts, which carry pain and temperature sensations from the opposite side of the body. The dorsal columns carry fine touch and co-ordination information from the same side of the body. Finally the cortico-spinal tracts control movements on the same side of the body.

If there is no sensory or motor activity this implies that there has been a total spinal cord lesion and this has a poor prognosis. An incomplete spinal cord lesion may recover to some extent so it is essential to be meticulous in the examination to detect any motor or sensory response. Sparing of sensation in the sacral dermatomes ('sacral sparing') may be the only sign of incomplete injury. The search for this must include sensory testing of the perineum and assessment of voluntary contraction of the anus.

Although there are many possible patterns of incomplete spinal cord injury, there are several common types.

ANTERIOR CORD SYNDROME

This is characterized by injury to the cortico-spinal tracts with severe motor loss, but the dorsal columns and therefore sensation are intact.

POSTERIOR CORD SYNDROME

The pattern of partial cord injury is opposite to that of anterior cord syndrome, with sensory loss and preservation of motor function.

BROWN–SEQUARD SYNDROME

This is very rare and usually results from penetrating cord injury. The presence of this syndrome indicates hemisection of the cord. On examination there is loss of fine sensation (dorsal columns) and movement (cortico-spinal tract) on the side of the lesion, with loss of pain and temperature sensation (spino-thalamic tract) on the opposite side.

CENTRAL CORD SYNDROME

Central cord syndrome is thought to result from ischaemia as a result of injury to the anterior spinal

artery or direct injury caused by impact from the ligamentum flavum. It classically occurs after an extension injury to the neck of a middle-aged or elderly patient and the X-rays do not show any obvious fracture or dislocation, although they may show some degenerative change. On examination there is tetraparesis with a patchy sensory loss. The upper limbs are affected much more than the legs, although the plantar reflexes are usually up-going. The anatomical basis of the condition is that there is injury to the central portion of the cord; cervical (central) fibres of the long motor tracts are affected but the lumbosacral (lateral) fibres are spared. The prognosis of this condition is usually good but paralysis may remain. No specific treatment is required other than the use of a cervical collar.

NEUROGENIC AND SPINAL SHOCK

It is very important to distinguish between these two phenomena, which are frequently confused with one another.

NEUROGENIC SHOCK

This is due to interruption of the descending sympathetic pathways in the spinal cord. It results in loss of vasomotor tone and sympathetic innervation to the heart. The clinical effects therefore include vasodilatation of blood vessels and hypotension. The heart cannot mount a sympathetic response and there may even be a bradycardia. Patients with pure neurogenic shock are classically well perfused peripherally and do not show the pallor, cold skin and sweating of other forms of shock. The combination of hypotension and bradycardia should alert the doctor to the possibility of neurogenic shock. It will not respond to fluid infusion alone but may require pressor agents to increase blood pressure, together with atropine to counter the bradycardia. A central venous line is invaluable in guiding treatment.

True cardiovascular shock in the presence of a spinal injury should always be assumed to be due to haemorrhage until proven otherwise, since any mechanism sufficient to cause a spinal injury is also likely to be sufficient to cause life-threatening injuries elsewhere.

SPINAL SHOCK

This is not a circulatory phenomenon and is not strictly a form of shock. It is the complete loss of neurological function that occurs shortly after a spinal cord injury and is manifest by flaccidity and loss of reflexes. Days or weeks later, the 'shock' disappears and spasticity may replace the flaccidity. Spinal shock might be considered as 'concussion of the spinal cord'.

SAFE HANDLING AND IMMOBILIZATION OF SPINAL-INJURED PATIENTS

It cannot be over-emphasized how vital it is to take all possible precautions when handling or moving patients with proven or suspected spinal injury. Ideally, such patients should be managed on a turning frame in order to avoid the development of pressure areas; however, this is rarely available in the emergency department. Whenever the patient is turned, the 'log-roll' technique described earlier should be used.

PREVENTION OF COMPLICATIONS IN SPINAL INJURIES

As stated previously, there is frequently little that can be done to improve the outlook in patients with spinal injury other than to prevent further harm. All care must be taken to avoid the development of bed-sores or decubitus ulcers, which begin to develop within hours of injury and usually involve the occiput, upper thoracic spine, sacrum and heels.

Steroids are of value to reduce further injury to the spinal cord and improve recovery if used early (within 8 h of the injury). Methyprednisolone should be given as an intravenous bolus of $30 \, mg \, kg^{-1}$ body weight over 15 min followed by an infusion of $5.4 \, mg \, kg^{-1} h^{-1}$ for 23 h. Before administering steroids the case should be discussed with the spinal or neurosurgeon who will be taking over the definitive care of the patient.

INTERPRETATION OF CERVICAL SPINE X-RAYS

Any patient with a suspected spinal injury must have a standard set of radiographs of the cervical spine. This comprises a lateral view (Fig. 22.6), an antero-posterior (AP) view (Fig. 22.7) and an open-mouth peg view (Fig. 22.8). If these are equivocal or show an injury CT scanning should be carried out. The film that gives the most information is the lateral view and a system for looking at this is given in Table 22.5. It should be remembered that a lateral view alone will miss approximately 15% of significant cervical spine injuries and therefore a full series of radiographs and clinical examination must be performed, as described above.

The X-ray should initially be checked for its adequacy. The occiput to the upper border of the

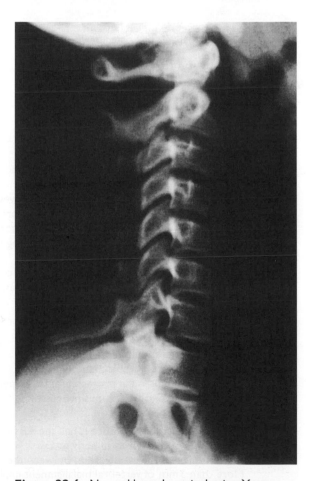

Figure 22.6: Normal lateral cervical spine X-ray.

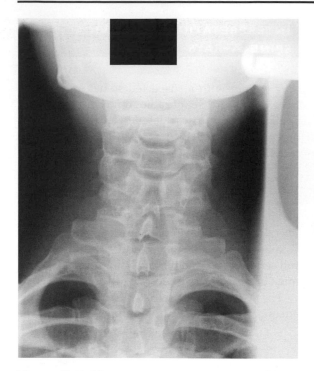

Figure 22.7: Normal antero-posterior view of the cervical spine.

first thoracic vertebra should be visible. The four lordotic curves of the cervical spine are then traced out (Fig. 22.9). These are the anterior borders of the vertebral bodies, the posterior aspect of the vertebral bodies, the junctions of the laminae and the spinous processes and the tips of the spinal processes. These should form smooth continuous lines. Next, each of the cervical vertebrae is examined for fractures. The cartilaginous spaces, particularly the gap between the odontoid peg and the arch of the atlas, the disc spaces, the facet joints

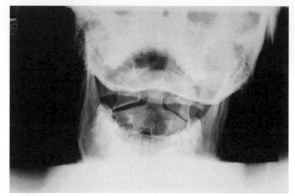

Figure 22.8: Normal open-mouth odontoid peg film.

Table 22.5: Looking at lateral cervical spine X-rays

A is for **Adequacy** and **Alignment**:
>   *Adequacy*: Are all seven cervical vertebrae and the top of the first thoracic vertebra visible? If not, the film is inadequate
>   *Alignment*: Check that the following four curves are all smooth (see also Fig. 22.8):
>>   1. The line joining the anterior borders of the vertebral bodies.
>>   2. The line joining the posterior borders of the vertebral bodies.
>>   3. The posterior spinal line, joining the posterior points of the laminae, where they meet in the mid-line.
>>   4. The line joining the spinous processes.
>>   If any of these curves is irregular, assume injury.

B is for **Bones**
>   Trace round each of the vertebrae looking for fractures and irregularities.

C is for **Cartilages** and soft tissue spaces:
>   The disc spaces should all be regular.
>   Look for prevertebral soft tissue swelling.
>   Is there any break in the prevertebral fat stripe, if present?
>   Distances between the spinous processes.

D is for **Distances**:
>   Normal prevertebral distance is half the AP diameter of the vertebral body at C3 and the full AP diameter of the vertebral body at C6.
>   In the adult there is usually 3 mm between the anterior arch of the atlas vertebra and the peg.
>   More than 3 mm of vertebral malalignment implies dislocation.

and the interspinous spaces are assessed. Finally, the prevertebral soft tissue thickness is measured. This should be a maximum of 3 mm at the lower border of the third cervical vertebra and the width of the vertebral body in the lower cervical spine.

If there is any doubt about the radiological appearances, the presence of a spinal injury should be assumed and full spinal immobilization maintained whilst a more senior opinion is sought. The emphasis for doctors working in emergency departments must be on the detection of abnormality rather than precise naming of injury and assessment of stability.

THORACIC AND LUMBAR SPINE INJURIES

These are common injuries that should be picked up during the secondary survey of the injured patient. Injuries to the lower thoracic and upper lumbar spines can cause paraplegia whilst sparing the upper limbs. The most likely sites to be injured are the cervico-thoracic and thoraco-lumbar junctions, where most movement can occur. Injuries to the relatively rigid thoracic spine imply massive forces in fit adults, although injuries can occur with much lower energy in the elderly with osteoporotic bones or in patients taking corticosteroids.

Radiographs of the thoracic and lumbar spines are indicated in the following situations:

- Any patient with a depressed level of consciousness who has sustained major trauma.
- Any patient with bony spinal tenderness.
- Any trauma victim with abnormal neurological findings.
- Any patient with major or multiple trauma who has distracting painful injuries.
- Any patient with a significant cervical spine injury.

X-rays of the thoracic and lumbar spines should be performed in the radiology department since films taken in the resuscitation room tend to be of poor quality.

SPECIFIC SPINAL FRACTURES

STABILITY AND COLUMNS OF THE SPINE

The spinal column can be regarded as being made up of three vertical columns. The anterior column consists of the anterior parts of the vertebral bodies, the discs in between them and the anterior longitudinal ligaments. The middle column consists of the posterior parts of the vertebral bodies and the posterior longitudinal ligaments. The posterior column consists of the spinous processes and the interspinous ligaments. If only one of these columns is disrupted the spine is usually stable, but damage to two or more of the columns usually produces instability and, consequently, cord damage in response to small amounts of movement is likely.

JEFFERSON FRACTURE OF THE ATLAS (FIG. 22.10)

This is a fracture of the atlas or first cervical vertebra. This vertebra is a diamond-shaped ring interposed

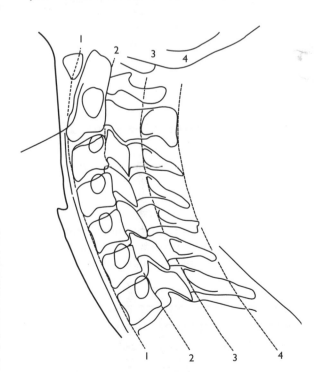

Figure 22.9: The lordotic curves of the cervical spine.

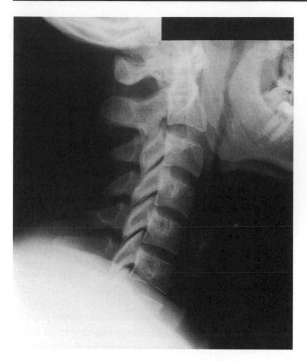

Figure 22.10: Jefferson fracture of the atlas.

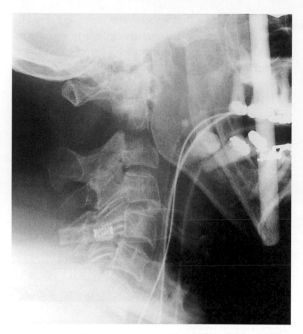

Figure 22.11: Odontoid peg fracture type II.

Table 22.6: Types of odontoid peg fracture

Type I: Above the base of the peg. Usually stable.
Type II: At the base of the peg. Very unstable.
Type III: Extending into the vertebral body of the axis. Unstable.

between the skull and the axis vertebra. It is commonly injured by axial compression forces (e.g. diving into an empty swimming pool, or a driver's head 'bullseyeing' a windscreen) which cause the ring to burst. (Imagine trying to break a Polo Mint in one place!)

Because the ring bursts and the fragments separate, there is relatively little risk of spinal cord compression. This is also suggested by Steel's rule of thirds: a third of the space within the ring is taken up by the odontoid peg, a third by the spinal cord and a third is relatively empty, leaving space for the injured cord to expand. These fractures are diagnosed on the lateral X-ray or peg view. They are unstable injuries but can be adequately treated by prolonged immobilization in a hard collar or Halo.

ODONTOID PEG FRACTURES (FIG. 22.11)

These are most commonly due to road traffic accidents and are of three types (Table 22.6).

All odontoid peg fractures can be very difficult to diagnose and CT scanning may be necessary to confirm the diagnosis. These patients should be cared for by spinal or neurosurgeons, and surgical stabilization is often required.

HANGMAN'S FRACTURE (FIG. 22.12)

This is a fracture through the posterior elements (laminae) of the second cervical vertebra. It is caused by extension in association with distraction or axial compression. It is the mode of death in judicial hanging and might more properly be called the 'hangee's fracture'! The injury is very unstable and often requires operative intervention.

CERVICAL FRACTURES AND FRACTURE-DISLOCATIONS (FIG. 22.13)

These can occur at any level in the neck; the most common site is the cervico-thoracic junction. The

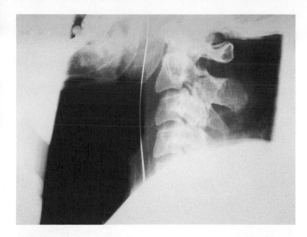

Figure 22.12: Hangman's fracture.

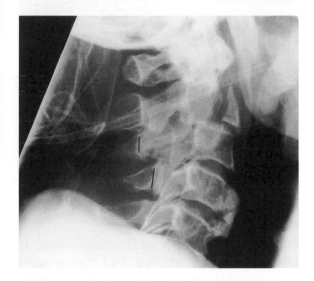

Figure 22.13: Unstable fracture of body of axis vertebra (C2).

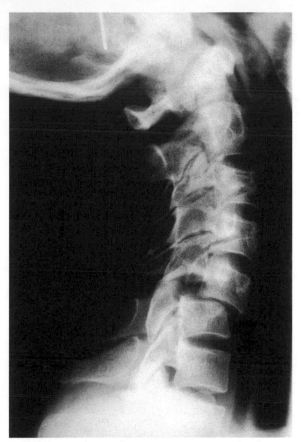

Figure 22.14: Bilateral facet joint dislocation, showing 50% slip.

causative event is usually a fall or a road traffic accident and the mechanism can involve any combination of flexion, extension, rotation and axial loading. Stability is often difficult to determine, especially in the emergency department, and all such patients should be referred to the relevant specialist team.

FACET JOINT DISLOCATIONS (FIG. 22.14)

One or both facet joints may be dislocated. The mechanism is usually a rotational force. On the lateral X-ray, the dislocation is probably unilateral if the upper vertebra is displaced on the lower by 25% or less of the AP diameter and bilateral if the displacement is 50% or more. Bilateral facet joint dislocations are unstable. All facet joint dislocations require traction for reduction.

TEAR-DROP FRACTURES (FIG. 22.15)

A small piece of bone avulsed from the superior aspect of the vertebral body represents an extension injury, is usually stable and requires only conservative treatment. On the other hand, a 'tear-drop' of bone avulsed from the lower border of the vertebral body is a flag to a much more serious injury, often with spinal cord damage. This injury requires further imaging and neurosurgical referral.

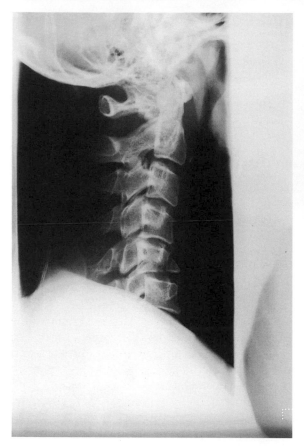

Figure 22.15: Tear-drop fracture.

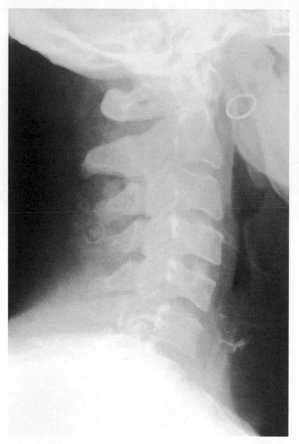

Figure 22.16: Clay-shoveller's fracture of the spinous process of C7.

CLAY-SHOVELLER'S FRACTURE (FIG. 22.16)

This is a fracture through the spinous process of the seventh cervical vertebra and nowadays is more commonly caused by a collapsing rugby scrum than by shovelling clay. It is often difficult to see on X-ray, owing to overlying soft tissue shadows. The injury is extremely painful but is stable and can be treated symptomatically.

COMPRESSION FRACTURES OF THE THORACIC AND LUMBAR VERTEBRAE (FIG. 22.17)

These injuries are usually due to hyperflexion or axial compression forces and wedge compression of the vertebral bodies occurs. These fractures are more common in those with osteoporosis. The amount of wedging is usually quite small. If, however, the anterior height of the vertebral body is more than 25% shorter than the posterior height, or if the angle exceeds 30%, internal fixation is usually indicated. Because the thoracic spinal canal is narrow relative to the cord, spinal cord injury is common in association with thoracic injuries.

THORACOLUMBAR INJURIES

These are common and due to flexion combined with rotation. They are often unstable. Because the spinal cord itself terminates at this spinal level, it is the nerve roots making up the cauda equina that are liable to injury. Injury here will therefore lead to bladder and bowel control problems along with sensory and lower motor neurone deficits in the lower limbs.

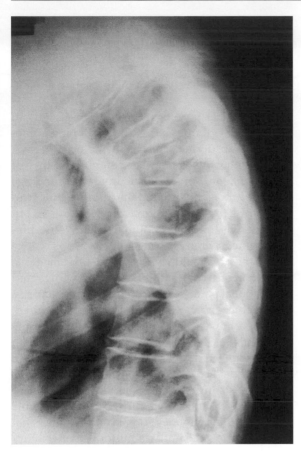

Figure 22.17: Wedge compression fracture of thoracic vertebrae.

TRANSVERSE PROCESS INJURIES

These are common in the lumbar area, their importance being as a marker of possible high-energy injury to the closely related kidney or ureter.

INTERVERTEBRAL DISC LESIONS

The intervertebral discs lie between the bodies of all vertebrae except the first and second cervical vertebra (the odontoid peg is part of C2 but represents the body of C1) and the sacrum (where the vertebrae are fused). The intervertebral discs consist of two parts: an outer fibrous ring or annulus fibrosus, and softer central material, the nucleus pulposus, which is like crabmeat in consistency. A 'prolapsed intervertebral disc' implies protrusion

Table 22.7: Signs suggesting entrapment of a lower lumbar nerve root

> Reduced straight leg raising on one side; this manoeuvre stretches the sciatic nerve and its constituent nerve roots and causes severe leg pain.
> Positive sciatic or femoral nerve stretch tests, depending on the level of the disc prolapse.
> Positive crossover test, where stretching the sciatic nerve on one side causes pain in the opposite leg.
> Reduced tendon reflexes and muscle weakness in the relevant motor nerve distribution.
> Reduced sensation in the corresponding dermatome.

of part of the nucleus pulposus into the spinal canal. Such an event is common in the lumbar spine, less so in the cervical spine and rare in the thoracic spine. The effects of such prolapse or disc herniation depend on how much of the nucleus pulposus is extruded and what it presses upon (the spinal cord or emergent nerve roots).

Disc herniation in the lumbar spine classically presents with fairly acute-onset back pain followed by unilateral leg pain, the leg pain being worse than the back pain. The typical onset is on rising from stooping, or during heavy lifting. The pain in the leg is often described as a sharp shooting pain down the back of the leg from the buttock. It may be associated with reduced or absent sensation, paraesthesiae or motor weakness. On examination there may be some tenderness in the back at the level of the disc involved, together with reduced movements of the lumbar spine. The crucial findings, however, are root tension signs indicating pressure on a nerve root (Table 22.7).

Central disc prolapse is an orthopaedic emergency. The root tension signs are accompanied by bladder or bowel sphincter disturbance. This implies that the spinal cord is being compressed by the disc material and emergency surgery to relieve compression is mandatory.

The investigation of disc prolapse is with CT or MRI scanning. Plain X-rays may show loss of disc space and can exclude bony pathology but are otherwise unhelpful in planning treatment. Some disc prolapses seen on MRI scanning are not clinically relevant, so the information from the scan must be tempered with clinical findings. The treatment of prolapsed lumbar discs is initially conservative, with gradual mobilization, physiotherapy and analgesia. Failure to settle with this regimen will require further intervention, possibly including surgical disc excision. Periods of complete bed rest are no longer recommended and have been shown to be associated with poorer recovery than early mobilization.

Cervical disc prolapse can be caused by sudden neck movement, classically flexion with rotation. The symptoms are neck pain together with abnormal neurological findings on the side of the compressed nerve roots. The discs most commonly affected are those either side of the sixth cervical vertebra, thus the 6th and 7th cervical nerve roots are those most frequently implicated. There is pain and paraesthesiae in the arm, but frequently motor function is normal. Investigation by MRI scan will confirm the diagnosis and exclude other pathology (e.g. tumours). The treatment ranges from conservative (rest, traction, analgesia) to surgical excision of the disc, usually by an anterior approach.

NECK SPRAINS

These injuries are due to acute flexion and extension closely following one another and classically occur in drivers and front-seat passengers of cars involved in road traffic accidents, where they are known as 'whiplash' injuries. The usual causative accident is where the patient's car is struck from behind or crashes into the vehicle in front.

The patient presents with neck pain, possibly a headache and variable neurological findings, although most commonly neurological examination is normal. As time goes on, the neck and head pain often persist and there may be problems with sleeping and concentration. Physical examination reveals tenderness over the neck itself, usually paravertebrally over the neck muscles, and reduced movements of the neck, especially rotation and lateral flexion.

Radiological investigation is controversial; an international group is currently developing guidelines to help decide which patients need X-rays. Those with bony tenderness, significant loss of movement or abnormal neurological findings should be imaged. X-rays of the cervical spine usually show a loss of the normal cervical lordosis but are otherwise normal (assuming there is no pre-existing degenerative changes).

Treatment should consist of good analgesia, using non-steroidal anti-inflammatory drugs and conventional paracetamol-containing formulations, neck mobilization with physiotherapy as required, and good advice about the natural history of the condition. Soft cervical collars are associated with more prolonged disability and recovery and should not be used. Recovery is slow, especially in patients with pre-existing cervical spondylosis. The patient should be encouraged to return as early as possible to their normal activities. There is no evidence that recovery is delayed until claims for personal injury have been settled.

FURTHER READING

Grundy, D. and Swain, A (2001) *ABC of Spinal Cord Injury*. BMJ Publishing, London.

Eismont, F., Garfin, S., Levine, A. and Zigler, J. (1998) *Spine Trauma*. WB Saunders, Philadelphia.

CHAPTER TWENTY THREE

THORACIC TRAUMA

- Introduction
- Mechanism of injury
- Primary survey

- Secondary survey
- Further reading

INTRODUCTION

Thoracic injury accounts for a quarter of all trauma deaths and contributes to a further half. The airway, breathing and circulatory components of the primary survey of resuscitation can all be affected by chest injury and therefore influence neurological disability through cerebral hypoxia and hypovolaemia. Most patients with unsurvivable thoracic injuries will die very soon after injury, before they can reach hospital. Patients who survive to hospital can usually be treated on basic principles and with simple procedures, such as chest drainage and analgesia. Only about 15% of cases require intervention by a cardiothoracic surgeon, more commonly after penetrating rather than blunt injury. It is therefore important to recognize and treat life-threatening conditions, and to know when help is required.

> Chest injury is a major cause of mortality and morbidity.

The outward appearance of the chest can be misleading when assessing thoracic trauma. Patients, especially children, can sustain severe internal injuries with few external signs. As a result it is essential to assess the patient thoroughly, taking account of the mechanism of injury and maintaining a high index of suspicion for major vessel and myocardial damage. The chest should never be considered in isolation and associated injuries, especially in the neck and abdomen, must be sought. In particular, it must be remembered

that any penetrating wound beneath the nipples must be considered to involve the abdomen as well as the chest until proven otherwise.

MECHANISM OF INJURY

The mechanism of injury will give important pointers as to what injuries are likely. Trauma team leaders must therefore obtain as much information as possible about the mechanism from the pre-hospital carers. Likely injuries can then be actively sought and excluded. Nevertheless, no injury should be missed as a consequence of a blinkered search for expected injuries.

BLUNT INJURIES

The type of blunt trauma is important, for example a fall or road traffic accident involving several vehicles, a pedestrian struck by a vehicle or a vehicle striking a tree. At a road traffic accident, the process of 'reading the wreckage' can give a large amount of information. Was the collision a head-to-head or a side impact (Fig. 23.1)? Where was the patient and were they restrained? Were there any other occupants of the same vehicle and what has happened to them? How much intrusion into the passenger space has there been? If the patient was the driver, was the steering wheel deformed?

If the mechanism suggests significant deceleration, great vessel or cardiac damage is possible with little or no external appearance of injury.

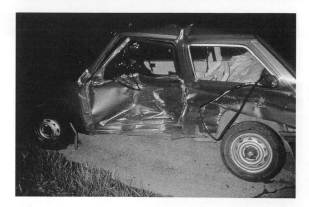

Figure 23.1: A side impact collision road traffic accident.

On the other hand, tyre or seat belt imprints on the chest wall signify a high level of force and must increase suspicion of serious internal injury.

PENETRATING TRAUMA

Surgical intervention is more likely (20–30%) to be needed in penetrating thoracic trauma than in blunt. The type of weapon, the range and direction of strike can again give the trauma team vital pointers. If the weapon is still *in situ*, it should not be removed. This should wait until the patient is in theatre, when any haemorrhage caused by the release of tamponade can be more easily controlled.

> Removal of knives from wounds should be carried out in an operating theatre.

In missile injuries, it is not immediately important as to whether a wound is an entrance or exit wound, and what the exact track of the missile was. Wrong assumptions can be made by premature labelling, and other injuries and projectiles missed as a result. The precise passage can be worked out later once the initial management is complete.

Penetrating injuries are likely to be the result of assault and therefore forensic and medicolegal aspects should be remembered.

BLAST INJURY

Patients involved in an explosion may have both penetrating and blunt trauma. In addition, the shock waves cause maximum damage at gas–tissue interfaces (see Chapter 29). The lungs are therefore particularly vulnerable and diffuse lung damage may develop up to 48 h later. Simple and tension pneumothoraces are frequent and air embolus can occur. Explosions are likely to be subject to intense criminal investigation and detailed notes must be kept.

PRIMARY SURVEY

The goal in the primary survey is to identify and treat any immediately life-threatening conditions as they are found. The six conditions that must be actively sought are shown in Table 23.1. The chest must be carefully examined in the usual sequence as part of the trauma primary survey.

> The immediately life-threatening chest injuries can be remembered using the mnemonic ATOMiC.

The neck, as well as the chest, must be examined at this time and the cervical collar may have to be removed while continuing to immobilize the spine manually. The collar may hide injuries and valuable information. If the patient already has a collar on, a limited examination should be possible through the cut-away section of the collar. A thorough and careful examination of the neck may reveal:

- tracheal deviation
- wounds
- surgical emphysema
- laryngeal disruption
- distended neck veins.

No wound penetrating the platysma should be explored in the emergency department. Thorough examination of all the structures in a deep neck wound must be performed in the operating theatre.

The examination of the chest should then proceed with inspection for wounds, flail segments, bruising and chest expansion. The chest is palpated for tenderness and surgical emphysema, then percussed and auscultated on each side in the second intercostal space anteriorly and in the sixth intercostal space in the mid-axillary line. Remember that a significant proportion of the chest wall is not

Table 23.1: Thoracic conditions to be diagnosed in the primary survey

> **A**irway obstruction
> **T**ension pneumothorax
> **O**pen pneumothorax
> **M**assive haemothorax
> **F**lail chest
> **C**ardiac tamponade

visible in the supine patient and the patient may have to be log-rolled early to search for wounds on the posterior chest wall.

The six immediately life-threatening thoracic injuries to be identified by clinical examination in the primary survey are now discussed.

AIRWAY OBSTRUCTION

The airway should be assessed and, if necessary, cleared and secured before moving on to the rest of the primary survey. Indicators of airway compromise include:

- hoarseness, change in voice quality
- noisy breathing, stridor or gurgling
- agitation
- reduced level of consciousness
- cyanosis (late)
- intercostal or subcostal recession
- accessory muscle use
- bilaterally decreased chest expansion.

The treatment of an obstructed airway begins with high-flow oxygen ($15\,l\,min^{-1}$) and cervical spine immobilization, with appropriate airway manoeuvres beginning simply and progressing to intubation or a surgical airway if necessary.

> All major chest injuries require high-flow oxygen.

TENSION PNEUMOTHORAX

Direct trauma to the lung or chest wall creates a one-way valve into the pleural space. Air accumulates in the pleural cavity, initially compressing the affected lung, then the other lung as the mediastinum is displaced. Another effect of mediastinal

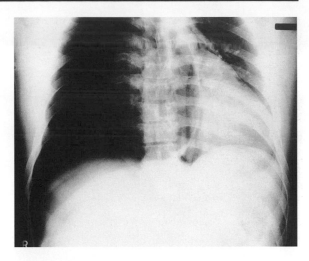

Figure 23.2: X-ray of a tension pneumothorax.

shift is decreased venous return to the heart, causing a drop in cardiac output and shock (Fig. 23.2).

A tension pneumothorax can be produced during resuscitation as a result of positive-pressure ventilation of the injured lung. The person ventilating the patient with a self-inflating bag will be aware of greater resistance to air flow. This diagnosis should be considered in any patient who has initially responded well but has then deteriorated, especially following intubation and ventilation. An open pneumothorax can be converted into a tension pneumothorax by completely sealing the wound with an occlusive dressing.

Figure 23.2 shows an X-ray of a tension pneumothorax, but it must be emphasized that tension pneumothorax is a clinical diagnosis and, if it is suspected, should be treated immediately without waiting for X-ray confirmation.

The classic signs of tension pneumothorax are:

- hyperinflation with decreased movement on affected side
- hyper-resonance on affected side
- absent or decreased air entry on affected side
- deviated trachea away from affected side
- distended neck veins
- shock.

Unfortunately, both distended neck veins and tracheal deviation are late signs and their absence does not exclude the diagnosis. In addition, distended neck veins will only occur if the patient is not already hypovolaemic from an associated injury.

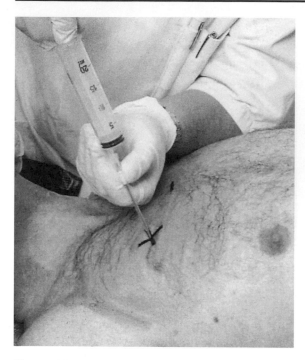

Figure 23.3: Needle thoracocentesis.

The immediate treatment of tension pneumothorax is needle decompression (needle thoracocentesis). A large-bore intravenous cannula connected to a syringe is inserted into the second intercostal space in the mid-clavicular line. The cannula is inserted *over* the third rib rather than *under* the second in order to avoid damage to the neurovascular bundle. If a tension pneumothorax is present, the plunger of the syringe will be driven back. If this fails to happen, air should be injected in order to dispel any possible tissue plug within the needle. Whether the diagnosis is confirmed or not, the cannula should be left in place. The trocar and syringe can be removed. Complications include pneumothorax (where the initial diagnosis was incorrect), lung laceration and local haematoma formation (Fig. 23.3).

Once a needle thoracocentesis has been performed, subsequent insertion of a formal chest drain is mandatory. The definitive treatment of a tension pneumothorax is a formal intercostal drain (Fig. 23.4a–d).

Before commencing the insertion, it is essential to ensure that all the necessary equipment is to hand and that the patient is correctly positioned (Fig 23.4a) with their arm abducted and the forearm

behind the head. In older patients, this position can be difficult to sustain for long periods.

The correct site, the fifth intercostal space just anterior to the mid-axillary line, is identified and cleaned. Insertion one space above or below this is acceptable if there is trauma at the normal site (Fig. 23.4b). The site is then draped and local anaesthetic injected. Local anaesthetic must be inserted as far as the pleura. It is also important to remember to inject local anaesthetic at the site of insertion of the retaining suture (see below). The fifth intercostal space is chosen for the following reasons:

- safety (absence of vital structures)
- ease of insertion (relatively thin part of chest wall)
- cosmetic result (discreet scar)
- patient comfort (ability to lie on back).

A 2.5–3 cm skin incision is made parallel to the rib (Fig. 23.4c), followed by blunt dissection down to the pleura using a pair of forceps and a gloved finger. Once the pleura is reached, it can be perforated using the same blunt forceps. A finger should then be inserted into the pleural cavity and swept around the margins of the hole in order to exclude adhesions (Fig. 23.4b). When this is done, care should be taken as fragments of broken rib can occasionally cause lacerations to the examining finger. The chest drain (usually about size 28) without a trocar can then be introduced in an upwards and backwards direction (Fig. 23.4c). A curved forceps can be used to guide the drain in the correct direction, and a second forceps is used to clamp off the drain during insertion (this is particularly useful in preventing blood spillage when draining a haemothorax) (Fig. 23.4d). Fogging of the tube during respiration will confirm its position. It is essential to ensure that all the side-holes on the drain are inside the pleural cavity. The drain can then be connected to an underwater seal or bag with one-way valve and the clamp removed. Rapid bubbling of air will occur. The connection between the drain and the drainage tube should be securely sealed with tape. The skin hole is then closed around the drain with mattress sutures and the drain held in place with strapping and suture (Fig. 23.4d). Purse-string sutures should not be used as they are difficult to close and cause an unsightly scar. Once the suturing is complete, 10-cm gauze pads are applied and the dressing taped in place. Once the drain is in place, a check chest X-ray

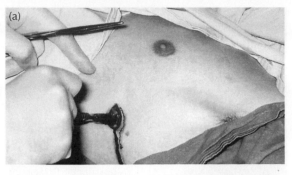
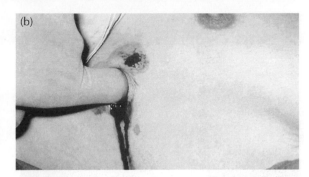
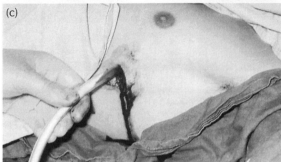
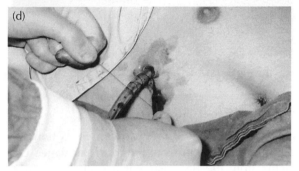

Figure 23.4: Insertion of an intercostal drain.

Table 23.2: Complications of intercostal drainage

Damage to the intercostal vessel or nerve
Damage to intrathoracic or intra-abdominal organs
Incorrect tube position (extrapleural)
Persistent air leak:
  Tracheo-bronchial rupture
  Leak at skin
  Leak in drainage system

should be taken. The complications of intercostal drainage are given in Table 23.2.

Although needle aspiration may be effective for spontaneous pneumothoraces, it should not be used for pneumothoraces that are traumatic in origin.

Intercostal drains should be inserted with a controlled open technique.

Once the drain is *in situ*, if an underwater seal is used the water level in the tube will rise and fall ('swing') with breathing. This will occur even if the lung is fully expanded. The only cause of a non-swinging water level is a blocked or displaced tube.

OPEN PNEUMOTHORAX

Large penetrating wounds to the chest which penetrate to the pleura will produce an open pneumothorax. The patient is likely to be in respiratory distress, and if the wound has a diameter more than two-thirds that of the trachea, air will pass preferentially through it on inspiration instead of ventilating the lungs. This is known as a 'sucking' chest wound (Fig. 23.5). A one-way valve effect may cause a rapidly developing tension pneumothorax if the air cannot escape in expiration.

The most effective emergency treatment for an open pneumothorax is an Aschermann Chest Seal® (Fig. 23.6). The older method of a sterile dressing fixed on three sides forming a valve in order to prevent a tension pneumothorax can also be used. A chest drain should be inserted away from the wound. The definitive treatment is surgical closure of the wound.

FLAIL CHEST

If two or more ribs are broken in two or more places, a segment of chest wall can become mechanically

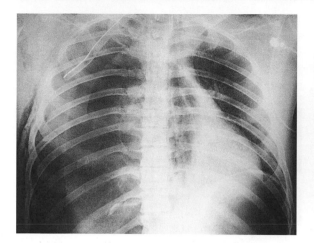

Figure 23.5: An open pneumothorax.

unstable. This can also occur with costochondral separation or fractures of the costal cartilages. On inspiration, the flail segment is sucked inwards, reducing the tidal volume (Fig. 23.7). The main contributor to respiratory compromise, however, is the underlying pulmonary contusion. Small flail segments can be extremely difficult to detect clinically, especially soon after injury. Paradoxical movement may be present although it may be masked by muscular spasm. Crepitus, pain and instability may be felt on palpation.

Treatment begins with the administration of high-flow oxygen. Analgesia, usually an intravenous opiate, will also be required but care should be taken to titrate the opiate carefully to prevent inhibition of ventilatory drive. Intercostal or epidural blocks can be considered at a later stage. Any associated haemopneumothorax should be drained. Fluid resuscitation should be cautious as the area of pulmonary contusion underlying the flail segment is vulnerable to fluid overload, and the arterial blood gases should be monitored regularly. Artificial ventilation is likely to be required if the blood gases are deteriorating, the respiratory rate rising, the patient is becoming exhausted or there are associated multiple injuries (particularly a head injury).

> Underlying pulmonary contusion is responsible for respiratory compromise in a patient with a flail chest.

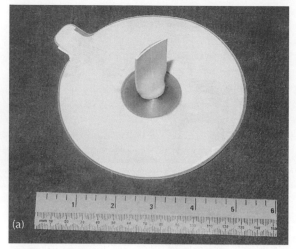

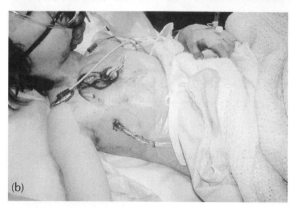

Figure 23.6: An Aschermann® Chest Seal (a) *in situ* (b).

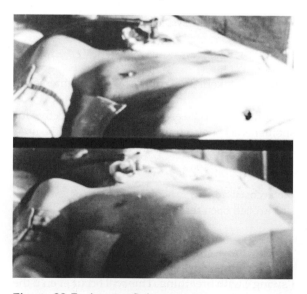

Figure 23.7: A major flail segment.

Massive haemothorax

A massive haemothorax is the collection of more than 1500 ml of blood in the pleural cavity due to injury to the great vessels, chest wall or lung. There is usally an associated simple (or occasionally tension pneumothorax). Massive haemothorax is a circulatory problem as well as a breathing one. Fluid resuscitation must be commenced before the insertion of a chest drain. Although re-expansion of the lung can reduce bleeding, the massive haemothorax may have established some tamponade of the bleeding site, which will be released by drainage, and this may precipitate torrential haemorrhage. The signs of massive haemothorax are:

- hypoxia
- shock
- dullness to percussion over affected side
- reduced air entry over affected side.

Two large-bore intravenous cannulae should be inserted before any attempt is made to drain the chest. Blood must be sent for cross-match and fluid resuscitation should be commenced. Once intravenous access has been achieved, a chest drain can be inserted. In general, a larger drain (size 36) than would be used for a pneumothorax should be used in order to prevent blocking. A drain inserted for a haemothorax should be inserted in the same location and in the same direction as for a pneumothorax.

Thoracotomy is indicated by initial blood loss into the chest drain of more than 1500 ml, continuing loss of more than 200 ml h^{-1} or the deteriorating physiological status of the patient.

Cardiac tamponade

The pericardium is a fibrous sac which cannot expand acutely. Blood leaking into it from injury (usually penetrating) to the heart will lead to an increase in intrapericardial pressure. Even small amounts of pericardial blood can cause reduction in ventricular filling and a drop in cardiac output. Similarly, the aspiration of only 20 ml can cause haemodynamic improvement. A high index of suspicion must be maintained if tamponade is to be recognized, as the clinical signs may be masked by other injuries or the environment of the resuscitation room. Cardiac tamponade should particularly be suspected in the shocked patient with a penetrating chest injury which does not respond to an intravenous fluid bolus.

Central venous pressure (CVP) measurement or echocardiogram may be useful in diagnosis but should not delay therapeutic aspiration if it is needed urgently. Pericardiocentesis in the resuscitation room should be reserved for seriously ill patients with suspected decompensated tamponade.

The diagnosis may be relatively straightforward if there is a penetrating wound to the chest or upper abdomen, otherwise it can be extremely difficult. It is characterized by Beck's triad:

- hypotension
- distended neck veins
- muffled heart sounds.

Muffled heart sounds as well as pulsus paradoxus and Kussmaul's sign (a raised jugular venous pressure (JVP) on spontaneous inspiration) can be extremely difficult to demonstrate in a noisy resuscitation room.

The treatment includes immediate fluid resuscitation and pericardiocentesis. The definitive treatment is thoracotomy and repair of the cardiac lesion. The technique of pericardiocentesis is given in Table 23.3.

The complications of pericardiocentesis include:

- pneumothorax
- coronary artery and vein damage
- myocardial damage
- cardiac dysrhythmias including ventricular fibrillation
- damage to other mediastinal structures.

Thoracotomy in the resuscitation room

This should only be attempted on patients with penetrating trauma to the chest who are in electromechanical dissociation on arrival. Even in the hands of experienced surgeons it has a poor chance of success. Victims of blunt trauma in cardiac arrest on arrival have a zero per cent chance of survival, and are not candidates for this procedure.

Table 23.3: Technique of pericardiocentesis

Ensure all equipment is to hand and attach patient to cardiac monitor

If time allows clean and drape skin and inject local anaesthetic

Attach 15-cm large-bore cannula to three-way tap and 20-ml syringe

Select entry site: 1–2 cm to the left and below xiphisternum

Direct cannula at 45° to skin, aiming for tip of left scapula and advance cannula slowly, aspirating continuously

Watch ECG for myocardial injury patterns – ST segment changes or dysrhythmias

Once blood is aspirated, aspirate to dryness

Watch ECG during aspiration

Withdraw needle leaving plastic cannula in place

Secure cannula and three-way tap

Reassess patient and response to procedure

Transfer for thoracotomy

Emergency room thoracotomy is indicated for patients with penetrating injury who have had signs of life documented by the paramedics or hospital staff.

A left anterior approach is usually used, after insertion of a chest drain on the right. This approach allows access to the heart and descending aorta. The incision is made through the fifth intercostal space from 5 cm lateral to the sternum to the posterior axillary line. This avoids the internal mammary artery. The incision is then opened with rib spreaders. The following actions are now possible:

- release of pericardial tamponade
- direct control of bleeding from the heart or other structures
- internal cardiac massage
- internal defibrillation
- direction of blood to the central circulation by compression of the descending aorta.

The decision to perform this procedure is for senior medical staff.

SECONDARY SURVEY

This head-to-toe examination of the patient should only be carried out once the primary survey

Table 23.4: Secondary survey chest injuries

Life-threatening:
  Pulmonary contusion
  Myocardial contusion
  Aortic rupture
  Diaphragmatic rupture
  Major airway rupture
  Oesophageal rupture
      (2 contusions + 4 ruptures)
Others:
  Simple pneumothorax
  Haemothorax
  Subcutaneous emphysema
  Traumatic asphyxia
  Rib and sternal fractures

---

has been completed and any immediately life-threatening injuries have been dealt with.

The chest should be fully reassessed in the usual progression – look, feel, percuss, listen. The life-threatening injuries that must be actively sought in the secondary survey are harder to identify and treat, but delay in diagnosis may have fatal results for the patient. Again a high index of suspicion and an appreciation of the mechanism of injury are essential (Table 23.4). An ECG, arterial blood gases and, where injuries allow, a chest X-ray (taken erect if possible) should be included in the secondary survey.

PULMONARY CONTUSION

Pulmonary contusion is the commonest of the life-threatening chest injuries. It appears on chest X-ray as diffuse shadowing (Fig. 23.8). In the early stages, however, the chest X-ray is often normal. Respiratory compromise increases insidiously as a ventilation/perfusion mismatch develops. The mechanism of injury is usually blunt but contusion can develop in the track of a high-velocity missile.

Pulmonary contusion is associated with flail chest. A degree of contusion should be assumed to be present under any rib fracture or mark on the chest wall, such as pattern bruising. Pattern bruising occurs when the thorax is compressed with such force that an imprint of the compressing object is left on the skin. In children and young adults, there may be significant pulmonary damage without any rib fracture or outward sign of

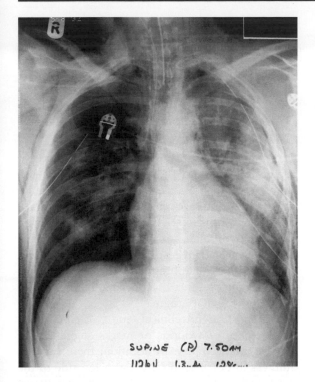

Figure 23.8: A chest radiograph of pulmonary contusion.

injury. The contused lung is very vulnerable to fluid shifts. Overload can lead to pulmonary oedema. Under-transfusion reduces pulmonary perfusion, causing tissue hypoxia and increased fluid leak from the alveolar membrane. Central venous pressure monitoring is advised.

Clinical features which suggest the possibility of pulmonary contusions include pattern bruising, tyre and seat-belt marks as well as evidence of tenderness and rib fractures. Hypoxia occurs and progresses despite oxygen therapy and resuscitation. As stated above, the chest X-ray shows progressive diffuse shadowing.

The immediate treatment of established or developing pulmonary contusion is high-flow oxygen. Serial arterial blood gas analyses and careful fluid resuscitation are essential. These patients may require intubation and ventilation as well as intensive and often prolonged medical support. The following features indicate the need to consider mechanical ventilation:

- multiple injuries, particularly head injury
- decreased level of consciousness
- falling PaO_2/rising $PaCO_2$

- transfer or surgery required
- elderly
- chronic lung or renal disease.

MYOCARDIAL CONTUSION

The severity of myocardial contusion ranges from minor bruising to necrosis as a result of coronary artery spasm, tissue oedema or intimal tears. The right ventricle, which lies anteriorly, is most often affected and rupture of chamber, septum and valve is possible. Myocardial contusion is easily missed but close attention to the prehospital report and associated injuries are useful pointers. A history of a deformed steering wheel and sternal bruising or fracture is a strong indicator of myocardial damage. It is worth remembering that an ischaemic infarct may have been the initial cause of the trauma.

The sequelae are similar to those of an ischaemic infarct – dysrhythmias, especially in the first 24 h; cardiac aneurysms, rupture and cardiac failure. Clinical features suggestive of myocardial contusion include heart failure, arrhythmias, ST segment changes on ECG, ventricular dysfunction on echocardiogram, a rise in cardiac enzymes and abnormal isotopes studies in recovery phase. In managing these patients acidosis must be avoided, as this will increase damage and potentiate arrhythmias. ECG monitoring is essential and a referral to cardiologists should be made early.

AORTIC RUPTURE

Aortic rupture is the result of severe deceleration and 85–90% of patients die from the resulting haemorrhage before reaching hospital. The aorta is vulnerable to this mechanism of injury as it is fixed at some points and mobile at others. The most common site of rupture is at the level of the ligamentum arteriosum. Patients who survive to reach hospital do so because haemorrhage is contained either within a mediastinal haematoma or by an intact adventitia forming a false aneurysm.

Those patients who survive to hospital can be treated by repair or grafting, provided the diagnosis is suspected and made. The mortality amongst survivors is 50% per day until operation. A high index of suspicion is vital to making the diagnosis

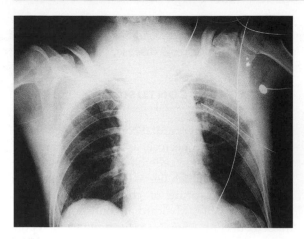

Figure 23.9: A chest radiograph of aortic rupture.

Table 23.5: X-ray signs of aortic rupture

Widened mediastinum
Deviation of trachea to the right
Elevation and rightward shift of the right main bronchus
Depression of the left main bronchus
Deviation of the oesophagus (nasogastric tube) to the right
Obliteration of aortic knob
Obvious double contour of aorta
Obliteration of the aorto-pulmonary window
Presence of a pleural cap
Abnormal left mediastinal stripe
Widened right paratracheal stripe

as there are few specific indicators on examination and chest X-ray. A widened mediastinum is the most reliable indicator on chest X-ray (Fig. 23.9) and other features are shown in Table 23.5. No single feature or combination of these is completely accurate in predicting the presence of this injury. The absence of all of these signs, however, has a high negative predictive value. The haemodynamically stable patient with suspected aortic rupture needs urgent further investigation. This should be at a hospital where any necessary operative cardiothoracic procedure can be performed. The investigation of choice is angiography or spiral CT, but trans-oesophageal echocardiography may be of use. Treatment is surgical.

Indicators of high-energy injury, such as fractures of the sternum, scapula, first or second rib, thoracic spine and multiple left rib fractures, may also be present.

A high index of suspicion should be maintained and the mediastinum should be positively cleared in any patient with a high-energy deceleration mechanism of injury.

DIAPHRAGMATIC RUPTURE

Diaphragmatic rupture can result from blunt or penetrating trauma. Blunt trauma tends to cause large lacerations and penetrating trauma smaller ones that progress over time. The right side of the diaphragm is relatively protected by the liver. Herniation of abdominal contents through the rupture can lead to respiratory compromise and strangulation. If diaphragmatic rupture is present it implies the presence of associated injuries above and below the diaphragm.

The most useful clinical clue will come from the presence of wounds or marks suggestive of diaphragmatic injury. In addition, there may be dullness to percussion on the affected side of the chest and decreased air entry with or without bowel sounds on chest auscultation. In many cases the diagnosis is made on the initial chest X-ray, where bowel or a nasogastric tube is seen in the chest (Fig. 23.10). Peritoneal lavage fluid may occasionally be aspirated from a chest drain. Contrast studies will provide further information.

The emergency treatment of a ruptured diaphragm is careful management of associated injuries with nasogastric drainage and suction. Definitive treatment is by surgical repair.

MAJOR AIRWAY RUPTURE

Like aortic rupture this is frequently fatal at the scene of trauma. Both penetrating and blunt trauma can cause airway rupture, the latter as the result of a direct blow or shearing forces. Laryngeal fracture is classically associated with injury caused by the neck of a cyclist striking a wire stretched across the road. The indicators vary depending on the level at which the rupture has occurred and can be subtle (Table 23.6). Associated injuries to other major structures must be excluded.

In many cases, intubation will be difficult or impossible owing to haematoma, emphysema or loss of continuity of the airway. In these cases, a

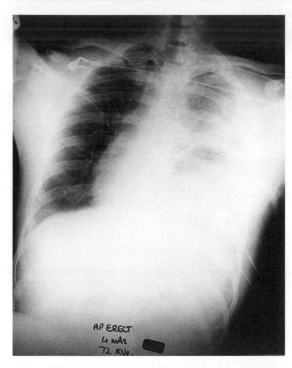

Figure 23.10: Diaphragmatic rupture on a chest radiograph.

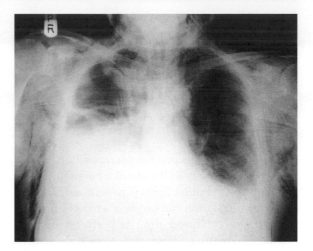

Figure 23.11: Oesophageal rupture on a chest radiograph.

Table 23.6: Signs of major airway rupture

Laryngeal:
Hoarseness, change in voice quality
Subcutaneous emphysema
Fracture may be palpable
Tracheal:
Noisy partially obstructed airway
Subcutaneous emphysema
Most common site is crico-tracheal junction
Bronchial:
Haemoptysis
Subcutaneous emphysema
Persistent large air leak from chest drain
Simple or tension pneumothorax
Most common site is within 2–3 cm of carina

surgical airway distal to the injury may be necessary. In injuries to the proximal major airways, expert anaesthetic or ENT assistance may be necessary. Where there is a pneumothorax, a formal intercostal drain should be inserted. In open tracheal rupture an endotracheal (ET) tube can be placed through the defect. Definitive management is by surgical repair following bronchoscopy.

OESOPHAGEAL RUPTURE

Oesophageal rupture is a rare consequence of trauma which produces few immediate signs but if missed can produce fatal complications. The usual mechanism of injury is penetrating, when associated injury to other major structures must be excluded. Blunt trauma to the upper abdomen can forcibly expel stomach contents into the lower oesophagus causing rupture similar to Boerhaave's syndrome.

Pain and shock are usually present disproportionate to obvious injuries, with a left pneumo/haemothorax in the absence of rib fractures or left chest trauma. Subcutaneous emphysema may be present. Food particles may be identified in the chest drain. The chest radiograph will demonstrate mediastinal air (Fig. 23.11).

The treatment of oesophageal rupture is surgical following endoscopy and other oesophageal imaging. Oral methylene blue appearing in the chest drain may be used to confirm the diagnosis. Prophylactic antibiotics must be given.

SIMPLE PNEUMOTHORAX (TABLE 23.7)

This may result from blunt or penetrating trauma, and should always be treated with an intercostal drain. A check radiograph should always be taken

Table 23.7: Signs of simple pneumothorax

Decreased expansion on affected side
Hyper-resonant percussion note on affected side
Decreased or absent air entry on affected side
Chest X-ray appearances (may be subtle if supine film)

Table 23.8: Causes of subcutaneous emphysema

Pneumothorax
Major airway rupture
Oesophageal rupture
Wounds
Blast injury

to confirm re-expansion and drain position. Where possible, the chest drain should be sited before mechanically ventilating the patient as positive-pressure ventilation can create a tension pneumothorax. The collapsed lung is perfused but not ventilated, creating a mismatch. A young fit patient may be uncomfortable but can often tolerate this with little respiratory distress. In an elderly patient with chronic lung disease and little respiratory reserve, a simple pneumothorax can be life threatening.

HAEMOTHORAX

Haemothoraces which are not immediately life threatening occur as the result of lacerations to the lung or intercostal blood vessels from blunt or penetrating trauma. They are normally self-limiting and have an associated pneumothorax. The diagnosis is usually made from the chest X-ray, but again a supine film may only demonstrate subtle changes of generalized opacification of the hemithorax, even with large quantities of pleural blood. An erect X-ray will show more classic appearances of pleural fluid. Insertion of a chest drain will re-expand the lung, which will help reduce bleeding. A large-calibre chest drain should be used to ensure the removal of as much blood as possible without blockage. Apparently minor haemothoraces must be carefully observed for continuing bleeding.

SUBCUTANEOUS EMPHYSEMA

Subcutaneous air does not require treatment unless there is an exceptional amount and respiration is compromised. It is a good indicator of underlying pathology (Table 23.8), which must be actively sought and treated.

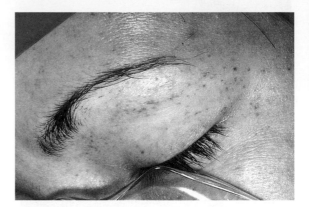

Figure 23.12: The petechial rash of traumatic asphyxia.

TRAUMATIC ASPHYXIA

Crush injury to the thorax prevents the patient expanding the chest and can cause temporary superior vena caval compression. Cardiac output is therefore reduced. Once the patient has been released, survival depends on treating the associated injuries. Respiratory distress may or may not be present; plethora and petechial haemorrhages in the distribution of the superior vena cava are characteristic (Fig. 23.12). Other signs include scleral haemorrhages, and a decreased level of consciousness. Associated injuries must be sought and treated and high-flow oxygen administered. Fluid resuscitation must be carefully monitored.

RIB AND STERNAL FRACTURES

Bony damage to the chest wall is a common result of trauma. Ribs fracture either at the site of trauma or laterally at the point of maximum curvature. The presence of a fracture implies underlying soft tissue damage. Palpation for tenderness, instability and crepitus is a more sensitive method for

Table 23.9: Rib fractures and associated injuries

Ribs 1–3:
  Protected by bony shoulder girdle
  Associated with severe injury to head, neck
    and chest
  High chance of major vessel or brachial plexus
    injury

Ribs 4–9:
  Pneumothorax
  Haemothorax
  Pulmonary contusion

Ribs 10–12:
  Right – liver laceration
  Left – splenic laceration

Sternum:
  Myocardial contusion
  Pulmonary contusion

---

identifying rib fractures than chest radiography, which may not detect undisplaced rib fractures and does not show costochondral separation. Chest X-ray can, however, show underlying damage such as pulmonary contusion or pneumothorax. The site of fracture determines the possible associated injuries (Table 23.9). The pain caused by a rib fracture, even if not associated with soft tissue damage, can restrict chest expansion and ventilation leading to pneumonia, especially in the elderly. Appropriate analgesia, which can be either systemic, or by intercostal or epidural block, is essential. Tape or any other form of external support must not be used as it reduces chest wall mobility and increases the risk of lung collapse and pneumonia.

Sternal fractures may be clinically obvious, with severe tenderness or occasionally a step in the sternal contour. Special radiographic views are necessary to demonstrate them adequately. Because of the association with severe trauma, the majority of patients with even apparently isolated sternal fracture should be admitted for observation. It is also essential that the rare sterno-clavicular dislocation is not missed, as backwards displacement of the medial end of the clavicle into the neck can cause airway compromise. Urgent elevation is then needed and expert surgical and anaesthetic assistance must be sought.

FURTHER READING

Westaby, S. and Odell, J. (Eds) (1999) *Cardiothoracic Trauma*. Arnold, London.

CHAPTER TWENTY FOUR

ABDOMINAL AND GENITOURINARY TRAUMA

INTRODUCTION

Assessment of the abdomen is a critical part of the examination of the trauma patient. The abdomen may be the site of massive blood loss and a cause of trauma deaths, especially if the injury is unrecognized or undertreated. A high index of suspicion for internal injuries must be maintained even in the face of a normal initial examination. The signs of haemoperitoneum and ruptured hollow viscus are often absent or subtle, and can be obscured completely by associated injuries, alcohol and illicit drugs. Adjuncts such as diagnostic peritoneal lavage (DPL), ultrasound (USS) and double-contrast computerized tomography (CT) are necessary to detect abdominal injury, particularly where the patient's conscious level is reduced.

The abdomen is vulnerable to trauma as most of it is not protected by the skeleton. Any patient with injuries above and below the abdomen must be assumed to have abdominal injuries, and any penetrating wound between the nipples and the knees must be treated as potentially involving the abdomen.

> The presence of injury above and below the abdomen indicates injury to the abdomen.

The haemodynamic state of the patient as well as the mechanism and site of injury will determine the timing of the formal abdominal assessment, but in the primary survey of a shocked patient the sites of occult haemorrhage must be checked. Early surgical involvement and frequent re-evaluation are mandatory.

Sources of concealed haemorrhage are:

- floor (external)
- chest
- abdomen
- pelvis and retroperitoneum
- thighs.

ANATOMY

A good knowledge of both external and internal anatomy is essential when assessing the patient with abdominal trauma (Fig. 24.1). In conjunction with an appreciation of the mechanism of injury, potential problems can be identified and treated early or excluded.

SURFACE ANATOMY

The surface of the abdomen can be divided into the following regions:

- Anterior abdomen: between the anterior axillary lines, from the inter-nipple lines to the inguinal ligaments and pubic symphysis.

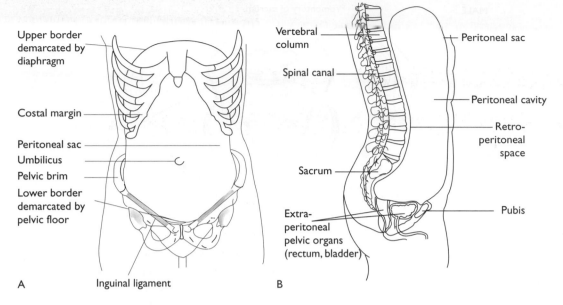

Figure 24.1: Anatomy of the abdomen and pelvis.

- Flanks: between the anterior and posterior axillary lines from the sixth intercostal spaces to the iliac crests.
- Posterior abdomen: from the tip of the scapulae to the iliac crests between the posterior axillary lines.

An area of all these regions is partly protected by the rib cage. Similarly, the posterior abdomen and flanks are covered by thick muscle layers affording some protection.

INTERNAL ANATOMY

The internal anatomy of the abdomen and pelvis is divided into three areas (Fig. 24.1).

Peritoneal cavity

The peritoneum is a serous membrane sac. It has two layers: the parietal layer covers the internal abdominal wall and the visceral the intraperitoneal organs. The layers are in contact with each other with a potential space in between. It is into this space that haemorrhage occurs following organ damage. The peritoneal cavity can be subdivided into two regions:

- *Intrathoracic or upper abdomen*: covered by the lower rib cage. Trauma to this area can cause both thoracic and abdominal injuries. Contents include the diaphragm, liver, spleen and gallbladder and biliary tree, as well as the stomach.
- *Lower abdomen*: contents include the small intestine, transverse and sigmoid colon.

Retroperitoneum

Injuries to the retroperitoneum are particularly difficult to recognize as its contents are not accessible to clinical examination. Bleeding is contained within this space and diagnostic peritoneal lavage will often be negative even with extensive haemorrhage. The retroperitoneum contains the aorta, inferior vena cava, most of the duodenum, pancreas, ascending and descending colon and upper urinary tract.

Pelvis

The contents of the pelvic cavity are protected by the bony pelvis: they include the iliac blood vessels, rectum, lower urinary tract and female reproductive organs. The anatomy of the bony pelvis is shown in Fig. 24.2.

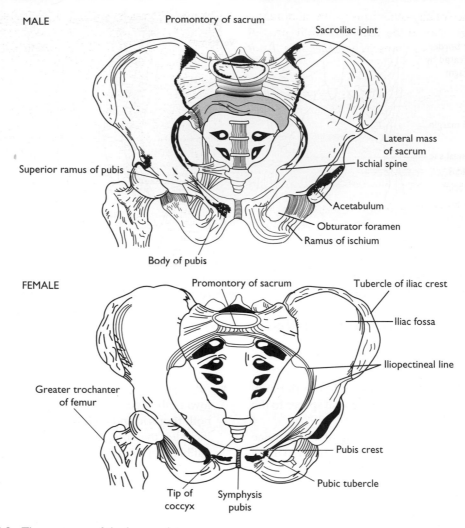

Figure 24.2: The anatomy of the bony pelvis.

MECHANISMS OF INJURY

It is vital that as much information as possible is obtained regarding the mechanism of injury. Different injury patterns are recognized and raising the index of suspicion will help the resuscitation team to avoid missing any possible diagnosis.

BLUNT TRAUMA

Physical examination is unreliable at identifying intra-abdominal pathology in blunt trauma, being correct in only 50–60% of cases. Information from the incident, for example the height of the fall or speed of the road traffic accident, will suggest the magnitude of the injury. Pattern bruising from seat belts or blunt weapons will also assist in diagnosis. The forces that may cause abdominal injury can be classified as follows. Severe direct trauma is usually responsible for solid organ injury such as liver, spleen and renal ruptures. Deceleration forces are most often associated with high-speed road traffic accidents and high falls. After the impact, organs continue to move forward on their points of attachment, tearing tissues and vessels. Examples include aortic and duodenal rupture. Shearing forces make tissue planes move over each other, tearing communicating structures and blood vessels.

If the patient with blunt trauma has unexplained shock and the chest and pelvic X-rays are normal, in the absence of any other cause, intra-abdominal haemorrhage should be assumed until proved otherwise. Proof of intraperitoneal bleeding is not a prerequisite for laparotomy.

> Organ-specific diagnosis is not required prior to laparotomy.

PENETRATING TRAUMA

In most of the UK penetrating trauma is relatively infrequent. Most penetrating abdominal wounds will require laparotomy, and all require at least local exploration. It is important to remember that any penetrating wound between the nipples and the knees should be assumed to potentially involve the abdomen until demonstrated otherwise. The damage caused will vary according to the weapon used.

Stab wounds are most commonly caused by knives but many other, often seemingly innocuous, implements have been used. Stab wounds are low-energy transfer injuries that cause direct tissue damage along a straight track. If the weapon is still *in situ*, it must be left until it can be removed in the operating theatre, where any resultant haemorrhage from tamponade release can be swiftly controlled (Fig. 24.3). Information from the prehospital carers regarding the type and size of the weapon, the time and angle of attack, the range at which it was thrown or fired (where appropriate), and the condition of the patient and blood loss at the scene may aid management.

In gunshot wounds (see Chapter 29), missiles may not follow straight tracks. Depending on the type of gun, the missile used and the range, there may be extremely high-energy transfer to the surrounding tissues causing cavitation. A large amount of dead tissue is created requiring extensive surgical debridement, especially since clothing and other foreign matter is carried into the wound. Secondary missiles can be formed if the initial missile fragments or bony splinters are produced.

Any patient with a penetrating wound causing hypotension or peritonitis must have an immediate laparotomy. Gunshot wounds traversing the peritoneum or retroperitoneum should also be explored at laparotomy. Haemodynamically normal patients with stab wounds who have no signs

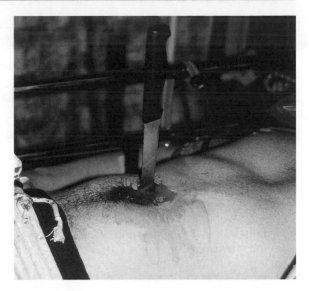

Figure 24.3: An abdominal stab wound. This wound was self-inflicted and the knife was removed in the operating theatre under general anaesthesia.

of peritonitis should have their wounds locally explored by a surgeon, who can extend the operation into a laparotomy if the abdominal fascia or peritoneum is breached. This is more likely with wounds to the anterior abdomen, as the flanks and posterior abdomen have thicker protective muscle layers. Stab wounds to the lower chest are difficult to explore and can be managed conservatively provided the patient remains well. The possibility of a small diaphragmatic wound should always be considered. This may initially be too small to allow herniation of abdominal contents, but over the years enlarge and eventually present as a result of strangulation of the contents of the hernia.

All patients should be admitted and observed with serial abdominal examinations. Other investigations include diagnostic peritoneal lavage for anterior abdominal wounds and contrast CT for flank and posterior abdominal wounds.

BLAST INJURIES

The intestines are vulnerable to the effects of blast because they have a large air/soft tissue interface. The shock front may cause contusion and rupture of the gut wall and haemorrhage into the lumen. The secondary and tertiary effects of the blast can also inflict a mixture of penetrating and blunt trauma on the abdomen.

PRIMARY SURVEY

The primary survey must follow the sequence of ABCDE. Each component is assessed and problems are treated as they are identified. Abdominal trauma predominantly affects circulation and control of haemorrhage, unless the diaphragm is ruptured or splinted. If the patient is in shock and there is no external haemorrhage then internal sites must be considered.

'Blood on the floor and four more'

- chest
- abdomen and retroperitoneum
- pelvis
- thighs (femoral fractures).

The patient must be exposed from the mid-chest to the knees, and the flanks and perineum (as well as the back and gluteal region during the log-roll) checked for pattern bruising and wounds. Palpation will localize pain, and the presence of guarding, rigidity and rebound tenderness should be established in the conscious patient. Percussion is usually difficult to hear in a noisy resuscitation room but the presence of rebound tenderness may be revealed. Auscultation for bruits and bowel sounds is rarely, if ever, of any value. Rectal examination will provide information on the presence and degree of sphincter tone, state of the bowel wall and the presence of bony fragments in the rectal lumen from pelvic fractures. In addition the position of the prostate and the presence of blood on the glove should be established. Blood on rectal examination usually indicates bowel injury and the requirement for laparotomy. Vaginal examination may also demonstrate the presence of bony fragments as well as blood.

Clinical examination and the trauma series of radiographs should reveal significant haemorrhage into the chest or due to pelvic and long bone fractures. A normal abdominal examination does not exclude significant pathology since signs may be absent, subtle or masked by drugs, alcohol and other injuries, especially in the early stages.

Table 24.1: Indications for immediate laparotomy

Hypotension with evidence of abdominal injury
Peritonitis – early
Persistent or recurrent hypotension despite adequate resuscitation
Air under the diaphragm on chest X-ray
Diaphragmatic injury
Penetrating trauma with bleeding from the stomach, rectum or genitourinary tract

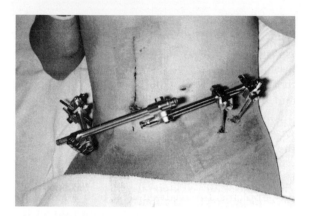

Figure 24.4: Emergency pelvic external fixation.

It is vital always to remember that laparotomy may be a part of resuscitation as a form of haemorrhage control. Aggressive fluid resuscitation in an attempt to stabilize the patient before theatre wastes valuable time and may exacerbate haemorrhage by disrupting clots and deranging clotting factors. The important procedure is 'turning the tap off'. The indications for immediate laparotomy are given in Table 24.1.

Laparotomy for abdominal bleeding must not be delayed.

If there is a pelvic fracture causing major haemorrhage, external fixation can be applied in the resuscitation room (Fig. 24.4) or, failing that, a sheet can be drawn around the pelvis pulling the fragments together or a pneumatic antishock garment applied and inflated.

Examination of the pelvic bones should be performed once only. If there is a fracture it will be painful if the patient is conscious and repeated examination may increase blood loss. Gentle compression of the pelvis from the sides and pressure in a posterior direction may be applied, but if one is positive (palpable instability, crepitus or pain) the other should not be performed. A pelvic X-ray can easily be performed without interrupting the resuscitation process.

SECONDARY SURVEY

The abdominal component of the secondary survey should be repeated regularly. An abnormal finding suggests intra-abdominal pathology. An apparently normal examination should be viewed with suspicion, especially if there are coexistent head or spinal injuries. The usual sequence of inspection, palpation, percussion and auscultation should be used, followed by rectal and vaginal examinations. A rectal examination is mandatory before a urinary catheter is inserted in order to check for a high-riding prostate suggesting posterior urethral rupture.

Normal clinical examination does not rule out abdominal injury.

Insertion of a nasogastric tube to decompress the stomach (orogastric if base of skull fracture is suspected) should be considered. This may provide diagnostic information, the presence of blood suggesting duodenal injury. Drainage of the stomach will also lessen the risk of vomiting and aspiration of the gastric contents. A urinary catheter should only be inserted when signs of urethral injury have been sought. If perineal bruising, meatal blood or a high-riding prostate are present there may be urethral injury and catheterization may cause further damage. Urological input is required. Once inserted, a urinary catheter will give diagnostic information, with haematuria suggesting upper urinary tract injury. Monitoring of the urinary output will provide a good index of tissue perfusion. Low urinary output suggests continued bleeding or inadequate fluid resuscitation.

Under no circumstances should the performance of these procedures be allowed to delay the provision of life-saving surgery. Sadly, all too often time is wasted in the performance of procedures which are not immediately necessary.

INVESTIGATIONS

BLOOD TESTS

In significant trauma, a full blood count and cross-match will be necessary and a clotting screen should be requested if significant amounts of transfused blood are likely to be required or the patient has, or is suspected of having, a clotting abnormality. Urea, electrolytes and amylase should also be requested, as should a pregnancy test in female patients of childbearing age. A raised amylase is a relatively insensitive and non-specific indicator of pancreatic injury.

RADIOGRAPHS

The chest X-ray in the initial trauma series may demonstrate gas under the diaphragm if it can be taken in the erect position (Fig. 24.5). Features of diaphragmatic rupture or low rib fractures should alert the doctor to the possibility of injury to the liver or spleen.

The pelvic X-ray is important in demonstrating a potential source of major haemorrhage, though it is not uncommon for pelvic fracture to coexist with a major abdominal injury.

ULTRASOUND (USS)

The use of ultrasound is increasing. Although it is operator dependent and not as sensitive or specific as CT or DPL, it is non-invasive and fast, especially as a scan can be done in the resuscitation room itself without transferring the patient to the X-ray department. The technique of FAST (Focused Abdominal Sonography for Trauma) is being developed as a rapid method of establishing the presence of free fluid in the abdomen by clinicians rather than radiologists. It is less important to know which organ has been injured once the diagnosis of haemorrhage has been established, as laparotomy is usually required. The pericardium can also be checked by ultrasound for developing tamponade. All these techniques are dependent on the experience of the operator but are likely to become increasingly common with the development of

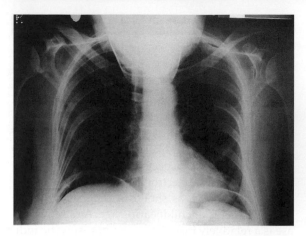

Figure 24.5: Gas under the diaphragm on an erect chest radiograph.

small hand-held ultrasound machines. A normal USS should be viewed in the same way as a normal clinical examination, with suspicion, and repeated regularly.

CT SCANNING

CT scanning requires transfer of the patient to the scanner suite and is time consuming as oral contrast needs to be administered prior to the scan. As a result, it is only suitable for haemodynamically normal patients. Patients with abdominal trauma are still inappropriately transferred for CT scans and die as a result. CT scanning is very specific but can miss diaphragmatic and pancreatic injuries.

Unstable patients die in the CT scanning suite.

DIAGNOSTIC PERITONEAL LAVAGE (DPL)

This invasive procedure can be rapidly performed in the resuscitation room. It should be done using the open method by the surgeon who will also carry out any subsequent laparotomy. The method for open peritoneal lavage is shown in Table 24.2. Peritoneal lavage is 98% sensitive for intraperitoneal bleeding but will not detect retroperitoneal haemorrhage and rarely detects bowel injury. A pelvic fracture may give a false positive result. USS

Table 24.2: Open method for peritoneal lavage

Insert nasogastric tube and urethral catheter to decompress stomach and bladder
Define site – midline, one-third of distance umbilicus to pubic symphysis
Clean and drape
Infiltrate the site with lignocaine and adrenaline
Make a small longitudinal incision and dissect down to peritoneum
Grasp and gently lift the peritoneum with forceps and make a small incision through it
Insert the catheter into the abdominal cavity, aiming for the pelvis
Attempt to aspirate through catheter – >5 ml fresh blood is positive
Infuse 1 l warmed Hartmann's and allow it to distribute
Lower the fluid bag and allow it to drain
Send a sample to laboratory for cell count and analysis

Note: if pelvic fractures are present or the patient is pregnant the catheter can be inserted a similar distance supra-umbilically

or CT after a DPL has been carried out is less accurate as residual lavage fluid makes identification of injury difficult.

Indications

The principal indication is an equivocal clinical examination, although an unreliable clinical examination due to head or spinal injury, alcohol or drugs should also be considered to be an indication.

Contraindications

The only absolute contraindication is the need for an immediate laparotomy. Relative contraindications include previous abdominal surgery, gross obesity, clotting disorders, cirrhosis and pregnancy.

Complications

Complications are rare with the open method, but include haemorrhage from the operation site, bowel or bladder perforation, injury to other intra-abdominal structures and wound infection

Positive results

A positive result is indicated by:

- 5 ml fresh blood on first aspiration
- red blood cells $>100\,000\,\mathrm{ml}^{-1}$ or white blood cells $>500\,\mathrm{ml}^{-1}$ in the aspirate
- presence of bile, bacteria or faecal material.

The presence of lavage fluid in a chest drainage bottle or urethral catheter bag suggests diaphragm or bladder rupture, respectively.

MANAGEMENT

After the initial phase of assessment and resuscitation, the secondary survey and any investigations, the final destination of the patient must be decided. In many cases of abdominal trauma, the secondary survey will only be performed after the patient has undergone emergency laparotomy. There is, however, an increasing trend to manage solid-organ injury in haemodynamically normal patients (particularly children) conservatively. All patients with suspected abdominal trauma but not requiring immediate surgical intervention must be admitted for close observation and repeated clinical examination, as signs of abdominal trauma may develop over a prolonged period.

Stab wounds that do not require emergency life-saving surgery can be explored. This should be done where an immediate laparotomy can be carried out should the need arise. Local anaesthetic is infiltrated and the wound track carefully followed. If it penetrates the peritoneum the patient is at higher risk of intra-abdominal injury and a DPL or exploratory laparotomy should be considered. A full list of indications for laparotomy is given in Table 24.3.

SPECIFIC ABDOMINAL INJURIES

SPLEEN

Injuries to the spleen may vary from avulsion of the spleen from its vascular pedicle at its hilum

Table 24.3: Indications for laparotomy

Hypotension with evidence of abdominal injury
Peritonitis – early or late
Persistent or recurrent hypotension despite adequate resuscitation
Air under the diaphragm on chest X-ray
Diaphragmatic injury
Penetrating trauma with bleeding from the stomach, rectum or genitourinary tract
Evisceration
Gunshot wounds traversing the abdominal cavity
Blunt abdominal trauma with positive DPL or ultrasound
CT evidence of injury to pancreas or intestine
CT evidence of specific injury to liver, spleen or kidneys
Extraluminal contrast on gastrointestinal/genitourinary studies
Persistent raised amylase

and massive shattering of the parenchyma to small capsular tears. Haemorrhage may be massive or minor. Splenic trauma is suggested by signs of injury to the left upper quadrant and may be associated with lower left rib fractures. Exsanguinating haemorrhage requires immediate surgical intervention. Minor degrees of injury, especially in children, may be managed conservatively, but the patient must be closely observed in an environment where they can be rapidly taken to theatre if there is any deterioration.

LIVER

Hepatic injury occurs as a result of blunt or penetrating injury to the right upper quadrant of the abdomen or right lower chest. Clinical signs may be obvious, with shock and abdominal tenderness and peritonism, but may be subtle or absent, particularly in the obtunded patient. The patient in shock will require laparotomy to control haemorrhage. Again, on occasions a selective conservative approach may be adopted by senior surgeons.

PANCREAS

Pancreatic injury occurs as a result of blunt trauma to the upper abdomen and is often associated with the wearing of a lap seat-belt in a frontal impact road traffic accident. Associated injuries include duodenal injury and thoracolumbar spine injury. Serum amylase is not a good predictor of pancreatic trauma and the injury is often only discovered on CT or at laparotomy.

SMALL BOWEL

As noted above, duodenal injury may occur as a result of blunt upper abdominal trauma. Suggestive findings include blood in the gastric aspirate and retroperitoneal air on X-ray. Rapid deceleration may cause injury to the jejunum and ileum, particularly with tears to the mesentery and its vessels, which may cause areas of bowel ischaemia and infarction. Small bowel is commonly injured by penetrating wounds to the abdomen. The detection of free gas on X-ray mandates surgical exploration.

LARGE BOWEL

Injury to the colon and rectum is rare and usually occurs as a result of penetrating injury. Again surgical exploration and repair is required.

PELVIC FRACTURES

An antero-posterior pelvic radiograph is part of the 'trauma series' of primary survey films. The bones and ligaments of the pelvis are very strong. Disruption of the pelvic ring suggests that high-energy forces have been involved in the mechanism of injury and other intra- and extra-abdominal injuries must be expected. Pelvic fractures can tear the presacral venous plexus and other blood vessels causing severe haemorrhage, but may not be the only bleeding point contributing to shock.

The mechanism of injury and the forces brought to bear on the pelvis will determine the pattern of fracture and associated injuries seen. Pelvic fractures can be classified into the following broad groups.

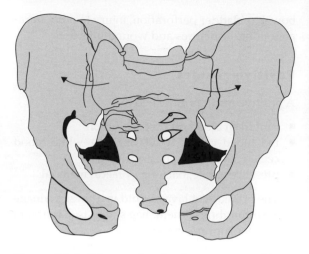

Figure 24.6: Diagram showing fractures caused by antero-posterior compression forces.

ANTERO-POSTERIOR COMPRESSION FRACTURES (FIG. 24.6)

Both the symphysis pubis and the sacroiliac joints can be disrupted. This causes the 'open-book' fracture and increases the pelvic volume. The presacral veins may be involved, causing life-threatening haemorrhage.

LATERAL COMPRESSION FRACTURES (FIG. 24.7)

These are caused by a sideways impact and cause one hemi-pelvis to internally rotate. As a result, the symphysis pubis may damage the bladder or urethra. The pelvic volume is decreased and severe haemorrhage is unusual.

FRACTURES DUE TO VERTICAL SHEAR FORCES (FIG. 24.8)

These fractures are often caused by a fall from height. Major bony instability and bleeding are likely.

Isolated fractures of one or more pubic rami are relatively common in the elderly after apparently trivial falls. Analgesia and mobilization, often after an initial period of rest, are usually all that is

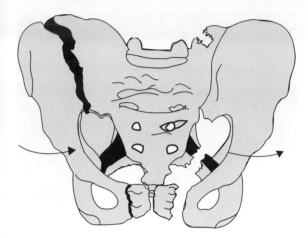

Figure 24.7: Diagram showing fractures due to lateral compression forces.

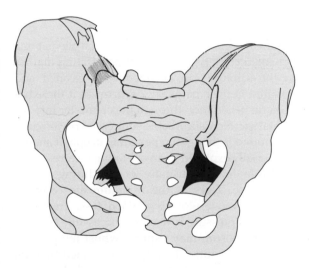

Figure 24.8: Diagram showing fractures due to shearing forces.

required. The so-called 'butterfly fracture' of all four pubic rami, however, can be associated with significant damage to the urethra and other structures.

EXAMINATION

Signs suggestive of pelvic fracture include bruising in the flanks, scrotum and perineum. The legs should be examined for equality of length and rotation. Rectal and vaginal examination may reveal bony fragments. The initial treatment of

pelvic fractures in order to reduce bleeding has already been discussed. Urgent orthopaedic referral for definitive management and prioritization of surgical and orthopaedic treatment is essential.

URINARY TRACT TRAUMA

Direct blows to the flanks and pelvic fractures are markers for potential genitourinary trauma. Haematuria is a poor indicator and may be absent in the most severe injuries, but its presence should not be ignored. Ultrasound, CT, intravenous urography (IVU) and other contrast studies are all useful investigative tools. Urological advice should be sought early. Operation is rarely required but delayed diagnosis will lead to increased long-term complications.

KIDNEYS

Avulsion of the kidneys from their blood supply is rare but will cause severe retroperitoneal bleeding and shock. If identified early the kidney may be saved by vascular repair. Most other renal injuries can be managed conservatively. If the patient has macroscopic haematuria they should be further investigated with a contrast CT scan or intravenous urography. In the absence of other signs of injury, if microscopic haematuria is present no further investigation is needed, though the patient should be reviewed and the urine regularly retested.

Renal trauma is predominantly treated conservatively.

URETERS

Injury to the ureters is rare since they are well protected by the peritoneum and the psoas muscle. Occasionally tears occur at the pelvi-ureteric junction.

BLADDER

The bladder lies within and is protected by the pelvis when empty but can rise as far as the umbilicus when it is full, and it is then vulnerable to trauma. Bladder rupture may occur as a result of direct trauma to the lower abdomen whilst the bladder is full or as a result of penetration by a spike of bone from a pelvic fracture. Rupture of the bladder may be peritoneal or extraperitoneal. Bladder rupture should be suspected if the bladder is empty on catheterization, and a cystogram will confirm the diagnosis and whether extravascation has occurred into the peritoneum. Intraperitoneal rupture always requires surgical repair.

URETHRA

The urethra is rarely injured in females owing to its short length. In males the posterior urethra (above the urogenital diaphragm) can be disrupted in anterior pelvic fractures and the anterior urethra in straddle injuries. If there is blood at the urethral meatus, bruising of the perineum or a high-riding prostate on rectal examination, the presence of a urethral injury should be assumed (Fig. 24.9). A urethrogram or retrograde urethrogram should be performed. If this is normal a gentle attempt at catheterization can be made. If the urethrogram is abnormal, a urologist should be consulted for a decision on bladder drainage and repair of the injury.

Always assess the patient for urethral injury prior to catheterization.

SCROTAL AND PENILE INJURY

Blunt injury to the scrotum may result in either scrotal haematoma or rupture of the tunica albuginea of the testis and extrusion of its contents. These conditions are difficult to distinguish clinically and an ultrasound scan is indicated. Rupture of the testis

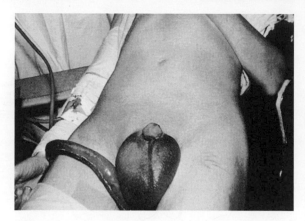

Figure 24.9: Scrotal bleeding in a patient with a ruptured urethra. (Reproduced with permission from L. Solomon, D.J. Warwick and S. Nayagam (eds), *Apley's System of Orthopaedics and Fractures*, 8th edition, published by Arnold, London, 2001.)

requires surgical repair, whereas scrotal haematoma is treated conservatively. Most penetrating injuries to the scrotum can be adequately cleaned and repaired in the emergency department if there has been no penetration through the cremaster into the scrotal sac. Non-absorbable sutures are preferred. If the wound is thought to penetrate deeply it should be formally explored in an operating theatre.

Penile injuries usually occur during sexual intercourse. Tears of the frenulum are common and may cause worrying blood loss. Treatment with local pressure is usually successful. The corpus cavernosum may rupture whilst the penis is erect in intercourse. Pain is accompanied by local swelling. Surgical repair is recommended.

FURTHER READING

Skinner D, Whimster F. *Trauma. A Companion to Bailey and Love's Short Practice of Surgery*. Arnold, London.

INJURIES TO THE LOWER LIMB

INTRODUCTION

Injuries to the lower limb are common and range in severity from minor sprains and lacerations to life-threatening injuries such as multiple long bone fractures. In this chapter, the common lower limb injuries are discussed together with practical advice on their management in the emergency department.

GENERAL PRINCIPLES

Airway obstruction and ventilatory inadequacy are always more important than limb injuries. Regardless of initial appearances, the primary survey should be carried out in sequence. A formal assessment of the lower limbs will begin under E for exposure and be completed as part of the secondary survey. Lower limb injury may, however, threaten life, usually due to shock as a result of fractures of the pelvis or femur, multiple long bone fractures or diffuse bleeding into the soft tissues of the thighs. When this occurs, the priorities under C of the primary survey are to control external bleeding and to splint the limb or pelvis (see Chapter 4). Only when resuscitation is under way and immediately life-threatening problems have been dealt with should limb-threatening injuries such as joint dislocation, open fractures, nerve or vascular injury and compartment syndromes be sought.

> Limb injuries may be life threatening or limb threatening.

Isolated lower limb injuries are most common and are usually self-evident. The patient will often be able to complain of wounds, pain, swelling, deformity and loss of movement following an injury.

HISTORY

Three key aspects of the history should be established:

- mechanism of injury
- events leading to the injury
- occupation and social circumstances (impact of injury).

Limb injuries can occur by direct violence, indirect transmission of forces or through chronic overuse. A clear history of the mechanism of injury allows the doctor to visualize the size and direction of forces and any likely deformity at the time of injury. There are clear patterns of lower limb and associated injuries that may be suggested by the history. This information can then guide examination and investigation. It is also important to establish why the injury occurred. A primary cardiac or neurological event may have precipitated the accident and should always be considered. It is also necessary to understand the patient's occupation and home circumstances in order to assess the likely impact of any injury. An ankle sprain in a professional footballer may have greater significance (and require different treatment and rehabilitation) than a similar injury in a bank clerk. A fractured neck of femur often signifies the end of independence for elderly patients.

The history of injury is an important component of the assessment of limb injury.

Elderly patients, young children and patients with learning difficulties can often present with non-specific symptoms, poorly localized pain and an uncertain mechanism of injury. These patients can be the source of clinical errors if they are not thoroughly examined. It is also important to have a low threshold for radiographic examination, temporary immobilization and out-patient clinic follow-up if there is doubt about the presence or severity of injury. Patient groups who are prone to falling, such as toddlers, may have their pain ascribed to a previous but unconnected injury. Other potential causes should always be sought.

EXAMINATION

Hurting the patient is often inevitable when examining limb injuries. If the patient expresses pain, then early analgesia (sometimes at the triage stage) should be given before a detailed examination is attempted. Examination should then be tailored to the needs of the patient. This may mean modification of the examination routine. Occasionally, provided significant injury can be excluded, detailed examination may have to be delayed until the patient returns for follow-up.

The traditional look–feel–move–test approach is well suited for examination of lower limb injuries. The injured limb should always be compared with the other side and a systematic approach is essential. Wounds, deformity, swelling, wasting, shortening and scars should all be sought, as should abnormal movement (indicating ligament injury) and bony tenderness. The most painful area should be left until last. The expression 'bony tenderness' refers to tenderness elicited when bone is palpated rather than tenderness over the general area of the injury. Active movements should be assessed before passive

Table 25.1: MRC system for grading muscle power

Grade 0	No movement
Grade 1	Flicker of movement
Grade 2	Movement when gravity eliminated
Grade 3	Movement against gravity
Grade 4	Movement against active resistance
Grade 5	Full and normal muscle power

movement (which may not then be necessary) is attempted. All the joints of the lower limb are at 0° when the body is in the anatomical position. The range of movement should be recorded in degrees from the anatomical position, with power graded using the Medical Research Council (MRC) scale (Table 25.1). This allows repeat assessments to be made and compared.

Most patients with fractures or joint injury will be reluctant to demonstrate active movements and unwilling to allow the examiner to test passive movements. If it is considered essential to examine passive movements before radiography, adequate analgesia should be provided. In most cases, however, sufficient information can be gleaned from inspection and palpation alone to allow the examiner to request appropriate radiographs. Once these have been obtained, careful examination of movements can then be performed.

Adequate analgesia aids assessment.

When an injury is of sufficient force to cause a fracture, all tissues around the point of injury will have been subjected to the same force. It is very easy to become focused on a bony injury and forget ligamentous instability, tendon rupture, muscle injury, nerve damage or vascular damage. Vascular damage may be indicated by classic signs of haematoma and distal ischaemia, or more subtle signs of venous congestion.

Circulation and sensation should be checked and documented distal to all injuries.

Nerve damage is often described in terms of neuropraxia, axonotmesis and neurotmesis (Table 25.2). In reality, there is often a complex pattern of injury. Any peripheral nerve may be damaged by

Table 25.2: Classification of nerve injury

Neuropraxia	Transient loss of function caused by compression. Rapid recovery
Axonotmesis	Loss of function but no loss of continuity. Recovery in weeks to months
Neurotmesis	Loss of function with division of nerve. No recovery unless repaired

injury but the most vulnerable nerves in the lower limb are the common peroneal nerve at the neck of the fibula and the sciatic nerve posterior to the hip joint. Screening of peripheral nerve function must be performed in all lower limb injuries.

Testing for ligamentous instability by stressing ligaments at the ankle and knee and looking for excess movement is often difficult in the acute phase because of pain and swelling. Depending on the injury, it may be appropriate to inject local anaesthetic prior to testing. In most cases, however, the patient should be brought back to clinic for formal testing once pain is controlled and swelling reduced. Tendon rupture may be evidenced by inability to complete movements such as extending the knee (failure of the extensor tendon apparatus) or plantar-flexing the ankle (ruptured tendo-achilles).

INVESTIGATION

The mainstay of investigation in lower limb injuries is plain radiography; however, radiographs will only reveal an underlying injury if they are accurately requested and directed. The most consistent diagnostic aid remains the history and examination. Radiographs should always be taken in at least two planes. In some cases additional views may be necessary but should normally only be carried out after discussion with a senior doctor. Most films will subsequently be reported by a radiologist, but decisions about management and referral are usually made by emergency department staff. It is therefore essential to have a good system of radiographic interpretation and a rapid follow-up process for undiagnosed or missed injuries.

Throughout this chapter, a systematic approach to radiographic interpretation is described for specific lower limb regions.

Radiographs do not show soft tissue disruption, nerve, muscle, tendon or ligament damage. In some cases, ultrasound examination by an experienced sonographer may be available and can be used to examine joints and soft tissues, particularly around the hip, knee and ankle.

TREATMENT

Definitive treatment for many lower limb injuries requires orthopaedic referral or follow-up. All fractures should be reviewed in fracture clinic according to local departmental policies. In general, urgent orthopaedic consultation is required for patients with open, complex or multiple fractures, major joint disruption and extensive soft tissue injury. Specific management guidance is provided for each injury described below.

Throughout this and subsequent chapters, reference is made to analgesia (see Chapter 8). Control of pain facilitates clinical examination, radiographic positioning, and effective treatment of limb injuries. It also gains the confidence of the patient. Pain should be controlled as early as possible and preferably before radiography. Non-pharmacological techniques such as supporting the injured limb, applying simple splints and covering wounds will help alleviate pain. In many cases, however, rapid control of pain with Entonox® or intravenous opioids may be necessary. In small children, oral or intranasal opiates may be used safely and effectively. Once acute pain is controlled, most patients will then require oral maintenance analgesia. For musculoskeletal injuries, the evidence supports the use of oral paracetamol, combined analgesics (e.g. paracetamol with codeine) or ibuprofen. A combination of paracetamol or a combined analgesic with a non-steroidal anti-inflammatory drug may be necessary. Where the oral route is not available, combinations of rectal paracetamol, intramuscular codeine and intramuscular or rectal diclofenac provide equivalent safe and effective alternatives. If pain is not controlled, the possibility of a missed diagnosis should be considered and the presence of complications such as arterial injury or compartment syndrome should be excluded.

PELVIC INJURIES

GENERAL PRINCIPLES

Pelvic injuries range in severity from stable uncomplicated avulsion fractures to major life-threatening disruption of the pelvic ring. The pelvis is formed by the two hip bones (each comprising ilium, ischium and pubis), the sacrum, the sacroiliac joints and the symphysis pubis. These form a strong bony ring. Stable pelvic injuries do not involve the ring at all or disrupt only one part of it. They are not associated with displacement. Such injuries include fractures of one or both pubic rami on the same side, fracture of the ilium (running into the sciatic notch) and fractures involving the sacroiliac joint on one side (Fig. 25.1).

In order to sustain a pelvic fracture, there must have been a significant compressive or transmitted force on the pelvis. It is therefore likely that there will be some disruption to another part of the ring. The pelvis has been compared to a Polo mint®: it is not easy to break a Polo mint in only one place. When two areas of disruption are present clinically or radiographically the injury is described as unstable. Varying degrees of instability can occur depend-ing on the forces involved. It is important to appreciate that a widened sacroiliac joint or symphysis pubis represents a fracture of the main pelvic ring. Thus, the combination of widening of the symphysis pubis and one sacroiliac joint is an unstable injury.

> A widened sacroiliac joint or symphysis pubis represents a disruption of the main pelvic ring.

When there is complete disruption of the ring, one half of the pelvis may rotate externally or, with more severe damage, be displaced in the vertical plane. Unstable injuries may thus be rotationally unstable but vertically stable, or both rotationally and vertically unstable. The latter represents the most severe disruption and is associated with high-energy transfer, multisystem trauma and high mortality. An average emergency department will see only two or three of these unstable fractures a year (Fig. 25.1). Their severity is therefore often underestimated.

Regardless of the classification, all suspected pelvic injuries seen in the emergency department should be regarded as unstable until proven otherwise. In the context of resuscitation, stability refers to the likelihood of further displacement, disruption of injured tissues and bleeding. The general management principles of suspected pelvic fractures are:

- early identification
- adequate resuscitation
- stabilization of the pelvis
- identification of complications.

Early identification can be achieved by maintaining a high index of suspicion in patients who have been subjected to high-energy trauma such as road accidents, falls from heights and crush injuries. Clinical examination will often reveal bruising

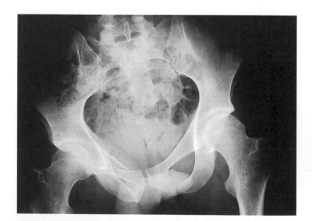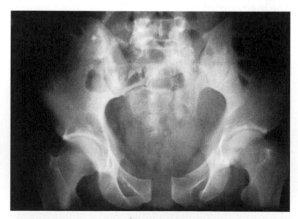

Figure 25.1: Pelvic fractures: a stable fracture (*left* – fractured pubic rami) and an unstable fracture (*right* – fractured rami and disrupted symphysis pubis).

spreading to the scrotum, buttock or anterior thigh if the pelvic floor is torn. The abdomen may be distended by a large retroperitoneal haematoma. In unstable injuries there may be differences in leg length and one or both legs may be externally rotated. One leg may be ischaemic if an iliac artery is damaged. If there is clinical evidence of pelvic disruption, no attempt should be made to confirm this by compressing or distracting the pelvis at the iliac crests. This will only cause further movement and disruption of haematoma. The diagnosis is usually confirmed by radiography.

PELVIC RADIOGRAPHS

There may be difficulty in interpreting initial pelvic radiographs. An important principle is that if only one fracture is seen, a search for the second fracture or disruption is essential. A systematic approach to radiographic interpretation is shown in Table 25.3.

> If only one fracture is seen, a search for the second fracture or disruption should be made.

EMERGENCY TREATMENT

Emergency treatment aims to reduce bleeding and identify the principal complications of pelvic injuries. These are:

- haemorrhage
- urethral injury
- visceral injury
- disruption of the acetabulum.

Table 25.3: Interpretation of pelvic radiographs

Look for:
Disruption to the inner or outer margin of the main bony ring
Disruption to the inner and outer margins of the obturator foramina
Differences in the widths of the sacroiliac joints
Horizontal alignment of the superior surfaces of the inferior pubic rami either side of the symphysis pubis
A symphysis pubis width of approximately 5 mm
Disruption to the margins of the sacral foramina (the arcuate lines)
Symmetrical appearance of each acetabulum

Haemorrhage

Because of the relatively low incidence of unstable injuries, there is a tendency to underestimate fluid losses. The pelvis is extremely vascular and blood loss of 3–4 l may occur. Hypovolaemic shock should therefore be anticipated in all but the most minor injuries (whether stable or unstable). Transient or no response to fluid resuscitation should prompt early stabilization of the pelvis by the application of traction, a pneumatic antishock garment or, preferably, an external pelvic fixation device (Table 25.4). A sheet wrapped around the pelvis and pulled tight to provide compression may be an effective temporary measure. Such measures may be required before radiography if bleeding is severe. Temporary fracture reduction will reduce pelvic volume, tamponade bleeding and allow blood clots to form.

Although bleeding is rarely isolated to one source, an attempt at selective embolization may be appropriate in uncontrolled shock; however, most pelvic fracture haemorrhage is venous and not amenable to embolization. An extreme measure is ligation of the internal iliac artery on one or both sides.

Urethral injury

Injury to the urethra is commonly associated with multiple fractures of the pubic rami or displacement

Table 25.4: Techniques for emergency stabilization of the pelvis

Simple manoeuvres:
Longitudinal traction of the leg in the vertically unstable pelvis
Internal rotation of the leg in the rotationally unstable pelvis
Sheet wrapped around the pelvis as a sling
Application of a vaccum mattress (acting like a sling)
Application of pneumatic antishock garment (PASG)
Application of an external pelvic fixation device:
Standard fixator with pins inserted into iliac crests joined by cross-connecting rods
C-clamp type fixator with pins inserted external to the sacro-iliac joints and joined by a single anterior bar

of the symphysis pubis. Clinical diagnosis is based on the presence of scrotal haematoma and blood at the urethral meatus. If urethral injury is suspected, a urological opinion should be sought and a urethrogram performed. Otherwise, it is reasonable to try to get the patient to void and check for blood in the urine. A clear urine is unlikely to be associated with urethral injury. Bloody urine may be associated with a urethral injury or a bladder tear. Although catheterization may convert a partial urethral tear into a complete one, it is acceptable for an experienced operator to attempt to pass a fine catheter. If this cannot be passed with ease, the attempt should be abandoned and suprapubic catheterization performed. This may also be difficult in a shocked patient with low urine output and suprapubic swelling associated with the fracture.

Visceral injury

Significant pelvic injury can damage the bladder, colon and uterus in the pelvis or the rectum, vagina and urethra as they pierce the pelvic floor. Injuries to the rectum or vagina represent open fractures and are associated with a high mortality. Vaginal and rectal examinations should be performed specifically to exclude such injury. Extraperitoneal rupture of the bladder frequently occurs and will produce haematuria. An early cystogram may be indicated to identify this complication. Because severe pelvic fractures result from high-energy injuries, simultaneous injury to other major viscera such as the liver or spleen is common and must be considered in the management of the shocked patient with a pelvic fracture.

PUBIC RAMUS FRACTURES

Pubic ramus fractures are generally associated with falls in the elderly. There is considerable pain and restricted mobility. There may be an associated vertebral crush injury. Subtle hip fractures (impacted subcapital fractures) may also be associated with pubic ramus fractures and it is essential to exclude these much more important injuries. If pain and circumstances allow, some patients may be managed at home. Most require only 2–3 days' bed rest with adequate analgesia and early mobilization. Many emergency departments experience considerable difficulty with admitting patients who cannot cope at home. A local policy for the management of these patients should be agreed between the orthopaedic, care of the elderly and rehabilitation services.

FRACTURES OF THE SACRUM AND COCCYX

Compression of the pelvis may fracture the ala of the sacrum on one side. Falls from a height on to a hard surface may fracture the sacrum in the transverse plane. In both injuries, undisplaced and uncomplicated fractures require symptomatic treatment with bed rest. Displacement of sacral fractures may compromise the sacral nerve roots. Perineal (saddle) anaesthesia, lower limb weakness (particularly plantar flexion) and incontinence should be excluded in all displaced fractures. Patients with neurological deficit must be referred urgently for orthopaedic review. In many cases, the nerve root function recovers.

Coccygeal injuries are common after falls in a seated position. Radiographic examination involves a high gonadal dose and should be avoided as it does not alter management. Tenderness over the coccyx or a palpable fracture is sufficient to make the diagnosis. Rectal examination should be performed in all patients to exclude the serious complication of a rectal tear. Severely displaced fractures should be referred for manipulation and possible excision. Most patients, however, can be allowed home with advice to use a ring cushion, avoid constipation and take adequate analgesia.

FRACTURES OF THE ILIAC BONES

The iliac crest and blade may be fractured by direct violence or as part of a more complex pelvic fracture. Isolated injuries of the crest and blade usually only require analgesia and bed rest, followed by early mobilization.

ACETABULAR FRACTURES

Fractures of the acetabulum may complicate pelvic fractures or may occur alone. They are usually

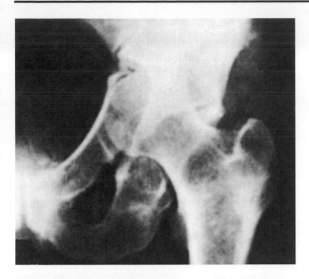

Figure 25.2: Radiograph showing central dislocation of the hip. (Reproduced with permission from L. Solomon, D.J. Warwick and S. Nayagam (eds), *Apley's System of Orthopaedics and Fractures*, 8th edition, published by Arnold, London, 2001.)

associated with forces transmitted along the femoral neck. There are many patterns of injury and radiographic appearances may be subtle. Central dislocation of the hip is an acetabular fracture where the head of the femur displaces the central part of the acetabulum medially (Fig. 25.2).

The anterior column refers to the mass of bone from the anterior inferior iliac spine to the superior pubic ramus. It includes the anterior part of the acetabular floor. The posterior column is the area from the sciatic notch to the ischial tuberosity that also includes the posterior part of the acetabular floor. Fractures may damage one or both of these columns and often require detailed radiographic assessment with oblique views (Judet views) and CT scanning. From an emergency department perspective, analgesia should be provided, the type of injury should be identified from standard anteroposterior (AP) and lateral hip views, and further injury to the pelvis and the neurovascular structures surrounding the acetabulum excluded. All acetabular fractures should be referred for immediate orthopaedic review.

Avulsion fractures

Avulsion fractures are commonly seen in adolescents. There is a history of sudden muscular

Table 25.5: Avulsion fractures of the pelvis

Fracture site	Muscle insertion
Anterior superior iliac spine	Sartorius
Anterior inferior iliac spine	Rectus femoris
	Quadriceps femoris
Inferior pubic ramus	Adductors
Ischial tuberosity	Hamstrings
Iliac crest	Oblique abdominal muscles
	Gluteus medius
	Erector spinae

contraction (such as kicking a football) followed by a sharp pain around the iliac crest or ischial area. The pain is worsened by resistance to contraction of the affected muscle group. Radiographs will often reveal avulsion fractures (Table 25.5). Adequate analgesia, rest and early mobilization are usually all that is required, although in some cases there is a risk of non-union. If there is no obvious avulsion fracture, the injury usually represents an apophysitis that will also settle with rest, analgesia and gentle return to activity. Physiotherapy is often of value.

INJURIES TO THE HIP

GENERAL PRINCIPLES

Elderly patients with fractured neck of femur account for the majority of hip injuries seen in emergency departments. Hip injuries in younger patients are relatively rare although there are a number of important conditions. The limping child is discussed in Chapter 39.

SPORTS INJURIES AROUND THE HIP

Sports injuries around the hip present to emergency departments as groin strains following exercise. The groin is the junction of the thigh and the abdomen and most strains represent tearing of the tendinous origins of the adductor muscles. The patient describes a sudden sharp pain in the groin following turning or rapid changes in direction with the hip abducted. Pain is exacerbated by adduction against resistance and bruising in the groin may be evident.

A more direct blow or twisting injury may cause a strain of the capsule of the hip joint. The pain radiates to the thigh and is worsened by movements that decrease the volume of the capsule (extension and internal rotation). Other causes of groin pain include iliopsoas tendinitis, pubic symphysitis and conjoint tendinitis. In all cases, more extensive injury should first be excluded. Once the likely diagnosis has been established, rest, analgesia and progressive return to activity with physiotherapy is indicated.

DISLOCATION OF THE HIP

The hip is a deep-socketed and naturally stable joint. Considerable force must be applied and soft-tissue damage occur for the hip to dislocate. The majority of dislocations are posterior although anterior dislocations also occur. Force transmitted along the femoral shaft with the hip flexed as when seated usually dislocates the hip posteriorly. This is most often seen in car occupants whose knees have impacted against the dashboard. The patient will be in severe pain and the hip is typically held slightly flexed, adducted and internally rotated (Fig. 25.3). A pelvic radiograph together with a lateral hip film will usually confirm the diagnosis. A careful search should be made for fractures of the posterior lip of the acetabulum and associated fractures of the femoral shaft, neck,

head and pelvis. There is also an association between posterior dislocation of the hip, sciatic nerve damage, ipsilateral posterior cruciate injury and fracture of the patella. These associated injuries should be actively excluded.

Anterior dislocation accounts for the minority of dislocations. The mechanism is wide abduction of the hip with or without transmission of force along the femur. This can occur in motorcyclists, athletes and horse riders. There may be groin swelling and bruising and the leg will be shortened and held in external rotation. Specific complications that should be sought include compression of the femoral vessels and femoral nerve damage.

The dislocated hip must be reduced as soon as possible to minimize the risk of sciatic nerve damage and avascular necrosis of the femoral head. A significant proportion of the blood supply to the femoral head is via the joint capsule. Dislocation both directly damages the capsule and stretches undamaged areas. The sooner the dislocation is reduced the lower the incidence of avascular necrosis of the femoral head. Reduction usually requires analgesia and deep sedation and is best performed under a general anaesthetic. If there is likely to be significant delay, experienced doctors may attempt initial reduction of posterior dislocations in the emergency department. The trolley is placed low to the floor and the hip and knee are flexed to right-angles. The deformity is increased and traction is applied in the long axis of the femur. The hip often reduces with a palpable give. Once reduced, check radiographs should be performed and the leg placed in a Thomas splint pending further orthopaedic management.

> Delay in reduction of the dislocated hip increases the risk of sciatic nerve injury and femoral head necrosis.

PROXIMAL FEMORAL FRACTURES

Below the age of 60 years, fracture of the femoral neck (hip) is generally associated with major trauma in men. With increasing age, however, falls in elderly women account for the majority of cases. Most of these fractures can be considered pathological because of the association with osteoporosis and the often trivial force required to sustain

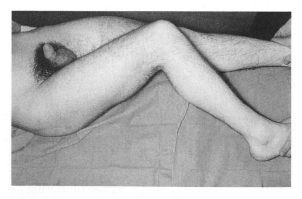

Figure 25.3: A patient with posterior dislocation of the hip showing shortening, internal rotation and flexion.

the injury. In some cases the fracture appears to precipitate the fall, implying that the injury is a stress fracture in osteoporotic bone rather than the result of trauma. Regardless of pathology, investigation of suspected femoral neck fractures represents a significant component of the emergency department workload and these injuries are associated with high mortality and major lifestyle changes. Approximately 10% of patients die within 6 weeks and 30% within 1 year. Of the remaining 70% who survive, one-third will be unable to return to their former level of independence or physical activity. Mortality and morbidity are high because of the frailty and co-morbidity associated with elderly patients, rather than the fracture itself.

The typical patient reports a minor fall or sudden giving way of the leg when turning abruptly or rising from a chair. There is well-localized pain and the patient is usually unable to bear weight. If the fracture is displaced, the leg will be shortened and externally rotated because the fracture allows iliopsoas (and gravity) to rotate the femur externally (Fig. 25.4). Pain is worsened by attempted rotation.

Radiographic examination must be performed in all elderly patients who have difficulty weight bearing and symptoms localized to the hip. An antero-posterior (AP) view of the whole pelvis and a lateral hip view on the affected side should be requested. Other pelvic injuries can mimic the pain of hip fracture and some fractures may only be visible on lateral views. Although most fractures are easily seen, a systematic approach to interpretation should be followed (Table 25.6).

There are many differences between the various proximal femoral and femoral neck fractures but they occur in the same group of patients. The most important distinction from an orthopaedic perspective is whether or not the fracture lies within the capsule of the hip joint. An intracapsular fracture can cut off the blood supply to the femoral head completely. Subcapital, transcervical and basicervical fractures are intracapsular. The common extracapsular sites of fracture are intertrochanteric (between the trochanters), pertrochanteric (involving both trochanters), subtrochanteric (beneath the trochanters) and avulsion of the greater trochanter (Fig. 25.5).

Fracture of the greater trochanter is a less serious injury and can occur following a violent adduction strain. The patient experiences severe pain over

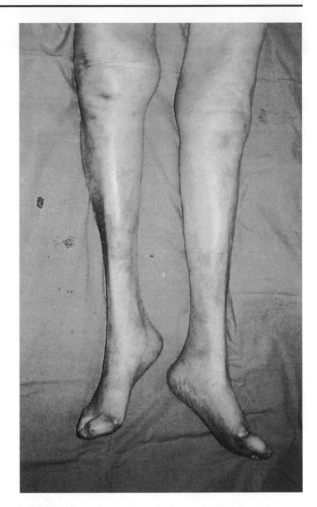

Figure 25.4: A patient with a proximal femoral fracture showing shortening and external rotation.

Table 25.6: Interpretation of hip radiographs

Use a bright light to assess the greater trochanter and the lateral view

Look for:
Fracture at the common fracture sites (basicervical, transcervical, intertrochanteric and pertrochanteric)
Uninterrupted cortices around the femoral neck and head
Symmetry of Shenton's lines (continuous arc from the inferior margin of the femoral neck to the inferior margin of the superior pubic ramus)
An uninterrupted trabecular pattern
Evidence of impaction (a dense white line crossing the femoral neck)
Pubic ramus and acetabular fractures
Angulation of the femoral head on the lateral view

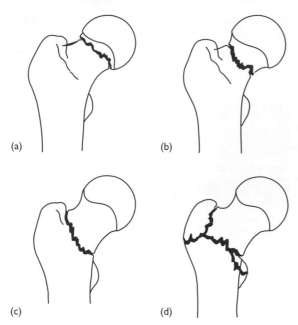

Figure 25.5: Diagram of proximal femur with common fracture sites. (a) Subcapital; (b) transcervical; (c) intertrochanteric; (d) pertrochanteric.

the trochanter, abduction is painful and, if they are able to bear weight, the Trendelenburg test (drooping of the pelvis below the horizontal on the injured side when the ipsilateral leg is raised) is positive. This is because the abductor muscles are separated from their bony attachment.

Most proximal femoral fractures are treated operatively. This should be done within 24 h to allow early mobilization. Optimum management in the emergency department involves:

- adequate analgesia (intravenous opiates)
- assessment of coexisting medical conditions
- rehydration
- protection from pressure sore risks
- transfer to a ward within 1 h.

Preoperative assessment can often be facilitated by routine ECG and chest X-ray before the patient is transferred to a ward. If there is a high level of clinical suspicion of a fracture, a chest X-ray should be performed at the same time as the pelvis and hip film. Fast-track admission procedures for patients with hip fractures should be in place. Decisions regarding the timing and nature of any operative intervention lie with the orthopaedic team. In general terms, prompt open reduction and internal fixation are indicated for younger patients

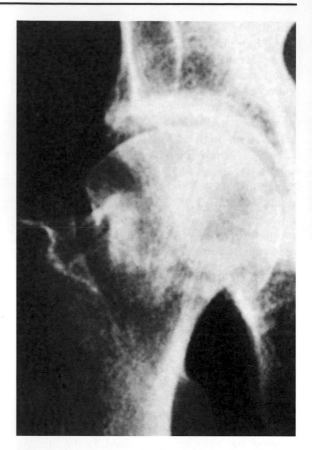

Figure 25.6: Radiograph of undisplaced femoral neck fracture. (Reproduced with permission from L. Solomon, D.J. Warwick and S. Nayagam (eds), *Apley's System of Orthopaedics and Fractures*, 8th edition, published by Arnold, London, 2001.)

with good bone quality and low fractures. In older patients, a hemiarthroplasty is probably more appropriate for fractures at risk of femoral head avascular necrosis.

Some patients may have an undisplaced (usually impacted) subcapital or intertrochanteric fracture. The patient may be able to weight-bear and the leg may be orientated normally. The radiographic appearances can be very subtle and these fractures may be missed until they become displaced days or weeks after the injury (Fig. 25.6). Patients who are being discharged from the emergency department should be advised to seek further medical advice if the pain persists or weight bearing becomes impossible. Good communication with nursing or residential homes and general practitioners is essential to ensure that these patients are appropriately followed up. Alternately, admission for rest and close supervision, further plain films, oblique views, tomography or even an isotope bone scan may be appropriate to exclude an impacted fracture if clinical suspicion is high. The patient who is non-weight bearing and definitely has no fracture also presents a problem. As with pubic ramus fractures, these patients usually require a short period of admission for analgesia, mobilization and assessment of home circumstances. A policy for the management of these patients should be in place.

> Patients with hip pain following a fall should be carefully followed up.

PROSTHETIC HIP PROBLEMS

An increasing proportion of elderly patients may have a hip prosthesis. These patients may have falls or other accidents and present to the emergency department with hip pain. The problems that may be associated with hip prostheses are:

- dislocation
- component failure
- loosening
- infection.

Dislocation

Following hip replacement, the fibrous capsule progressively thickens and strengthens. Within the first few months, however, minimal force may dislocate a recently fitted or poorly aligned prosthetic joint. When this occurs, patients experience pain and are unable to stand. The leg is shortened and externally roated (similar to a hip fracture). The diagnosis is confirmed by radiographs in two planes which will clearly show the dislocated joint. Urgent orthopaedic referral for reduction and treatment is required. Sciatic nerve damage should be excluded as with any other hip dislocation.

Component failure

Although this is rare with new prostheses, any of the components of a prosthetic hip may fail. All patients who have a history of trauma and report pain around the hip should have radiographs to exclude component failure or damage. These are best interpreted by experienced orthopaedic surgeons and it may be appropriate to refer the patient for routine orthopaedic review once acute injury has been excluded radiographically.

Loosening and infection

Loosening may be the result of infection and occurs at the interface between cement and bone. It is commonest in the femoral stem and leads to pain and impaired function. These patients should have radiographic assessment of the joint and be referred for orthopaedic follow-up. If there is no acute problem, it is best to refer patients to the orthopaedic team who performed the original procedure.

SLIPPED FEMORAL EPIPHYSIS

Acute slip of the femoral epiphysis in children is the anatomical equivalent to an intracapsular fracture of the neck of femur in adults. Although it may result from direct trauma, it more commonly represents an acute-on-chronic problem. Weakening of the epiphyseal plate and soft tissues by the hormones of adolescence is one of many factors that are thought to predispose to this condition. Others include genetic factors and obesity. The condition is most common in overweight adolescent boys. Those who are weight bearing will have an antalgic gait, external rotation of the leg and possibly referred knee pain. More often the child will not weight-bear after a twist or fall, and the leg lies shortened and externally rotated.

> Always consider the diagnosis of slipped upper femoral epiphysis in adolescents presenting with knee pain.

Radiographic examination will usually reveal the displacement. An AP pelvis film will show if there is any evidence of chronicity (new bone formation buttressing the neck) and exclude a subclinical epiphyseal slip on the other side (Fig. 25.7). The lateral view provides the earliest signs of displacement. If no slip is present, a line drawn up the centre of the neck of the femur should bisect the epiphyseal base of the femoral head.

Acute injuries caused by direct violence require urgent reduction and stabilization to prevent avascular necrosis of the femoral head. No attempt should be made to manipulate a slipped femoral epiphysis in the emergency department.

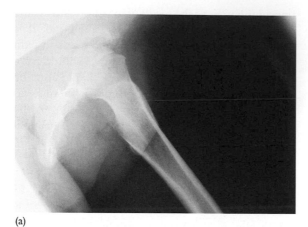

(a)

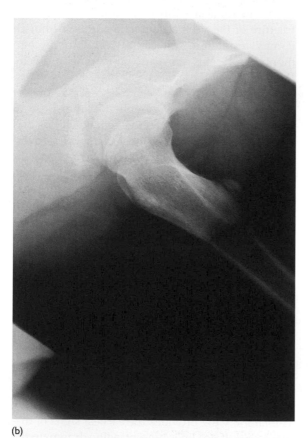

(b)

Figure 25.7: Radiograph showing slipped upper femoral epiphysis (a) compared with normal lateral hip view (b).

INJURIES TO THE THIGH AND FEMUR

SOFT TISSUE INJURIES

The large muscle mass of the thigh is prone to injury following blunt trauma or strenuous activity. Acute injuries result in bruising and partial or complete rupture of muscles. The injury may be extrinsic (such as a 'dead leg' from a blow to the thigh) or intrinsic (a ruptured hamstring muscle). Rupture of the rectus femoris is caused by sudden violent contraction of the quadriceps. Similar forces can cause rupture of the quadriceps tendon. Rupture of a hamstring muscle is common following sprinting. In all cases, the patient feels sudden severe pain and the ruptured part of the muscle is tender. A defect can sometimes be felt in completely ruptured muscles.

Immediately after injury the traditional treatment is RICE (rest, ice, compression, elevation) to reduce pain and swelling. Further oral analgesia should be provided if necessary, although it is illogical to give anti-inflammatory drugs for acute injuries as inflammation is part of the repair process. The need to repair a complete rupture will depend on which muscle is involved. Rectus femoris rupture rarely requires repair even if a palpable gap is present. In contrast, surgical repair is indicated in quadriceps tendon rupture to prevent the defect from widening.

Aspiration of a thigh haematoma secondary to either a muscle rupture or an extrinsic injury is often unsuccessful; patients with significant muscle rupture or large haematomas should be referred for orthopaedic review. Less significant injuries should be referred for physiotherapy to restore function and prevent shortening.

FEMORAL SHAFT FRACTURES

The femur is the largest and strongest bone in the body. It can be fractured by direct trauma, twisting, or a blow to the front of the flexed knee. These high-energy injuries are commonly associated with multiple trauma (such as road accidents, falls from a height and ballistic injury). The most common associated limb injuries are ipsilateral femoral neck, patellar and tibial fractures, posterior dislocation of the hip and ligament disruption in the knee. These must all be actively excluded. If there is no major trauma then pathological fracture secondary to osteoporosis or metastases should be considered.

The diagnosis is usually obvious, with severe pain, swelling and deformity in the thigh. Weight bearing is impossible and there is abnormal mobility at the fracture site. Spasm of the large adductor and hamstring muscles and loss of longitudinal stability result in shortening and external rotation of the leg. This shortening allows sequestration of large amounts of blood in the thigh and patients are frequently shocked. Blood loss of 3–5 units (1–2 l) can easily occur in a closed fracture.

Open femoral shaft fractures are relatively common although the large soft-tissue mass surrounding the femur tends to reduce their severity. The fractures are usually open 'from within out', with a wound on the front or lateral aspect of the thigh. These wounds require meticulous debridement in the operating theatre and should be photographed and covered in the emergency department as soon as possible to minimize further contamination. A traction splint will reduce blood loss, help relieve pain and prevent further soft tissue injury by movement at the fracture site. Antibiotics and antitetanus treatment should be given as for any open fracture.

Arterial and nerve injury is uncommon. Acute ischaemia due to femoral artery damage almost always resolves with traction and reduction of the fracture. Nerve palsy tends to be axonotmesis. Operative exploration should be performed if there is any suspicion of vessel or nerve division. Neurovascular examination should also be repeated following any manipulation or application of traction. Loss of sensation or of pulses is an indication for loosening and reapplying traction.

The emergency management of femoral shaft fractures involves control of bleeding and application of traction. Traction splints used by ambulance services vary in their mechanism of traction and release. If a patient arrives with a traction splint in place, the position and traction should be checked but the splint should not be removed by inexperienced staff. Ideally, the splint should not be removed until after analgesia has been provided and either a Thomas splint has been prepared or the patient taken to theatre for definitive treatment of the fracture.

All patients require analgesia. A femoral nerve block will provide excellent analgesia to the anterior of the thigh and the periosteum of the middle third of the femur (Chapter 8). A more extensive block (the 'three-in-one' block) can be achieved if volumes of 20–30 ml of local anaesthetic are used and pressure is applied with the palm of the hand to the femoral sheath distal to the block during and after injection. The local anaesthetic will track up the femoral sheath to anaesthetize the obturator nerve and the lateral cutaneous nerve of the thigh as well as the femoral nerve. This provides analgesia for the hip as well as the anterior and lateral aspects of the thigh and femur. Traction reduces bleeding, pain and the risk of fat embolism; it also allows other more urgent injuries to be treated. It can be applied manually as soon as the injury has been identified. Temporary traction splints for adults and children can then be applied very rapidly and should be readily available in the emergency department. Radiographs of the whole femur and pelvis can then be taken whilst analgesia is taking effect. It is possible to miss a femoral neck fracture if the proximal femur is obscured on the radiograph by the traction splint.

Isolated femoral shaft fractures can be treated as a planned procedure. In the multiply injured patient, stabilization of the fracture within 24 h decreases the incidence of pulmonary complications, systemic infection and mortality. In most cases the Thomas splint remains the mainstay of treatment in the intervening period. This can be applied using skin traction or, where large open wounds exist, skeletal traction via a pin in the proximal tibia (Table 25.7). Urgent orthopaedic

Table 25.7: Application of Thomas splint

Apply and maintain manual traction throughout

Clean, photograph and dress any wounds

Measure circumference of proximal thigh on uninjured side to determine appropriate Thomas splint ring size (allow some room for swelling)

Apply skin traction or insert pin

Place a large pad directly beneath the fracture to act as a fulcrum

Pull on the cords connected to either the skin traction tapes or the metal loop attached to the pin to maintain traction

Slide the Thomas splint up the leg (whilst traction is maintained) until the ring reaches the ischial tuberosity

Tie the cords to the end of the splint and use a Chinese windlass (tongue depressor or metal rod) to take up the slack

Reassess neurovascular function

Check regularly for thigh swelling and tightness of the ring

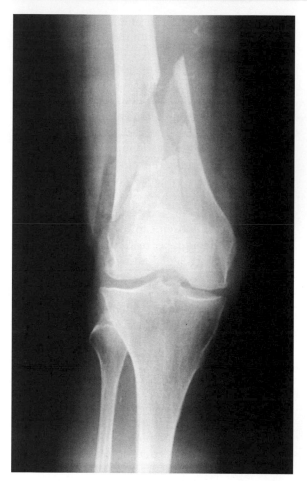

Figure 25.8: Radiograph of supracondylar fracture.

consultation is required for all patients with femoral shaft fractures.

SUPRACONDYLAR FRACTURES OF THE FEMUR

Supracondylar fractures of the femur are relatively common in elderly patients following a fall on to the flexed knee. Similar fractures in younger patients are associated with high-energy trauma and there may be significant fracture displacement, with open wounds and associated injuries. The equivalent injury in a child is a displaced lower femoral epiphysis. The limb is shortened and angulated at the fracture site. If the distal fragment is intact, it is pulled backwards by the action of gastrocnemius. This may endanger the popliteal artery and distal neurovascular function should be

carefully assessed. Traction splints may increase this deformity and should be applied with a pad behind the fracture to allow slight flexion.

Radiographs should be carefully studied for displacement and intra-articular extension (Fig. 25.8). Fractures that extend to the intercondylar notch can separate one or both condyles away from the femoral shaft, or follow an oblique line. The normal relationship of the condyles is essential for knee function: even a millimetre of displacement may result in deformity and interfere with flexion. All patients should therefore be discussed with the orthopaedic team.

INJURIES TO THE KNEE

GENERAL PRINCIPLES

It is often difficult to establish an accurate diagnosis at the initial presentation of acute knee injuries. Although most settle with conservative treatment, there are some important injuries that require urgent intervention. Allowing patients to rest for 2 weeks with review in clinic 'once swelling has subsided' may actually cause further harm by allowing muscle wasting, delaying repair of ligament and tendon injuries, and allowing haemarthroses to clot and organize. Thus every effort must be made to identify major ligamentous injury, intra-articular fractures, acute haemarthroses and extensor mechanism damage.

> The clues to the underlying diagnosis are mainly in the history.

Most patients will accurately describe the mechanism of injury and direction of the forces involved. Patients often report hearing or feeling a pop or crack at the time of the injury when complete ligament rupture has occurred. If the patient reports feeling something break then both a fracture and a major ligament injury must be excluded.

Pain may help to localize the site of injury but is often non-specific. Rapid swelling indicates soft-tissue injury or, more importantly, an acute haemarthrosis due to an intra-articular fracture or rupture of the anterior cruciate ligament (ACL). In contrast, a gradual onset of swelling is more likely to represent a reactive traumatic effusion. Locking refers to inability to extend the knee fully. Blocking is probably a better term because some flexion is still possible. Locking may be true locking caused by intra-articular loose bodies of meniscal, cartilaginous or bony origin, or it may be due to pain behind the knee. Giving way is a sign of instability or meniscal injury. Early instability may indicate complete ligament rupture or a loose intra-articular structure, but it may also be the result of pain. The patient's experiences of giving way, locking, swelling and pain can all be confirmed on clinical examination.

Examination should follow the basic look–feel–move–test principles. Of particular importance is the presence of a joint effusion, the patient's ability to straight leg-raise and the presence of any ligamentous laxity on stress testing.

The four cardinal symptoms of significant knee injury:

- pain
- swelling
- giving way
- locking.

A set of decision rules has been developed which can help in deciding who requires radiographic examination (Table 25.8). These 'Ottawa knee rules' have not been validated in patients aged less than 18 years or older than 55 years. In all cases, AP and lateral films should be requested. A system for reviewing knee films is shown in Table 25.9. Most fractures are obvious but a normal radiograph does not exclude major ligamentous injury. Subtle signs include a lipohaemarthrosis (Fig. 25.9) and minor displacement or impaction of the lateral tibial plateau (Fig. 25.10). A pure chondral fracture cannot be seen on a radiograph.

There is frequently only a sliver of bone attached to an osteochondral fracture, which is therefore difficult to see on a radiograph. There will, however, be a haemarthosis. If a tibial plateau fracture is suspected but not apparent on the AP film, oblique views are necessary to exclude the diagnosis. Similarly, oblique or skyline views may be necessary to exclude a patellar fracture that is not clearly seen on the AP film.

If there is no convincing evidence of bony or major ligamentous injury, the patient should be reassured and a provisional diagnosis of knee sprain

Table 25.8: Decision rules for knee X-ray

AP and lateral views are only required in patients who:
  Have isolated bony tenderness of the patella **or**
  Have bony tenderness at the head of the fibula **or**
  Are unable to flex the knee to 90° **or**
  Are unable to weight-bear both immediately after the injury and on examination

(weight bearing is defined as taking four steps and transferring weight twice on to each leg)

Table 25.9: Interpretation of knee films

On the AP film:
  Uninterrupted cortices around the femur, tibia, fibula and patella
  A step in the articular margins of the femur or tibia
  Fragments within the joint space
  Avulsion fractures of the tibial spines, biceps and collateral ligaments
  An area of increased bone density in the proximal tibia (impaction)
  Loss of vertical alignment between the outer margin of the tibia and the femoral condyles
  Fracture of the fibular neck
  Fracture of the tibial spines

On the lateral film:
  Uninterrupted cortices around the femur, tibia, fibula and patella
  A fat–fluid level (lipohaemarthrosis) in the suprapatellar bursa

(with or without a traumatic effusion) made. Correctly applied compressive bandage, circular woven bandage (Tubigrip®) or simple crepe bandage can be provided to reduce swelling. Advice regarding rest and adequate analgesia, partial weight-bearing crutches and a review clinic appointment in 2–5 days are also required. Whether knee injuries are reviewed in emergency or orthopaedic clinics often reflects local policies and practices. In general terms, knee injuries are best reviewed weekly by those with an interest in knees. Where an orthopaedic knee service exits, this should be utilized.

SOFT-TISSUE INJURIES

The knee has a restricted range of movement (from 0° to 150° of flexion and extension) and depends

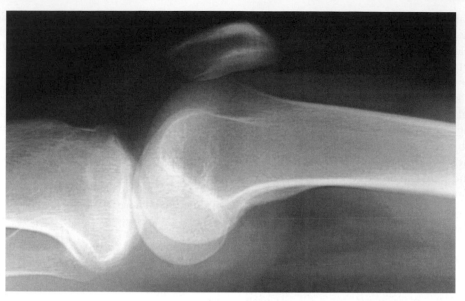

Figure 25.9: Radiograph of lateral (horizontal) knee film with lipohaemarthrosis highlighted. (The fat–fluid level in the suprapatellar bursa indicates release of marrow from an intra-articular fracture – even if no fracture is visible.)

primarily on the cruciate and collateral ligaments for stability. Any of these ligaments may be partially or completely ruptured. With partial rupture, stressing a ligament will produce pain but no laxity. With complete rupture, stressing the ligament may not be painful at the ligament site but there will be laxity. In the acute setting, it is sufficient to determine whether there is anterior, posterior, medial or lateral laxity. If there is doubt, stress radiographs are helpful but should only be requested after examination by an experienced doctor.

Anterior cruciate ligament (ACL) rupture

Anterior laxity indicates ACL rupture. The ACL limits forward movement of the tibia on the femur and is most often ruptured by a sharp twisting movement of the femur relative to the tibia. Injuries are often caused by a rugby or football tackle from behind, which forces the upper tibia forwards. ACL rupture is the commonest major ligament injury. A haemarthrosis will develop very quickly and approximately a quarter of patients will also have a medial collateral ligament injury or a torn meniscus (O'Donohue's triad refers to injury to all three structures). ACL laxity can only usually be demonstrated immediately after injury (before swelling and muscle spasm become prominent). It is tested

with the knee at 90° (the anterior drawer test) and 20° of flexion (Lachman's test). Patients often hold the knee in slight flexion because of the tight effusion, so Lachman's test is generally more accurate and easier to perform in the acute phase.

Approximately one-third of patients with ACL rupture recover completely and have no further difficulties (even with sports). In another third the knee remains unstable and the patient is plagued by frequent giving way. The remaining third lie somewhere between the two extremes, with intermittent symptoms. Because the outcome for any individual patient cannot be predicted, routine orthopaedic follow-up and conservative management are usual. This is in contrast to the patients with displaced avulsion fractures of the tibial spine, who are candidates for immediate repair. Undisplaced tibial spine fractures can be immobilized in a plaster cylinder and referred to fracture clinic.

Posterior cruciate ligament (PCL) rupture

The PCL can be ruptured by hyperextension or a blow to the upper tibia when the knee is flexed. This injury is typically seen in association with major trauma to the lower limb, such as occurs in motorcyclists and front-seat occupants of cars involved in collisions. There will be backward sag of

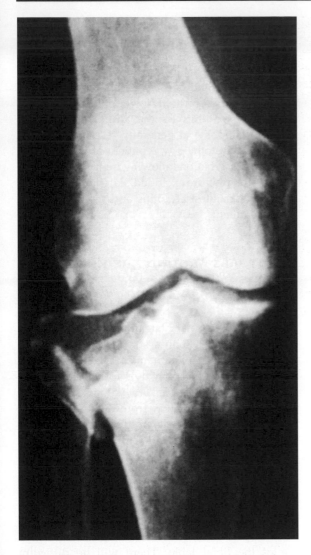

Figure 25.10: AP radiograph of knee with lateral tibial plateau fracture. (Reproduced with permission from L. Solomon, D.J. Warwick and S. Nayagam (eds), *Apley's System of Orthopaedics and Fractures*, 8th edition, published by Arnold, London, 2001.)

the tibia relative to the femur and a haemarthrosis. In contrast to acute ACL rupture, patients tend to make an excellent recovery from PCL rupture without surgical treatment. None the less, acute injuries should be discussed with the orthopaedic team.

Collateral ligament injury

Medial and lateral laxity should be tested at 20°–30° of flexion to negate the action of the anterior cruciate ligament. If there is significant laxity when the knee is in full extension then the ACL must also be damaged. Isolated tears of the medical collateral ligament (MCL) are caused by a blow to the lateral side of the knee (a pure valgus strain) or a combination of external rotation and valgus strain. The knee is held flexed and extension is limited by pain. There will be tenderness along the ligament. Isolated lesions usually heal well with rest, analgesia and graded quadriceps exercises. Depending on the degree of pain, long leg splintage or plaster may be appropriate pending routine clinic review.

The lateral collateral ligament (LCL) joins the femoral condyle to the head of the fibula and is part of a ligament complex incorporating fascia lata and the biceps tendon. It is less important for stability than the other ligaments. Injury may result from a twisting injury or blow to the medial side of the knee causing a varus strain. Patients with suspected LCL tears can be treated symptomatically and reviewed routinely in clinic unless there is gross instability. Common peroneal nerve palsy may be associated with LCL injuries as the nerve passes around the neck of the fibula.

Meniscal injury

Meniscal injuries are usually caused by a clearly defined incident of rotational stress in the partially flexed, weight-bearing knee. The meniscus is torn by compression between the femoral and tibial articular surfaces. Pain is immediate and the patient cannot continue the activity. Weight bearing is also difficult and painful. There may be an acute haemarthrosis following a tear of the vascular periphery, but usually there is minimal swelling as most of the meniscus is avascular. The joint line on the affected side will be tender. Medial meniscal injuries are five times more common than lateral injuries. Acute tears are usually vertical splits in the substance of the meniscus but may extend into a bucket handle (by anterior extension) or a flap tear (by radial extension). Both can cause a springy block to full extension by jamming in the anterior segment of the joint. Smaller tears cause recurrent clicking, catching and joint line pain.

If there is no locking, the patient can be safely reviewed in clinic once pain and swelling have subsided (usually 2–4 weeks). Analgesia, advice regarding quadriceps exercises and partial weight-bearing crutches can be provided in the interim.

A locked knee requires urgent orthopaedic review.

Haemarthrosis

Bleeding into the knee is caused by major ligament injury, intra-articular fractures and rupture of the capsule. Although most patients with a haemarthrosis have an ACL injury, the other causes must be excluded. A haemarthrosis is therefore an indication for further investigation. Ideally, the knee should be washed out in the operating theatre and an arthroscopic examination performed. This relieves pain, prevents the synovitis that may result from the irritant effect of blood and reduces adhesions. Recovery and rehabilitation are thus much more rapid if the knee is washed out. If arthroscopy is not available, blood should be aspirated under aseptic conditions and the aspirate examined for fat. The presence of fat in the aspirate indicates a likely intra-articular fracture. If the diagnosis remains unclear the patient should be referred for early orthopaedic review.

A haemarthrosis indicates a significant intra-articular injury.

CHRONIC KNEE PAIN

Patients often attend an emergency department to seek advice about chronic knee pain. A wide range of conditions, most secondary to overuse, can cause pain and patients should initially be advised to rest, take adequate analgesia, and continue non-weight-bearing exercises. The most common complaint is anterior knee pain that is usually not associated with injury. The pain is poorly localized and aggravated by weight bearing on a flexed knee as well as prolonged sitting. There may be crepitus, weakness and an effusion, although clinical examination is usually normal. Causes include malalignment, osteochondral injury, degenerative change and chondromalacia patellae. The majority of patients improve with physiotherapy and symptomatic management. Those that do not should be referred to orthopaedics.

Osgood–Schlatter's disease is a tibial tubercle apophysitis in active children characterized by pain, swelling and radiographic fragmentation of the tibial tubercle. It usually resolves with symptomatic treatment. The Sinding-Larsen–Johansen syndrome is a similar condition at the lower pole of the patella. Insertional tendinitis is the adult equivalent of these conditions and generally responds to analgesia and physiotherapy. A patient presenting with an acute exacerbation following injury should have an avulsion fracture excluded. Patellar tendinitis is similar to Achilles tendinitis and responds to the same treatment.

FRACTURES AROUND THE KNEE

Tibial plateau fractures

Fractures of the tibial plateau are caused by axial loading combined with a strong valgus or varus force. The collateral ligaments act like a hinge and the tibial condyle is crushed or split by the opposing femoral condyle. Severe valgus stress (displacement of the leg away from the mid-line) will impact the mass of the lateral femoral condyle on to the lateral tibial plateau. This is the most common tibial plateau fracture and approximately half occur in road accidents. Fractures of the medial tibial plateau are uncommon but do occur. A range of fracture patterns can be found. Most represent either splitting of the tibial plateau with downward displacement of the tibial fragment or crushing of the tibial table. There will be difficulty weight bearing, pain and tenderness over the lateral joint line, a haemarthrosis, and bruising over the lateral side of the knee. Symptoms and signs may be surprisingly subtle and weight bearing has a high discriminatory value. AP, lateral, and occasionally oblique radiographs will confirm the diagnosis (see Fig. 25.10). A vertical line drawn at the outer margin of the femoral condyles should pass within 5 mm of the outer margin of the tibial plateau. If it does not, then a plateau fracture should be suspected.

Tibial plateau fractures require urgent orthopaedic assessment. Although minimally displaced fractures (<2–3 mm) can be treated conservatively, full assessment of the knee requires an examination under anaesthesia and arthroscopy, or further imaging may be required to determine the true

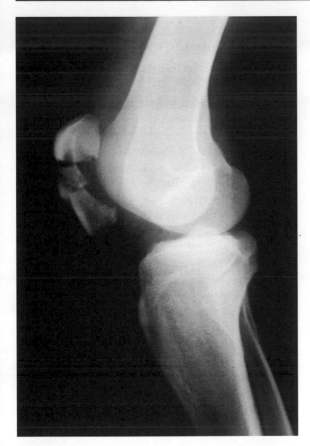

Figure 25.11: Fractured patella on a lateral knee radiograph.

extent of the fracture. A plaster cast will provide stability and comfort in the interim.

Patellar fracture (Fig. 25.11)

The patella lies within the quadriceps tendon in the centre of the extensor mechanism and is surrounded by a fibrotendinous capsule. It acts as a pulley carrying the extensor mechanism around the knee during flexion. It may be fractured by direct violence (a fall on the knee or a road accident) or following sudden muscle contraction (a stumble or partial fall). Fractures resulting from direct trauma may be incomplete, stellate or comminuted. Fractures resulting from sudden contraction tend to be transverse. Treatment depends on the nature of the fracture and whether the extensor mechanism is intact (demonstrated by full active extension of the knee against gravity). Surgery is not indicated for undisplaced fractures where the extensor mechanism is intact. Thus if the patient is able to straight leg raise, the fractured patella will heal within its 'capsule'. Only analgesia and aspiration of any haemarthrosis may be required. If swelling allows, a long leg plaster cylinder can be applied in the emergency department and the patient reviewed in fracture clinic.

Although it is important to preserve the patella where possible, any irregularity of its articular surface will cause osteoarthritis in later life, so comminuted fractures are referred for reduction or excision. A damaged extensor mechanism also requires referral for orthopaedic review and surgical repair. A transverse fracture tends to split the quadriceps expansions on either side and will require repair to prevent widening of the fracture.

Avulsion of the quadriceps tendon from the patella, avulsion of the patellar tendon from the tibial tuberosity, avulsion fracture of the tibial tuberosity and rupture of the quadriceps and patella tendons may also occur with the same mechanism of injury. These conditions may easily be misdiagnosed by assuming that the inability to straight leg raise is due to pain. These injuries generally require surgical repair and should be referred.

Knee dislocation (Fig. 25.12)

Dislocation of the knee joint is rare and is often associated with major injuries to all the ligaments. The tibia is most often displaced anteriorly and reduction is best effected by gentle but sustained longitudinal traction. There can be additional injury to the popliteal vessels and nerves. An angiogram should be performed to exclude an intimal flap tear of the politeal artery and reduce the risk of late occlusion. Orthopaedic teams should be involved in the care of these patients from the outset. Following reduction and immobilization, reconstruction of a dislocated knee can be attempted electively.

> Dislocation of the knee is associated with popliteal artery injury and requires vascular assessment.

Patellar dislocation

Dislocation of the patella may occur singly or as a recurrent problem. The patella can be dislocated by a sharp, twisting movement of the knee in slight flexion. It is common in female adolescents and is

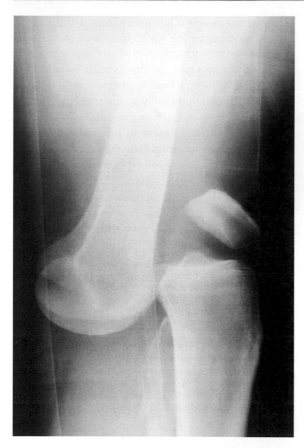

Figure 25.12: Dislocated knee on a lateral radiograph.

often associated with abnormal patellofemoral anatomy. If spontaneous reduction has occurred, the patient will describe seeing the 'kneecap' lying on the lateral side of the knee. If still dislocated, it can be reduced under Entonox® by applying medial pressure and gently straightening the knee. The knee will remain swollen from local swelling and a haemarthrosis. There will be tenderness on the medial side of the patella. Radiographs may show a haemarthrosis and sometimes an osteochondral fracture on the medial side of the patella.

The torn medial expansion needs to be rested in a plaster cylinder for 4 weeks. If there is no haemarthrosis and minimal swelling, this can be arranged in the emergency department and the patient brought back to fracture clinic. For patients who have recurrent dislocation, the chance of adequate healing is remote and they may need later operative repair.

INJURIES TO THE LEG

SOFT-TISSUE INJURIES

Minor soft-tissue injuries of the calf and shin are common. One of the most important injuries in the leg is a pretibial laceration in an elderly patient. Its importance lies in its frequency and the risk of complications. The typical laceration has a distally based flap with fragile, poorly viable skin. Very occasionally mattress sutures are required to oppose the wound edges, but excellent results can usually be obtained by applying adhesive wound tapes and a light pressure dressing once the wound has been cleaned. Patients should be advised to keep the limb elevated and return to the clinic in 5 days for wound inspection. Large, poorly viable flaps and complex lacerations may require plastic surgical review and it is essential to consider this early.

Rupture of gastrocnemius occurs during racket sports, jumping and sprinting. The medial head is most commonly injured and the symptoms are similar to those of a ruptured Achilles tendon. Once this has been excluded, treatment is with analgesia, gentle stretching, and strengthening exercises under the supervision of a physiotherapist. Repair is only indicated in the athlete with major disruption and wide separation of the muscle and aponeurosis.

Patients may present with shin pain that is associated with sporting activities or running. This is often described as 'shin splints'. The differential diagnosis of shin pain is wide and includes tibial periostitis, stress fractures of the tibia and chronic compartment syndromes. They can be very difficult to distinguish and are essentially chronic overuse injuries.

Both the tibia and fibula are sites of stress fractures. Stress fractures are characterized by gradual onset of pain, localized swelling and tenderness. The most frequent sites are the junction of the middle and distal thirds of the tibia and just above the inferior tibiofibular ligament in the fibula. Hairline cracks or endosteal or exosteal callus may be visible on plain radiographs, but there are often no radiographic features and bone scanning may be required to confirm the diagnosis. Rest, analgesia and physiotherapy usually alleviate symptoms of both stress fractures and tibial periostitis. Chronic muscle compartment syndromes are mainly confined to the anterior and deep posterior compartments of the leg. Pain is produced by running and the diagnosis can be difficult to confirm without compartment pressure measurement during exercise. This is usually only available to specialist sports injury services.

FRACTURES OF THE TIBIA AND FIBULA

Isolated fractures of the tibia or fibula may occur from direct violence. Indirect forces tend to cause fractures of both bones. Isolated fractures, of the tibia can occur as a result of direct trauma, twisting and repeated stress. They are frequently associated with ligamentous injuries of the knee. The fracture is treated in the same way as a fracture of both bones.

The fibula can be fractured by a direct blow to the outer side of the leg or by twisting. These injuries cause transverse or spiral fractures, respectively. An isolated spiral fracture at the upper end of the fibula may be associated with a fracture of the tibia at the ankle that is easily overlooked (Fig. 25.13). The ankle must therefore be examined carefully in every patient with an apparently isolated fracture of the fibula. Similarly, the neck of the fibula should be examined in every patient with a significant ankle injury. It is essential that the combination of a fibular fracture with diastasis of the inferior tibiofibular joint and rupture of the medial ligament of the ankle (the Maisonneuve injury, see below) is not overlooked.

If a fibula fracture is undisplaced and the tibia is intact, the patient can be allowed to weight-bear and no immobilization is required unless movement is painful. A below-knee plaster can always be used if pain is severe. These patients should be reviewed in fracture clinic. Common peroneal nerve injury should be excluded and any impairment documented.

Fracture of both the tibia and fibula is common. These injuries are amongst the leading causes of disability in young adults. The patient cannot weight-bear and is usually in severe pain. Signs include swelling and bruising over the anterior border and angular and rotational deformity of the limb. Bony tenderness will be obvious in conscious patients. Evidence of open fracture may be subtle, with only a small 'from within out' puncture wound visible.

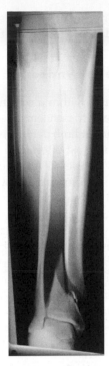

Figure 25.13: Radiograph showing spiral fibular fracture associated with medial malleolar fracture.

Any wounds should be photographed then covered with sterile dressings. These should not be disturbed again until the patient reaches the operating theatre (ideally within 6 h of injury). Antibiotic therapy should be commenced according to local antibiotic policy for all open fractures. The popliteal artery is anchored under the upper third of the tibia and is susceptible to damage in proximal fractures. Distal circulation should therefore be checked carefully. AP and lateral views to include the knee and ankle joints are the only radiographs necessary.

Uncomplicated tibial fractures will require manipulation and immobilization in a long-leg cast with the knee slightly flexed. The ankle should be at right-angles. This dorsiflexion of the ankle must be achieved by traction on the heel and not by dorsiflexing the forefoot and forcing the tibial fragment posteriorly. All patients will require hospital admission for observation and elevation.

The two major complications of tibial fractures are compartment syndrome and infection in open fractures. Osteomyelitis complicates as many as 10–20% of open tibial fractures and is reduced by meticulous debridement, early restoration of soft tissue cover and stable fixation of the fracture.

Compartment syndrome

Increased pressure within a confined fascial compartment may lead to ischaemia, necrosis, contractures and permanent limb deformity. Compartment syndromes occur most often with fractures of the tibia and crush injuries of the foot. Despite this, clinical evidence of compartment syndrome should be sought in all injuries of the lower limb. Other causes include haematomas and swelling after athletic exertion or operation. The diagnosis is based on symptoms and signs, and can be confirmed by direct measurement of the compartment pressure. The patient complains of severe pain (not relieved by analgesia or splinting), localized tenderness, pain with movement and paraesthesiae. Pallor, paralysis and pulselessness are late signs and irreversible muscle necrosis will already have taken place.

> Passive stretching of the muscles within the compartment will elicit severe pain and is a sensitive test.

The immediate treatment of suspected compartment syndrome includes splitting any plaster or bandages and elevating the limb to the level of the heart. Irreversible damage to the limb will occur if the compartment is not decompressed by fasciotomy within 4 h. The symptoms and signs are usually sufficient grounds for decompression. However, direct measurement of compartment pressure may be helpful. A single pressure reading of greater than 45 mmHg is an indication for fasciotomy. A 30 mmHg gradient between compartment pressure and diastolic blood pressure is required to maintain normal metabolic function. It may be possible to measure the pressure continuously and relate it to diastolic blood pressure in equivocal cases. Despite this, measurement of pressures can be misleading and should never override clinical judgement. Urgent orthopaedic review is indicated.

> Compartment syndrome is largely a clinical diagnosis.

INJURIES TO THE ANKLE

GENERAL PRINCIPLES

The ankle joint is described as a mortice joint with the two malleoli and the articular surface of the tibia forming a socket for the talus. The talus is held in the mortice on the medial side by the strong deltoid ligament. On the lateral side it is held by the lateral ligament complex. The fibula and tibia are tightly bound by the tibiofibular ligaments. As with the pelvis, the ankle may be regarded as a ring-like structure composed of bones joined together by ligaments. As a general principle instability results when the ring is broken in two places, because of either two fractures or a combination of a fracture and ligament damage.

Injury occurs when the talus is moved within the rigid mortice. Ankle joint structures then fail in predictable ways according to the magnitude and direction of the forces involved. In general a traction force (a pull by intact ligaments) on a malleolus results in a transverse fracture, and a pulsion or rotation and pulsion force results in an oblique or spiral fracture. Four basic mechanisms of injury (external rotation, abduction, adduction and vertical compression) account for the majority of ankle sprains and fractures.

Inversion of the heel when walking over rough ground causes external rotation of the talus. The talus rotates against the lateral malleolus and causes injury to the lateral ligaments. If the forces are great enough, the lateral malleolus fractures obliquely. If the force progresses further, the medial ligaments may be disrupted or the medial malleolus may be pulled off. This bimalleolar fracture is unstable. Continuation of the rotation pulls on the posterior tibiofibular ligament and avulses a posterior malleolar fragment. This is now a trimalleolar fracture. Dislocation of the ankle may also occur (Fig. 25.14).

Adduction of the talus results from striking the inverted foot on the ground. If the forces are slight, a partial tear of the lateral ligament occurs. With greater energy there will be complete rupture of the lateral ligaments and possibly an avulsion fracture of the lateral malleolus. With yet further force the talus drives medially, knocking off the medial malleolus.

Abduction of the talus will occur if the medial side of the heel and foot strikes the ground. As the

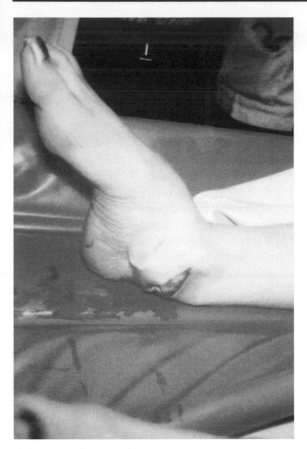

Figure 25.14: Ankle dislocation.

foot everts, the talus drives laterally and tears the medial ligaments (or pulls a medial malleolar fragment off). The tibiofibular ligaments are then stressed and the talus may push a fibular fragment off.

Vertical compression injuries may occur in road accidents (floor hitting foot) and falls from heights. Forces are transmitted vertically through the talus and into the tibia. The talus is often dorsiflexed during vertical compression injuries and its wide anterior part is forced into the mortice, shearing off the medial malleolus. The anterior tibial margin is next to be fractured (usually a crush fracture), followed by the lateral malleolus. With even greater forces the distal tibia may become grossly comminuted. This is an unstable injury that may require internal fixation.

SOFT-TISSUE INJURIES

A sprained ankle is one of the most common reasons for attending an emergency department.

Table 25.10: Ottawa ankle rules for use of radiography in acute ankle injuries

An ankle series (AP mortice view and lateral) is only required if:
  There is malleolar pain **and**
  The patients is aged 55 years or over **or**
  There is inability to weight-bear both immediately and in the emergency department **or**
  There is bony tenderness in the posterior half of the distal 6 cm of the medial malleolus **or**
  There is bony tenderness in the posterior half of the distal 6 cm of the lateral malleolus

A foot series is only required if:
  There is pain in the mid-foot area **and**
  The patients is age 55 years or over **or**
  There is inability to weight-bear both immediately and in the emergency department **or**
  There is bony tenderness at the base of the fifth metatarsal or at the navicular

Clinically, there is localized swelling and tenderness and early bruising may be apparent. The pattern of injury is related to the position of the foot at the time and the direction and magnitude of the forces involved. Patients will often clearly describe the mechanism and will be able to demonstrate the direction of deformity using the other leg. An audible snap or crack may be reported by the patient at the time of the injury but is rarely associated with specific injury. The specific mechanisms that lead to ligament rupture and fracture are discussed above.

The key issues for the doctor at this stage are whether there is likely to be an underlying fracture, and provision of the appropriate advice and follow-up. The Ottawa ankle rules are a set of decision rules that help the doctor judge whether radiographic examination is likely to reveal a fracture (Table 25.10). A guide to interpreting ankle radiographs is given in Table 25.11. The AP mortice view is taken with the foot internally rotated 15° to show the entire joint space and the presence of any shift or tilt of the talus (Fig. 25.15).

Sprains and partial ligament tears are best managed by protected mobilization. The RICE regimen for the treatment of soft-tissue injuries should be followed. A firm elastic support provides sufficient compression. The use of anti-inflammatory drugs reduces the time to recovery. The pain settles substantially after 10 days, but patients should be warned that the ankle will be uncomfortable for as long as 3 months. Physiotherapy should be provided for all patients as soon as pain allows. Many departments have limited access to physiotherapy so the resources of the patient's general practitioner

Table 25.11: Interpretation of ankle radiographs

Look for:

On the AP mortice view:
  A uniform joint space all the way round the talus
  An intact talar dome with no evidence of
    osteochondral fracture
  Fragments within the joint space
  Epiphyseal plate fractures

On the lateral view:
  Uninterrupted cortices around the medial,
    lateral and posterior malleolus (posterior tibia)
  An intact calcaneum
  A normal Bohler's angle (30°–40°, see text)
  A fracture of the base of the fifth metatarsal

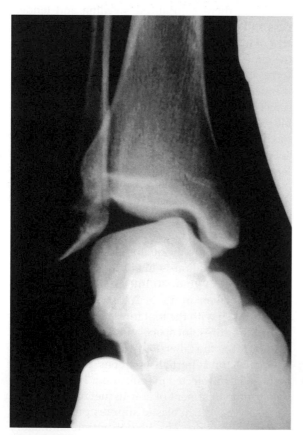

Figure 25.15: AP mortice view of the ankle showing talar shift due to disruption of the lateral ligament complex of the ankle.

should be utilized where possible. Some patients may require a few weeks of rest before they can tolerate physiotherapy. The treatment of complete ruptures of the lateral ligament is controversial, but consideration should be given to surgical repair.

RICE – Rest, Ice, Compression, Elevation.

A specific injury is rupture of the interosseous membrane and tibiofibular ligaments with a diastasis (widening between the tibia and fibula) and a high spiral fracture of the fibula (the Maisonneuve fracture). The importance of this injury is that the radiographs of the ankle may not reveal a fracture despite the severity of the injury. The diastasis requires operative correction.

The Achilles tendon is susceptible to inflammation as a result of overuse, and to acute partial or complete rupture (Fig 25.16). Of particular relevance to emergency department practice is distinguishing acute tendon rupture from Achilles tendinitis or bursitis. The tendon is ruptured by the same movements that can tear the head of gastrocnemius (typically sudden plantarflexion against resistance). Classically, the patient reports a feeling of being kicked or otherwise hit in the back of the leg or heel. Pain, weakness and swelling may only be moderate. Active plantar flexion will be intact owing to the action of other posterior tendons. On examination, however, a gap between the two ends of the tendon can usually be palpated and Simmonds' test reveals no plantar flexion on squeezing the calf on the affected side. This test will be negative in partial ruptures and tendinitis. Complete ruptures should be treated by application of a

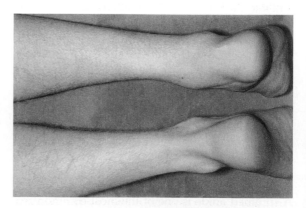

Figure 25.16: Right Achilles tendon rupture.

full below-knee cast in plantarflexion (an equinus plaster). Patients who present late (more than 7 days after injury) have a high rate of rerupture and orthopaedic referral for operative management is indicated. Achilles tendinitis produces pain localized to the tendon itself and is attributed to a recent increase in use rather than a specific event. The tendon is tender but intact. Analgesia and relative rest will usually suffice.

FRACTURES ABOUT THE ANKLE

Significant ankle fractures occur in three places:

- the medial malleolus of the tibia
- the lower end of the fibula, including the lateral malleolus
- the 'posterior malleolus', or posterior margin of the tibia.

The mechanism for these fractures is described above. Stable, undisplaced fractures of the lateral malleolus may be treated conservatively in a below-knee cast. The patient can subsequently be reviewed in fracture clinic. Undisplaced bimalleolar fractures may be treated the same way and reviewed after 1 week. Unstable fractures should be discussed with the orthopaedic team. Ankle fractures are intra-articular injuries and the aim of treatment is reduction to restore the normal ankle mortice. Pain, instability and osteoarthritis will result if an accurate reduction is not achieved. Manipulation under anaesthesia (by an orthopaedic surgeon) and application of a cast may be used, but more commonly open reduction and internal fixation are appropriate to achieve anatomical reduction. Check radiographs are essential in interpreting the success of reduction. All of the following radiographic criteria should be met:

- fibular length is restored
- joint space all the way round the talus is uniform
- the talus sits squarely in the mortice with parallel articular surfaces
- there is no tibiofibular diastasis.

DISLOCATION OF THE ANKLE

The ankle may dislocate if the mortice becomes unstable. This is usually associated with significant ligamentous and bony injury, although dislocation without fracture can occur. The acutely dislocated ankle should be reduced as soon as possible to preserve skin viability and distal neurovascular function. If it is possible to take plain radiographs without incurring delay (while titrating analgesia to effect), then it is valuable to do so (see Fig. 25.14). These initial views can convey the degree of deformity and displacement even if no fracture is present. Reduction is achieved by traction on the heel and the leg can then be placed in a plaster back-slab pending further orthopaedic review.

> Ankle dislocations should be urgently reduced to prevent ischaemia of soft tissues overlying the injury.

INJURIES TO THE FOOT

FRACTURES OF THE TALUS

Fractures of the talus are unusual and associated with high-energy mechanisms of injury. The talus plays an important role in the ankle joint, the subtalar joint and the mid-tarsal (talonavicular) joints. It is largely covered by articular cartilage. Fractures may involve the dome, the neck, the body or the smaller processes of the talus. The commonest fracture is of the neck of the talus following road accidents and falls from heights. The talus is forced against the anterior tibial margin as the foot is forcibly dorsiflexed. The diagnosis is confirmed on radiographs (Fig. 25.17). The talus, like the scaphoid, receives its blood supply from distal to proximal and there is a significant risk of avascular necrosis. Displaced fractures should therefore be referred for urgent orthopaedic review. Undisplaced fractures may be treated in a below-knee non-weight-bearing cast, with orthopaedic follow-up. Fractures of the talar dome are osteochondral fractures that are usually caused by inversion injuries of the ankle and can be diagnosed by plain radiographs.

CALCANEAL FRACTURES

The calcaneum is fractured by a direct blow to the heel, most often caused by falling from a height.

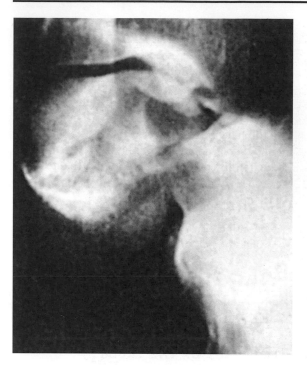

Figure 25.17: Radiograph of fractured talus. (Reproduced with permission from L. Solomon, D.J. Warwick and S. Nayagam (eds), *Apley's System of Orthopaedics and Fractures*, 8th edition, published by Arnold, London, 2001.)

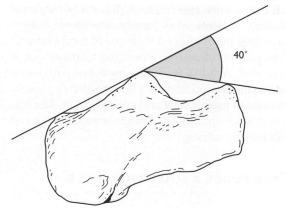

Figure 25.18: Böhler's angle.

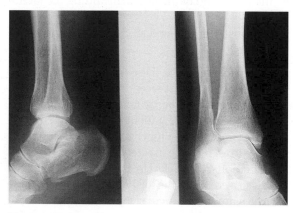

Figure 25.19: Lateral radiograph showing a calcaneal fracture.

Fractures are therefore often bilateral and associated with thoraco-lumbar wedge fractures. Because the calcaneum is made of cancellous bone, it is crushed at the moment of impact and the heel may appear wider, shorter and flatter. There is usually marked swelling and tenderness, with inability to weight-bear. Radiographic assessment of the calcaneum involves a lateral and an axial view. Measurement of Böhler's angle will reveal flattening of the fracture (measured by drawing a line from the posterior aspect of the calcaneum to its highest midpoint. A second line is drawn from this point to the highest anterior point. The angle between these two lines is Böhler's angle) (Fig. 25.18). A number of different types of fracture have been described and there are a number of treatment options. Of greater importance, however, is whether the subtalar joint has been involved. Major fractures destroy the subtalar joint and cause stiffness of the subtalar and midtarsal joints. This leads to disabling pain when walking on rough surfaces. All calcaneum fractures should be referred for orthopaedic review. If subtalar joint involvement

is suspected, further imaging is used to assess the degree of displacement of the articular surface (Fig. 25.19).

TARSAL FRACTURES AND DISLOCATIONS

Minor extra-articular fractures in the foot require only ice, elevation and early mobilization with the aid of physiotherapy. Any intra-articular fractures should be referred to the orthopaedic surgeons. The tarsal bones are hard, solid bones that are difficult to fracture. They may, however, dislocate at either the mid-tarsal or tarsometatarsal joints. The mid-tarsal joint lies between the talus and the calcaneum posteriorly and the navicular and cuboid anteriorly. A mid-tarsal dislocation may be

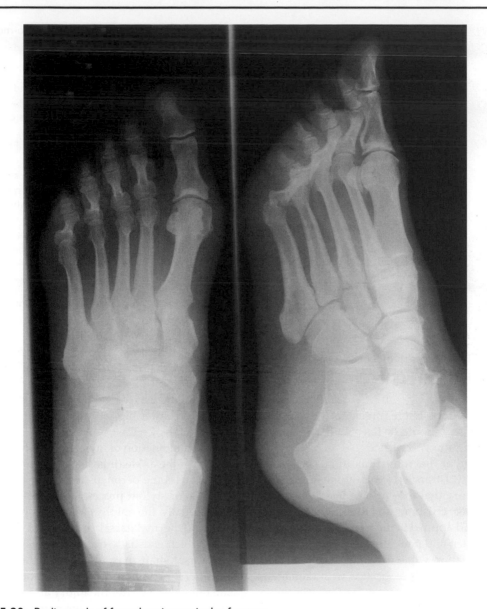

Figure 25.20: Radiograph of foot showing navicular fracture.

associated with fracture of any of the tarsal bones, crush injuries to the foot and twisting injuries of the forefoot. The dislocation may be to the medial (adduction dislocation) or lateral (abduction dislocation) side. These injuries can be missed both clinically and radiographically. If they are not correctly diagnosed and accurately reduced the dislocation becomes permanent, and a disabling deformity may result.

Fractures of the cuboid occur as a result of lateral subluxation of the mid-tarsal joint with longitudinal compression of the cuboid. This rarely causes significant displacement and treatment is by immobilization in a cast.

Fractures of the navicular may involve the tuberosity, the body or the dorsal lip. The tuberosity may be avulsed in an eversion injury (by the tibialis posterior tendon). Where the tuberosity is significantly displaced it should be reduced. Fractures of the cuboid and navicular may coexist. Fractures of the body of the navicular are often associated with injuries involving the mid-tarsal joint and result from high-energy trauma (Fig. 25.20). Avulsion fractures of the dorsal cortex are caused by forced

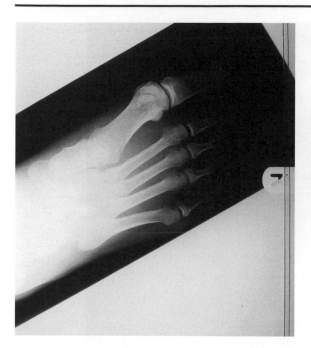

Figure 25.21: Radiograph of foot showing tarso-metatarsal dislocation.

Table 25.12: Radiographic signs of tarso-metatarsal fracture dislocations

Look for:
Diastasis between the first and second metatarsal shafts
Small fracture fragments of the bones comprising the mid-tarsal joint
Residual subluxation of the metatarsal bases seen on the lateral projection
The medial margin of the base of the second metatarsal should line up with the medial margin of the middle cuneiform on the AP view
The medial margin of the base of the third metatarsal should line up with the medial margin of the lateral cuneiform on the oblique view

eversion of the foot. Large fragments (>25% of the articular surface) should be fixed. Otherwise, plaster immobilization will suffice.

Dislocation or fracture–dislocation of the tarsometatarsal (Lisfranc's) joint of the foot is an important injury that may also be overlooked. It is caused by direct crushing, an indirect twisting force or an axial load applied to the trapped foot. The foot appears swollen and pain is exacerbated by supination and pronation while the subtalar joint is held. Severe displacement is associated with damage to the dorsalis pedis artery and forefoot ischaemia. Radiographic signs may be subtle, requiring a high degree of clinical suspicion (Fig. 25.21). AP, oblique and true lateral projections are required (Table 25.12). Treatment requires prompt anatomical reduction by applying traction in the line of the metatarsals and pressure over their bases.

METATARSAL FRACTURES AND DISLOCATIONS

Metatarsal fractures may result from crush injuries to the forefoot. Although there may be little evidence of significant neurovasular damage, the margin of safety for soft-tissue swelling is much lower in the foot than elsewhere in the leg and a careful watch for compartment syndrome is warranted. Patients should be referred for admission if swelling is considerable. Otherwise, rest, ice, elevation and a cast is often all that is necessary. In cases where there are multiple displaced fractures, orthopaedic intervention may be required to ensure that the normal relationship of the metatarsal heads is restored (Fig. 25.22).

The combination of inversion and forced plantar flexion at the ankle (mis-stepping on the edge of a step) causes the peroneus brevis tendon to avulse the base or styloid process of the fifth metatarsal. Occasionally, the epiphysis that lies parallel to the shaft of the metatarsal is confused with a fracture (which is usually transverse) (Fig. 25.23). The metatarsal shaft may also be fractured. There is considerable pain and tenderness of the fracture site immediately after the injury and a below-knee cast may be needed to relieve pain. Some patients can manage well with just a firm crepe bandage and will recover faster.

The metatarsals are also prone to stress fractures ('march fractures'). The neck or the shaft of the second or third metatarsal is usually affected. The history is of prolonged exercise (or marching). There is a gradual onset of pain in the forefoot, with local tenderness and swelling on the dorsum of the foot. Radiographs often do not show the fracture initially but if repeated will demonstrate the appearance of a haze of callus at the fracture site. If pain is severe the patient may require a below-knee walking plaster, but mild cases require only a period of rest of the part.

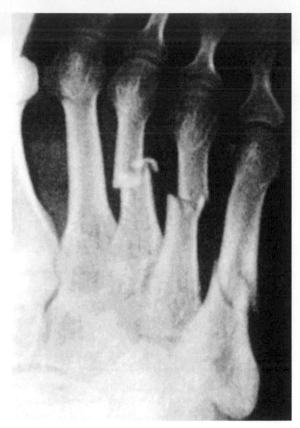

Figure 25.22: Radiograph of foot showing multiple metatarsal fractures. (Reproduced with permission from L. Solomon, D.J. Warwick and S. Nayagam (eds), *Apley's System of Orthopaedics and Fractures*, 8th edition, published by Arnold, London, 2001.)

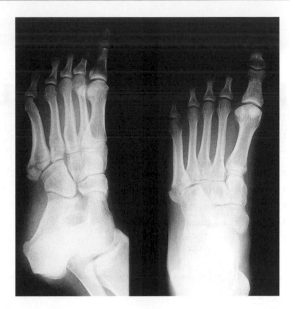

Figure 25.23: Contrasting radiographs of fifth metatarsal fracture (*left*) and epiphysis (*right*).

TOE FRACTURES AND DISLOCATIONS

The phalanges of the toes are vulnerable to crushing and stubbing injuries. Toes are also at risk of more severe open injuries, such as when the blade of a lawn mower clips them. There is often significant nail and soft tissue damage and a fracture that extends into the interphalangeal joint.

Many emergency departments will avoid radiographs of toes (other than the great toe) if there is no evidence of open wounds, dislocation, angulation or rotation, on the basis that the radiograph will not change the doctor's management. On the other hand, certain knowledge that a toe is not broken may fundamentally alter the patient's approach to their symptoms and activities, and thus clearly affects the patient's management of themselves. Plain radiographs should therefore always be considered.

Wounds and crush injuries of the distal phalanges should be treated as soft-tissue injuries without regard to bony continuity. Severely contaminated open fractures should be treated like any other open fracture. The wound should be thoroughly cleaned and the nail plate retained as much as possible (if only as a splint). Analgesia should be provided and the foot elevated until swelling has subsided. Closed fractures of the phalanges rarely require treatment other than reduction of rotational or angular deformity and strapping to an adjacent toe for 3–4 weeks. If there is obvious dislocation or displacement, this should be reduced. Orthopaedic follow-up need only be sought for injuries to the great toe that involve the proximal phalanx or are intra-articular.

FURTHER READING

Greaves, I., Porter, K. and Burke, D. (1997) *Key Topics in Trauma*. Bios, Oxford.

McRae, R. (1994) *Practical Fracture Treatment*. Churchill Livingstone, London.

CHAPTER TWENTY SIX

INJURIES TO THE UPPER LIMB

- Introduction
- General principles
- Brachial plexus injuries
- Injuries to the shoulder
- Injuries to the arm

- Injuries to the elbow
- Injuries to the forearm
- Wrist injuries
- Further reading

INTRODUCTION

Injuries to the upper limb account for a high proportion of patients presenting to emergency departments. The disabling effect of upper limb injury in the longer term can be out of proportion to the extent and life threat of the initial injury. Accurate diagnosis and treatment are therefore essential. This chapter provides a practical approach to the assessment and management of traumatic injury to the upper limb.

GENERAL PRINCIPLES

Many of the general principles that were discussed in relation to history, examination, investigation and treatment of lower limb injuries (Chapter 25) apply equally to the upper limb. In the seriously injured patient, the primary survey should always precede any formal assessment of limb injury. The priorities for management of the severe limb injury are then to control bleeding, provide immobilization and analgesia, and identify limb-threatening injuries such as major joint dislocation, open fractures, nerve or vascular injury and compartment syndromes.

Fractures in the upper limb are common. They are also commonly missed. To avoid this, particular attention must be paid to the mechanism of injury, the likely forces involved and the likely deformity of the limb at the time of injury. Knowledge of the typical presenting features associated with specific fractures is required to guide the effective use of radiography. As with lower limb injuries, there are clear associations and patterns that are often suggested by the history. A fall on the outstretched hand, for example, can be associated with characteristic wrist, elbow and shoulder injuries, depending on the position of the hand and arm at the time of the fall. Frequently missed fractures include greenstick fractures and fractures of the humeral neck, radial head, distal radius and carpal bones. Another key aspect of the history is the patient's occupation and home circumstances. The disability caused to an elderly patient with a fracture of the distal radius of the dominant hand may be so great as to prevent the patient from cooking, shopping, bathing and using their mobility aids. Such patients are at further risk from accidental injury and should be carefully assessed before considering discharge. General principles of examination are given in Table 26.1.

All the joints of the upper limb are at 0° when the body is in the anatomical position. There is often confusion over the movements of the thumb. Unlike the remainder of the upper limb, movements of the thumb are not in the true sagittal or coronal planes: they are in a plane which is angled some 30° forward from the coronal.

As with lower limb injuries, urgent orthopaedic consultation is required for patients with open,

Table 26.1: General principles of upper limb examination

If the patient expresses pain then provide analgesia early
Tailor the examination to the needs of the patient
Follow the look–feel–move–test approach
Always compare limbs with the other side
Look for abnormal contour, deformity, swelling, wasting, scars and wounds
Feel for swelling, abnormal movement, crepitus and bony tenderness
Leave the most painful area until last
Observe active movements before attempting passive movement
Record range of movement in degrees from the anatomical position
Grade power according to the Medical Research Council scale
Always assess circulation and sensation distal to the injury

Table 26.2: Aide-mémoire for neurological examination of the upper limb

	Motor	Sensory
C5	Shoulder abduction	Lateral arm
C6	Elbow flexion	Thumb
C7	Elbow extension	Middle finger
C8	Wrist flexion	Little finger
T1	Little finger abduction	Ulnar aspect of forearm

complex or multiple fractures, major joint disruption and extensive soft-tissue injury. All other fractures should be reviewed in clinic according to departmental policies. Specific management guidance is provided below.

Nerve injuries in the upper limb range from major brachial plexus lesions to isolated peripheral nerve injuries. They are potentially disabling and must always be carefully sought and excluded. Common injuries occur to the axillary nerve at the shoulder, the radial nerve round the humeral shaft, the ulnar nerve at the medial epicondyle, the median nerve at the wrist and the digital nerves in hand wounds.

Table 26.2 provides an aide-mémoire for the neurological examination of the upper limb: it should be remembered that C5 has no exclusive dermatome, so injuries may not be associated with sensory loss.

BRACHIAL PLEXUS INJURIES

Brachial plexus injuries can give complex patterns of clinical signs and are generally divided into upper and lower lesions. Upper brachial plexus lesions affect the upper roots (C5, 6) and cords. They are caused by excessive separation of the neck and shoulder such as in falls from motorcycles, cycles or horses, where the patient lands on the upper aspect of the shoulder and the head and shoulder are forced apart. They can also occur when the shoulder hits an immovable object while the body is still in motion. Wounds to the neck and contact sports may produce similar injuries. Signs and symptoms depend on which part of the plexus is involved. Careful neurological examination must be documented. There may be varying degrees of paralysis, altered sensation and anaesthesia.

Lower brachial plexus lesions occur when the arm is suddenly pulled superiorly, such as when falling from a height and grasping something to prevent the fall. The inferior trunk is injured (C8, T1), with possible avulsion of the spinal nerves. Sensation and muscle power in the ulnar nerve distribution are most commonly affected.

In any suspected brachial plexus lesion it is important to define the anatomical injury on the basis of neurological symptoms and signs. In particular, the presence of a Horner's syndrome may indicate a preganglionic and irreparable lesion. The precise location of the injury may be very difficult to establish with certainty in the emergency department and all patients with suspected brachial plexus lesions should be referred for early orthopaedic opinion.

INJURIES TO THE SHOULDER

GENERAL PRINCIPLES

The shoulder is designed for mobility rather than stability and it is vulnerable to a range of acute

Table 26.3: Screening test for shoulder movements

> The patient is instructed to:
>   Place their hands on the top of the head
>   (abduction)
>   Place their hands on the back of the neck
>   (external rotation and abduction)
>   Place their hands behind back (internal rotation,
>   adduction and extension)

Table 26.4: The rotator cuff muscles

> Supraspinatus – initiates arm elevation and abducts
>   the shoulder
> Infraspinatus – external rotator
> Teres minor – external rotator
> Subscapularis – internal rotator

and chronic injuries. Their are four articulations (glenohumeral, acromioclavicular, sternoclavicular and scapulothoracic), all of which are involved in the normal range of movement. The most important of these are the glenohumeral and the acromioclavicular joints. Examination of the acutely injured shoulder should initially focus on these.

Patients with acute shoulder injuries will often present with the shoulder adducted and supported by the other arm. Inspection of the shoulder from the front, side and back will reveal any abnormality of contour when compared to the other side. For example, if the tip of the acromion can be joined to the lateral epicondyle by a straight line then the glenohumeral joint is likely to be dislocated. Similarly, a complete acromioclavicular joint disruption will allow the shoulder to hang and make the lateral end of the clavicle very prominent. Palpation will reveal a step or tenderness. Abnormalities of peripheral sensation or circulation should be readily identifiable if there is damage to the axillary or brachial arteries. In many cases, radiography can then be requested without attempting to move the injured joint. With less severe injuries, a simple screening test can be employed to assess the range of movement (Table 26.3).

When testing individual movements it is important to separate scapulothoracic from glenohumeral movement. When testing abduction, compensatory movements of the shoulder girdle and spine can be eliminated by holding the palm downwards. This will allow the range of glenohumeral abduction to be observed. To test flexion, the palm should be facing medially. Horizontal flexion is tested with the arm abducted to 90° and rotation tested with the elbows flexed and tucked in at the waist. Extension is the least important movement.

ROTATOR CUFF INJURIES

The head of the humerus is held against the glenoid by a cuff of specialized muscles known as the rotator cuff (Table 26.4). These all originate on the scapula, traverse the glenohumeral joint and insert on the proximal humerus. Repetitive impingement of the subacromial bursa and the rotator cuff muscles and tendons produces a syndrome of acute inflammation progressing to chronic inflammation, degeneration and eventual tearing of the rotator cuff. This spectrum of impingement injury includes subacromial bursitis, rotator cuff or supraspinatous tendinitis and rotator cuff tears.

Acute rotator cuff tears may be due to direct trauma, such as traction on the arm or a relatively minor fall on a background of chronic impingement.

In patients who present to the emergency department with acute shoulder pain following a sports injury or fall, it may be impossible to distinguish an acute rotator cuff tear (partial or full thickness) from rotator cuff tendinitis or subacromial bursitis. In general terms, bursitis and tendinitis tend to affect younger patients who have a short history of repetitive activity with the arm abducted. Tears tend to occur with significant acute injury or in older patients with a history of a previous injury and chronic shoulder pain.

On examination, differences in the range of active and passive movements may help identify a rotator cuff problem. Active abduction and external rotation worsen the pain and patients are generally unable to hold the arm at full abduction (tending to hunch the shoulders instead). There may be a painful range of movement (often described as a painful arc). Passive movements tend to be easier because the rotator cuff muscles are relaxed and impingement is reduced.

Well-localized subacromial tenderness and pain on stressing the individual rotator cuff muscles may also provide further information. It is, however, notoriously difficult for the non-specialist to make an accurate diagnosis. Radiographs may be normal or reveal evidence of chronic impingement (non-specific sclerosis of the humeral head, degenerative changes in the glenohumeral and acromio-clavicular joints and osteophytes). Once fracture and dislocation have been excluded, analgesia and a sling should be provided and the patient should be followed up within a week. Stiffness can be problematic if the patient keeps the shoulder immobile for any significant length of time. The patient should be warned that pain from shoulder injuries is often worse at night and that they should tailor their analgesia to reflect this.

FRACTURES OF THE SCAPULA

Scapular fractures are rare. They can be divided into three broad categories: fractures of the muscle-covered body, fractures of the acromion and coracoid process, and fractures of the glenoid and neck. Despite being embedded in a large muscle mass, the body of the scapula is most often fractured. This results from high-energy direct blows or crush injuries and is frequently associated with underlying chest injuries and injuries of the spine and pelvis. Motorcyclists and patients ejected from vehicles in road accidents typically have these fractures. Fractures of the acromion and coronoid process tend to occur following direct blows, and fractures of the glenoid and neck of the scapula are often associated with subluxation or dislocation of the shoulder.

In the multiply injured patient, a fracture of the body of the scapula should be positively excluded on the chest radiograph (Fig. 26.1). Otherwise, these patients tend to have a shoulder series performed because of pain localized to the shoulder. Fractures of the scapula may still be overlooked, particularly fractures of the glenoid. A true antero-posterior (AP) view, an axillary view and a lateral scapular or 'Y' view may be necessary to exclude a fracture.

If a fracture of the body of the scapula is found, there should be a low index of suspicion for pulmonary contusion. It is wise to assess baseline arterial blood gases and admit these patients for observation regardless of how well they appear. Despite the forces involved, the displacement of the fracture itself is minimal and healing is usually quick and uncomplicated. Treatment is with a

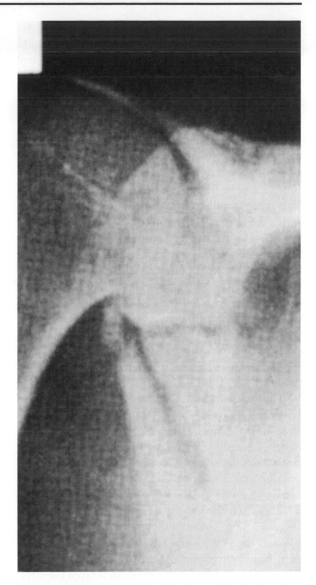

Figure 26.1: Fracture scapula seen on a chest X-ray. (Reproduced with permission from L. Solomon, D.J. Warwick and S. Nayagam (eds), *Apley's System of Orthopaedics and Fractures*, 8th edition, published by Arnold, London, 2001.)

broad arm sling and analgesia followed by gentle mobilization.

> Fractures of the body of the scapula may be associated with significant intrathoracic injury.

It may be possible to treat patients with fractures of the glenoid and acromion as out-patients. However, large articular steps in the glenoid cavity, substantial fragments (>25% of the articular surface) and associated subluxation or dislocation are indications for urgent orthopaedic referral rather than routine fracture clinic review.

FRACTURES OF THE CLAVICLE

The clavicle is the most commonly fractured bone in the body. Most injuries result from a fall directly on to the shoulder or on to the outstretched hand. The patient will support the injured arm with the other hand and there may be obvious deformity and swelling at the fracture site. The commonest site of fracture is the middle third. With complete separation of the bone ends, the medial fragment is pulled upwards and backwards by the clavicular head of sternocleidomastoid and the lateral fragment is pulled downwards, forwards and medially by the weight of the arm. The bone fragments may then overlap and there will be shortening. Most movements of the shoulder will cause considerable but well-localized pain.

The clavicle is not routinely radiographed in two projections: a single AP view will usually confirm the diagnosis (Fig. 26.2). It is important to check carefully for a greenstick fracture in children. Injuries to the acromioclavicular, sternoclavicular and shoulder joints should be excluded. Neurovascular function in the arm should be documented although, despite the proximity of the clavicle to the subclavian vessels and brachial plexus, there is rarely any injury. Occasionally, a communicating vein passing anterior to the clavicle is ruptured. This may produce a large subcutaneous haematoma anterior to the fracture site. This does not indicate subclavian vessel injury.

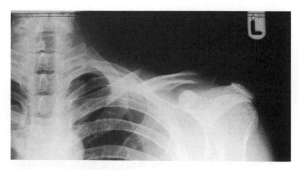

Figure 26.2: AP radiograph of clavicle fracture with overlap of fragments.

A broad arm sling and analgesia should be provided immediately. Patients with compromised or tented skin, open fractures, abnormal neurological or vascular signs in the arm and fractures associated with torticollis (possible cervical spine facet joint dislocation) must be discussed with senior staff. Otherwise there is little indication for reduction (even with comminution and extensive deformity) and the patient can be reviewed in fracture clinic.

A collar and cuff which allow the arm to pull the lateral fragment down should not be used since they do not provide support for the weight of the arm and act to distract the bony ends. Figure-of-eight bandages or other elaborate slings should not be used by the non-specialist. Immobilization should be for only as long as pain persists, in order to prevent stiffness at the shoulder and elbow (1–2 weeks). Thereafter, gentle mobilization within the limits of pain should be advised. Healing will take place over 6–10 weeks. The patient should be warned that there may be a prominence at the fracture site, much of which will resolve with time.

ACROMIOCLAVICULAR (AC) JOINT INJURIES

The clavicle is attached to the acromion by the AC and coracoclavicular ligaments. Falls on to the point of the shoulder, such as in a fall from a horse or bicycle, commonly sprain or rupture the AC ligament as the shoulder moves downwards but the clavicle is restrained by the first rib. With greater forces, all the ligaments may be ruptured and the clavicle completely separated from the acromion. In both cases there is marked pain and tenderness at the AC joint. The outer end of the clavicle will appear prominent and it may be possible to temporarily reduce a subluxation or dislocation by lifting the arm while pushing down on the clavicle. When the clavicle is no longer attached, the shoulder may appear deformed and the outer end of the clavicle will not move with the acromion when the abducted shoulder is moved anteriorly and posteriorly (horizontal flexion).

Specific radiographs should be requested when AC joint injury is suspected. Subluxation is detected as a step between the inferior surfaces of the acromion and the clavicle on an erect AP radiograph. These inferior surfaces should be

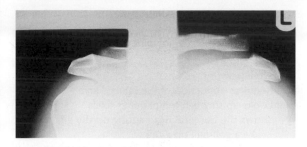

Figure 26.3: Comparative radiographs of AC joints before and after weight bearing, showing widening of the AC joint.

in a straight line. If the appearances are equivocal, further radiographs can be taken with the patient holding weights in both hands so that both AC joints can be compared (Fig. 26.3).

Where there is complete dislocation of the AC joint in the dominant hand in a patient whose work involves strenuous upper limb use, an orthopaedic opinion should be sought regarding open reduction. However, most cases can be treated initially by taking the weight off the joint with a broad arm sling and providing analgesia. Despite persistent deformity most patients achieve excellent functional results with minimal treatment.

STERNOCLAVICULAR (SC) JOINT INJURIES

Injuries to the SC joints are rare. A fall or blow to the front of the shoulder may transmit forces through the clavicle, disrupting the SC joint. Sprains may be complicated by rupture of the SC and costoclavicular ligaments, with anterior or retrosternal displacement of the medial end of the clavicle. The clavicle is most often forced forwards and downwards, leaving the patient with intense local pain, marked tenderness over the joint and an asymmetrical appearance of the suprasternal notch. Radiographs are rarely helpful. Again, the weight of the arm should be supported with a broad arm sling and the patient provided with simple analgesia. The patient should be warned that some prominence of the medial end of the clavicle may persist. Otherwise, pain will settle with time and avoidance of heavy lifting, and there is rarely any resultant instability. A much more serious but less common injury is retrosternal

displacement of the medial end of the clavicle. The structures in the thoracic inlet may be compressed in these patients and they should all be referred for further investigation (usually CT) and, if necessary, reduction under anaesthesia.

DISLOCATION OF THE SHOULDER

The glenohumeral joint may be dislocated in three directions: anterior, posterior and true inferior (luxatio erecta). Anterior dislocation is most common and results from forced abduction and extension of the arm, or forced external rotation such as occurs in a fall where the hand is fixed on the ground and the body rotates internally. The humeral head rotates externally out of the glenoid and comes to lie anteriorly and medially, to give the classic appearance of squaring of the shoulder (Fig. 26.4). There is variable damage to the anterior

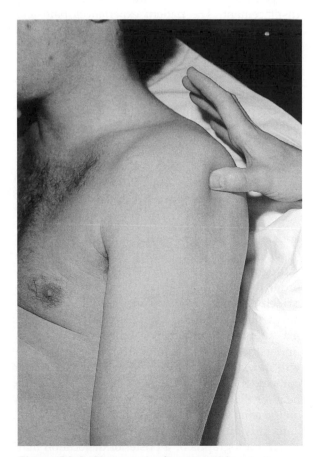

Figure 26.4: Photograph of patient with anterior shoulder dislocation showing squaring of the shoulder.

joint capsule and rotator cuff. There may also be a fracture of the greater tuberosity of the humerus or the anterior lip of the glenoid.

Anterior dislocation is often easy to identify and clinical examination should be directed at excluding lower brachial plexus lesions (radial portion of posterior cord), axillary nerve and axillary artery damage. The axillary nerve may be injured as it winds round the surgical neck of the humerus. Paralysis of the deltoid and anaesthesia over the lateral part of shoulder result, but it may be impossible to determine deltoid function in the acute phase.

Posterior dislocation is less common than anterior dislocation and easily missed. It may be caused by a direct blow on the front of the shoulder or a fall on the outstretched, internally rotated hand. It should be specifically excluded in patients who have been electrocuted or suffered generalized seizures. The head of the humerus is displaced posteriorly but there is little medial displacement. The patient experiences pain and the contour of the shoulder is abnormal when looked at from the side.

True inferior dislocation is rare. The humeral head slips inferiorly and becomes lodged beneath the glenoid with the arm fully abducted. The patient presents with their arm fully abducted and held above their head. There may be significant neurovascular damage.

Radiographs should always be obtained before attempted reduction. An AP view is standard and may show anterior dislocation clearly. In all cases, however, a second view should be taken. Patients with dislocated shoulders experience a lot of pain and are reluctant to allow the shoulder to be moved at all. Thus, analgesia should be provided before radiography, as some movement is inevitable in order to obtain appropriate views. There are two principal types of second view: axial or 'armpit' and Y view (Table 26.5). It is essential that the normal anatomy on whichever second view is used is understood. Radiographs of an anterior dislocation will show the head of the humerus lying under the coracoid process on the AP view (Fig. 26.5), the head of the humerus lying anterior to the glenoid on the axial view (Fig. 26.6) and the head displaced anteriorly on the Y view (Fig. 26.7).

AP radiographs of a posterior dislocation may initially appear normal. Internal rotation of the humeral head may, however, alter the shape of the

Table 26.5: Shoulder radiography

An AP view should be obtained in all patients (Fig. 26.5)

An axial view (Fig. 26.6):
   Requires abduction of the injured arm
   Looks up through the patient's axilla
   Shows the humeral head sitting on the glenoid like a golf-ball on a tee
   Shows the acromion and coracoid processes (which point anteriorly)

A Y view (Fig. 26.7):
   Is a lateral scapular view
   Does not require the arm to be moved
   Shows the scapula posteriorly and the ribs anteriorly
   Shows the blade of the scapula (stem of Y)
   Shows the coracoid and acromion (limbs of Y)
   Shows the humeral head overlying the centre of the glenoid (centre of Y)

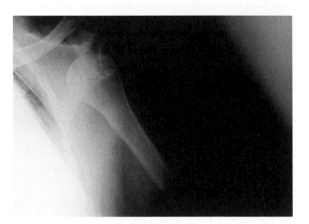

Figure 26.5: Typical appearance of anterior dislocation on AP radiograph.

humeral head on the radiograph and give it a 'light- bulb' appearance (Fig. 26.8). The head of the humerus will lie posterior to the glenoid on the axial view and be displaced posteriorly on the Y view.

Dislocations without fractures should be reduced in the emergency department. Orthopaedic or senior medical advice should be sought for fracture/ dislocations before attempted reduction. Reduction requires adequate analgesia, the correct environment, adequate personnel and the correct manoeuvre. No single method will work for all dislocations, but the most commonly used technique

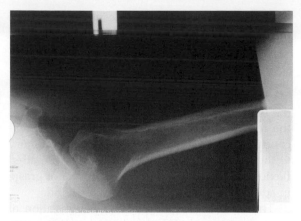

Figure 26.6: Axial X-ray of posterior dislocation.

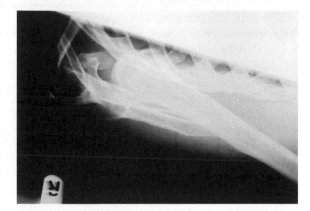

Figure 26.7: Y-view (lateral scapula) radiograph of anterior dislocation.

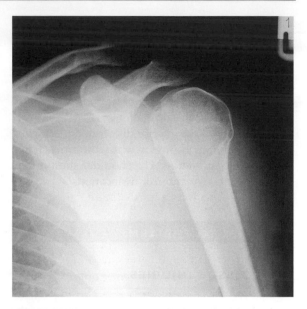

Figure 26.8: AP radiograph of posterior dislocation with 'lightbulb' shape of humeral head (compare with Fig. 26.5).

Table 26.6: Reduction of anterior dislocation of shoulder – Kocher's method

Provide adequate analgesia and sedation if necessary
Apply traction along the arm with the elbow flexed
Slowly rotate the arm externally
If muscle resistance felt, stop for a moment then continue
Once 90° external rotation reached, shoulder may reduce
If pain and spasm prevent external rotation then provide further analgesia and consider referral
If external rotation achieved but shoulder has not reduced, maintain traction and adduct the shoulder (bring elbow across chest)
Then rotate the shoulder internally to bring the hand towards the opposite shoulder
If unsuccessful, repeat all stages
Repeat radiography after reduction

for anterior dislocations is Kocher's method (Table 26.6). An often forgotten alternative is to use gravity and lie the patient face down on the couch with a fluid bag or sandbag under the clavicle. The arm is then allowed to hang freely (weights can be added) and the patient is pro-vided with analgesia. As the muscles relax, the dislocation will often reduce spontaneously. In a busy department there is no reason why patients with anterior dislocations cannot lie in this position during the inevitable wait for formal reduction.

Radiography should be repeated after all reductions. Once reduction has been achieved, the patient should be provided with a collar and cuff and advised to wear appropriate clothing so that external rotation is prevented. A further examination of the neurovascular status should be made and documented. An alternative is to provide a body bandage or stocking, but many patients find this uncomfortable. All dislocated shoulders should be reviewed in fracture clinic.

Reduction of a posterior dislocation is achieved by applying traction to the abducted shoulder and rotating the arm externally. If the reduction appears stable then the patient can be provided with a collar and cuff, analgesia, and a routine fracture clinic appointment. Uncertainty regarding stability should warrant urgent orthopaedic review. Instability may occur because of damage to the posterior joint capsule, and patients with unstable injuries may require plaster immobilization in abduction and external rotation.

Reduction of true inferior dislocation is achieved by traction in the position in which the arm is lying, followed by adduction. The shoulder should then be managed as for anterior dislocations.

INJURIES TO THE ARM

SOFT-TISSUE INJURIES

Wounds in the upper arm may damage the brachial artery, the median, ulnar or radial nerves and the tendons of the muscles that act at the shoulder and elbow. Wounds that extend beyond the deep fascia should be referred for appropriate surgical review depending on local policy. Incised wounds and lacerations can often be cleaned and closed provided there is no evidence of glass or other foreign bodies. A low threshold for soft-tissue radiography should be maintained.

The triceps tendon may rupture spontaneously or after injury. There is usually well-localized pain of sudden onset and a defect can be felt in the tendon. There will be weakness of resisted extension at the elbow. Distal biceps rupture may also occur after a single traumatic event and is usually a sports injury associated with heavy lifting or sudden forced contraction of the biceps. There is sudden pain in the antecubital fossa and weakness of elbow flexion and supination. A defect will also be palpable. The long head of biceps can also rupture at its proximal insertion following sudden heavy lifting or pulling. Rupture may be associated with chronic impingement and bicipital tendinitis. In these cases, relatively little force may be required to cause rupture. The ruptured biceps muscle will bulge in the arm.

The median nerve arises from the lateral and medial cords of the brachial plexus and runs with the brachial artery to the antecubital fossa, where it lies deep to the bicipital aponeurosis and the median cubital vein (medial to the brachial artery). There are no branches in the arm. Damage to the median nerve in the arm will cause weakness of pronation of the forearm and flexion of the wrist, in addition to the classic features of median nerve damage seen in the hand.

The ulnar nerve is the terminal branch of the medial cord of the brachial plexus and it runs with the brachial artery deep within the arm. It enters the forearm by passing between the medial epicondyle of the humerus and the olecranon. Injury to the ulnar nerve in the arm will cause impaired flexion and adduction of the wrist and poor grasp, in addition to ulnar nerve signs in the hand.

The radial nerve is the direct continuation of the posterior cord of the brachial plexus. It passes around the body of the humerus in the radial groove and then anterior to the lateral epicondyle, where it divides into deep and superficial branches. The deep branch is entirely muscular. Injury to the radial nerve proximal to the origin of triceps results in weakness of triceps, brachioradialis, supinator and extensors of the wrist, thumb and fingers. When the radial nerve is injured in the radial groove by a humeral shaft fracture, the triceps is not completely paralysed. Wrist drop is the characteristic clinical sign in the hand.

FRACTURES OF THE PROXIMAL HUMERUS

Fractures of the proximal humerus are often caused by a direct blow to the anterior or lateral part of the arm, a fall on the side of the body or a fall on the outstretched hand in an elderly osteoporotic patient. In younger patients, these are high-energy injuries that result from contact sports, heavy falls or road traffic accidents. The patient will support the arm with the other hand. There will typically be severe pain in the upper arm that is aggravated by movement. There may also be gross deformity or bruising gravitating down the arm, particularly if presentation is delayed.

There are many different patterns of proximal humerus fractures but these can be grouped into four main types in adults:

- avulsion fractures of the tuberosities
- impacted fractures of the surgical or anatomical neck
- displaced comminuted fractures
- fracture–dislocations.

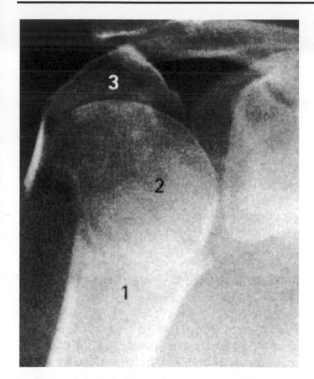

Figure 26.9: AP radiograph of three-part proximal humeral fracture. (Reproduced with permission from L. Solomon, D.J. Warwick and S. Nayagam (eds), *Apley's System of Orthopaedics and Fractures*, 8th edition, published by Arnold, London, 2001.)

These are usually diagnosed by AP and lateral radiographs (Fig. 26.9) and are commonly described by the specific injury or the number of fragments involved (e.g. 'three-part fracture'). In children, the common injuries are a greenstick fracture of the surgical neck or proximal epiphyseal separation.

Proximal humerus fractures can, as with shoulder dislocations, cause neurovascular damage. The axillary neurovascular bundle is immediately anteromedial to the glenoid and may be compressed or disrupted by the fracture. If the humeral shaft is displaced medially, the lower cords of the brachial plexus may also be damaged. Neurovascular examination is essential to exclude these complications.

Correct shoulder function relies on the orientation of the rotator cuff muscle insertions (tuberosities) and the humeral head. It is therefore important to obtain early orthopaedic advice about the management of these injuries, and all patients should be seen in fracture clinic unless there is an indication for immediate referral. While awaiting clinic review, patients with undisplaced avulsion fractures of the tuberosities and undisplaced or impacted fractures of the neck can be treated with a sling and analgesia. Displaced or angulated fractures of the neck may benefit from the gentle traction applied by the weight of the arm in a collar and cuff. Where disimpaction is unnecessary, a broad arm sling should be used. Dislocations with fracture of the greater tuberosity should be treated like uncomplicated dislocations of the shoulder and reduced. The greater tuberosity will usually return to its normal position. Failed reductions, displaced fractures of the tuberosities and complex fracture dislocations should all be referred urgently for orthopaedic review.

HUMERAL SHAFT FRACTURES

Fractures of the humeral shaft may result from either direct forces such as blows to the arm or falls on to the side, or indirect forces such as a twisting fall or a fall on an outstretched hand. The humerus is also a common site for pathological fractures. The patient will be unable to move their elbow or shoulder and will be supporting the injured arm against the torso with the other hand. There may be detectable mobility at the fracture site, although deliberate attempts should not be made to elicit this.

Radiographs in two projections will show the true relation of the fragments. In fractures involving the upper third, the upper fragment will be pulled medially by pectoralis major. In middle third fractures the upper fragment tends to be abducted, owing to deltoid pull. The radiograph therefore frequently reveals a displaced and angulated fracture. The radial nerve may be injured in middle third fractures as it spirals round the humerus. It may be transected, trapped between the fragments, impaled on a bone spike or simply contused. Evidence of radial nerve palsy (weak extensors of the wrist) should be sought.

Simple fractures may be treated by analgesia and a collar and cuff. A hanging plaster or a U-slab may enhance traction in moderately displaced fractures. Open fractures, fractures with comminution, marked angulation or displacement, and patients with radial nerve injury should be referred immediately for orthopaedic review.

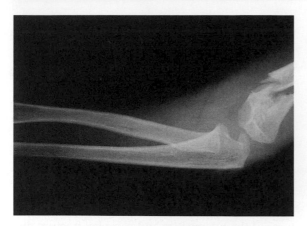

Figure 26.10: Radiographic appearance of a supracondylar fracture of the humerus.

FRACTURES OF THE DISTAL HUMERUS (FIG. 26.10)

A fall on the outstretched hand or on to the point of the elbow may result in a supracondylar fracture of the humerus. These fractures of the distal humerus are more common in children than in adults. They should be excluded in all children who have pain, swelling and restriction of movement around the elbow following injury. On examination, there may be marked swelling and deformity with tenderness over the distal humerus. The radial, anterior interosseous, median and ulnar nerves and the brachial artery can be damaged as the distal fragment is displaced (usually posteriorly) during the injury.

AP and lateral radiographs of the elbow will reveal the majority of fractures, although greenstick fractures can be difficult to identify and up to a third of fractures will be undisplaced. The fracture line is usually transverse and lies just proximal to the trochlea and capitellum. The complexity of the epiphyseal arrangement around the elbow in children and difficulties with radiographic positioning in all patients can lead to difficulty interpreting the films (see Table 26.7). Comparison views of the other elbow are justified if there is diagnostic difficulty.

Provided neurovascular damage has been excluded, pure posterior, lateral or medial displacement of less than 50% of bony contact and greenstick fractures without angulation can often be managed conservatively. Undisplaced fractures in adults can

be held in an above-elbow back slab with a sling, or treated with only a collar and cuff in children. The radial pulse must be checked after applying the cast. If this has been lost, the dressings from in front of the elbow should all be cut and the arm extended slightly until pulse is restored (a pulse oximeter on the finger during application of the plaster can be a useful way of monitoring the pulse waveform). It is often advisable to refer children with displaced supracondylar fractures for a period of observation, given the risk of neurovascular damage.

Urgent operative reduction is generally indicated if there is evidence of arterial obstruction, off-ending of the fracture or significant angulation (e.g. a tilt of greater than 15° from the normal 45° relationship between the articular surfaces of the humerus and the humeral shaft).

In adults, a direct blow or a fall on to the point of the elbow with the elbow flexed may cause fractures which, in contrast to children, commonly involve the articular surfaces and split the distal humerus. Intra-articular fractures bleed into the joint capsule and cause swelling and stiffness in the elbow. Operative repair may be required if the fragments are large, but conservative management often suffices. Nevertheless, orthopaedic advice should be sought.

INJURIES TO THE ELBOW

SOFT-TISSUE INJURY ABOUT THE ELBOW

The elbow is injured relatively infrequently compared to other upper limb joints. Soft-tissue injuries tend to represent over-use rather than acute sprains or tendon rupture. The most frequent of these are medial and lateral epicondylitis and olecranon bursitis. Wounds around the elbow can damage the brachial artery and any combination of the radial, ulnar and median nerves, but these are uncommon.

Lateral epicondylitis is commonly referred to as tennis elbow. It is caused by inflammation at the insertion of the common extensor origin. Patients present with pain and tenderness over the lateral epicondyle which may radiate down the arm. This may follow acute injury or, more commonly, a period of unaccustomed activity that puts tension on the common extensor tendon. Tennis and other racquet sports are good examples but not the only cause of this condition. The pain is reproduced by both active extension and passive flexion of the wrist (with the elbow held straight). Treatment involves rest, activity modification as appropriate and analgesia. Physiotherapy may also be required. More rarely resistant cases may require local steroid injection or even surgery. An avulsion fracture of the lateral epicondyle should be excluded if there has been an injury.

Tennis elbow is *lateral* epicondylitis.

Medial epicondylitis is commonly referred to as golfer's elbow. It is caused by inflammation of the common flexor origin. Patients present with pain and tenderness over the medial epicondyle that may also radiate down the arm. As with lateral epicondylitis, this may follow acute injury or a period of any unaccustomed activity that puts tension on the common flexor tendon. Tennis, golf and other activities involving repetitive wrist flexion and pronation may be responsible. The pain can be reproduced by both active flexion and resisted extension of the wrist. The ulnar nerve may be involved in the inflammatory process in two-thirds of patients and ulnar nerve signs should be sought. Treatment also involves rest, activity modification, analgesia and physiotherapy. An avulsion fracture of the medial epicondyle should be excluded if there has been a specific injury.

Golfer's elbow is *medial* epicondylitis.

Olecranon bursitis is inflammation of the superficial olecranon bursa following blunt injury or repetitive stress. It may also be a manifestation of gout or rheumatoid arthritis (see Chapter 31). The bursa is enlarged and may be pain free. There is usually little or no restriction of elbow movement. Tenderness and erythema associated with systemic symptoms suggest a septic bursitis. This should be excluded by aspiration and urgent microscopy of the aspirate. Simple bursitis can be treated with rest and activity modification. Patients with septic bursitis should be investigated further and treated with antibiotics. These patients should be followed up to ensure resolution of symptoms.

PULLED ELBOW

Pulled elbow is a specific upper limb injury frequently seen in young children (usually under 4 years old). When the child is suddenly lifted by the wrist or hand with the elbow extended and the forearm pronated, the radial head is pulled out of the annular ligament. The child experiences pain and subsequently refuses to use the affected arm. The elbow is typically held partially flexed and pronated. There may be tenderness over the lateral side of the elbow. If there is a clear history of sudden traction and the appearances are characteristic, it is generally acceptable to attempt reduction during initial examination. This is achieved by placing the thumb over the radial head then, with the other hand, supinating and pronating the forearm fully with the elbow flexed to 90°. The child will often cry out and the radial head will be felt to reduce. Following a successful reduction the child should start using the arm and hand, although it may be necessary to wait for about an hour. Failure to use the arm after this merits an X-ray to exclude a fracture. However, some small children will not use their arm for up to 48 h following successful reduction of a pulled elbow and if the X-ray is normal, clinic review in 24 h is appropriate. In some cases, reluctance to move the arm may be due to failure of reduction: in these cases review at 24 h is also appropriate and very often the pulled elbow will have reduced spontaneously before clinic review.

In cases where the history is uncertain, elbow radiographs should be obtained to exclude a fracture before attempting reduction. A pulled elbow is often reduced by the radiographer positioning the elbow at 90° for a lateral radiograph.

FRACTURES AROUND THE ELBOW

Falls on to the point of the elbow and the outstretched arm may cause fractures around the elbow. Typically, these are either distal humeral (supracondylar fractures) or fractures of the olecranon or radial head. However, the medial and lateral epicondyles may be avulsed and complex intra-articular fractures of the humeral condyles may occur.

Almost all patients will complain of severe pain and will support the injured elbow. There is often

Table 26.7: Radiographic interpretation of elbow views

Look for:
On the AP film:
   Uninterrupted cortices around the ulna, radial
      head and neck and distal humerus
   An abnormal radiocapitellar line (a line drawn
      along the centre of the shaft of the proximal
      radius should pass through the capitellum)
   The ossification centre of the trochlea and, if
      that is present, the ossification centre of the
      medial epicondyle
On the lateral:
   A visible posterior fat pad (always abnormal)
   A displaced anterior fat pad (may be normal
      unless displaced)
   Uninterrupted cortices around the ulna, radial
      head and neck and distal humerus
   An abnormal radiocapitellar line
   An abnormal anterior humeral line
      (approximately one-third of the capitellum lies
      anterior to a line traced along the anterior
      cortex of the humerus)
   The medial epicondyle lying within the joint

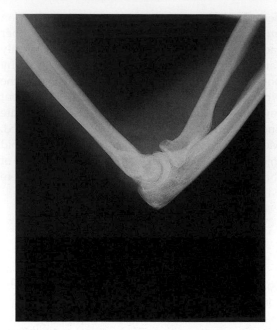

Figure 26.11: Lateral radiograph of elbow showing abnormal anterior and posterior fat pads.

considerable swelling and the elbow is held partially flexed. There is often little to be gained from clinical examination other than localization of tenderness and reassurance that neurovascular function remains intact. AP and lateral radiographs will usually identify the fracture (Table 26.7).

A useful clue to the presence of a subtle fracture is the presence of a visible posterior fat pad and a displaced anterior fat pad on the lateral view. These fat pads are in close association with the joint capsule and appear as black streaks adjacent to the surrounding grey soft tissues. A joint effusion or haemarthrosis displaces the fat pads away from the bone. A visible posterior fat pad is always abnormal. An anterior fat pad may be visible in normal films but it should not be displaced (Fig. 26.11). Other radiographic features to suggest injury are given in Table 26.7.

A common problem is the patient with a history of direct or indirect elbow injury following a fall, a reduced range of movement on examination and visible fat pads but no fracture on radiographic examination. The effusion may be felt as a bulging of the joint capsule mid-way between the lateral epicondyle and the olecranon process. There is likely to be a radial head or other intra-articular fracture

in these patients and they should be reviewed in clinic. Repeat films may subsequently reveal the fracture if there is little clinical improvement.

The medial epicondyle may be avulsed or fractured by sudden contraction of the forearm flexors or a direct blow. In most cases there is bruising and pain around the medial epicondyle, with symptoms similar to medial epicondylitis (although more severe). There may be ulnar nerve injury as well. Radiographs will usually reveal the fracture in adults, although there may be considerable difficulty in children because of the variable development of ossification centres. Paradoxically, minor displacement may be more obvious than major displacement (when the avulsed fragment may come to lie within the elbow joint). Undisplaced fractures may be treated with analgesia, collar and cuff and routine fracture clinic follow-up.

The medial epicondyle usually ossifies by 6 years of age although this may be variable. A useful rule of thumb is therefore to look for the ossification centre of the trochlea on the radiograph. This invariably ossifies after the medial epicondyle. Thus if the trochlea is visible, the medial epicondyle should also be visible somewhere on the radiograph. If it is not where it should be, then it has been avulsed (Fig. 26.12).

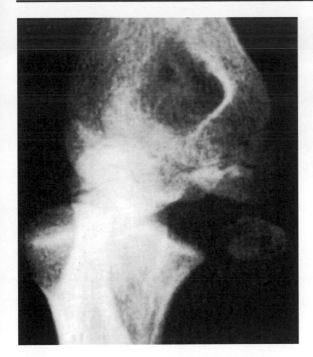

Figure 26.12: Avulsion fracture of the medial epicondyle in a child. (Reproduced with permission from L. Solomon, D.J. Warwick and S. Nayagam (eds), *Apley's System of Orthopaedics and Fractures*, 8th edition, published by Arnold, London, 2001.)

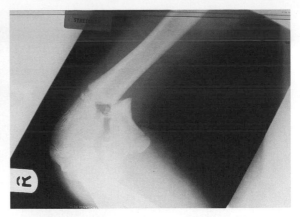

Figure 26.13: Radiograph of complex elbow fracture.

During dislocation of the elbow, the medial epicondyle may also be avulsed. It may subsequently become lodged within the joint when the elbow is reduced. This diagnosis may be made radiographically by identifying whether the medial epicondyle is visible on the lateral film. If it is, then it is lying within the joint. These patients require manipulation under anaesthesia and possibly open reduction.

The lateral epicondyle is much less frequently injured than the medial epicondyle. Fracture may follow a varus strain and the fragment may be displaced. Rarely, it may become lodged within the joint. Symptoms and signs resemble those of lateral epicondylitis. The ossification centre for the lateral epicondyle appears much later than that for the medial epicondyle and there is rarely the same degree of diagnostic difficulty as in medial epicondyle injuries.

Fracture of the condyles, capitellum and trochlea, intercondylar fractures and comminuted fractures may all cause intra-articular fragments (Fig. 26.13) and long-term elbow problems. These complex injuries should all be referred for orthopaedic opinion.

Fractures of the olecranon tend to follow a fall on the point of the elbow. They may become displaced owing to the pull of the triceps tendon. Less frequently, the fracture may represent an avulsion fracture caused by forced contraction of triceps (or resisted extension of the elbow). In minimally displaced fractures, it is reasonable to place the arm in an above-elbow back slab and refer the patient to fracture clinic. There is, however, a risk of further displacement. Displaced fractures require immediate orthopaedic referral.

Radial head and neck fractures are considered here because they often present as elbow stiffness and pain. In a fall on the outstretched hand, the radial head impacts with the capitellum and may fracture in a number of ways. The patient will present with a painful elbow with restricted extension. Supination and pronation are often preserved. In some cases, tenderness will not be elicited until the radial head is rotated under the examiner's thumb. The fracture is usually visible on the standard elbow radiographs but additional radial head views may be required (Fig. 26.14). Undisplaced fractures should be mobilized early. The patient will require analgesia and a sling, together with advice about maintaining mobility of the elbow. It may take several months for full extension to be restored. Displaced fractures will restrict pronation and therefore require orthopaedic review. Grossly displaced or comminuted fractures are best treated by early excision and mobilization and should therefore also be referred urgently.

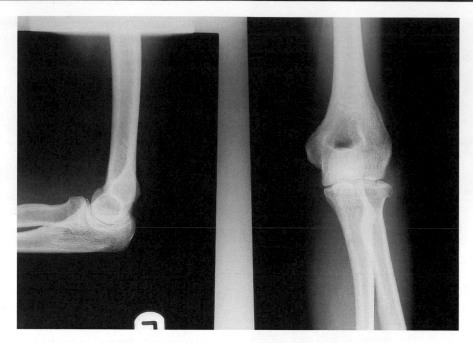

Figure 26.14: Radiograph showing a radial head fracture.

DISLOCATION OF THE ELBOW

Dislocation of the elbow is frequently caused by a fall on to the outstretched hand with the elbow partially flexed. The patient is in great pain and will support the arm. On examination there is often marked swelling and deformity, with loss of the normal contour of the olecranon and epicondyles. A dislocated elbow can be distinguished from a supracondylar fracture by the relationship between the epicondyles and the olecranon. These structures normally form an equilateral triangle when looking at the flexed elbow from behind. This relationship is distorted when the elbow is dislocated. This distinction is rarely of any value given that both injuries will be clearly identified radiographically (Fig. 26.15). Associated fractures of the humeral condyles, epicondyles, coronoid process and radial head may also be seen. The radius and ulna are most often dislocated posteriorly and laterally relative to the humerus. Occasionally, the ulna or radius may be dislocated in isolation. These injuries are always associated with accompanying injuries to the radius and ulna, and further radiographs should be obtained to identify these (see below). The brachial artery, radial and ulnar nerves

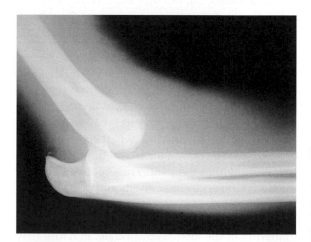

Figure 26.15: Radiograph showing dislocation of the elbow.

are then vulnerable to damage, and this should be excluded in every case.

Reduction can be achieved by applying traction along the limb with the elbow in slight flexion. The elbow often reduces with a definite 'clunk'. An assistant can greatly assist the reduction by placing their hands around the arm from behind and pushing on the olecranon with the thumbs. Once reduced, repeat radiographs should be obtained and the elbow placed in an above-elbow plaster back slab at 90°. All dislocations with associated fractures should be discussed with the orthopaedic team. Uncomplicated dislocations may be reviewed in fracture clinic.

INJURIES TO THE FOREARM

SOFT-TISSUE INJURY

The forearm is a common site for wounds, crush injuries and fractures. Considerable anxiety is caused by forearm wounds that involve profuse arterial bleeding. Bleeding can always be controlled by both direct pressure and elevation or, if this cannot be tolerated by the patient, application of pressure or a tourniquet over proximal arteries. A sphygmomanometer can be used as an above-elbow tourniquet. Attempts at clamping or tying the severed artery often damage the vessel further and may result in excessive blood loss. Once bleeding has been controlled, the patient can be treated for shock and referred urgently for exploration and surgical repair.

As with the upper arm, any wound that penetrates the deep fascia should also be referred for surgical review. More superficial wounds can often be managed in the emergency department. Of particular importance are injuries involving glass and those that may lead to the development of a compartment syndrome.

All wounds caused by glass should have soft tissue radiographs to exclude retention of glass in the wound.

This should be the case for all wounds, regardless of how convinced the patient and doctor are that there is no glass in the wound. If glass is found then the patient should be referred for surgical review, given the danger of damaging other structures in the forearm during removal. 'Blind' removal of foreign bodies is rarely successful and a formal attempt with a bloodless field and image intensification where necessary is much more appropriate.

There is a high incidence of compartment syndrome in forearm injuries. As discussed in Chapter 25, increased pressure within confined fascial compartments may lead to ischaemia, necrosis, contractures and permanent limb deformity. Although the forearm compartments are most vulnerable, fascial compartments in the arm may also be affected and clinical evidence of compartment syndrome should be sought in all upper limb injuries. Compartment syndromes may occur shortly after the initial injury or several hours later. The typical symptoms are persistent pain that is disproportionate to the severity of the injury (and poorly responsive to analgesia or splinting), a tensely swollen and tender muscle compartment, and worsening of the pain on passive stretching of the muscles within the compartment. There may be subtle sensory impairment and paraesthesiae as nerves passing through the compartment become hypoxic. The intracompartmental pressures rarely rise sufficiently to obstruct the brachial or radial arteries so the pulse is usually maintained and the hand remains warm.

The presence of a distal pulse does not exclude compartment syndrome.

As with the lower limb, immediate treatment includes splitting any plaster or removing bandages and elevating the limb. A clinical diagnosis is usually sufficient to arrange urgent fasciotomy and decompression, although many surgeons measure compartment pressure directly. Urgent orthopaedic review is required for any patient with a suspected compartment syndrome.

The median, ulnar and radial nerves may be damaged by injury to the forearm. These injuries are usually caused by incised wounds that may result from deliberate self-harm or, more often, by accidents in the kitchen or falls while holding a glass. The median nerve supplies most of the anterior compartment muscles of the forearm before becoming relatively superficial at the wrist. At the wrist it lies medial to the flexor carpi radialis tendon and deep to palmaris longus (which is absent in about 20% of people). It is most commonly injured at the wrist just proximal to the flexor retinaculum and carpal tunnel. In the hand the median nerve gives off motor fibres to the three thenar muscles (abductor pollicis brevis, flexor pollicis brevis and opponens pollicis) and the first and second lumbrical muscles.

Injury to the median nerve around the elbow results in weakness of pronation and flexion of the wrist and fingers as well as loss of thumb movements and impaired sensation in the hand. Flexor tendon injuries are frequently associated, as the median nerve lies deep to the flexor tendons in the forearm. Injury to the median nerve at the wrist will result in classic hand signs such as inability to oppose, abduct or flex the thumb and loss of sensation in the lateral portion of the palm, the palmar surface of the thumb and the radial two and a half fingers. Simple tests of median nerve motor function are to ask the patient to make a fist, and to resist attempts to press the abducted thumb into the plane of the hand with the back of the hand lying flat on a table.

The radial nerve is occasionally injured with deep wounds of the forearm. The radial nerve passes into the forearm anterior to the lateral epicondyle and divides into deep (posterior interosseous) and superficial (radial nerve) branches. The posterior interosseous branch supplies most of the extensor muscles in the forearm and the superficial radial nerve continues on the radial side of the forearm lateral to the radial artery. It supplies sensation to the dorsum of the thumb, first web space and hand. Injury at the elbow (or to the deep branch) results in weakness of wrist, thumb and finger extension and loss of sensation on posterior surface of forearm, hand and proximal phalanges of lateral three and a half digits. The sensory innervation overlaps with the median and ulnar nerves and is so variable that normal sensation does not indicate an intact radial nerve.

The ulnar nerve enters the forearm between the olecranon and medial epicondyle and is particularly vulnerable to both elbow injuries and wounds along the ulnar border of the forearm. It lies relatively superficially in the distal forearm just medial to the ulnar artery and supplies the small muscles of the hand. The characteristic clinical sign of ulnar nerve damage is inability to adduct or abduct the medial four digits (weak interosseous muscles). This can be demonstrated by asking the patient to hold a piece of paper between the ring and little fingers with the fingers extended. Flexion of the ring and little fingers and sensation over the ulnar one and a half digits and the ulnar half of the palm is also impaired.

All patients with suspected nerve injury should be referred urgently for surgical review. Early repair is possible and may restore a great deal of useful function.

RADIAL AND ULNAR FRACTURES

The bones of the forearm are often fractured following direct blows or in falls where the forearm is subjected to twisting forces. Adults tend to have either isolated fractures of the ulna or complex angulated and displaced fractures of both bones. Children more commonly have greenstick fractures where the cortex on one or both bones remains at least partially intact and there is angulation but no displacement. In all cases, patients with visible deformity of the forearm require early analgesia and splinting in a position of comfort before radiography. The distal pulses and sensation must always be checked and the development of compartment syndrome considered.

Fractures of the forearm bones are often associated with radio-ulnar joint dislocations and axial or rotational deformity. The radius and ulna are bound together at the elbow and wrist, as well as throughout their length, by the interosseous membrane. Thus any injury to one of these bones is frequently associated with an injury to either the other bone or to the ligaments that bind them. If isolated fracture of the radius or ulna occurs with angulation or displacement but no dislocation, then there must also be shortening of the forearm and the other bone must be dislocated at either the elbow or the wrist. The commonest combination of this type is a fracture of the ulna with dislocation of the radial head. This combination is often referred to as the Monteggia fracture–dislocation and is typically caused by forced pronation. The characteristic radiographic abnormality is disruption of the radio-capitellar line on the AP or lateral elbow views (Fig. 26.16). This is a line drawn through the centre of the shaft of the radius. It should always pass through the capitellum on both views. If it does not, then the radial head is dislocated.

Monteggia fracture: fracture of the ulna with dislocation of the radial head.

The mirror image of this injury is a fracture of the radial shaft with dislocation of the ulna at the distal radio-ulnar joint (Fig. 26.17). This is referred to as the Galeazzi fracture–dislocation. The distal end of

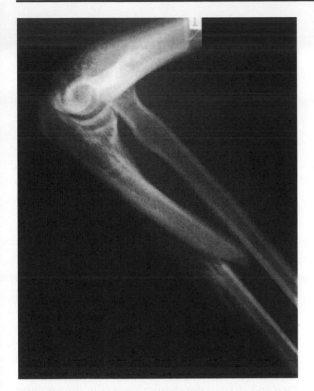

Figure 26.16: The Monteggia fracture–dislocation: fracture of the ulna with dislocation of the radial head.

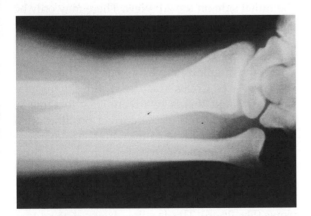

Figure 26.17: The Galeazzi fracture–dislocation: fracture of the radial shaft with dislocation of the ulna at the distal radio-ulnar joint.

the ulna (excluding the ulnar styloid) should lie just proximal to the articular surface of the radius on AP radiographs of the wrist. If it extends further distally then the joint is disrupted. Both of these injuries should always be excluded in patients with isolated radial or ulnar fractures. Radiographs of the forearm must therefore include the whole length

of the radius and ulna together with the elbow and wrist joint in both AP and lateral views.

> Galeazzi fracture: fracture of the radial shaft with dislocation of the ulna at the distal radio-ulnar joint.

> Dislocation at the proximal or distal radio-ulnar joints should always be excluded in patients with isolated radial or ulnar fractures.

Axial rotation occurs in forearm fractures if the fracture line allows the pronators of the forearm to work independently of the supinators. This is more common in fractures involving the upper third of the radius, where the proximal fragment is supinated by the action of biceps and the distal fragment is pronated by pronator teres and quadratus. Axial rotation occurs in addition to any angulation or displacement caused by the fracture. Rotational deformity may be evidenced on plain films by loss of the normal relationship between bony landmarks on lateral or AP films. In extreme cases, a lateral forearm radiograph may show a lateral view of the elbow but an AP view of the wrist. Because of the complexity of these injuries and the fact that they invariably require internal fixation, orthopaedic review should be sought in every case.

Direct blows can result in isolated transverse fractures of the radius or ulna, but fracture or dislocation of the other bone must still always be excluded. The ulna is most often fractured in isolation, as the forearm is used to defend against direct blows. An undisplaced fracture of the ulna can be treated with an above-elbow plaster (with the hand in mid-pronation) and a broad arm sling. Routine fracture clinic review can then be arranged.

In children, the fractures are frequently buckle or greenstick fractures. In buckle or torus fractures, there is often a subtle buckling of one or both cortices of the distal radius or ulna. These are essentially compression fractures and they are rarely displaced. They heal without complication and can be treated symptomatically (Fig. 26.18). A short period in a below-elbow plaster may be required to control pain. These fractures are very commonly missed. Greenstick fractures in the forearm are usually angulated but, because at least one cortex is intact, are not displaced (Fig. 26.19). Whether manipulation is required or not depends on the degree of angulation. Angular deformities of less

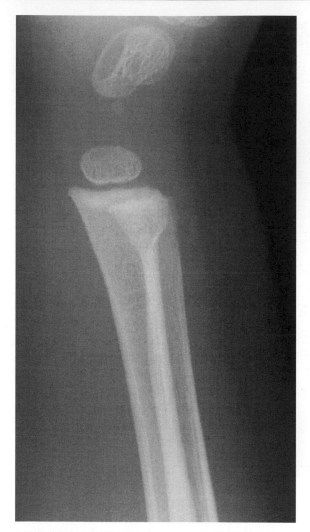

Figure 26.18: Radiograph of wrist showing buckle or torus fracture.

than 10° rarely require manipulation. However, the presence of intact periosteum and cortex at the concavity of the fracture can cause further angulation. It is often necessary to overcorrect the deformity to reduce it and great care is required in applying the plaster. These fractures should therefore be discussed with the orthopaedic team.

DISTAL RADIAL FRACTURES

Fractures of the distal radius are amongst the commonest limb fractures seen in the emergency department. They are caused by falls on to the outstretched

hand with the hand itself in various positions, the most common being a Colles' fracture. A Colles' fracture is a fracture of the distal radius within 2.5 cm of the wrist joint which results in dorsal angulation and displacement of the distal fragment towards the dorsum and the radial side (Fig. 26.20). There is accompanying damage to the inferior radio-ulnar joint and the ulnar styloid may be avulsed by the triangular fibro-cartilage as the distal radial fragment displaces. It is predominantly seen in middle-aged to elderly women who have fallen on to the pronated outstretched hand (so-called 'fall on outstretched hand' or FOOSH).

The patient has a painful and often obviously deformed wrist (described as the dinner-fork deformity). However, much more subtle presentations can arise and all patients with pain and tenderness of the distal radius after a fall should have AP and lateral wrist radiographs.

The fracture is usually obvious on the films but may be missed if impaction has rendered the fracture line difficult to see. In these cases, it is useful to measure the angles between the articular surface and shaft of the radius. Normally, the articular surface of the distal radius is tilted forward on the lateral view and approximately 20° forward on the radial side on the AP view. There may only be a reduction of these angles with a subtle buckle in the cortex over the dorsal aspect of the distal radius, or a very slight increase in bone density where the fragments have impacted.

A displaced Colles' fracture requires manipulation. Although this is relatively easy to achieve, holding the fracture in the correct position often causes problems. In deciding whether to manipulate the fracture, the degree of deformity, the presence of an ulnar styloid fracture or a backward tilt of 10° or more on the lateral radiograph may be used as a guide. Any clinically obvious deformity requires manipulation. Fractures of the ulnar styloid indicate significant disruption of the radio-ulnar joint and backward tilt of greater than 10° will affect future wrist flexion and hand function. If there is doubt about whether to manipulate a fracture, senior advice should be sought.

Colles' fractures are much less common in younger adults and do not occur in children. The same mechanism of injury tends to be associated with comminuted fractures of the distal radius or fractures of the radial styloid in young adults. Where the distal radial fragment is comminuted

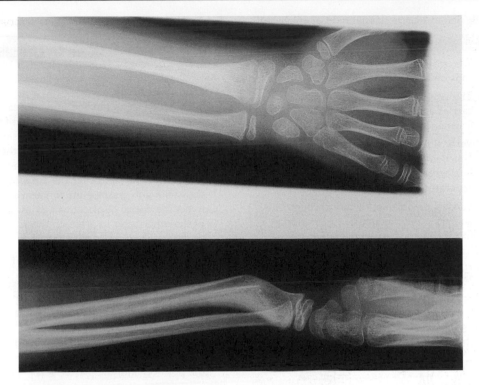

Figure 26.19: Radiograph of forearm showing angulated greenstick fracture.

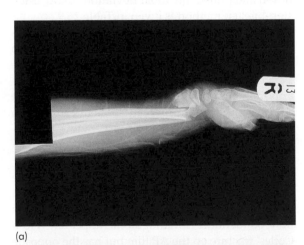

(a)

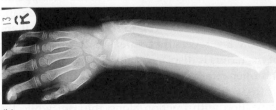

(b)

Figure 26.20: Colles' fracture. (a) Lateral and (b) AP radiographs.

and the fracture line extends into the joint, it is important to seek orthopaedic advice regarding the need for open reduction and internal fixation. A dinner-fork deformity in children indicates an angulated fracture of the distal radius or, more often, an epiphyseal fracture. The Salter–Harris classification of epiphyseal injuries should be used to describe these fractures (Table 26.8 and Fig. 26.21). One of the commonest epiphyseal fractures in children is that of the distal radius and the commonest type is a Salter–Harris type II.

Anaesthesia must be provided in order to reduce distal radial fractures. Options include intravenous regional anaesthesia (Bier's block), haematoma block and general anaesthesia. Haematoma blocks are often more successful if the anaesthetic is correctly placed and sufficient time (at least 20 min) is allowed to pass before manipulation is attempted. It is often forgotten that the ulnar styloid will not be included in the haematoma block and will require a separate local anaesthetic injection.

Whichever anaesthetic method is chosen, manipulation involves preparation, disimpaction, correction of dorsal displacement and angulation, correction of radial displacement and application

Table 26.8: Salter–Harris classification of epiphyseal injuries

Type I	The whole epiphysis separates from or slips off the shaft (metaphysis)
Type II	The whole epiphysis separates and carries a small triangular metaphyseal fragment
Type III	Vertical fracture through the epiphysis which joins with fracture through epiphyseal plate (only part of epiphysis separates)
Type IV	Vertical or oblique fracture through epiphysis and metaphysis (separation of part of epiphysis with metaphyseal fragment)
Type V	Crushing of part or all of the epiphysis

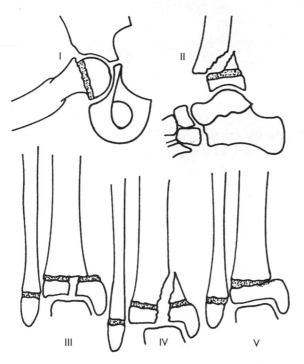

Figure 26.21: Salter–Harris classification of fractures.

Table 26.9: Manipulation of Colles' fracture

Provide adequate analgesia and anaesthesia
Prepare a bandage and plaster slab
Ask an assistant hold the elbow flexed and provide counter traction
Apply traction along the line of the forearm by grasping the thumb, index and middle fingers
Maintain traction until the fragments disimpact (confirm this by palpation with the other hand)
Extend the elbow and maintain traction by placing the heel of one hand over the dorsal surface of the radius and grasping the forearm and wrist
Correct the dorsal displacement by using the heel of the other hand to press on the volar surface of the forearm proximal to the fracture site
Correct the radial displacement by using the heel of the other hand to press on the radial side of the hand and forearm distal to the fracture site
Apply the plaster slab while maintaining traction through the thumb, index and middle fingers again
Position the wrist in slight palmar flexion and full ulnar deviation with the plaster on and maintain the position until the plaster sets

flexed and pulled into ulnar deviation. A suggested step-by-step method is given in Table 26.9.

As with all reductions, check radiographs should be taken to ensure an acceptable reduction has been achieved. If the position is acceptable, the patient can be provided with a sling and a review appointment for the following day. Provided there are no complications then, the patient can be seen in fracture clinic in a week with a view to completing the plaster and assessing any change in position.

Falling on to the outstretched hand with the wrist flexed rather than extended may cause a Smith's (or reverse Colles') fracture (Fig. 26.22). This may be identical in radiographic appearance to a Colles' fracture on the AP film but has the opposite deformities on the lateral film (volar angulation and displacement to the volar and ulnar side). If the fracture line enters the joint so that the anterior lip of the radius is displaced proximally with the hand it is often referred to as a Barton's fracture.

Reduction of a Smith's fracture requires disimpaction with traction along the arm while the elbow is extended and the forearm supinated. Once disimpaction has been achieved, the wrist is extended, pulled radially and held in this position

of a plaster back slab. Following manipulation, the forearm should be fully pronated with the wrist slightly palmar flexed and in full ulnar deviation. There are several techniques for manipulating a Colles' fracture. In simple terms, the hand is pulled distally to disimpact the fracture, then the wrist is

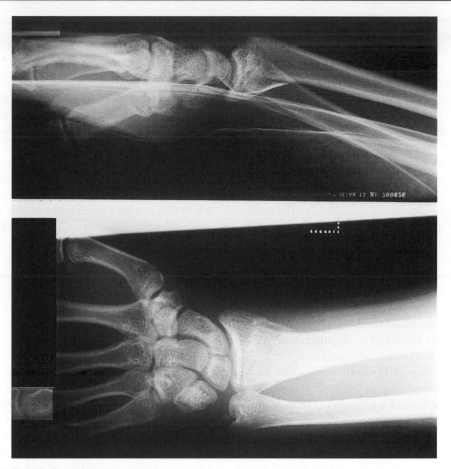

Figure 26.22: Smith's fracture.

while plaster is applied. The forearm should be fully supinated and the wrist fully extended. This is a difficult position to maintain and open reduction and internal fixation is often the preferred option. Comminuted or intra-articular fractures should be referred to orthopaedics prior to any attempt at manipulation.

WRIST INJURIES

SOFT-TISSUE INJURIES

Wrist pain is a common presenting complaint to emergency departments. The wrist acts as a stable platform for the hand and is intimately involved in hand movements. Significant disability can therefore result from acute soft-tissue wrist injuries.

Patients will often report a fall on to a hyperflexed (palmar flexion) or hyperextended (dorsiflexion) wrist, or a similar mechanism such as stopping a football with the palm of the hand. There will usually be some soft-tissue swelling and restriction in movement. A simple screening test for dorsiflexion is to ask the patient to place the palms together (as in prayer) and then bring the hands down the front of the body to extend the wrists. Placing the backs of the hands together will reveal the extent of palmar flexion possible. Gentle passive circular movements will often give a feel for the severity of injury. If movements are relatively preserved, there is rarely a major injury to the wrist and a sprain can be diagnosed. In all cases, however, the possibility of distal radial and scaphoid fractures should be considered. If there is any doubt then radiographs should be obtained.

The precise anatomical diagnosis of wrist sprains may be very difficult. Pain that is well localized to the ulnar side of the wrist may indicate a triangular fibrocartilage complex injury. The pain will be exacerbated by ulnar deviation and palmar flexion. If pain is aggravated by pronation and supination then the distal radio-ulnar joint may be involved. In all cases a period of rest, immobilization and analgesia will provide effective treatment for the acute injury. It is important to remember that some patients may come to rely on wrist braces and recovery can be prolonged.

Tendinitis and tenosynovitis may occur in any of the flexor or extensor tendons that cross the wrist. Tenosynovitis is inflammation of the tendon sheath and it commonly occurs after repetitive activity. Patients complain of a pain over the affected part of the wrist following the activity. They may relate the onset of symptoms to an acute event. The wrist will have a slight reduction in range of movement and there will be signs of acute inflammation. The individual tendons or tendon sheaths involved may be localized by detailed examination although this is not usually necessary. In many cases, palpable or even audible crepitus can be detected on clinical examination. One of the most common examples is De Quervain's tenovaginitis. Repetitive pinching motion may cause inflammation around the abductor pollicis longus and extensor pollicis brevis tendons. Patients complain of well-localized pain from the radial styloid to the metacarpophalangeal joint of the thumb. This pain is exacerbated by ulnar deviation of the hand and flexion of the thumb.

Treatment of tenosynovitis involves activity modification, rest in a thumb spica or wrist brace with thumb extension, and non-steroidal anti-inflammatory drugs until the inflammation subsides. If the pain is very severe, rest in a plaster of Paris may, rarely, be necessary. The most important differential diagnosis is suppurative or pyogenic tenosynovitis. If there is any doubt about the possibility of infection, a septic screen should be performed and the patient reviewed by a senior doctor.

Any process that significantly reduces the size of the carpal tunnel (inflammation, anterior dislocation of the lunate, arthritis, tenosynovitis) may compress the median nerve. The patient may present with wrist pain from the primary injury and paras-thesiae or diminished sensation in the digits. These median nerve signs must be recognized and the cause of the carpal tunnel compression identified.

CARPAL FRACTURES AND DISLOCATIONS

A fall on an outstretched hand may cause a fracture or dislocation involving any of the carpal bones. These are arranged in two rows that are bridged by the scaphoid. The scaphoid is therefore the most vulnerable to injury during dorsiflexion of the wrist, and over 90% of carpal fractures involve the scaphoid. It is commonly fractured across its waist (Fig. 26.23). The patient will complain of pain and tenderness in the wrist, with a reduced grip. Although there may be some fullness in the anatomical snuff-box, there is usually no deformity or bruising. On examination, there is tenderness in the snuff-box, weakness of pinch grip and pain on dorsiflexion. Other signs include pain on axial compression of the thumb metacarpal and tenderness over the palmar aspect of the scaphoid. These are all non-specific signs. Fractures of the radial styloid, severe wrist sprains and fractures of the thumb metacarpal will all have similar features. Thus radiography is required in all cases. A guide to interpretation of wrist radiographs is given in Table 26.10.

Fractures of the scaphoid are often hairline and very difficult to see. To reduce the chance of missing the injury, therefore, two oblique views are taken in addition to the AP and lateral of the wrist. Displaced fractures should be referred immediately to the orthopaedic team. Undisplaced fractures may be placed in a scaphoid plaster and referred routinely to fracture clinic. A scaphoid plaster is applied with the wrist fully pronated, radially deviated and moderately flexed with the thumb in mid-abduction (opposite the ring finger). The position of this plaster is important and advice should be obtained if there is uncertainty.

If there is pain and tenderness but no radiological abnormality, the patient should be provided with analgesia and a review clinic appointment for approximately 10 days after the injury. It should be explained to the patient that there may be a fracture that is not visible on the initial film and that it will be necessary to repeat the films. The use of some form of immobilization, such as a scaphoid plaster or a simple wrist brace with thumb extension, depends on the pain experienced by the patient. When the patient returns to clinic, the brace or plaster should be removed and further scaphoid

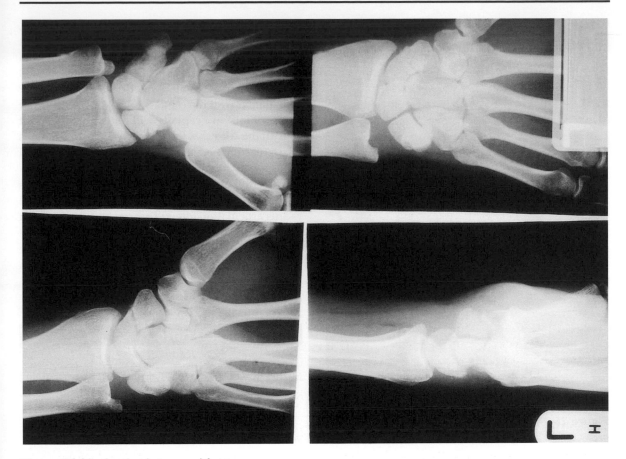

Figure 26.23: Scaphoid views and fracture.

Table 26.10: Interpretation of radiographs of the wrist

> Look for:
> *On the AP view*:
>   Uninterrupted cortices around the eight carpal
>   bones – particularly the scaphoid
>   Uniform joint spaces between the carpal bones
>   (approximately 1–2 mm)
>   Uninterrupted cortices around the distal radius
>   and ulna
>   Uninterrupted cortices around the distal
>   metacarpals
>
> *On the lateral*:
>   The straight line through the centres of the
>   radius, lunate and capitate
>   The capitate lying within the concavity of the
>   lunate
>   Uninterrupted cortices around the radius and
>   ulna

radiographs taken. The fracture line should be more easily visible following bone resorption. If there is still no fracture despite persisting symptoms then a further 2 weeks of analgesia and immobilization are required. If there is still pain after further review then a bone scan should be arranged as an out-patient and immobilization continued. In some centres, MRI scanning is being used as an alternative to nuclear bone scanning.

Fractures through the bodies of other carpal bones are rare. Minor avulsion or 'flake' fractures of the carpal bones may be associated with dorsiflexion and palmar flexion injuries (wrist sprains). Occasionally, such fractures result from a direct blow. The exact origin of the flake is often difficult to determine radiographically. These injuries require symptomatic treatment only. They often represent significant soft tissue injury and benefit from subsequent physiotherapy.

There are a number of carpal dislocations and fracture dislocations. The most important of these

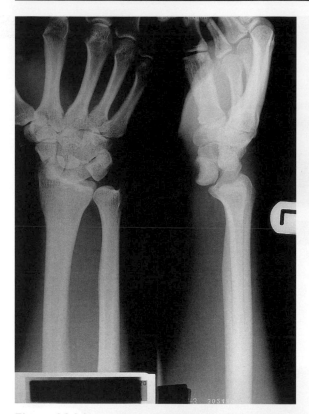

Figure 26.24: Lunate dislocation.

the concavity of the lunate. In a lunate dislocation, the patient is in considerable pain and movement at the wrist will be minimal. There is often median nerve compression. The lateral radiograph will reveal the lunate rotated anteriorly and no longer articulating with the capitate (Fig. 26.24). The centre of the radius and capitate will remain in a straight line. In the AP view, the dislocated lunate becomes triangular shaped and the margins of the carpal joints are no longer uniform.

In perilunate dislocation the whole of the carpus is dislocated posteriorly, leaving the lunate and radius articulation intact. This severe injury is often associated with a scaphoid fracture. Both lunate and perilunate dislocations should be referred to the orthopaedic team for urgent review and reduction under anaesthesia.

FURTHER READING

McRae, R. (1994) *Practical Fracture Treatment*. Churchill Livingstone, London.

are lunate and perilunate dislocations. These may be easily overlooked. The radius, lunate and capitate articulate with each other and lie in a straight line on the lateral radiographs. The capitate sits in

THE HAND

INTRODUCTION

Hand injury, infection and inflammation are common presentations to the emergency department, and are all too often treated insufficiently seriously by doctors. This leads to a greater likelihood of incorrect diagnosis and suboptimal treatment that can result in prolonged morbidity for the patient.

The objectives in this chapter are to discuss the salient features in the assessment of the hand, and the general principles of managing hand problems. Common pathologies presenting to emergency departments are described, subdivided into soft-tissue injuries and infections, tendon, ligamentous, nerve and bony injuries.

ANATOMY OF THE HAND

A basic knowledge of the anatomy of the hand is essential for the correct management of hand conditions and injuries.

NERVES

The cutaneous nerve supply of the hand is illustrated in Figure 27.1. It is important to note that the cutaneous nerve supply does vary between individuals and in particular the ulnar nerve may cover the ulnar two and a half digits. The nerve supply to the small muscles of the hand is given in Table 27.1.

Each digit is supplied by two digital nerves. The digital nerves to the fingers run in close association with the digital arteries on the volar aspects to the radial and ulnar sides of the digit.

TENDONS

There are two flexor tendons to each finger, the flexor digitorum profundus (FDP), which attaches to the proximal part of the distal phalanx and flexes the distal interphalangeal joint (DIPJ), and the flexor digitorum superficialis (FDS), which attaches to the proximal part of the intermediate phalanx and flexes the proximal interphalangeal joint (PIPJ). The deep flexor emerges from under the superficial flexor (which divides into two slips) at the intermediate phalanx. The thumb has one long flexor, flexor pollicis longus (FPL), which attaches to the distal phalanx and flexes the interphalangeal joint (Fig. 27.2).

There are two extensor tendons to the index and little fingers and one each to the middle and ring fingers. The action of the extensor tendons is to extend the metacarpophalangeal joints (MCPJ) and the interphalangeal joints. Each tendon divides into a central slip and two lateral slips. The central slip inserts into the base of the intermediate phalanx and extends the PIPJ. The lateral slips insert into the base of the distal phalanx and extend both PIPJ and DIPJ. The extensor tendons to the thumb are the extensor pollicis longus (EPL)

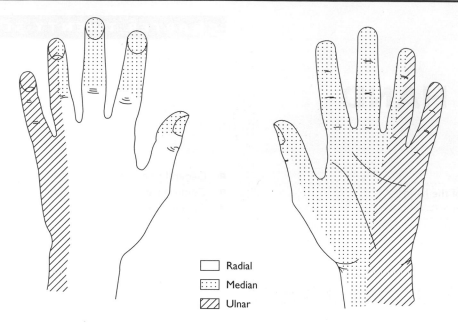

Radial

Median

Ulnar

Figure 27.1: Sensory nerve distribution of the hand.

Table 27.1: Nerve supply of muscles of the hand

Nerve	Muscle	Action
Median nerve	Abductor pollicis brevis	Abduction of the thumb
Ulnar nerve	Adductor pollicis	Adduction of the thumb

and extensor pollicis brevis and, with the abductor pollicis longus, these tendons form the borders of the anatomical snuff-box. The EPL inserts into the base of the distal phalanx and extends the interphalangeal joint of the thumb. The extensor pollicis brevis and abductor pollicis longus abduct and extend the thumb.

Bones

The bones of the wrist and hand are illustrated in Fig. 27.3. Injuries of the wrist are dealt with in Chapter 27.

Blood supply

The blood supply to the hand arises from the radial and ulnar arteries, which form the palmar

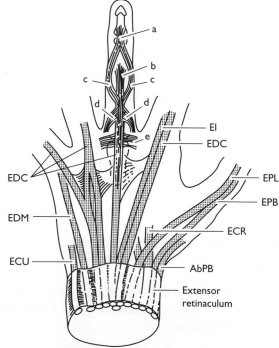

a	Extensor insertion into distal phalanx	EDC	Extensor digitorum communis
		EDM	Extensor digitorum minimi
b	Central slip	ECU	Extensor carpi ulnaris
c	Lateral slip	EI	Extensor indicis
d	Slips from lumbrical and interossei	EPL	Extensor pollicis longus
		EPB	Extensor pollicis brevis
e	Sagittal bands	ECR	Extensor carpi radialis
		AbPB	Abductor pollicis brevis

Figure 27.2: Extensor tendons of the hand.

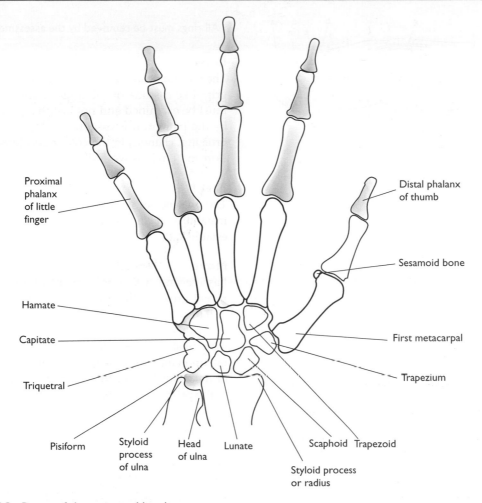

Proximal
phalanx
of little
finger

Distal phalanx
of thumb

Sesamoid bone

Hamate

Capitate

First metacarpal

Triquetral

Trapezium

Pisiform

Styloid
process
of ulna

Head
of ulna

Lunate

Scaphoid Trapezoid

Styloid process
or radius

Figure 27.3: Bones of the wrist and hand.

arch. Each finger has two digital arteries, which arise from the palmar arch and pass along the sides of the fingers adjacent to the digital nerves. The blood supply to the thumb is more complex.

FINGER TIP AND NAIL BED

The anatomy of the finger tip and nail bed is shown in Figure 27.4.

ASSESSMENT

The assessment should be structured and methodical. It is divided into history, examination and appropriate investigations.

HISTORY

Essential background information regarding hand dominance, occupation and hobbies or pastimes should be clearly recorded. Previous significant injuries or illness affecting the hand or other joints should be noted.

The patient should be asked about the main complaint. A clear history relating to the main complaint must be elicited. Exactly what happened should be clearly recorded, including how it occurred and when it happened, together with any associated or subsequent symptoms. The environment in which the injury was sustained should be recorded. In workplace accidents, details of any machinery involved and whether the correct protection and accident prevention procedures were being followed at the time of the injury should be

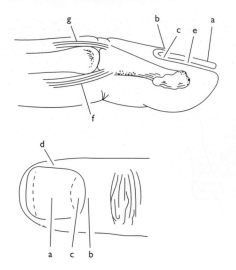

a Nail plate
b Eponychium (nail fold)
c Lunula (overlies germinal matrix)
d Paronychium
e Sterile matrix (nail bed)
f Insertion of FDP
g Insertion of extensor tendon

Figure 27.4: Anatomy of the finger tip and nail bed.

noted. This information may be required for sub-sequent legal reports.

In patients without a history of trauma the story is often longer and less precise and greater acumen is required to identify the correct diagnosis. It is important to ask about factors that exacerbate or relieve the main symptoms in such patients and to record any relevant past history related to tetanus status, allergies and current medication.

EXAMINATION

It is important to be aware of the possibility of associated injury elsewhere, and especially to the ipsilateral shoulder, elbow or wrist when examining the hand. All rings must be removed by the assessment nurse. Patients who are unwilling to have their rings removed must sign a form indicating their responsibility for this course of action. A methodical approach must be followed:

- look
- feel
- move.

All rings must be removed by the assessment nurse.

LOOK

The natural position of the hand reveals a 'racquet-grip'-like cascade of the fingers. The whole hand must be examined and not just that part indicated by the patient. It is essential to look for swelling, bruising, changes in the colour and tension of the skin and obvious wounds.

FEEL

The presence of warmth, tenderness, crepitus and instability of any of the affected parts should be established.

MOVE

Passive and active movement of the hand will reveal gross pathology. In the injured hand pain will be an obvious limiting factor.

At this stage it may be possible to reach a primary or short list of differential diagnoses. Depending upon the site of the injury or illness one or more of the following specific tests will confirm or add to the primary diagnosis.

Tendons

The examination of the important tendons of the hand is summarized below:

- Flexor digitorum profundus (FDP). With the palm up, the patient is asked to 'bend the tip of your finger' whilst the proximal interphalangeal joint (PIPJ) is held immobilized.
- Flexor digitorum superficialis (FDS). The other fingers are immobilized (thus immobilizing the deep flexors) in full extension on a flat surface and the patient is asked to bend the injured finger. Flexion of the PIPJ confirms that the FDS tendon is intact.
- Flexor pollicis longus (FPL). The patient is asked to bend the tip of the thumb against resistance.
- Extensor tendons. The patient is asked to straighten fingers fully against resistance from flexion at the level of the proximal phalanx.
- Extensor pollicis longus (EPL). The hand is placed flat on the table (palm down) and the patient is asked to lift only the thumb. EPL will become prominent as the dorsal border of the anatomical snuff-box.

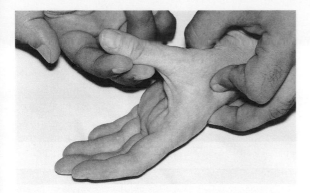

Figure 27.5: Testing the ulnar collateral ligament of the thumb.

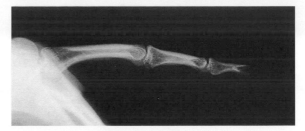

Figure 27.6: Volar plate avulsion fracture.

Ligaments

THE ULNAR COLLATERAL LIGAMENT (UCL) OF THE METACARPOPHALANGEAL JOINT OF THE THUMB

The UCL of the thumb is tested by grasping the thumb metacarpal firmly between the thumb and index finger of one hand. With the other hand the thumb is abducted with the joint in 30° of flexion. The ulnar collateral ligament must always be compared with the uninjured side as there is considerable variation between individuals. An intact UCL is confirmed by a firm end point (Fig. 27.5). An ill defined, 'spongy' end point suggests likely UCL rupture.

COLLATERAL LIGAMENTS (CL) OF THE INTERPHALANGEAL JOINTS

Interphalangeal joints are stabilized by the collateral ligaments laterally and a fibro-cartilaginous volar plate on the flexor aspect. The collateral ligaments are tested in 30° of flexion. Each collateral ligament that may have been damaged should be stressed, bearing in mind the mechanism of the injury. Injury to the ligament is recognized by abnormal movement at the joint with a soft end point in comparison with uninjured joints.

Damage to the volar plate will often be recognized radiologically as a small avulsion fracture from the base of the intermediate phalanx (Fig. 27.6).

Nerves

The motor and sensory supply to the hand is via a combination of the median, ulnar and radial nerves (see Table 27.1 and Fig. 27.1).

SENSORY

The history will provide the first clue of injury. Blunt trauma to the hand may induce 'numbness' but this is due to neuropraxia and the patient can be reassured. Where a laceration is present (especially where glass was involved) the patient should be assumed to have nerve injury and this should be positively excluded. Any laceration involving glass should be X-rayed.

In assessing for nerve injury the most useful examination is for abnormalities of light touch and pin-prick sensation, which are usually more apparent when comparing an abnormal with a normal area. A useful technique is to instruct the patient to close their eyes and say 'yes' when they feel the touch stimulus. In addition, loss of sympathetic innervation leads to absence of sweating in the distribution of the injured nerve which may be detectable on examination.

MOTOR

The median nerve is assessed by testing its thenar motor branch. This is performed by assessing the strength of opponens pollicis or flexor pollicis brevis. Palpable contraction of the muscles in the thenar eminence indicates intact median nerve motor function.

The ulnar nerve's motor function can be assessed by testing the strength of the intrinsic muscles using finger abduction by asking the patient to cross their fingers. Alternatively, Froment's test can be used which tests the function of the adductor pollicis. Normal ulnar nerve function allows a piece of paper to be held between the thumb and index finger with the thumb extended at the interphalangeal joint (Fig. 27.7a). Weakness due to ulnar nerve injury will result in flexion of the interphalangeal joint of the thumb (Fig. 27.7b).

The radial nerve has no motor supply in the hand.

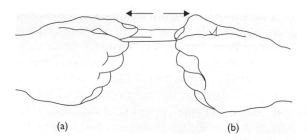

Figure 27.7: Froment sign indicating (a) normal and (b) abnormal ulnar nerve function.

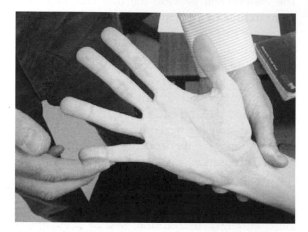

Figure 27.8: Testing ulnar nerve function.

Despite a nerve being divided examination may initially be normal due to conduction of impulses across the site of nerve injury. After 24–48 h, axonal degeneration occurs and neurological signs of injury become obvious.

Vascular supply

Examination must include assessment and documentation of the blood supply distal to the injury.

INVESTIGATIONS

X-ray examination is commonly carried out for trauma, foreign body demonstration or to exclude osteomyelitis. Rare diagnoses of metabolic or inflammatory diseases (sarcoid, gout) or arthropathies can also be made.

When ordering investigations it is important to be as specific as possible about the required

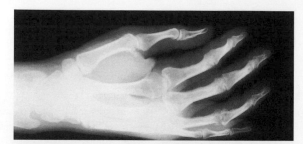

(a)

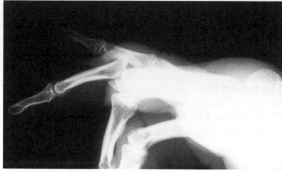

(b)

Figure 27.9: Adequate (a) and inadequate (b) radiographs.

films rather than, for example, requesting 'hand, wrist and scaphoid'. Adequate films in two planes are essential and the purpose of the film (e.g. identification of foreign body) should be made clear on the request form (Fig. 27.9).

GENERAL PRINCIPLES OF HAND MANAGEMENT

Adherence to a number of basic principles will lead to the patient's hand injury being properly managed. There are three main phases in the management of such patients that will, if carried out correctly, result in the best possible outcome for the patient:

- immediate treatment
- a period of immobilization, elevation and rest
- aggressive physiotherapy and rehabilitation.

ACUTE TREATMENT

All the structures that may be involved in a hand injury must be individually examined. In the case of penetrating wounds each structure must be seen to be intact as well as to be functioning normally, in order to ensure that partial injuries do not subsequently progress to loss of function.

Pain may significantly affect the likelihood of achieving an informative examination. Good local anaesthetic blockade, therefore, may be important for both diagnosis and treatment. It is important to make sure that sensation is recorded prior to blockade.

All wounds should be fully explored once they are anaesthetized. In deep wounds or extensive wounds, when local anaesthesia cannot be achieved or damage to involved structures excluded, formal exploration in an operating theatre by a surgeon will be required. Adequate debridement and irrigation of fresh wounds is mandatory for good healing. If the wound is dirty it may sometimes be necessary, following surgical debridement, to leave the wound to heal by secondary intention. Alternatively, delayed primary closure may be used. These patients should be discussed with a senior doctor. The hand has an excellent blood supply that encourages rapid healing. Straightforward, clean wounds should be closed with 4.0 or 5.0 monofilament non-absorbable suture. Adhesive wound tapes should not be used for the closure of lacerations involving the flexor or extensor surfaces.

Following reduction of any dislocated joints and manipulation of fractures repeat X-ray is essential to determine the effect of the intervention.

In general, antibiotics are recommended for contaminated wounds, human and animal bites, open fractures, and old (>12 h) wounds. The urinary sugar or BM Stix® and temperature should be checked in patients with signs suggestive of infection.

> Do not forget to record tetanus status and immunize if necessary.

IMMOBILIZATION

Wounds will range from those that can be left open to those that will require dressing with a combination of non-adherent paraffin gauze, gauze swabs and bandages. Elevation of the hand in a high arm sling for 24 h in any significant injury where swelling is likely, is necessary in order to minimize oedema and enhance healing. Adequate analgesia is also essential.

A variety of basic splint techniques are available to immobilize all or part of the hand for a short period of time. These include neighbour (buddy) strapping, Bedford splints, metal and foam combination Zimmer splints, mallet splints and plaster of Paris (PoP). They are discussed in the relevant sections below. It is important only to immobilize that part of the hand that requires it and to give the patient clear guidance on the period of splintage. Follow-up with the appropriate specialist is vital.

REHABILITATION AND PHYSIOTHERAPY

All significant hand injuries must be referred back for emergency department review clinic, the orthopaedic fracture clinic or a specialist hand clinic. Rehabilitation with a combination of self- and formalized physiotherapy may be prolonged. However, even injuries that do not need specialist follow-up in a hospital will require simple commonsense advice on early self-physiotherapy in order to gain full and early function.

COMMON AND IMPORTANT HAND PATHOLOGIES

In the following sections the hand service refers to the hospital specialist who deals with hand injuries. He or she may be a specialist hand surgeon, an emergency physician with an interest in hand injury, an orthopaedic surgeon or a plastic surgeon.

SOFT-TISSUE INJURIES AND INFECTIONS

Nail-bed injuries

These are common, especially in children, and often occur as a result of catching a digit in a door. In adults, a misplaced hammer blow is a common method of injury. There are four grades of severity (Table 27.2).

SUBUNGUAL HAEMATOMA
The nail-bed injury manifests only as a subungual haematoma. This can be inordinately painful but is

Table 27.2: Classification of nail-bed injuries

Subungual haematoma
Sprung nail
Nail-bed laceration
Open fracture of the terminal phalanx

satisfyingly relieved by trephining the nail using a heated paperclip and releasing the underlying pressure if performed early. There is no value in trephining a subungual haematoma which is more than 24 h old as the blood is likely to have clotted.

SPRUNG NAIL

When the nail base comes to lie above the nail fold, the term 'sprung nail' is used. There is usually an associated subungual haematoma. In such patients the nail should be repositioned under the nail fold using a local anaesthetic ringblock (see Chapter 8). This may require mobilization of the nail from the underlying matrix and repair of any associated laceration.

NAIL-BED LACERATION

A laceration may be confined to the nail bed or extend into the surrounding skin. In children the laceration may be deep enough to cause a partial amputation. The best cosmetic result is obtained by formal repair under tourniquet and ring block. The nail is removed and the nail bed repaired with absorbable 6-0 sutures. The remaining wound is also sutured and the nail replaced to act as a temporary splint. In some cases the use of multiple adhesive wound tapes may be an effective method of closing finger-tip lacerations, particularly those to the pulp.

OPEN FRACTURE OF THE TERMINAL PHALANX

In these cases a deep nail-bed laceration is associated with a fracture of the terminal phalanx. Formal repair of the laceration is again recommended. The nail should be replaced *in situ* as a splint for the fracture.

Antibiotics (flucloxacillin or erythromycin) should be given if there is a bony injury in association with the nail-bed injury or in association with a subungal haematoma requiring trephining. Trephination in the absence of a fracture is not an indication for antibiotics. Follow-up should be arranged at 1 week and the patient advised that

although a new nail will grow back there may be a ridging to the nail plate.

Finger-tip injuries

These injuries may be due to slicing, producing a relatively clean laceration, or crushing, resulting in partial or complete amputation of the tip of the finger. They can be classified as follows:

- Pulp loss alone less than $1\,cm^2$. These can be treated conservatively by cleaning the wound and applying a non-adherent dressing. Regular review is usually necessary.
- Pulp loss greater than $1\,cm^2$ with or without bone exposure should be referred to the hand service. Skin closure can be achieved either by the formation of flaps, by skin grafting or by terminalization (shortening of the terminal phalanx to achieve adequate skin cover).

In children conservative treatment is generally recommended even where there is bony involvement. This decision should be left to experienced staff.

Antibiotics are indicated where an open, bony injury is confirmed on X-ray. Non-adherent dressings (e.g. paraffin gauze) should be used, although all dressings become adherent after a few days of drying. Follow-up to review cosmetic results and instigate appropriate exercises for the finger tip is important.

Bites

Bite injuries may be caused by a variety of animals, including other humans. Patients presenting with lacerations over the extensor aspect of the metacarpophalangeal joint may have sustained the injury by punching another person in the mouth. Examination will reveal an abrasion or ragged laceration over the extensor aspect of the metacarpal head. X-ray may reveal a fracture of the metacarpal head (classically of the little finger) and possibly retained tooth fragments from the opponent. The main concern is the variety of bacteria present in the wound (commonly streptococci and mixed anaerobes). Small abrasions and lacerations require an aggressive surgical scrub, debridement and prophylactic antibiotics (usually co-amoxiclav).

All such wounds should be explored down to the MCPJ space. Any suggestion of joint involvement mandates referral to the hand service for formal exploration. If the wound is not deep, the edges should be debrided and the wound left open for delayed closure or allowed to heal by secondary intention. Follow-up should be arranged at 1–2 days. The hand must be elevated in a high arm sling and appropriate prophylactic antibiotics provided. Patients should be advised to return if they develop spreading cellulitis, lymphangitis or the systemic symptoms of infection. Any indication of failure to control infection is an indication for admission and intravenous antibiotic therapy.

Other bite injuries are commonly caused by dogs or cats. *Pasteurella multocida* is a common pathogen. Bites from cats should be X-rayed to exclude the presence of tooth fragments. Wounds from large dogs should be X-rayed to check for underlying fractures and tooth fragments. Aggressive surgical debridement and cleansing of the wound in combination with penicillin therapy is appropriate. Abrasions, however, require cleaning only and antibiotic prophylaxis is not indicated. Wounds should be left open, as immediate closure is likely to result in sepsis. Always check tetanus status and provide further immunization if required.

Glass lacerations (Fig. 27.10)

Injuries to the hands associated with glass merit particular mention. The exact mechanism of the injury must be elucidated and documented. The wound must always be examined carefully as it may be deeper than it initially appears. A major structure is often involved despite an innocuous appearance of the wound. The wound must always be X-rayed. However, not all glass is opaque and exploration of the wound may also be required.

> All glass wounds must be X-rayed.

High-pressure injection injury

High-pressure injection injuries are rare but important. They are easily misdiagnosed and the end result may be catastrophic (potentially amputation). They occur as a result of high-pressure injection of paint or sealant from a spray gun. A detailed history is essential. The wound initially looks benign with no physical signs apart from a tiny puncture. If diagnosis is delayed, the inoculum travels along

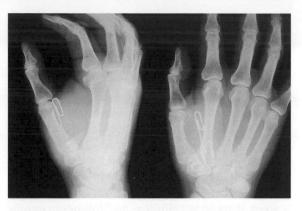

Figure 27.10: X-ray of a retained glass foreign body.

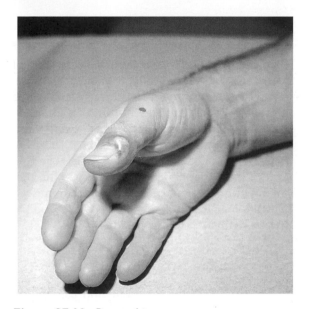

Figure 27.11: Paronychia.

the tendon sheath into the palm, setting up an intense inflammatory tenosynovitis which can extend into the forearm. X-rays may show a radio-opaque inoculum. The hand should be elevated and the patient referred immediately to the hand service for urgent surgery. Formal exposure and irrigation from the finger tip into the palm or even more proximally is required.

Paronychia (Fig. 27.11)

Paronychia is a common infection involving the tissues surrounding the nail. It is common in those whose occupation involves chronic exposure to water. There are two broad categories. Early paronychia manifests as a cellulitis affecting the nail fold but with no signs of pus formation. Treatment with antibiotic therapy against staphylococcus is usually successful. Established paronychia will demonstrate fluctuance around the nail fold, with a collection of pus that may extend under the nail. A digital nerve block is essential. Management consists of drainage of the pus through an incision over the point of maximal fluctuance and irrigation, leaving the wound open. On occasions, removal of the nail is required to drain the pus completely. Flucloxacillin (or erythromycin if the patient is allergic to penicillin) may be required for a week if there is cellulitis, and follow-up can be arranged with the patient's GP.

Pulp space infection

This is an infection of the terminal volar pad of the finger, usually as a result of a puncture wound. Pus collects within the tense fibrous septa of the pulp space. A patient presents with an intensely painful throbbing finger and a tense swollen finger tip, suggesting the presence of pus. These are often not fluctuant. Management consists of a ring block of the finger and surgical drainage through a lateral pulp incision. Late presentation or missed diagnosis may lead to osteomyelitis of the terminal phalanx, with long-term morbidity.

Palmar space infections

Palmar space infections are rare and usually follow a penetrating injury to the palm that has been neglected by the patient or misdiagnosed by the doctor. The two main potential spaces in the hand are the palmar space (lying between the flexor tendons and metacarpals of the ulnar three fingers) and the thenar space (between the flexors of the index and adductor pollicis). Severe pain and tenderness in the palm are the predominant features. There may also be a loss of the normal concavity and curvature of the palm as well as dorsal swelling. Management consists of intravenous antibiotics and urgent referral to the hand service for formal incision and drainage.

Web space infection

This is typically due to a penetrating injury. Presentation, especially if delayed, is of pain with swelling of the web on dorsal and volar aspects. Intravenous antibiotics should be given and the patient referred to the hand service for incision and drainage.

Tendon sheath infections

These are easily missed, leading to long-term morbidity. The wound may initially be innocuous and often occurs on the volar aspect of the finger tip. Progression of the infection along the flexor tendon will lead to the finger being held in flexion, with tenderness progressing into the palm. Pain at this stage is severe and exacerbated by attempted passive extension of the finger (Kanavel's sign). Management consists of elevation, intravenous antibiotics and urgent referral to the hand service for incision, drainage and irrigation of the entire sheath.

Septic arthritis

This classically occurs as a consequence of a penetrating injury although it may occasionally result from haematogenous spread of infection. Patients present with pain swelling and erythema of the hand and a misdiagnosis of uncomplicated cellulitis may be made. However, the pain is usually focused around a joint and is severe when any attempt is made to move the joint. Management consists of elevation, intravenous antibiotics and referral to the hand service for incision and drainage. Appropriate X-rays should be performed.

Nerve injury

Recognition of nerve injury in the hand relies upon obtaining a clear history and performing an appropriate examination. Inability to do this (e.g. in intoxicated patients) should be managed by simple wound dressing and reassessing the patient when they are sober. Objective sensory disturbance in the hand should always be referred to the hand service for exploration. Depending upon the level of the nerve injury, repair or debridement to prevent neuroma formation will be required. This decision should be made by a member of the hand service. In general, lacerations distal to the distal interphalangeal joint (DIPJ) that result in sensory loss are not suitable for surgical repair.

Burns

Burns to the hand are extremely common and usually result from contact with a hot surface or liquid. The area of the burn should be recorded on a simple diagram and the depth of burn indicated (see Chapter 28). Full-thickness burns of the hand should be referred to the burns or hand service. Partial thickness burns may be treated in a 'Flamazine®' bag' or with paraffin-gauze-based dressings. Paraffin-based dressings will require regular changes and the patient is usually best reviewed after 24 h. When a 'Flamazine® bag' is used this should not be routinely changed after 24 h unless a large amount of exudate has accumulated in the bag. Although 'Flamazine® bags' are easy to apply they are less convenient for the patient, who should also be warned about the macerated appearance of the hand when the bag is removed. In due course the bag should be replaced by paraffin-gauze-based dressings. In all cases moderately strong analgesia such as codydramol will be required, and early mobilization of the hand must be encouraged.

TENDON AND LIGAMENTOUS INJURY

Mallet finger

A mallet deformity of the finger results from a seperation of the insertion of the terminal extensor slip from the base of the distal phalanx. Such injuries are commonly due to an impaction injury or a blow to the end of the finger, for example from a cricket ball. In elderly patients there may be no clear history of trauma. Examination reveals a 'droop' to the terminal phalanx, with the patient able to flex at the DIPJ but not extend (Fig. 27.12). X-ray should always be performed as a proportion will avulse a fragment at the terminal phalanx as well.

Treatment consists of a well-fitting mallet splint that immobilizes the DIPJ in full extension but should not impair movement of the PIPJ (Fig. 27.13). The patient should be taught how to remove and reapply the splint on a flat surface to prevent flexion. Review is arranged for 2 weeks to resize the splint once oedema has settled. The splint is applied for up to 6 weeks in those with associated bony injury and 8 weeks where tendon rupture alone has occurred. Mallet deformity with an associated avulsion fracture tends to have a better outcome.

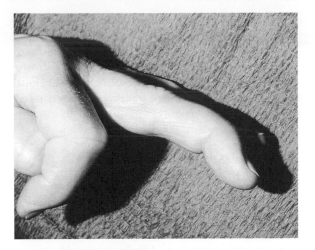

Figure 27.12: Mallet finger.

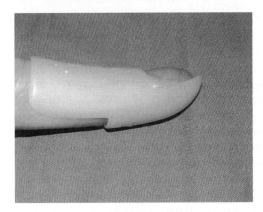

Figure 27.13: Mallet finger treated in a mallet splint.

Mallet finger with an associated laceration can be managed in a similar fashion once the laceration has been sutured. If both ends of the tendon can be clearly identified, repair to the tendon should be carried out by the hand service.

Boutonnière deformity

This results from rupture of the central slip of the extensor tendon over the PIPJ of the finger, such that the PIPJ 'herniates' through the lateral slips. It may occasionally present as an open injury. Mechanisms include landing on the knuckles on hard ground or lacerations on glass. The classic appearance is of flexion of the PIPJ; an inability to fully extend the fingers may not become obvious for a few days, owing to general swelling of the PIPJ. As a consequence, this is an injury that can easily be missed.

The acute presentation is with a swollen PIPJ and possible Boutonnière deformities should be reviewed in 3–5 days. Patients with a confirmed Boutonnière deformity should be referred to the hand service for either closed splintage or surgical repair. Open Boutonnière injuries will need referral for surgical repair.

UCL rupture ('gamekeeper's thumb')

Rupture of the UCL occurs as a result of a hyperabduction injury to the thumb. Sport, in particular skiing (often on dry ski slopes), seems to be the main culprit nowadays. Misdiagnosing the injury as a 'sprain' will inflict significant morbidity on the patient (Fig. 27.14).

It is essential to listen carefully to the patient regarding the precise mechanism of injury. Examination has been outlined above in the section on ligament examination. Management in confirmed cases consists of referral to the hand service for early repair. If the presence of rupture is suspected but unconfirmed, review in 3–5 days for reassessment is appropriate when swelling has reduced. Ultrasound examination may also be used to assess the integrity of the UCL.

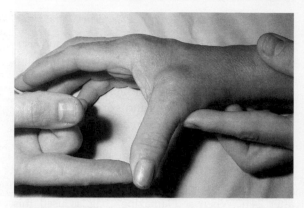

Figure 27.14: Gamekeeper's thumb.

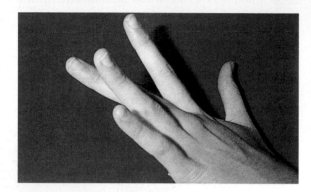

Figure 27.15: An extensor tendon injury.

Flexor tendon injury

The commonest cause is penetrating injury to the hand. The exact mechanism of the laceration must be clearly identified. Examination may reveal an obvious division of the tendon. It is essential to formally test the integrity of both the FDS and FDP. Seemingly normal clinical examination must always be followed by careful inspection of a well-anaesthetized wound with a tourniquet in good light to exclude partial tendon division. One should remember that a tendon injury may not be at the same level as the laceration. X-ray is essential to exclude foreign body or bony injury.

If a partial or complete rupture is suspected or found the patient must always be referred to the hand service. Antibiotics and tetanus cover should be given as appropriate.

Closed rupture of the flexor digitorum profundus may also occur. This classically happens in rugby players who grasp an opponent's jersey as he pulls away. The patient presents with severe pain or the appearance of a lump along the track of the flexor tendon and inability to flex at the DIPJ. This is a significant injury that requires urgent referral to the hand service.

Extensor tendon injury (Fig. 27.15)

Extensor tendon injury is usually associated with a laceration. Diagnosing extensor tendon injury relies on identifying the mechanism of injury and careful evaluation of the wound. X-ray examination is essential to exclude foreign bodies or associated bony injuries. Confirmation of a complete or partial tear should result in referral to the hand service. Antibiotics and tetanus cover should be given as appropriate.

BONE AND JOINT INJURIES

Fractures and dislocations involving the bones of the hand provide due warning of significant associated soft-tissue injury and the likelihood of prolonged rehabilitation, especially if the initial care is poor.

Adherence to the basic principles of obtaining a clear history, careful examination and the appropriate X-rays will set the patient on the correct path leading to a short period of immobilization followed by early rehabilitation. Most fractures and dislocations can be managed conservatively.

Details of the mechanism of injury will give an indication of the forces involved in causing the injury. Examination will reveal signs of possible bony injury, including bruising, swelling, crepitus, deformity, or in some cases just significant tenderness at the fracture site. X-rays must then be ordered. Inadequate views of the injured joint or bone all too often lead to misdiagnosis.

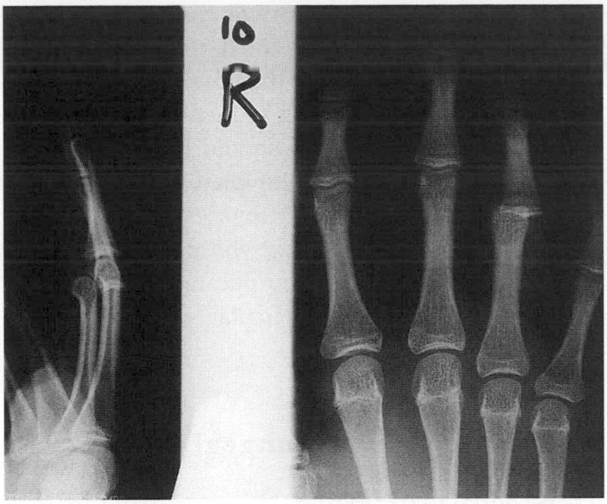

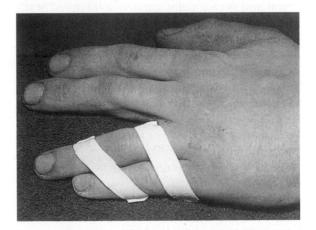

Figure 27.16: Dislocated interphalangeal joint.

Dislocations

These are most commonly of the PIPJ or DIPJ of the finger, although occasionally of the metacarpophalangeal joints (MCP) or the interphalangeal joints (IPJ) of the thumb. Mechanisms include end-on impact or hyperextension injury. Clinical examination usually confirms an obvious dislocation. Digital nerve blockade and an X-ray to exclude associated fracture are essential.

If X-ray confirms dislocation alone, longitudinal traction will usually result in relocation. In certain circumstances where there is an associated fracture or where the volar plate has interposed itself into the joint space, closed reduction will not be achieved. Such patients should be referred to the hand service for open reduction. Once reduction has been achieved it is essential to reassess the joint, ensuring that the collateral ligaments are checked and that reduction has occurred. AP and lateral X-rays should be performed (Fig. 27.16).

A stable joint can be neighbour strapped (also called buddy or companion strapping: Fig. 27.17) or a Bedford splint (Fig. 27.18) can be applied: the patient should be encouraged to start mobilization in 4–5 days and reviewed in clinic at 2 weeks. An unstable joint requires a dorsal splint with the MCPJ at 70° and the PIPJ at 30° in the first instance. The patient should be referred to the hand service for follow-up.

Dislocation of the DIPJ will respond similarly to longitudinal traction. The flexor and extensor insertions to the terminal phalanx must be assessed.

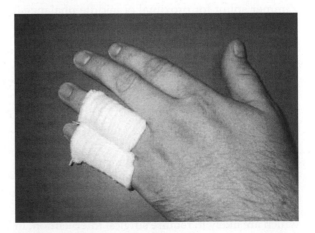

Figure 27.17: Neighbour (buddy) strapping.

Figure 27.18: Bedford splint.

If the joint is stable, treatment consists of neighbour strapping the fingers for 10–14 days.

Testing the integrity of the ulnar collateral ligament is essential following reduction of the MCPJ of the thumb. The thumb should be immobilized in a cast for 14 days. Volar plate injury is commonly associated with IPJ injuries. Close follow-up and early physiotherapy will prevent stiffness and contracture. More complicated fracture dislocations involving the articular surfaces require referral to the hand service.

Non-articular phalangeal fractures

It is essential to distinguish the fracture of the phalanx which is stable and will go on to rapid bony union from the fracture which is unstable and that will lead to delayed union or to surgery. Oblique, spiral and occasionally transverse fractures of the middle and proximal phalanges, especially where rotation or significant displacement has occurred, are unstable.

Rotational deformity must be corrected before application of splintage. This can be assessed by making sure that the ends of the nails are aligned when viewed end-on. If the fracture is comminuted or open this will also complicate or delay bony union. All such unstable fractures should be referred to the hand service in the hospital.

Stable fractures of the phalanges can have appropriate conservative treatment instituted in the emergency department if local joint guidelines have been agreed with the hand service. Treatment options include neighbour strapping, mallet splint for terminal phalangeal fractures or flexion block Zimmer splint for proximal or middle phalangeal fractures. Fractures classified as unstable but where rotation has been corrected may also be managed conservatively in the first instance with a flexion block splint (Fig. 27.19) and referred to the hand service.

Articular fractures

These range from small chip fractures associated with dislocations, commonly of the PIPJ, which are managed conservatively by splintage, to fractures involving more than 25% of the articular surface which are likely to require surgical intervention. In certain circumstances where there is associated

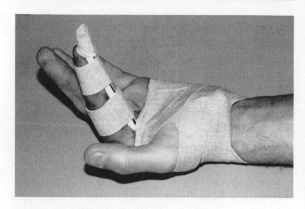

Figure 27.19: Zimmer splint *in situ*.

dorsal subluxation on the true lateral X-ray, these may be managed conservatively by a technique of closed reduction with extension block splintage for a period of time. However, these will require close follow-up.

In children, articular fractures are classified using the Salter–Harris classification (see Chapter 39). Fractures involving the epiphysis and resulting in angulation will require manipulation under regional anaesthesia to achieve a true alignment. This can be achieved using a pen as a fulcrum (Figs 27.20 and 27.21).

Bennett's fracture (Fig. 27.22)

This is an unstable intra-articular fracture of the carpometacarpal joint of the thumb. The fragment is left in joint but the abductor pollicis longus pulls the metacarpal shaft out of position. The injury is inherently unstable. These fractures should be referred to the hand service for closed reduction and fixation or even open reduction.

Metacarpal fractures

The commonest metacarpal fractures are of the little and ring metacarpal heads and these usually result from the patient punching someone or something (often a wall). It is, however, not unusual for the patient initially to deny the true mechanism of injury. Associated abrasions are often from teeth, and significantly increase the risk of infection. The majority of these fractures can be treated conservatively, usually by neighbour strapping of the associated fingers, although in some centres a 'boxing glove' splint around a rolled bandage is used or a

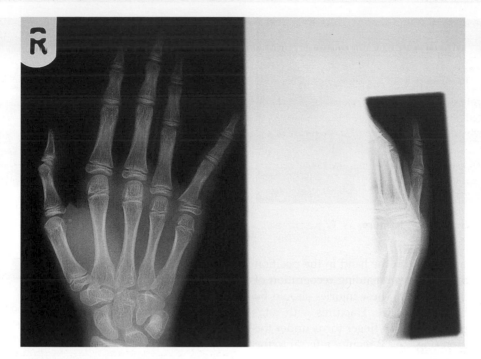

Figure 27.20: An angulated epiphyseal fracture.

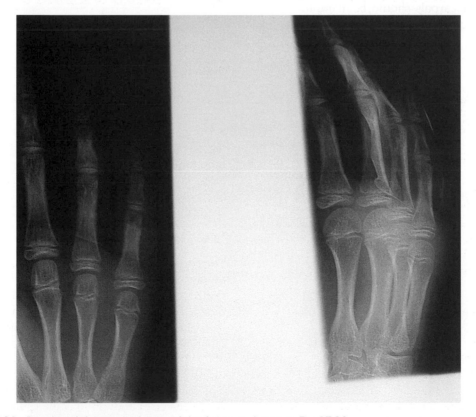

Figure 27.21: Results of the manipulation of the fracture shown in Fig. 27.20.

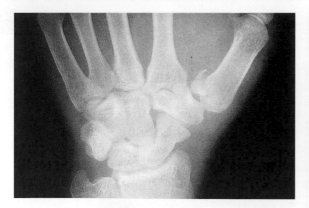

Figure 27.22: Bennett's fracture.

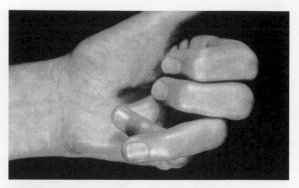

Figure 27.23: Little finger metacarpal fracture with rotational deformity.

volar cast is applied with the hand in the position of function. Similar rules regarding recognition of unstable fractures apply. These injuries should be referred to the hand service. Fractures with rotational deformity where one finger turns under the others on flexion (Fig. 27.23) require referral to the hand service.

Angulation of 30° or more for the index and middle metacarpals and 60° or more for the 4th and 5th metacarpals should be manipulated, but may well require surgical fixation.

FURTHER READING

Wilson, G.R. Nee, P.A. and Watson, J.S. (1997) *Emergency Management of Hand Injuries.* Oxford Handbooks in Emergency Medicine. Oxford University Press, Oxford.

CHAPTER TWENTY EIGHT

BURNS

- Introduction
- Major burns
- Smaller burns
- Infection and burns

- Burns in special places
- Burns and children
- Further reading

INTRODUCTION

Many doctors never forget their first patient with a major burn. These patients have a unique emotional impact on all who are involved with them. Fortunately, the majority of burns presenting to emergency departments are not life threatening. However, correct management of minor burns is important to speed return to full function and ensure the best possible cosmetic result.

MAJOR BURNS (FIG. 28.1)

A major burn is present when 15% or more of the total body surface area (TBSA) is burned beyond simple erythema. Children tolerate burns less well and 10% of the TBSA is an indication for active

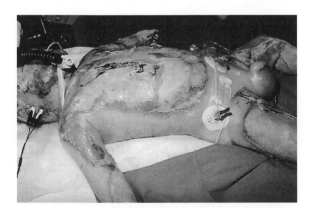

Figure 28.1: A major burn.

resuscitation with intravenous fluids. Major burns are frequently associated with other significant injuries. A patient may jump from a height to avoid flames or receive blast injuries (see Chapter 29) as a result of an associated explosion.

> Burned patients may sustain further injury in escaping from the fire.

FIRST AID FOR A MAJOR BURN

In the prehospital environment, the first priority is to ensure that it safe to approach the burn victim. The patient must be removed from risk of further injury. Burning clothes should be extinguished as quickly as possible. Flames travel upwards and will continue to burn the upright patient. The patient should therefore be lain flat and face down, and the actively burning area should be smothered with a heavy coat or rug. Smouldering clothes should be doused with water. Hot wet clothes should then be removed. The patient must be transferred to hospital as quickly as possible. Time spent on active cooling and elaborate dressings is wasted. If clingfilm is available, this makes a good field dressing. Clean plastic bags are useful for hands. Burnt clothes that are adherent to the skin should be left as attempts to remove them may cause further injury.

Chemicals causing corrosive burns should be removed as quickly as possible. If the corrosive is a dry powder, it should be brushed off. More often the corrosive is liquid or gas. In these cases, there should be prolonged irrigation with water. Particular attention should be paid to irrigating the face and the eyes. The name of the corrosive and any related information should accompany the patient to the hospital since this may affect management. Further information is often available from the Regional Poisons Unit.

As with all trauma, the history and the mechanism of injury is important. In particular, it is important to ascertain:

- The nature of the burning agent. Flame burns have a high risk of inhalational injury; hot water burns do not.
- If flame burns are involved, whether there was entrapment in a confined space, increasing the risk of inhalational injury.
- Whether there was loss of consciousness, suggesting carbon monoxide poisoning.
- Whether associated injuries are possible.

HOSPITAL MANAGEMENT

Airway

Resuscitation should follow the ABC system. The airway is frequently mismanaged in major burns. Early endotracheal intubation, using a gaseous induction, is recommended if there is evidence of inhalational injury. There is no place for observation and conservative management of a compromised airway. Over hours tissue swelling develops, making delayed intubation increasingly difficult.

> The burned airway should be secured with an endotracheal tube *before* problems occur.

Airway assessment should include the factors that suggest inhalational injury (Table 28.1).

Table 28.1: Factors associated with inhalational burns

Flame burns (hot water burns may compromise airways but this is rare and usually the result of hot fluid aspiration)
Facial burns
A hoarse voice (ask the patient whether their voice seems normal for them)
Carbonaceous sputum
Burns in the oropharynx
Confusion or agitation
Stridor
Entrapment in a burning environment

Pulse oximetry is useful in assessing oxygenation but should be interpreted cautiously, since carbon monoxide poisoning will result in falsely high saturations in the presence of significant tissue hypoxia. If there is any possibility of cervical spine trauma, the neck should be immobilized with a rigid collar, sandbags and tape.

Breathing

Once the airway has been secured, breathing can be assessed. Circumferential full-thickness burns of the chest can cause restricted chest excursion and subsequent respiratory embarrassment. However, this does not occur acutely and escharotomy is rarely required in the early stages. The incisions required for an adequate chest escharotomy are shown below (Fig. 28.2). Since full-thickness burns are insensate, analgesia is not necessary. The incision is of adequate depth if it bleeds or fat is visible, and the edges of the wound will be seen to part as the tension is released.

Smoke inhalation may coexist with a respiratory burn or occur in isolation. It results in the deposition of soot in the distal airways which damages the mucosa and cilia and may obstruct smaller calibre airways. Irritation of the airway may also result from products of combustion, resulting in laryngospasm and bronchospasm of varying severity. Most patients will respond well to treatment with a nebulized β_2-agonist such as salbutamol. A small number of severely affected patients may go on to develop a pneumonitis and pulmonary oedema over the next 48 h.

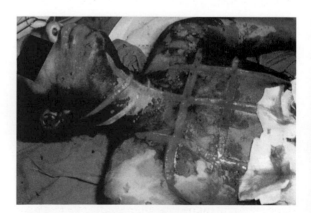

Figure 28.2: Chest escharotomy.

Carboxyhaemoglobinaemia (or carbon monoxide poisoning) should be suspected whenever there is entrapment in a burning environment. Peak carboxyhaemoglobin levels (COHb) levels of less than 20% are usually asymptomatic; higher levels cause headache (20–30%), confusion (30–40%) and coma (40–60%). Levels greater than 60% are usually fatal. There is, however, poor correlation between the measurements made in the emergency department and symptoms, as levels will have declined, depending on the length of time that has elapsed since the patient was removed from the source of poisoning and whether oxygen has been administered.

Treatment is with high-flow oxygen. Increasing the inspired oxygen concentration as much as possible (use a well-fitting face mask with a rebreathing bag) dramatically increases the dissociation of carbon monoxide from haemoglobin. Hyperbaric oxygen is often considered and physiologically sound. However, there is no real proven benefit and the logistics of arranging hyperbaric care may make it impractical. Individual cases should be discussed with the nearest hyperbaric unit.

> The cherry-red appearance of carbon monoxide poisoning is rarely seen in live patients.

Cyanide poisoning should be suspected when there has been exposure to fumes from burning polyurethane (furniture padding), wool, silk or vinyl. Hydrogen cyanide gas is released when these substances are burnt. Cyanide is a cellular poison that prevents oxygen utilization. Clinical pointers include extreme anxiety, a depressed level of consciousness, respiratory distress without cyanosis and a metabolic acidosis. Venous oxygen saturation is high (40% is normal) and values of greater than 90% have been reported in cyanide poisoning. Diagnosis is based on the findings of severe metabolic acidosis with a raised anion gap and serum lactate. Treatment is with dicobalt edetate, and 300 mg should be given and repeated if there is no rapid clinical improvement. The diagnosis must be clear in these cases since these treatments have a considerable risk. Expert advice from a poisons unit is essential. Increasing evidence favours high-dose vitamin B_{12} as a less toxic alternative.

Circulation

Inadequate treatment of the fluid losses occurring in major burns continues to be a preventable source of mortality and morbidity. Two secure, short, wide-bore intravenous cannulae should be inserted and rapid intravenous fluid infusions should be started. Blood should be taken for investigations, including baseline haematocrit and urea and electrolytes. Burnt overlying skin is not a contraindication to cannulation. If simple intravenous cannulation proves impossible then an ankle venous cut-down should be established. Performing a cut-down through burnt skin is often an effective way of gaining intravenous access unless the skin is deeply charred. The cosmetic effect of a cut-down through burnt skin is unimportant and underlying veins may be spared. Central access should be avoided where possible as these cannulae have low flow rates.

Once fluids are up and running a calculation should be made as to the fluid requirement for the first 8 h. The amount of fluid required is related to the weight of the patient, the burn surface area and the time elapsed since the burn. The aim should be to provide $4 \, \text{ml} \, \text{kg}^{-1}$ of body weight of Hartmann's solution per % total body surface area. This volume is given in the first 24 h from the time of burn. Half the volume is given in the first 8 h, the other half in the remaining 16 h (the Parkland formula). An example of a calculation of fluid requirement is given in Table 28.2.

All timings are calculated from the time of the burn, not the time of arrival in hospital. As with all fluid therapy, the correct volume is reflected by adequate urine flow rates. The urine output should be at least $0.5 \, \text{ml} \, \text{kg}^{-1} \text{h}^{-1}$ in adults, $1 \, \text{ml} \, \text{kg}^{-1} \text{h}^{-1}$ in children and $2 \, \text{ml} \, \text{kg}^{-1} \text{h}^{-1}$ in those aged under 1 year. If urine output is inadequate, additional

Table 28.2: Worked example of fluid replacement for burned patient

An 80 kg patient suffers a 70% burn and arrives 1 h after the accident.

Requirement in the first 24 h =
$4 \times 70 \times 80 = 22\,400 \, \text{ml}$

In the first 8 h after the burn = 11 200 ml

As 1 h already elapsed initially requires 1600 ml per hour for next 7 h fluids should be infused. It is important to note that intravenous fluid maintenance requirements should be added to these amounts, which are designed simply to replace fluid lost from the burn wound.

> Adequacy of fluid replacement should be assessed by monitoring urine output.

There are many different formulae for calculating burns fluid requirement and the choice of fluid is controversial: low molecular weight colloid solutions such as Haemaccel® or Gelofusine® are often used in the UK. These probably have no significant advantage over crystalloid solutions. Hartmann's solution is an increasingly popular choice and is the recommended fluid if using the formula given above. Whatever fluid is used it should be warm and there should be enough of it.

Obese patients should have their fluid requirement calculated using their ideal weight. Elderly patients and those with cardiac disease present a difficult fluid management problem. A central venous catheter may be useful to monitor venous pressure, but should not be used as an infusion line and should not be inserted in the emergency department.

Disability

Disability should be assessed in the conventional way using the Glasgow Coma Scale pupillary reactions.

Exposure

The area of the burn should be estimated. The 'rule of nines' (Fig. 28.3) is easily remembered and very useful for rapid assessment. It does, however, lead to over-estimation of the burn surface area.

As a rough guide, the palmar surface of the patient's hand, *including the adducted fingers*, can be considered to represent 1% of the TBSA. This is also useful for estimating the total area of multiple small burns. A more accurate estimation of the burn surface area can be made at this stage by using the Lund and Browder charts (Fig. 28.4).

Burn size is often over-estimated in the initial assessment as a result of including simple erythema in the burnt area.

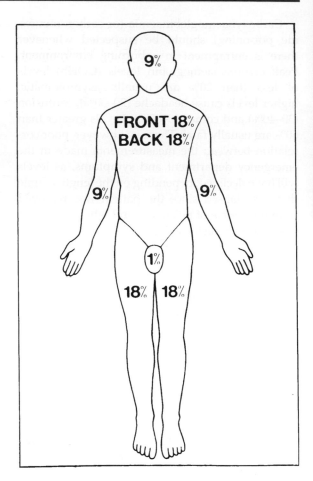

Figure 28.3: The rule of nines.

> Simple erythema is not counted as part of the burnt area.

Circumferential full-thickness burns should be specifically noted. Around the trunk, neck, limbs and digits burnt skin contracts, producing a tourniquet effect that can cause distal ischaemia in the limbs or restriction of respiration. This should be relieved as soon as possible and certainly within 3 h by longitudinal incisions through the burnt skin along its full extent. Since full-thickness burns are insensate, analgesia should not be necessary.

Hypothermia should be anticipated and avoided. Burnt patients may rapidly become hypothermic. The on-scene first aid may result in rapid cooling as a result of cold water hosing and the application of wet blankets. The removal of clothing and loss

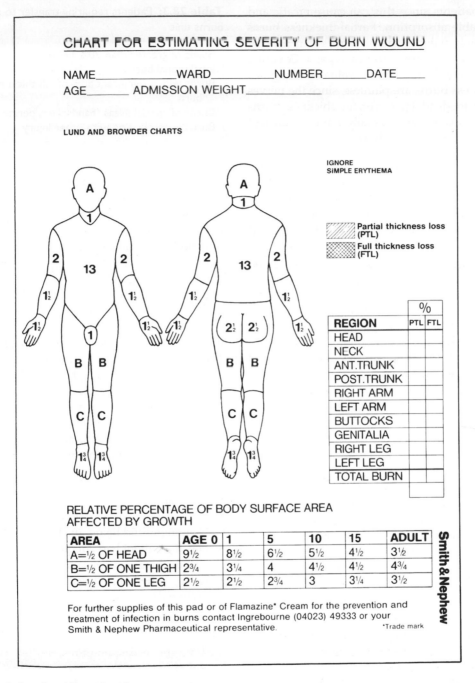

CHART FOR ESTIMATING SEVERITY OF BURN WOUND

NAME_____WARD_____NUMBER_____DATE_____
AGE_____ ADMISSION WEIGHT_____

LUND AND BROWDER CHARTS

IGNORE
SIMPLE ERYTHEMA

Partial thickness loss (PTL)
Full thickness loss (FTL)

REGION	%	
	PTL	FTL
HEAD		
NECK		
ANT.TRUNK		
POST.TRUNK		
RIGHT ARM		
LEFT ARM		
BUTTOCKS		
GENITALIA		
RIGHT LEG		
LEFT LEG		
TOTAL BURN		

RELATIVE PERCENTAGE OF BODY SURFACE AREA
AFFECTED BY GROWTH

AREA	AGE 0	1	5	10	15	ADULT
A=½ OF HEAD	9½	8½	6½	5½	4½	3½
B=½ OF ONE THIGH	2¾	3¼	4	4½	4½	4¾
C=½ OF ONE LEG	2½	2½	2¾	3	3¼	3½

Smith & Nephew

For further supplies of this pad or of Flamazine* Cream for the prevention and
treatment of infection in burns contact Ingrebourne (04023) 49333 or your
Smith & Nephew Pharmaceutical representative.   *Trade mark

Figure 28.4: Lund and Browder chart.

of the normal thermoregulatory function of the skin reduce protection. Rapid infusion of cool fluid can further exacerbate the problem. Steps should be taken from the patient's arrival in hospital onwards to keep them warm.

Analgesia must be given. Intravenous opiates are ideal, in small boluses titrated to effect, with an antiemetic, for instance 2.5 mg of morphine every 2–3 min in an adult. Subcutaneous and intramuscular injections should be avoided in potentially shocked patients since this can cause erratic and unpredictable absorption. Partial-thickness burns are extremely painful: the presence of air passing over them can cause significant pain. Covering and dressing a burn provides valuable analgesia. Full-thickness burns are painless, since the nerves to the skin are dead. However, full-thickness burns are rarely isolated and usually have an area of adjacent partial-thickness burn.

Secondary survey

Once appropriate resuscitation is established, a thorough examination of the whole patient should be carried out. This must include a search for occult injuries. A chest X-ray should be obtained and pelvic and cervical spine X-rays may be necessary depending on the clinical setting. A urinary catheter should be passed if there is no evidence of urethral disruption. A sample of the urine should be dip-tested for blood and sent for microscopy. A positive test for blood on dipstick with clear urine on microscopy implies the presence of myoglobin. This should be specifically sought, and if it is found therapy should be initiated in consultation with the intensive care unit in order to prevent acute renal failure.

A nasogastric tube should be inserted to decompress the stomach, as gastric stasis and vomiting are common. The burns should be photographed with a Polaroid camera and the images stored in the patient's notes. The burns should initially be covered with a dry non-absorbent material. Clingfilm has the advantage of transparency; sterile towels are also useful. Clingfilm must never be wrapped circumferentially around a limb since subsequent swelling may result in distal ischaemia: it should be carefully laid in sheets over the area of the burn wound. Absorbent dressings may be necessary for areas of bleeding following escharotomy. Creams such as Flamazine® must never be applied to major burns.

Do not cover a major burn in cream.

The patient's tetanus status should be ascertained if possible, and, if there is any doubt, immunization and immunoglobulin should be given.

Table 28.3: Patients requiring transfer to a burns unit

Burns of greater than 20% TBSA
Inhalational burns
Burns with a significant area of full-thickness burn
Burns of special areas (hands, feet, perineum)
Burns in association with other injury

There is no place for administering prophylactic antibiotics. Infection can convert a partial-thickness burn to a full-thickness burn, but prophylactic antibiotics merely encourage resistant bacteria. Infection risks can be minimized by keeping the burn covered and encouraging staff to wear sterile gloves.

Major burns require referral to a burns unit and some smaller burns will also benefit from the expertise of such a unit (Table 28.3). In most cases this requires interhospital transfer of the patient. The decision to transfer burns with associated injuries will depend on the availability of other specialities at the hospital with the burns unit. It is vital to ensure that the patient is adequately resuscitated prior to transfer and that all relevant notes are photocopied and accompany the patient. Care is improved if the following questions are asked before transfer:

- Is the airway clear?
- Is there good vascular access?
- Is enough fluid being given?
- Has the patient had adequate analgesia?
- Has the bladder been catheterized?
- Have other life-threatening injuries been excluded?

SMALLER BURNS

Minor burns is a misleading term. They are certainly not minor to those who suffer them. Smaller burns is a more accurate term. Inappropriate management will delay return to normal function and impairs the cosmetic outcome. This section discusses first the diagnosis of the burn and then the management.

HISTORY AND EXAMINATION

The nature of the burning agent should be ascertained, and the circumstances leading to the burn described. If a doctor cannot visualize the mechanism of injury then the history is incomplete. The time-lapse since the accident is important. A brief medical history should be taken to look for:

- allergies, particularly to antibiotics
- tetanus status
- other illnesses, such as diabetes or epilepsy.

A social and occupational history should be taken. This has more significance at the extremes of age. Elderly patients living alone with a burn to the dominant hand may require help from social services. Neglect or even non-accidental injury should be considered in children and in the elderly.

The burn should be examined, and if possible, a Polaroid photograph should be taken. Burns are classified into the following types.

Simple erythema

Simple erythema heals well and requires no treatment other than analgesia.

Superficial partial-thickness burns

Superficial partial-thickness burns extend no further than the germinal layer of the skin (sited between the epidermis and the dermis). These burns appear red and raw, with thin-walled blisters. These usually heal well with dressings and analgesia. The cosmetic result is usually excellent, provided infection is avoided.

Full-thickness burns

Full-thickness burns extend through the dermis into the subcutaneous tissues. They are insensate on testing with a sterile pin. There is a characteristic leathery, hard look and coagulated vessels may be seen. Again the dead germinal layer makes healing from the base of the wound impossible and grafting is usually necessary unless the burn is

small (usually less than $1\,\text{cm}^2$), in which case slow healing may occur from the wound edges.

The burn should be measured and these findings documented on the patient's record.

CAUSES OF BURN

Hot water burns are the commonest burns in emergency department practice. Elderly patients often spill hot drinks into their lap and children pull boiling kettles on to themselves. Most domestic hot water burns are superficial partial-thickness burns. However, steam has the ability to cause full-thickness burns rapidly. Industry often uses super-heated steam and this can cause greater damage. Boiling oil, most commonly from deep-fat frying pans, is hotter than water and the damage caused is consequently greater.

Direct thermal burns are also common, for example from burnt clothing. These burns are more likely to be full-thickness or deep partial-thickness than are hot water burns.

Electrical burns are fortunately less common. The systemic state of the patient should be considered and it should be noted that the electric shock may have thrown the patient some distance, resulting in other injuries. Loss of consciousness suggests an arrhythmia and the need for cardiac monitoring. A normal ECG without loss of consciousness probably excludes significant cardiac injury. Electric shocks can also damage joints, notably classically but rarely causing posterior dislocations of the shoulder, and tetanic contraction of the hands may delay release of the electrical source.

The burn damage and depth are usually greater than the superficial appearance would suggest. The entry wound is usually small and full-thickness. Exit wounds should be looked for. The ipsilateral elbow is a common site from a burnt hand. Electrical burns across the head have the ability to cause early and late ophthalmic injuries such as cataract and glaucoma. Electricity is preferentially conducted through tissues such as muscle and nerves. Underlying damage to the muscles around the burn site is common and is often not immediately apparent. Compartment syndrome is possible and should be anticipated. If there is the possibility of any injury worse than superficial burns, specialist advice should be sought.

Electrical burns are often worse than they look, with severe underlying tissue damage.

Chemical burn severity depends on the contact time and chemical agent. If the chemical's characteristics are unknown, advice should be sought from the Regional Poisons Unit. Whatever the chemical agent is, dry powders should be brushed off and wet chemicals should be washed off with copious amounts of water. Irrigation should be prolonged for at least 15 min. Neutralizing agents must not be used as the neutralization process often results in the generation of further heat, worsening the burn wound.

Neutralizing agents for chemical burns are generally of no use.

Cement is a common cause of chemical burns, classically involving the knees. The lime component combines with water to form calcium hydroxide. This is a strong alkali and penetrates the skin, causing deep burns that may only become apparent when clothing is removed. Initial treatment consists of brushing off any visible dry powder followed by sustained powerful irrigation by water. Clothing containing cement dust should be washed before it is worn again. These burns should be followed up in clinic, as burns that are initially superficial may become deeper over a couple of days.

Hydrofluoric acid causes particularly unpleasant burns and systemic effects. It is used widely for etching and frosting glass and in the production of fuels, electronics, dyes, and for cleaning stone and brick buildings. Rapid penetration of the skin causes local and systemic effects. The systemic release of fluoride ions alters calcium, magnesium and potassium homoeostasis. The increased potassium permeability causes nerve depolarization and subsequent pain. Hypocalcaemia should be treated with intravenous calcium chloride.

The immediate management is copious irrigation; ice applied to the burn provides good analgesia. Topical calcium gluconate gel has been used in the past and intralesional calcium gluconate injections ($0.5 \, ml \, cm^{-2}$ of burn) can provide rapid analgesia. Senior staff and poisons units should be involved in making treatment decisions in these patients. Significant (greater than 2%) hydrofluoric acid burns should always be admitted.

Phenol (carbolic acid) is a corrosive agent widely used in industry. It causes necrosis of the skin resulting in a white or brown painless coagulum. Systemic effects are uncommon, but renal failure should be considered. The initial treatment is as for any other chemical burn.

Radiation burns are rarely seen in emergency departments. Simple sunburn usually produces erythema only, but in severe cases there may be partial-thickness burns that require dressing.

TREATMENT OF SMALLER BURNS

Initial first aid consists of placing the affected part under a cold, running tap. This provides analgesia and stops the burn process. Rapid cooling of this type should be used cautiously in children with torso burns, since hypothermia is a real possibility.

The aims of treatment are to:

- prevent infection
- treat any infections as they occur
- create an optimal environment to promote healing
- identify patients who need further specialist help
- ensure rapid return to function.

Large thin-walled blisters should be aspirated with a sterile needle (if left they will usually rupture, soaking the dressings with oedema fluid); smaller blisters may be left intact. There is no point in removing the surface of a blister ('deroofing'), since all that will be left is a painful raw surface to which dressings will stick. The intact blister leaves a sterile, moist environment in which the burn will heal well. The wound should be dressed and advice should be sought regarding departmental policy; experienced nurses are usually happy to advise. The functions of the dressing are to prevent infection, provide a moist environment for healing and provide analgesia. There are many ways of dressing a burn and practice will vary from department to department. A 'traditional' burns dressing consists of four layers:

- a moist non-adherent layer
- a dry non-adherent layer

- an absorbent layer
- a bandage to secure the dressing in place.

A paraffin gauze preparation is the most common choice for the inner layer. Preparations containing antiseptics such as chlorhexidine have no additional benefit and may stimulate an allergic reaction. Two or three sheets of the first layer should be applied. A simple non-adherent dressing makes a good second layer. The purpose of this layer is to prevent burn exudate reaching the absorbent layer and providing a track for infection. Burn exudate reaching the third layer indicates that the protective function of the dressing has been lost and the dressing should be replaced. Simple gauze is a good third layer.

The burn wound should be inspected at regular intervals. Every 3–5 days is usually sufficient, though each time the dressing is completely removed healing epithelial cells are stripped from the surface of the healing wound and the infection risk is increased. The aims of follow-up are to:

- accurately diagnose the depth of the burn
- identify those patients who will need skin-grafting
- identify infections early and provide treatment
- change part of the dressing.

Changing the whole dressing for the sake of change is not necessary. The outer three layers should be removed. If the wound is clean and healing well, then there is no merit in removing the inner layer.

INFECTION AND BURNS

A severe infection can convert a partial-thickness burn to a full-thickness burn. Treatment of infections should start from the first dressing. Covering the wound provides an important barrier. There is, however, no place for systemic, prophylactic antibiotics. Infection is not prevented and all that occurs is later infection with resistant bacteria. There is one exception to this rule. Early infection of a burn with beta-haemolytic *Streptococcus* is life-threatening, especially in a child, and can result in a toxic shock syndrome. If the burn patient has a sore throat, a throat swab should be taken.

If beta-haemolytic *Streptococcus* is isolated, then benzyl penicillin should be given.

Prophylactic antibiotics are rarely indicated for burns.

If a burn appears to be infected at follow-up then the dressing should be removed and the burn swabbed and redressed. Systemic antibiotics should be given and the usual infecting agents are *Staphylococcus aureus* and *Streptococcus*. Flucloxacillin is a reasonable first-choice antibiotic although it may need to be changed depending on swab results. Admission for intravenous antibiotics may be necessary in cases where there is systemic illness or oral therapy is unsuccessful. Burns are tetanus-prone wounds: if there is any uncertainty about the immune status of the patient immunization should be given.

BURNS IN SPECIAL PLACES

Common causes of facial burns (Fig. 28.5) include release of steam and hot water from car radiators or flashbacks from gas appliances. The possibility of airway involvement (see above) should always be considered. The eyes must be carefully examined for any injury. The visual acuity should be recorded and fluorescein used to identify any corneal damage. Ocular burns require ophthalmology referral. Burns involving the eyelids and lip margins should be referred to a plastic surgeon.

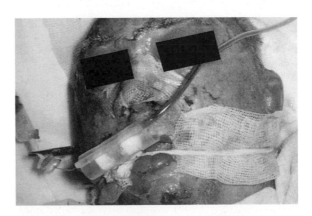

Figure 28.5: Facial burns.

Contractures, particularly of the eyelids, can occur within 24 h. Less significant burns can be managed in the emergency department. Dressing facial burns is usually difficult or impossible and leaving the burn open to the air is usually the best option in simple uncomplicated facial burns. The patient must be instructed to keep the area clean and return at the first sign of infection. Applying creams and ointments to the burn is generally of little benefit. Flamazine® cream must never be applied to the face as it can result in permanent black discoloration, owing to its silver content (Flamazine® contains silver sulphadiazine).

Never apply Flamazine® to facial burns.

The hands are a common site for burns. The most important concern with burnt hands is not cosmesis but minimizing the loss of function that can occur. Flexion deformities can result from contractures secondary to deep partial-thickness or full-thickness burns.

Immobilization results in stiffness of fingers and mobilization of the hand should occur as soon as pain permits. Adequate analgesia will promote mobilization. Specialist referral is often necessary despite the small areas involved.

Patients with hand burns should be encouraged to mobilize the hand early.

Dressing the hand can often be an involved and time-consuming process. The Flamazine® bag (Fig. 28.6) is a good initial treatment. The hand is liberally coated in ointment and placed inside a waterproof bag. This is sealed at the wrist. The hand is then elevated in a high arm sling. The bag needs to be changed every day. The patient should be warned that the hand will become swollen, white and unsightly, partly from being in a moist warm environment. After a few days the extent of the burn will be more apparent and less cumbersome dressings can be applied. After a few days, the dressing can be changed for a standard paraffin-gauze-type dressing. Flamazine® bags are often not robust enough for use in small children, and small localized areas of burn to the hands can be treated with local application of a paraffin-based dressing which may be less incapacitating to the patient.

The soles of the feet are occasionally burnt. Patients with burns to both feet usually require admission for elevation and dressings. Similarly, burns to the genitalia and perineum are not uncommon. These areas are difficult to dress and prone to infection. Admission may be necessary if the area cannot easily be dressed, and treatment involves exposure of the burn in a clean environment. Specialist referral is usually necessary for further management in these cases.

BURNS AND CHILDREN

Children's skin is more delicate than adult skin; as a consequence, hot water that may be merely

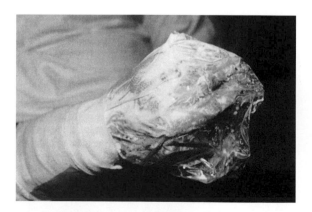

Figure 28.6: Flamazine® bags.

Table 28.4: Factors suggesting non-accidental cause of burn injury

Delay in presentation: burnt children usually scream and demand immediate attention in a way that is hard to ignore
If the reported mechanism of injury is inconsistent with the physical findings
If there is a 'dipping injury': both legs are burnt as if the child has been dipped into hot water. This is particularly suspicious if the buttocks are spared; this implies that the child was pushed on to the cooler floor of the bath
If the burn is on the dorsum of the hand: curious children touch hot objects with the palmar aspect of the hand
If the burns could have been caused by a cigarette

uncomfortable to an adult can cause scalds in children. Burning is a regrettably common form of non-accidental injury (Chapter 39). The suspicion of child abuse should be raised in the presence of any of the factors listed in Table 28.4.

FURTHER READING

Settle J. (1986) *Burns: The First Five Days*. Smith & Nephew Pharmaceuticals, Romford, Essex.

CHAPTER TWENTY NINE

BLAST AND GUNSHOT INJURY

- Introduction
- Blast injury
- Gunshot injury

- Clinical management
- Further reading

INTRODUCTION

With the growth of terrorism on a national and international scale, incidents involving injuries caused by bombs, bullets and other projectiles are becoming increasingly common (Fig. 29.1). The prevalence of the drug culture in many of our inner cities also provides an environment within which the use of firearms is common and brings the threat to the doors of our emergency departments. Therefore, it is now important that all doctors who might have to deal with the victims of such incidents are aware of the features of the injuries these weapons cause.

The first priority for any doctor in these circumstances is to avoid becoming a victim themselves. If called to the scene it is important to follow the instructions given by the security services precisely, otherwise more people may become involved in attempts to rescue the hapless good Samaritan. In the emergency department it should not be forgotten that dangerous weapons may still be on the body of the victim and that it is not unknown, even in this country, for a 'gangland battle' to continue within the department.

BLAST INJURY

A list of recent UK terrorist explosions is given in Table 42.2. It should not be forgotten, however,

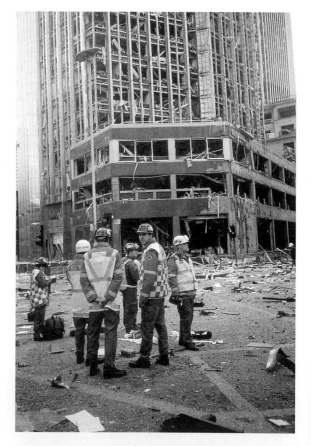

Figure 29.1: The City of London bomb.

that injuries due to blast also occur in industrial situations, and may bring with them problems specific to that environment, such as chemical contamination.

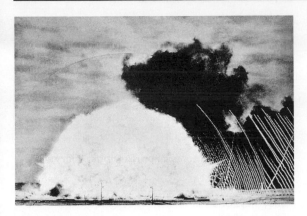

Figure 29.2: The shock front following the detonation of high explosive.

THE NATURE OF BLAST

Shock wave (Fig. 29.2)

Explosives are substances that produce large volumes of gases at high temperature and pressure when detonated. So-called *low explosives*, such as gunpowder, burn on ignition and only explode if confined. *High explosives*, however, do not need to be confined, but require a small detonating charge ('detonator') to initiate the explosion.

As the gases expand they compress the surrounding air, creating a shock wave (or shock front) with an almost immediate rise in pressure, which moves out from the source of the explosion as a rapidly expanding sphere of high-pressure gas. The velocity of the shock wave, at over $3000\,\mathrm{m\,s^{-1}}$ in air, is initially faster than the speed of sound, but this rapidly declines depending on the amount and nature of the explosion and the surrounding environment. As the shock wave moves away from the source, the pressure difference generated falls away and is briefly replaced by a period of relative negative pressure. The shock wave is responsible for the primary blast injury. When blast waves meet an object such as a wall, they are reflected (like ripples meeting the side of a pond) and the reflected wave reinforces the original (incident) blast wave, producing even higher pressure and potentially devastating injuries. This is an important factor in many terrorist bombings of public houses and similar settings and accounts in part for the appalling injuries received in such confined spaces.

Table 29.1: Blast injuries

Primary (blast wave): ears, lungs, abdomen
Secondary (fragment injuries)
Tertiary (displacement, leading to impact injuries and amputations)
Burns
Crush injuries
Psychological effects

Blast wind

The shock wave produces an area of rapid turbulent movement of displaced air, the blast wind or dynamic overpressure. This movement of a large volume of air (equal to the volume of gases produced by the explosion) has potentially devastating effects. It is the blast wind that is responsible for the traumatic amputations, bodily disintegrations and fragment injuries of secondary and tertiary blast injury.

EFFECTS OF BLAST (TABLE 29.1)

Primary blast injury

Primary blast injuries result from the effects of the shock wave. It must be emphasized, however, that the injuries described rarely occur alone and are almost invariable found together with the more obviously dramatic secondary and tertiary blast effects.

When blast waves meet a body, two types of wave result:

- stress waves
- shear waves.

Stress waves are similar to sound waves and travel through the body at very high speeds. Very large local forces produced by the passage of the waves produce small but very rapid distortion of the tissues. These are stress waves and are particularly important in areas where tissues of different densities meet. The greater the difference in density, the greater the effect.

At the same time, *shearing forces* are created by the different accelerations imparted to tissues of different densities by the shock wave.

The blast wave also compresses and heats small areas of air (e.g. the alveoli) which expand, creating further shock fronts (*implosion*). Within the body, the blast wave will be reflected off denser structures in its path causing very significant local forces by summation. The final primary blast effect is direct *compression* of the body of the victim by pressure waves encircling the body.

The organs most effected by primary blast effects therefore are the lungs, abdominal organs and tympanic membranes.

Injury to the ears

The ears are the most sensitive organs to primary blast injury and rupture of the tympanic membrane can occur at pressures above about 15 kPa. The effects of blast vary from congestion of the tympanic membrane to complete disruption of the ossicles of the middle ear. Whilst it is undoubtedly true that patients rendered deaf by blast have suffered significant blast effects and should be observed for other potential injuries, ear injury is extremely unpredictable as it depends largely on the orientation of the auditory canal to the shock front and may therefore be absent in patients at serious risk of injuries elsewhere.

Deafness is a sign of significant blast exposure.

Lung injury

Injury to the lung occurs at pressures above 175 kPa. The term blast lung is usually used to refer to a syndrome of alveolar damage with haemorrhage and consolidation, pulmonary oedema and airway haemorrhage. These changes are due to the transmission of the shock wave through the wall of the thorax rather than via the upper airways. Other problems include acute pulmonary oedema, pneumothorax, haemothorax or pneumomediastinum, and a syndrome resembling adult respiratory distress syndrome (ARDS) (Table 29.2).

The injuries seen in lungs as a consequence of blast are thought to be due to the initial rapid acceleration imparted to the chest wall by the shock wave. The lung changes in so-called blast lung are very similar to those seen in conventional traumatic lung contusion.

The symptoms of lung injury due to blast are given in Table 29.3. Breathlessness and hypoxia occur, with possible progression to acute respiratory

Table 29.2: Primary blast effects on the lungs

Alveolar haemorrhage with consolidation
Acute pulmonary oedema
Pneumothorax, haemothorax or
    pneumomediastinum
Adult respiratory distress-like syndrome

Table 29.3: Symptoms of primary blast injury to the lungs

Shortness of breath
Dry cough
Chest pain
Restlessness
Confusion/agitation

failure in a minority of cases. Frank blood or blood-stained pulmonary oedema fluid may be aspirated from the upper airways. The chest radiograph may be normal or show diffuse or localized shadowing typical of alveolar consolidation as well as pneumothorax, haemothorax or pneumomediastinum and rib fractures.

Currently, the only effective treatment for progressive respiratory failure is respiratory support in intensive care. However, lung injury is uncommon and the majority of victims appear to suffer short, self-limiting symptoms without progression to respiratory failure. It is usually found in patients who were close to the initial explosion and all such patients, irrespective of apparent absence of physical injury, should be admitted for observation, as a very small proportion will subsequently develop ARDS-like syndrome. In practice, the vast majority of victims who are sufficiently close to the blast to sustain primary blast injuries will also have sustained serious, if not fatal, secondary and tertiary injuries.

High-flow oxygen should be given to all blast victims.

Pneumothorax, haemothorax and pneumomediastinum require the insertion of an intercostal drain, and all patients who receive mechanical ventilation should be very carefully observed for the development of these complications. The use of prophylactic chest drains should be considered in patients who are to be mechanically ventilated.

Table 29.4: Primary effects of blast on the abdomen

Immediate perforation
Intestinal wall haemorrhages with delayed
  perforation
Mesenteric tears
Retroperitoneal haemorrhage
Solid organ damage

All blast victims should be monitored by pulse
oximetry.

Fluid replacement in blast victims should always be carefully monitored as there is no doubt that over-enthusiastic infusion of large amounts of fluid increases pulmonary oedema, producing hypoxia and worsening the prognosis.

Abdominal injury

Injuries to gas-containing intra-abdominal organs occur at higher pressures than cause injury to the lungs. The primary effects of blast on the abdomen are summarized in Table 29.4. These injuries are relatively uncommon in explosions in air, although they occur more frequently with explosions under water.

Intestinal perforation presents in the same way as any other perforation, with peritonitis. Laparotomy and surgical repair is usually required. Haemorrhage may also occur into the retroperitoneum, from solid organs and from mesenteric tears.

The initial treatment of primary blast injury to the abdomen, like that of primary lung injury, relies on careful attention to the primary survey sequence of airway, breathing, circulation, disability and exposure. Symptoms and signs suggestive of abdominal injury include abdominal tenderness and distension, rectal bleeding (a sign of intramural haemorrhage) and abdominal pain. Testicular pain is common but does not require any specific treatment.

Any patient who has any evidence of abdominal injury requires urgent surgical review and is likely to require laparotomy. If there are any victims of an explosion, a wait and see policy may be instituted for patients with equivocal findings.

Sudden death

A small proportion of the victims of blast die without any evidence of external injury. It has been

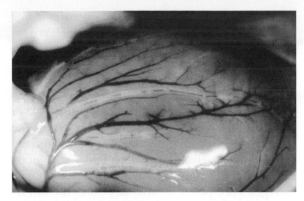

Figure 29.3: Air emboli in the coronary arteries following exposure to blast.

suggested that these deaths are due either to cardiac arrhythmia or to air emboli (Fig. 29.3).

Secondary blast injury

Secondary blast injuries result from fragments displaced by the blast wind. These may be fragments of the bomb (bomb casing or nails) or materials from the environment such as glass, masonry or wood. The size and number of fragments varies dramatically, as do the injuries – from massive non-survivable wounds to multiple superficial lacerations. All these wounds can be assumed to be heavily contaminated with bacteria. Tattooing of exposed skin with dirt is a problem in these patients.

It should also be remembered that it is in this group of patients that primary blast injuries are also most likely to occur.

Management of these patients follows the standard system of primary and secondary survey, and the devastating nature of some of these injuries should not distract from careful attention to such a systematic approach.

Tertiary blast injuries

Tertiary blast injuries result from the blast wind. The mass rapid movement of air causes the devastating injuries so commonly associated with terrorist incidents. Victims standing very close to the explosion may suffer complete disintegration. Slightly further away, traumatic amputations occur, producing ragged amputations usually through a long bone rather than a joint. These are avulsive amputations and the tissue damage, which is usually extensive, will be found to extend proximally from the amputation stump where tendons and other tissues are avulsed. It is possible that these amputations follow damage to the limb from the initial shock wave. The blast wind also causes movement of bodies through the air, giving the opportunity for further injuries on impact with the environment. These appalling-looking injuries require careful surgical toilet (reimplantation is rarely, if ever, possible) after any other life-threatening injuries have been identified and dealt with (Figs 29.4 and 29.5).

Burns

Flash and flame burns occur in explosions. Flash burns usually occur at the time of detonation. Although the results may look dramatic (like very severe sunburn) they are usually superficial and

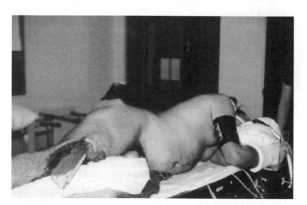

Figure 29.4: Secondary blast injuries.

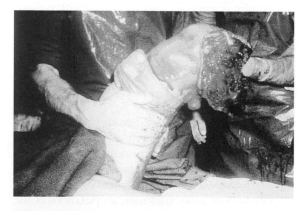

Figure 29.5: Amputations due to blast.

healing is rapid, without scarring. Flame burns usually only occur if the explosion has caused the environment to ignite. The treatment of burns due to explosion is identical to that of other burns although particular attention must be paid to the presence of possibility of other injuries.

Crush injuries

Crush injuries are relatively common following explosions and crush asphyxia is a common cause of death amongst victims recovered from the ruins of buildings. Intensive respiratory support is likely to be needed for those patients who have sustained crush injuries to the chest. Abdominal crush injuries may require laparotomy. The possibility of electrolyte disturbances following the relief of pressure on trapped muscle should not be overlooked. Hyperkalaemia can cause cardiac arrest and released myoglobin can contribute to renal failure. A good urine output should be maintained by appropriate fluid replacement.

Psychological

Both the victims of blast explosion and the rescuers are at risk of suffering psychological sequelae from their experiences. Factors in the development of a post-traumatic stress reaction include the preincident mental state and 'support systems' available, the nature of the experience and the support and leadership given during the incident. Feelings of guilt occur in survivors (especially those who have lost relatives) as well as in rescuers who have been involved in unsuccessful actions. There is no doubt that the terrible nature of the injuries that result from explosions can be particularly devastating for some people. Coupled with this is the indiscriminate nature of the terrorist bomb. Emergency service personnel and medical and nursing staff function more effectively and suffer less psychological damage if they see themselves as performing a valuable role as part of a team, and are kept well informed and perceive strong but concerned leadership. All those involved in such an incident should be involved in a 'hot' debrief at the end of the incident and also encouraged to attend a more detailed debrief a short time after the incident, as well as to talk about their experiences with colleagues and family or friends.

GUNSHOT INJURY

INTRODUCTION – MISSILES

Missiles, including bullets, are effective at causing damage because they have kinetic energy given by the formula:

$$KE = 1/2\, M\, V^2$$

where KE is the kinetic energy, M the mass of the projectile and V^2 the square of the velocity of the missile.

The effectiveness of bullets in causing damage to tissues depends on how much of the available energy is transferred to the tissue. Thus if a bullet is stopped by tissue, all the available energy is transferred to work upon the tissue to cause damage. If a bullet passes straight through tissue without any significant slowing, very little damage may be done, as the energy given up is only proportional to the difference between the initial and final velocities.

Thus, the old concept of high- and low-velocity missiles has been replaced by the concept of energy *transfer*. It is this that determines the damage produced. The wounds are more usefully divided into *high-energy transfer* and *low-energy transfer* rather than high- and low-velocity. It should also be remembered that the same amount of damage will produce different effects depending on the tissue involved – a gunshot wound to the heart will have immediate devastating effects compared to one producing equal damage to the muscle of the thigh.

HIGH- AND LOW-ENERGY TRANSFER WOUNDS

Clinically, the most important difference between high- and low-energy transfer wounds is that in low-energy transfer wounds the tissue damage is largely confined to the track of the missile, whereas in high-energy transfer wounds injury extends radially for some distance from that track. This is because of the formation of a *temporary cavity* (Fig. 29.6).

Temporary cavitation occurs when the missile transfers large amounts of energy, causing the tissue to accelerate away from the path of the missile. The cavity lasts a few milliseconds, then collapses. The temporary cavity formation results in negative pressure, which sucks dirt and debris into the wound, producing gross tissue contamination and destruction.

Factors affecting the amount of energy transferred may be divided into two groups:

- features of the missile
- features of the tissue.

FEATURES OF THE MISSILE

Greater amounts of energy are transferred by a bullet to tissue if the area of the bullet that strikes the tissue is increased by deformation (the principle behind the notorious 'dum-dum' bullet with its soft nose) or fragmentation. Military bullets, including many of those used by terrorists, are required by law (under the Hague Declaration of 1899) to have a 'full metal jacket' in order to reduce the likelihood of fragmentation or deformation and hence to reduce 'superfluous wounding'. Many bullets used by the police or sportsmen (hunters) have an exposed core at the tip designed to ensure maximum energy transfer and hence stopping power, whilst minimizing collateral damage as a result of complete penetration of the intended victim by the bullet.

The rifling that is found in rifle (and some handgun) barrels is designed to give stability to the bullet in flight. In practice all bullets are unstable, and demonstrate deviation along their long axis, or yaw, whilst in flight (Fig. 29.7(a)).

This effect is increased when the bullet enters a denser medium such as soft tissue, causing the

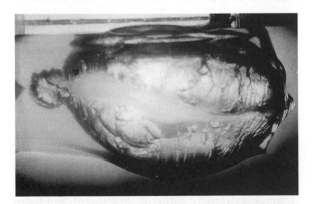

Figure 29.6: Temporary cavitation in a high-energy transfer wound. This photograph, taken using a high-speed camera, is of a simulation using a bullet fired into a block of gelatine.

(a)

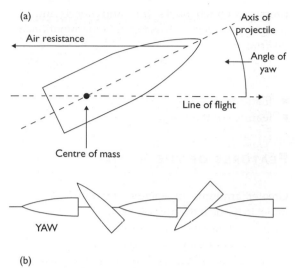

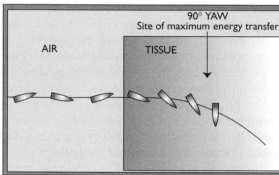

(b)

Figure 29.7: (a) Yaw and (b) tumbling.

bullet to tumble. The effect of this is to increase energy transfer. Retardation of a bullet is greatest when its long axis is at 90° to the axis of its travel.

FEATURES OF TISSUE

As stated above, when a missile strikes a very dense substance such as bone, rapid slowing results in the transfer of large amounts of energy together with bony destruction and the formation of secondary fragments of bone, which in turn can cause further damage. A further effect of striking bone is to change the direction of the path of the missile: this makes clinical prediction of likely damage extremely difficult. In general, the more dense the tissue penetrated, the greater the energy transfer. The effects of the energy transfer will vary to some extent on the type of tissue involved. Cavitation within an organ such as the liver is

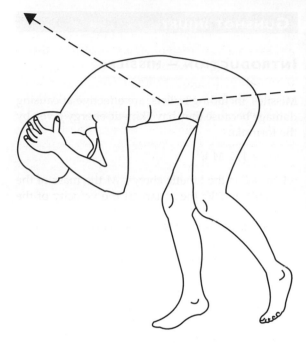

Figure 29.8: Missile track and position at time of wounding.

likely to cause devastating damage to the friable tissue, particularly as it is contained within a non-distensible capsule. Injury to skeletal muscle may well be more extensive than is clinically apparent owing to stretching of the muscle tissue.

> The track of a bullet cannot be predicted from the entry wound.

It is vital that it is always remembered that a major determinant of the track of a missile is the position of the victim at the time of wounding (Fig. 29.8). As a consequence of this it is possible for missiles entering the shoulder to cause abdominal injury, or missiles entering the thighs to penetrate the thorax.

Fracture of bone may also occur distant from the track of a bullet owing to the transfer of large quantities of energy to the tissue immediately surrounding the missile track.

TYPES OF MISSILE

Bullets

In clinical practice, unless the bullet was fired from a weapon belonging to the police or military, it is likely that the precise type both of the weapon and of the bullet will not be known to the clinician. In any case, such information should not lead to the clinician drawing unjustifiable conclusions regarding the nature of the injury based on erroneous assumptions and lack of clinical experience in this field.

In general, handguns fire jacketed lead bullets producing low-energy transfer wounds and injury along the track of the projectile. The significance of the injury will depend to a large extent on the organs involved in the wound. A wound to the heart involving low-energy transfer is still almost certain to be lethal.

As mentioned above, police and hunting weapons are usually partially jacketed, deform on impact and produce high-energy transfer wounds. Modern bullets designed for military use (which are in widespread use amongst terrorists) have a full metal jacket and are intended not to deform or fragment. Complete penetration of a body is possible unless very dense tissue is struck. However, tumbling and fragmentation can also occur, producing devastating high-energy transfer wounds.

Baton rounds

The baton round (Fig. 29.9), usually referred to as a 'rubber bullet' or 'plastic bullet', presents a large area of impact and is designed to cause painful soft-tissue injury in order to discourage further involvement in civil disturbance. Penetration does not occur; however, fatalities have occurred when rounds have struck the abdomen, chest or head. Injuries tend to be more severe in children.

Airguns

Airgun injuries produce single low-energy wounds, which in the majority of cases are not associated with significant injury. Their effects can be serious in small children or when penetration of the eye with intracranial involvement occurs. As a consequence these injuries must always be taken seriously. In the majority of cases, without complications, referral or simple removal under image intensification is appropriate (Fig. 29.10).

Shotguns

Shotguns are designed to fire multiple pellets varying in size from birdshot (the smallest) to buckshot.

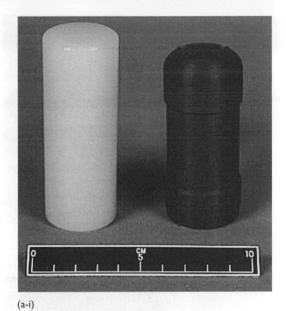

(a-i)

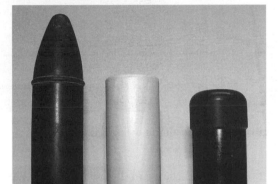

(a-ii)

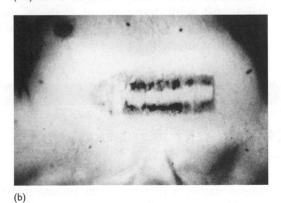

(b)

Figure 29.9: Baton rounds: (a) round; (b) skin marking.

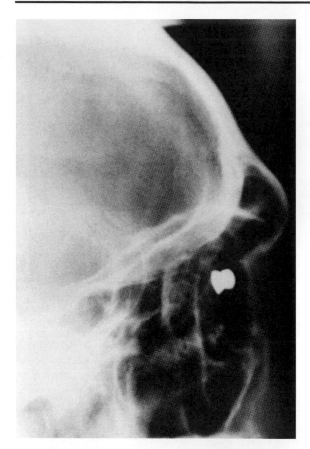

Figure 29.10: An airgun pellet in the orbit.

At ranges of less than 5 m the pellets may act as a single missile, producing a large entry wound and a high-entry transfer wound which may be lethal. At longer ranges, individual pellets result in multiple low-energy transfer wounds with varying depths of penetration. Close-range shotgun wounds are contaminated with fragments of clothing and wadding from the cartridge and are consequently at high risk of infection.

CLINICAL MANAGEMENT

MANAGEMENT IN THE EMERGENCY DEPARTMENT

The resuscitation of all patients with ballistic injury must follow the principles of the primary survey. It is vital that clinicians are not distracted by the cause of the patient's injury.

Resuscitation always follows the system of primary and secondary survey.

Life-saving surgery should not be delayed. Wounds should be covered with moist sterile dressings, not impregnated with iodine.

Victims of both explosions and shootings are by definition victims of crime and a full forensic investigation will be necessary. It is essential therefore that clinicians do not damage evidence that might subsequently be of value. Clothing should be cut, if necessary, away from rather than through holes made by fragments or bullets, and should be handed over to the police. If bullets are removed from wounds, gloved fingers should be used as forceps can damage the rifling marks that may link the bullet to a particular weapon.

It is widely stated that entrance and exit wounds can be identified because the latter tend to be larger and more ragged than the former. Although in general this is true, unfortunately it is not invariably the case and a mistaken approach along these lines can lead to significant errors in clinical management. Furthermore, because of deflection of bullets by bone, fragmentation and through-and- through penetration, the presence of missiles within the body can only be safely established by appropriate radiographs taken in two planes.

REGIONAL INJURIES

Chest injury

A plain chest X-ray should be performed, in order to identify any of the injuries listed in Table 29.5, and the location of any missile present. If there is any possibility of mediastinal injury, CT scanning with contrast should be performed. Other useful investigations *in the stable patient* include oesophageal contrast studies and echocardiography.

In patients in whom there is no evidence of injury to the mediastinum, conservative management following the insertion of an intercostal drain is appropriate in the majority (85%) of cases.

Penetrating ballistic injury to the thorax requires intercostal drain insertion.

Table 29.5: Chest X-ray findings in gunshot injury to the chest

Pneumothorax/tension pneumothorax
Haemothorax
Fractures
Lung tissue injuries
Diaphragmatic injuries
Mediastinal injuries
Missile/missile fragments

Occasionally, fragments of a missile may cross the mediastinum, causing injury on the opposite side of the chest without external evidence of injury.

Major haemorrhage will require urgent thoracotomy. Other indications for surgery include evidence of mediastinal damage, major chest wall injury and persisting air leak from an intercostal drain. Very occasionally, emergency room thoracotomy should be considered for patients with no cardiac output as a result of massive haemorrhage or cardiac tamponade.

Unless there is evidence of mediastinal injury, conservative management is appropriate in the majority of cases of chest injury.

Abdominal injury

All patients with penetrating ballistic trauma to the abdomen will require urgent laparotomy and there is therefore no role for complex radiological investigations that will result in unnecessary delay in transferring the patient to theatre. Plain X-rays in two planes may provide useful evidence regarding the missile track and location of any foreign body. The presence of gas under the diaphragm does not necessarily signify visceral perforation as gas can be introduced at the time of peritoneal perforation.

Penetrating ballistic trauma to the abdomen mandates laparotomy.

Rectal examination, which is mandatory, may reveal evidence of bleeding into the gastrointestinal tract.

Spinal injuries

As with all spinal injuries, the essence of good management is the prevention of further damage by restriction of unnecessary movement, together with prevention of further tissue deterioration by maintenance of optimal tissue perfusion and oxygenation. Late-onset paralysis may occur due to thrombosis of arterial blood supply to the spinal cord. In the presence of a neurological deficit, high-dose methylprednisolone should be administered after consultation with the appropriate specialty.

Limb injury

Ballistic injuries to the limbs may be life threatening or limb threatening owing to damage to major vessels. Vascular damage requires initial control of haemorrhage and adequate resuscitation followed by reconstructive surgery. All soft-tissue wounds of the limbs require surgical exploration and wound toilet, in order to ensure that all foreign material and dead and non-viable tissue that might act as a focus for infection is removed.

ANTIBIOTIC THERAPY

All ballistic wounds must be assumed to be bacterially contaminated. Tissue necrosis in an anaerobic environment makes life-threatening infection a significant possibility. All patients should receive broad-spectrum antibiotic cover together with tetanus prophylaxis. Third-generation cephalosporins are appropriate for limb injuries, with the addition of metronidazole where leakage of bowel organisms is likely.

FURTHER READING

Greaves, I. and Porter, K. (Eds) (1999) *Pre-hospital Medicine: The Principles and Practice of Immediate Care.* Arnold, London.

Ryan, J.M., Rich, N.M., Dale, R.F. *et al* (1997) *Ballistic Trauma: Clinical Relevance in Peace and War.* Arnold, London.

PART FOUR

JOINT AND SOFT TISSUE

EMERGENCIES

CHAPTER THIRTY

SOFT-TISSUE AND WOUND INFECTIONS

- Introduction
- Primary soft-tissue infection

- Wound-related infection
- Further reading

INTRODUCTION

Soft-tissue infections can be broadly divided into primary soft-tissue infection and those associated with wound management. The general principles of wound management are covered in Chapter 5. Specific issues related to the prevention, recognition and treatment of wound infection are discussed here. The practical management of other forms of primary soft-tissue infection are also covered.

PRIMARY SOFT-TISSUE INFECTION

The term primary soft-tissue infection is used here to differentiate between infections associated with the management of traumatic injury and those which either present without a history of wounding (such as furuncles and paronychia) or arise following minor defects in the skin, such as cellulitis. Although most soft-tissue infections arise following some form of dermatological insult, the division is useful and aids discussion of their management.

CELLULITIS, ERYSIPELAS AND IMPETIGO

Cellulitis refers to soft-tissue inflammation secondary to bacterial invasion of the skin. Streptococci (principally *Streptococcus pyogenes*) are the most common cause, although staphylococci and, in younger children, *Haemophilus influenzae* may cause the same condition. Cellulitis may develop anywhere in the body from a small puncture wound or in an area of skin that is damaged in some other way (such as dermatitis). There is localized tenderness, skin warmth, swelling and erythema over the affected area. The irregular border is often poorly defined. When the calf is involved, there may be difficulty differentiating cellulitis from deep vein thrombosis or phlebitis. Streptococcal cellulitis may be followed within a relatively short period by bacteraemia or septicaemia.

Cellulitis around the eye is not uncommon. It is usually caused by *Staphylococcus*, *Haemophilus* or *Pneumococcus* species (which also cause bacterial conjunctivitis). The risk of spread of infection to the orbit behind the eye is great and these patients should be urgently referred to the ophthalmology team.

Erysipelas is a rare but characteristic streptococcal infection that is localized to the dermis or epidermis in the face, leg or arm. Pain, burning and redness are preceded in many cases by a prodrome of headaches, malaise and fevers. There is typically a well-defined hot, red plaque with an irregular raised and well-defined margin. Facial erysipelas extends in a butterfly distribution and may affect the forehead and scalp (Fig. 30.1). As the infection progresses, vesicles and bullae appear and there is marked oedema. The vesicles rupture and become crusted. Desquamation occurs as the rash fades. Erysipelas is more superficial than cellulitis and has a sharper demarcation.

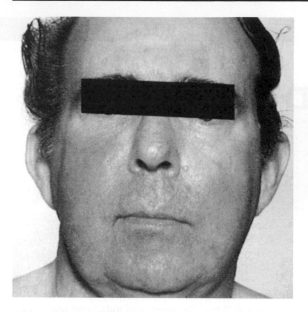

Figure 30.1: Erysipelas.

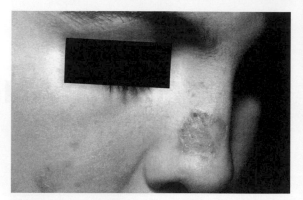

Figure 30.2: Impetigo.

Swabbing of the skin or aspiration at the edge of the infection may allow a microbiological diagnosis to be made but this is rarely successful in either cellulitis or erysipelas.

Uncomplicated cellulitis can be treated with oral penicillin and flucloxacillin and the patient either referred to their general practitioner or followed up in clinic. Before discharge, the edge of the cellulitic area should be clearly marked on the skin and the patient told not to erase the mark. This aids the determination of improvement or spread, especially if the review is by another doctor. The patient should be advised to return straight away if he develops any systemic symptoms, the cellulitis continues to spread or there are signs of 'tracking' up the limb. Erysipelas can be treated with penicillin alone unless staphylococcal infection is also suspected. An appropriate alternative antibiotic should be given if there is penicillin allergy.

Patients with cellulitis or erysipelas who are systemically unwell should be referred for in-patient care and intravenous antibiotics commenced after blood cultures. Systemic antibacterial treatment is more appropriate than topical antibiotics because the infection is too deeply seated for adequate penetration of topical preparations. Options include phenoxymethylpenicillin with flucloxacillin (or erythromycin alone if penicillin-allergic), or co-amoxiclav alone.

Impetigo is a highly infectious superficial skin infection caused by streptococci or staphylococci. It may involve normal skin or complicate pre-existing skin problems (such as eczema or psoriasis). There is blistering with a yellow crusting exudate (Fig. 30.2). Lesions are often first visible around the mouth and nose before spreading to other parts of the body. Streptococcal impetigo is superficial and does not affect the dermis. The lesions are heaped up and may be crusted spots or red papules. Staphylococcal impetigo tends to produce larger, blistering lesions that also become crusted. There may be bullae with pus.

Impetigo may be treated by topical application of fusidic acid or mupirocin or, if widespread, with oral administration of flucloxacillin or erythromycin. Topical treatment for 7 days is usually adequate. Mupirocin is not related to any other antibiotic in use and is particularly effective for skin infections due to Gram-positive organisms. To avoid the development of resistance, mupirocin should not be used in hospital or for longer than 10 days.

ABSCESSES

An abscess is a localized collection of pus. Abscesses take a variety of forms and are referred to by a variety of different names. In general terms, however, all present with similar features. The patient complains of localized pain and swelling and there is a tender, fluctuant mass on examination. If the patient is systemically unwell and there is evidence of cellulitis, lymphadenitis and regional lymphadenopathy, then the infection may be becoming disseminated. These patients warrant

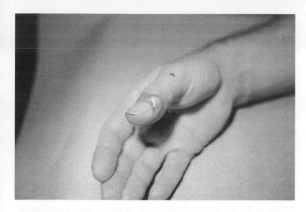

Figure 30.3: A paronychia of the thumb.

Table 30.1: Incision and drainage of an abscess

Clean the surrounding skin
Anaesthetize and drape the area
Make an incision which conforms to skin creases and fold
Incise along the length of the abscess cavity
An elliptical incision will prevent premature closure and reaccumulation of pus
Probe the cavity with a blunt instrument to gently break down any loculations
Do not compress the surrounding tissues
Send sample for culture
Place loosely packed antiseptic (usually iodine-based) wick in cavity

early referral. Most patients who attend the emergency department will, however, have a well-localized and uncomplicated cutaneous abscess. Despite this, it is prudent to bear in mind that this may be the first manifestation of an underlying condition such as diabetes, inflammatory bowel disease or HIV infection.

Abscesses are caused by a variety of organisms and arise in a variety of skin types and appendages. Folliculitis is a superficial infection of the hair follicle that is commonly caused by *Staphylococcus aureus*. Deep-seated infections around the hair follicle are called furuncles (boils). They occur in the head, neck, axillae, thighs and buttocks. When a number of adjacent hair follicles are involved, a carbuncle develops with a large indurated area and multiple draining sinuses. This commonly occurs on the back or back of the neck. It is very often associated with diabetes.

Another common cause of an abscess is an infected sebaceous cyst. There is obstruction of the ducts of a sebaceous gland and formation of a sterile cyst. This may be present for many years. Should the cyst contents become infected, however, an abscess rapidly forms. Most of these abscesses occur in the trunk and extremities and are caused by *Staphylococcus aureus* or *Escherichia coli*, *Klebsiella* and *Proteus* species.

Perirectal, genital, inguinal and buttock abscesses are predominantly caused by anaerobic bacteria. Abscesses in the axillae may be associated with apocrine sweat glands infected with *Proteus*, *Staphylococcus aureus* or *Streptococcus viridans*. A paronychia is a superficial abscess over the lateral nail fold of a finger or toe (Fig. 30.3), commonly caused by anaerobes or staphylococci.

Whatever the location or causative organism, the mainstay of treatment for abscesses is incision and drainage (Table 30.1). In most cases, incision and drainage is all that is required. Simple abscesses which are well localized and can be readily anaesthetized using field or regional blockade can be treated in an appropriate treatment room within the emergency department. Complex abscesses, those that are close to underlying neurovascular structures and those which are difficult to anaesthetize, should be referred for surgical consultation. This is particularly important for carbuncles, perirectal abscesses, pilonidal sinuses and abscesses in the face, mouth, breast, hand, axilla, groin and perineum. Children should also generally be referred.

There is sometimes uncertainty about the fluctuance of an abscess. In these cases it is worth attempting to aspirate pus in order to guide treatment decisions. Ultrasound may also help to confirm the presence of pus. If pus is present, the abscess should be incised and drained. The aspirated pus can be sent for microscopy and culture. If no pus is obtained, the patient can be treated with antibiotics and reviewed. Once the abscess is drained, antibiotics are rarely required in otherwise healthy patients. Antibiotics are only indicated if the patient is systemically unwell or the infection shows signs of spreading. Patients with infected sebaceous cysts will require follow-up for removal of the cyst capsule.

Following excision and drainage, early follow-up will be required for dressing and wick changes.

Soft-tissue infections in the hand and face merit special mention. Those in the face may rapidly progress to involve the cavernous sinus and should therefore be referred urgently. Collections of pus in the hand tend to have throbbing pain and local tenderness without the classic sign of fluctuance. Hand infections can rapidly spread through the fascial spaces and cause long-term damage. Pus may collect in the finger pulp space, the thenar space or any of the web spaces. A collection of pus in one of the web spaces of the hand should be drained in theatre by a specialist surgeon through a vertical dorsal incision. These can all be difficult to distinguish and should be referred urgently. The hand should be elevated and systemic antibiotics commenced.

Suspected deep hand infections require urgent surgical referral.

LIFE-THREATENING SOFT-TISSUE INFECTION

Any soft-tissue infection may, if untreated, progress to cause a generalized bacteraemia or septicaemia. Of particular importance in the emergency department are rapidly progressive soft-tissue infections which require urgent treatment and referral.

Necrotizing fasciitis is a term used to describe soft-tissue infection which spreads rapidly along fascial planes. *Streptococcus pyogenes* and *Staphylococcus aureus* are usually involved. The infection starts in an arm or a leg. There is swelling, redness, pain and fever followed by bronze discoloration of the limb. Haemorrhagic blisters and necrosis of skin and soft tissues then occur within a few days. With mortality reaching 40% at this stage, antibiotics combined with surgical removal of the necrotic tissue can be life saving.

Staphylococcal scalded skin syndrome (Fig. 30.4) is a rare disease caused by an exotoxin of *Staphylococcus aureus*. It is characterized by the sudden onset of extensive erythema followed by bulla formation and desquamation of large areas of skin which then resembles scalds. The exotoxin cleaves the epidermis and renders the patient susceptible to bacterial superinfection. This condition affects children more often than adults and may progress to a toxic shock syndrome with fever, hypotension and renal failure. Treatment is supportive, with intensive care and antibiotics to eliminate the toxin-producing staphylococcus. Both staphylococcal

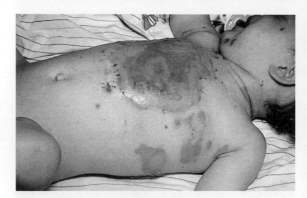

Figure 30.4: Staphylococcoal scalded skin syndrome.

scalded skin syndrome and toxic shock syndrome should be differentiated from toxic epidermal necrolysis. Despite the similar names, toxic epidermal necrolysis is regarded as a severe form of erythema multiforme following hypersensitivity to chemicals or drugs. It primarily affects older children and adults. Patches of tender erythematous skin suddenly appear and become loose. There is then separation of the dermis from the epidermis and extensive mucous membrane involvement. Dehydration and infection then become the major risks. It is not caused by infection or exotoxins but may appear very similar clinically.

WOUND-RELATED INFECTION

Although all wounds are colonized by bacteria, only approximately 10% of wounds treated in emergency departments will become clinically infected. The risk of a wound becoming infected depends on the mechanism of wounding, the anatomical site, the degree of contamination and the level of host susceptibility. Wound management therefore involves assessment and reduction of the risk of infection as well as repair of tissues (see Chapter 5).

PREVENTION OF WOUND INFECTION

The important components of wound management in preventing infection are shown in Table 30.2.

With regard to wound cleaning and irrigation, the method of cleaning is perhaps more important

Table 30.2: Measures to reduce wound infection

Aseptic wound management
Skin cleansing
Wound cleansing and irrigation
Removal of debris
Debridement
Prophylactic antibiotics
Delayed closure
Wound dressings

Table 30.3: Prophylactic antibiotics – factors to consider

Compound fractures
Deep puncture wounds
Mammal bites
Heavily contaminated wounds
High-risk occupation (farmer, gardener, fisherman etc.)
Delayed presentation
Extensive wound
Necrotic tissue
Tetanus risks (see below)

than the agents used. Irrigation and gentle scrubbing will considerably reduce the bacterial load. Bacterial proliferation occurs within the first 6 h so thorough wound irrigation should be performed as soon as possible. Low-pressure irrigation will remove large particles of debris in the wound, but higher pressures (such as through a 21 gauge needle) may be required in untidy wounds with deep contamination and small particles of debris. Scrubbing will help to remove embedded debris and is best performed with a surgical scrubbing brush or high-porosity sponge. Given the paucity of evidence to suggest that any cleaning or irrigation fluid is superior to normal saline, some emergency departments use normal saline to clean and irrigate simple uncomplicated wounds. Regardless of the type of irrigation fluid, sufficient quantities must be used.

Wound cleaning can be painful and distressing for the patient. In order to ensure that it is done effectively, adequate analgesia and local anaesthesia should be provided. In some cases, it may be better to get the patient to clean the wound themselves (under guidance).

When a patient attends with an untidy, heavily contaminated wound, decisions regarding prophylactic antibiotics are often only considered after cleaning, debridement and repair. It has long been recognized in elective surgical practice that prophylactic antibiotics are more effective if given before the procedure rather than after. Thus, if antibiotics are to be used they should be given early, initially as an intravenous bolus prior to handling and manipulation of the wound itself.

In deciding whether to use prophylactic antibiotics, a number of factors should be considered (Table 30.3). Particular attention should be paid to patients who are at risk of endocarditis, have indwelling prosthetic devices or who are immunosuppressed (e.g. are diabetic or on corticosteroids).

Flucloxacillin alone is usually sufficient for prophylaxis unless specific risk factors indicate an alternative (co-amoxiclav for mammal bites and anaerobes, metronidazole for serious anaerobic risk). Most patients do not require any form of antibiotic prophylaxis.

Debridement, delayed closure and wound dressings are considered in more detail in Chapter 5.

To reduce the risk of infection, a wound should not be closed if it is not clean.

TREATING INFECTED WOUNDS

Wounds that have received a high inoculating dose of bacteria may become infected regardless of the use of good wound management techniques and prophylactic antibiotics. Clinically significant infection is classically revealed by:

- pain and tenderness at the wound site
- redness and heat in the area surrounding the wound
- purulent exudate
- general malaise with raised temperature.

A challenge in emergency department practice is to identify early wound infection before all of these classic features become obvious. Streptococcal infections tend to cause an early spreading cellulitis and ascending lymphangitis. There is spreading erythema and pitting oedema. The wound should be opened to ensure that there is no localized abscess and then cleaned and left open. A skin marker should then be used to delineate the extent of the erythema. After an initial intravenous dose of benzyl penicillin, the patient should commence oral penicillin and flucloxacillin pending review in 2 days. Before prescribing any penicillin, a drug history should be taken. If there is a history of an allergic reaction to any penicillins, erythromycin or clarithromycin should be used as an alternative. If the history is unconvincing, a penicillin can be given but the patient should be warned of the potential risk and be closely monitored for the first 4 h after administration.

Staphylococcal infections often result in local pus formation. Throbbing pain that disturbs the patient is an early sign and often indicates abscess formation. If a local abscess is suspected, all sutures or staples should be removed and all pus and dead material debrided. Swabs should be sent for culture and any specimen of pus sent for Gram staining. Blood cultures may be appropriate if the patient appears systemically unwell.

The wound should be cleaned and irrigated and allowed to heal by secondary intention. Systemic antibiotics, an appropriate dressing and daily inspection will be required. Patients who are systemically unwell, pyrexial (temperature greater than 38°C) and have regional lymphadenopathy or spreading cellulitis should be referred for in-patient management.

The choice of antibiotic will vary according to local policy and prevalent organisms. It should be assumed that staphylococcal infections will be resistant to penicillin and that flucloxacillin will also be required. Ciprofloxacin and co-amoxiclav have been advocated for wound infections but Gram-positive organisms, which are much more likely to cause skin and soft-tissue infections, respond less well to ciprofloxacin. Co-amoxiclav is effective but is expensive and has not been directly compared with flucloxacillin. Doses of all antibiotics should be checked with the current formulary, particularly when treating children. A common error is to prescribe too small a dose for too short a period. All patients with wound infections should be reviewed within 1–2 days.

INFECTIONS DUE TO BITES

Wound infections which occur within 24 h of animal bites are often caused by the Gram-negative bacillus *Pasteurella multocida*. Dogs and cats are often responsible and the infection is characterized by an intense and rapid inflammatory response. There is an acute onset of redness, swelling, pain and regional lymphadenopathy within hours of the bite. Occasionally, the patient may present with life-threatening sepsis. If more than 24 h has elapsed since the bite, it is likely that the wound infection is caused by staphylococci or streptococci. In either case, wound swabs should be taken and the patient commenced on co-amoxiclav or penicillin and flucloxacillin. Patients who are allergic to penicillin should be given erythromycin or clarithromycin.

LIFE-THREATENING WOUND INFECTION

Simple wounds can lead to life-threatening sepsis if they are not managed correctly. Of particular importance are clostridial and uncontrolled staphylococcal infections. The clostridia are anaerobic Gram-positive spore-forming organisms. Their natural habitat is the soil or the intestinal tract of animals and humans. Wound infection with clostridial species can produce gas gangrene or tetanus.

Tetanus

Clostridium tetani spores are worldwide in distribution in the soil and in animal faeces. It is not an invasive organism and infection remains very strictly localized to the wound which has become contaminated with spores. The spores germinate and develop in devitalized tissue. The incubation period ranges from 4–5 days to several weeks and the inoculating dose may be very small. The organisms then produce a toxin called tetanospasmin, which interferes with neuromuscular transmission. The disease manifests as muscular spasms and stiffness around the wound, followed by trismus, tetanic seizures and respiratory failure. Although it is a rare disease, most cases occur in elderly, non-immunized patients and the mortality is approximately 50%. Prevention of tetanus depends on effective immunization, proper care of wounds contaminated with soil and prophylactic use of antitoxin. All patients should have their tetanus immunization status clearly determined.

Appropriate wound management is the most effective way of preventing wound infection.

Tetanus vaccination is offered routinely to babies in combination with diphtheria and *Bordetella pertussis* as a triple vaccine (DTP). The triple vaccine gives protection against tetanus in childhood. Subsequent booster doses of tetanus vaccine are offered at school entry and school leaving.

Wounds are considered to be tetanus prone if:

- they more than 6 h old
- are puncture-type
- have devitalized tissue
- are septic
- are contaminated with soil or manure.

Patients with tidy wounds that are more than 6 h old should have a booster dose of adsorbed tetanus vaccine if the primary course (or any previous booster) was given more than 10 years previously. If the patient has never been immunized, the first dose of the full course of tetanus immunization should be given in the emergency department and the patient instructed to consult their GP for the remainder of the course (two further doses at 4-week intervals). If the patient is a school-age child then, provided more than 10 years have elapsed since the school-entry booster, tetanus vaccine should be given. It is important to then notify the GP that this booster has been given so that records can be updated and the school-leaving booster be omitted.

The addition of a dose of human tetanus immunoglobulin and antibiotic prophylaxis (with benzyl penicillin, co-amoxiclav or metronidazole) should be considered for tetanus-prone wounds. In general terms, the decision to provide immunoglobulin will depend on whether the patient has ever been immunized (many elderly patients may not have completed immunization), whether the patient has received a dose of tetanus vaccine within the previous 10 years, and whether the risk of infection is considered to be very high (such as in contamination with faeces). These cases should be discussed with a microbiologist. Patients with any features suggestive of tetanus should be referred urgently.

Gas gangrene (clostridial myonecrosis)

Gas gangrene is a rapidly progressive limb- and life-threatening wound infection. Many different toxin-producing clostridia can cause invasive infection if introduced into damaged tissue. The commonest is *Clostridium perfringens* (formerly called *Clostridium welchii*). Once a wound is contaminated, the spores germinate and the bacteria multiply. They ferment carbohydrates in the tissues and produce gas within 1–4 days. The resulting distention of tissues, along with release of other damaging toxins, allows spread of infection. Tissue necrosis extends, there is increased bacterial growth and generalized sepsis follows. Clinically, there is severe pain and swelling at the wound site, with generalized toxicity, crepitus in the subcutaneous tissues and a malodorous serosanguinous discharge from the wound. Severe muscle injuries and deep wounds of the thighs and buttocks are often affected.

As with tetanus, appropriate wound care and prophylactic antibiotics and antitoxins in heavily contaminated wounds will prevent clostridial infections. Prompt and extensive surgical debridement may be required for patients who present with old wounds and early evidence of infection. Gas gangrene is typically a mixed infection with proteolytic clostridia, Gram-negative organisms and other bacteria present. Broad-spectrum antibiotics (including Gram-negative cover), hyperbaric oxygen and surgery form the basis of treatment of established cases.

FURTHER READING

Barkin, R., Rosen, P., Hockberger R. *et al.* (Eds) (1998) *Emergency Medicine Concepts and Clinical Practice*, 4th Edn. Mosby, St Louis.

CHAPTER THIRTY ONE

THE PAINFUL JOINT

- Introduction
- Approach to the patient
- Differential diagnosis of painful joints

- Important conditions
- Further reading

INTRODUCTION

This chapter concerns the assessment, diagnosis and treatment of patients with pain or swelling in or around joints that appears to be unrelated to injury. Traumatic injury involving the joints is covered in Chapters 25 and 26. A wide range of conditions may cause joint pain and this chapter provides a structured approach to the most important of these in the emergency department.

APPROACH TO THE PATIENT

Traumatic injury is often easier to assess and treat than symptoms that appear to be unrelated to injury. In the former, a focused history and examination can be rapidly conducted and effective treatment initiated. In contrast, joint pain unrelated to trauma may be a manifestation of complex and severe underlying systemic disease. It is therefore important to approach these patients holistically and with an understanding of the common diseases that may present with joint pain.

> In all cases, the differential diagnosis should include infection and referred pain.

Ideally, on completion of the assessment, it should be possible to characterize the joint pain as articular or non-articular in origin and inflammatory or non-inflammatory in nature (Table 31.1).

Table 31.1: Assessment of patients with joint pain

> Determine whether it is acute or chronic (more than 6 weeks)
> Localize the complaint (articular or non-articular)
> Determine the pathological process (inflammatory or non-inflammatory)
> Formulate a differential diagnosis

Given the chronic nature of many rheumatological and musculoskeletal disorders, it may not be possible to establish a clear diagnosis in the emergency department. None the less, a logical approach to the history, examination and investigations will ensure that important conditions are identified and referred appropriately.

HISTORY

Patients may present complaining of pain in any joint. They may have little appreciation of the significance of repetitive activity, minor injury in the recent past or other apparently unrelated symptoms. A clear and detailed history is thus essential. Many patients may have no recollection of injury, but will recognize a temporal relationship between their symptoms and possible precipitating events when prompted. Common examples include the painful wrist after painting the bedroom, a painful shoulder after moving house and pain in the knee following a short gastrointestinal illness. Equally, the patient may ascribe their pain to a coincidental and unrelated minor injury.

Certain diagnoses are more frequent in specific age groups. Reactive arthritis (Reiter's syndrome) is more common in the young, whereas osteoarthritis is most often a condition of the elderly. When considering elderly patients, the impact of existing medical conditions and treatment should be considered. Drug-induced gout is, for example, more common in the elderly. Some diseases are also more common in a particular gender or race. Gout and reactive arthritis occur more often in men, whereas rheumatoid arthritis is commoner in women.

The chronology of the complaint (onset, evolution and duration) is important. Acute-onset joint pain tends to be infectious, crystal-induced or reactive. It is these patients who more often present to the emergency department. Non-inflammatory and immune-related joint conditions such as osteoarthritis and rheumatoid arthritis are often chronic. Chronic symptoms are generally defined in rheumatology as those lasting for more than 6 weeks. Most of these patients consult their general practitioner. Joint pain may also be described as intermittent (gout) or migratory (gonococcal or viral arthritis).

Determining if joint pain is articular in origin requires careful evaluation. Articular disorders are associated with pain and a restricted range of both active and passive motion. Non-articular joint pain (from associated muscles, ligaments, bursae and tendons) is generally worse on active movement. Stiffness is common in all musculoskeletal disorders. However, morning stiffness related to inflammatory disorders lasts several hours and is usually improved with activity and anti-inflammatory medicines. The stiffness associated with non-inflammatory conditions, such as osteoarthritis, is intermittent, short-lived, and tends to be exacerbated by activity.

> Morning stiffness is typical of an inflammatory arthropathy.

The number and distribution of involved joints should be noted. Articular disorders are described as monoarticular (one joint involved), oligoarticular, pauciarticular (up to three joints involved) or polyarticular (more than three joints involved). Joint pain secondary to septic arthritis or gout is typically monoarticular, whereas rheumatoid arthritis is polyarticular. Joint involvement tends to be symmetric in rheumatoid arthritis but is often asymmetric in reactive arthritis and gout. The upper extremities are frequently involved in rheumatoid arthritis, whereas lower extremity arthritis is characteristic of early Reiter's syndrome and gout.

A systems review should reveal systemic features such as fever, rash (Reiter's syndrome), myalgia and weakness (polymyalgia rheumatica) and morning stiffness. In addition, some conditions are associated with involvement of other organ systems, including the eyes (Reiter's syndrome) and gastrointestinal and genitourinary tracts (gonococcal arthritis).

EXAMINATION

Examination should not be limited to the affected limb or joint as is often the case following injury. Many rheumatological conditions have systemic or extra-articular manifestations and a full general examination is usually indicated for non-traumatic joint pain. Specific examination of the affected joint should follow the traditional look–feel–move–test sequence. The aim is to establish whether the pain is articular or non-articular in origin and inflammatory or non-inflammatory in nature. Comparison should always be made with the unaffected side when examining limbs.

> In joint examination – look, feel, move, test.

Articular disorders are often associated with swelling of the whole joint caused by an effusion, bony enlargement or synovial proliferation. There may be deformity of the joint. Non-articular disorders are associated with focal areas of tenderness which are often remote from the joint margins. There is seldom any deformity. It may be difficult to distinguish true articular swelling caused by effusion or synovial proliferation from non-articular or periarticular swelling and inflammation (such as bursitis). The latter usually extends beyond the normal joint margins. Bursal effusions overlie bony prominences and are fluctuant with sharply defined borders. A distended joint may be obviously swollen but this may only be revealed in full extension. The patient may attempt to minimize pain by keeping the joint partially flexed. This is the position of least intra-articular pressure and greatest volume.

A restricted range of motion is frequently caused by effusion, pain, deformity or contracture.

Table 31.2: Inflammatory and non-inflammatory causes of joint pain

Inflammatory:
  Infection (*Staphylococcus aureus*, *Neisseria gonorrhoeae*)
  Crystal-induced (gout, pseudogout)
  Immune-mediated (rheumatoid arthritis, systemic lupus erythematosus)
  Reactive (rheumatic fever, Reiter's syndrome)
Non-inflammatory:
  Trauma (rotator cuff tendinitis)
  Degenerative change (osteoarthritis)
  Synovial hyperplasia (pigmented villonodular synovitis)
  Mechanical joint pain (degenerative meniscal tear)

Table 31.3: Aspiration of synovial fluid

Revise the anatomy
Clean the skin
Anaesthetize the skin and subcutaneous tissues
Insert a large-bore needle into the site of maximal fluctuation or by the route of easiest access
Empty the joint space as completely as possible
Examine synovial fluid for appearance and viscosity
Send fluid for urgent cell count, microscopy and Gram staining

Contractures may reflect previous episodes of synovial inflammation. Crepitus may be felt during palpation or movement and may be prominent in osteoarthritis. Joint deformity usually indicates a long-standing or aggressive pathological process. Deformities may result from ligamentous destruction, soft-tissue contractures, bony enlargement, ankylosis, erosive disease or subluxation. A careful examination for sources of musculoskeletal pain or pain of soft-tissue origin should be undertaken when a complaint of joint pain is not supported by any objective findings referable to the joint capsule. Non-articular conditions such as a carpal tunnel syndrome, enthesitis (such as Achilles tendinitis) and bursitis should be readily identified.

The underlying pathological process may be inflammatory or non-inflammatory (Table 31.2). Inflammatory disorders are suggested by the cardinal signs of inflammation (erythema, warmth, pain and swelling), the presence of well-defined systemic symptoms (morning stiffness, fatigue, fever), or biochemical evidence of inflammation (elevated acute-phase proteins). Non-inflammatory causes of joint pain are rarely associated with acute inflammation or systemic illness.

INVESTIGATIONS

An initial differential diagnosis of the cause of joint pain can be made following the detailed history and clinical examination. A number of features may indicate that further investigation is warranted in the emergency department. Any acute monoarthritis requires further investigation, as does joint pain associated with neurological signs or systemic manifestations of serious underlying disease. Where there is doubt about the role of investigations, advice should be sought from a senior clinician. Orthopaedic teams tend to manage suspected septic arthritis, whereas general medical or rheumatology services tend to manage the other forms of arthritis. Early referral is often more appropriate than arranging a selection of screening tests with little predictive value. Such referrals need not be on an emergency basis if the problem is long-standing and infection has been excluded.

Investigations that may influence management in the department are a full blood count and measurement of an acute-phase protein such as the C-reactive protein (CRP) or erythrocyte sedimentation rate (ESR). These are characteristically raised in inflammatory conditions such as rheumatoid arthritis but are normal in osteoarthritis and non-inflammatory conditions.

A raised serum uric acid is a good confirmatory test for gout but is not diagnostic.

A low level of uric acid excludes acute gout. It is more commonly used to monitor treatment. Specialist serological investigations such as rheumatoid factor, antinuclear antibodies and complement levels should only be performed after discussion with the appropriate specialist. These tests should not be used for screening.

Aspiration and analysis of synovial fluid is always indicated in acute monoarthritis or when an infectious or crystal-induced arthropathy is suspected (Table 31.3). The shoulder, wrist, knee and ankle may all be aspirated in the emergency

Table 31.4: Synovial fluid analysis

Non-inflammatory:
  Clear, viscous and amber-coloured
  White cell count <2000 μl^{-1}
  Predominance of mononuclear cells

Inflammatory:
  Turbid and yellow with reduced viscosity
  White cell count 2000–50 000 cells μl^{-1}
  Predominance of polymorphonuclear leucocytes

Infection:
  Turbid and opaque with reduced viscosity
  White cell count usually >50 000 μl^{-1}
  Predominance of polymorphonuclear leucocytes
    (>75%)

department if a suitably experienced clinician is available. Relative contraindications to aspiration are cellulitis or impetigo at the injection site and coagulopathy.

Synovial fluid analysis may be crucial in distinguishing between non-inflammatory and inflammatory processes. This distinction can be made on the basis of the appearance, viscosity and cell count of the synovial fluid (Table 31.4). Haemorrhagic synovial fluid may be seen with a 'bloody' (traumatic) tap, neuropathic arthropathy, haemarthrosis or following injury. Synovial fluid should always be sent for Gram staining, microscopy and culture. Cellularity and the presence of crystals are assessed by light and polarizing microscopy. If gonococcal arthritis is suspected, immediate plating of the fluid on appropriate culture medium may be required and microbiological advice should be sought.

In terms of imaging, plain radiographs are useful when there is a history of trauma, chronic infection is suspected, there is a chronic, progressive disability, or in any acute monoarthritis. In most inflammatory disorders, early radiography may only reveal soft-tissue swelling or juxta-articular demineralization. Calcification (of soft tissues, cartilage or bone), joint space narrowing, erosions, bony ankylosis, new bone formation (sclerosis, osteophyte formation or periostitis) or subchondral cysts may suggest specific underlying conditions. Ultrasound is useful in the detection of some soft-tissue abnormalities. These include synovial cysts (Baker's cysts) in the knee, rotator cuff tears and major tendon injuries.

TREATMENT

The aim of treatment in the emergency department is to relieve pain, prevent further injury and treat the underlying condition. The fundamentals of treatment are:

- treatment (or referral for treatment) of the underlying cause
- rest or activity modification
- analgesia
- temporary splintage
- physiotherapy.

Corticosteroid injections are often used by orthopaedic surgeons, rheumatologists and general practitioners to treat established causes of joint pain (such as impingement syndrome). It is generally inappropriate to commence such treatment in an emergency department setting unless the diagnosis is clear.

DIFFERENTIAL DIAGNOSIS OF PAINFUL JOINTS

THE PAINFUL SHOULDER

Rotator cuff tendinitis (impingement syndrome), chronic rotator cuff tears, bicipital tendinitis, subacromial bursitis, calcific tendinitis, acromioclavicular joint arthritis, adhesive capsulitis and septic arthritis may all present with shoulder pain. However, the commonest cause of non-traumatic shoulder pain is referred pain from the neck. A history of restricted shoulder movement, pain at either the extremes of movement or on specific movements, and pain which tends to be worse at night tends to localize pathology to the shoulder. Referred pain from the cervical spine tends to be worse during activity and better at night and does not usually restrict shoulder movements. None the less, mid-cervical disc or nerve root disease may produce pain very similar to rotator cuff pathology, so an examination of the neck and a simple neurological examination of the limbs is indicated in all patients presenting with non-traumatic shoulder pain. Other sources of referred pain are the chest wall, diaphragm (liver and gallbladder) and intrathoracic lesions.

Always consider the cervical spine as a possible source of shoulder pain.

The shoulder joint has the greatest mobility of all peripheral joints (Table 31.5). It is therefore

Table 31.5: Range of movement at the shoulder

Movement	Normal
Abduction	180°
Adduction	45°
Flexion	180°
Extension	60°
Internal rotation (arm at side)	100°
Internal rotation (arm abducted)	80°
External rotation (arm at side)	70°
External rotation (arm abducted)	90°

vulnerable to a range of traumatic and non-traumatic conditions. The importance of shoulder stability and strength in controlling upper limb movements is reflected by the degree of disability experienced by patients with painful shoulders. A simple screening test for shoulder movement is to ask the patient to abduct both arms (full abduction) then place both hands behind the neck with elbows out to the side (external rotation and abduction), then place both hands behind the small of back (internal rotation). If these active movements are restricted, then the patient should be asked to indicate the precise site of pain and passive movement should be tested.

Most non-traumatic shoulder pain is a consequence of chronic impingement. In understanding the spectrum of impingement syndrome, it is important to appreciate the anatomy of the coracoacromial arch (Fig. 31.1). This is formed by the

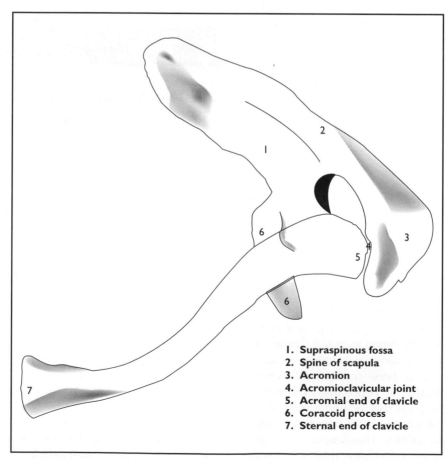

1. **Supraspinous fossa**
2. **Spine of scapula**
3. **Acromion**
4. **Acromioclavicular joint**
5. **Acromial end of clavicle**
6. **Coracoid process**
7. **Sternal end of clavicle**

Figure 31.1: Anatomical diagram of the coracoacromial arch.

coracoid process anteriorly and the acromion posteriorly. The coracoacromial ligament forms the roof of the arch and the humeral head provides the floor. This arch defines the space within which the muscles of the rotator cuff (supraspinatus, infraspinatus, teres minor and subscapularis), the subacromial bursa and the tendon of the long head of biceps must fit. Impingement syndrome refers to the pathological changes that occur in these structures owing to repetitive mechanical impingement between the humeral head and coracoacromial arch. This is caused by narrowing of the space under the arch by acromioclavicular joint arthritis or repetitive use of the arm above the horizontal. Oedema and haemorrhage eventually lead to chronic inflammation, fibrosis and rupture of the rotator cuff. Impingement syndrome is also referred to as painful arc and supraspinatus syndrome. It covers a spectrum of conditions, including subacromial bursitis, rotator cuff tendinitis and rotator cuff tears.

The subacromial bursa lies lateral to and immediately beneath the acromion. Subacromial bursitis is essentially early impingement and tends to occur in younger patients. There is a dull aching pain deep within the shoulder that can often be related to activity. It improves with rest. There may be tenderness over the lateral aspect of proximal humerus or on deep palpation of the subacromial space. Pain may be experienced between 60° and 100° of abduction (a painful arc) but there is usually a full range of movement. Patients should be advised to avoid activities that reproduce the symptoms and reviewed either in the emergency department or by their GP in 7–10 days. Physiotherapy, corticosteroid injections or alternative diagnoses may then be considered.

Rotator cuff tendinitis most commonly affects supraspinatus. Patients frequently have a history of episodes of shoulder pain (possibly an episode of subacromial bursitis) and complain of a deep, aching discomfort that interferes with normal daily activities. It also affects sleep. There will be pain and tenderness on the lateral aspect of the deltoid and proximal humerus, which is worse with active abduction (but not passive abduction). Crepitus may be felt when movement is attempted. Movement will generally be restricted. The best way to reproduce impingement is by passive abduction or rotation of the shoulder across the patient's body with the arm abducted to 90° and the elbow flexed to 90°. The patient should be warned that this movement may produce pain. Reduction in pain by at least 50% after injection of 10 ml of 1% lidocaine into the subacromial space can help distinguish pain of impingement from other causes of shoulder pain. Plain radiographs may show acromioclavicular joint arthritis but are often normal. If tendinitis is considered to be the likely diagnosis in the emergency department, then the aim of treatment is to reduce pain and inflammation and prevent further progression. Rest and activity modification combined with analgesia and anti-inflammatory drugs may initially suffice but patients should be advised to consult their GP if symptoms progress.

Acute rotator cuff tears are considered in Chapter 25. Chronic impingement accounts for most chronic tears and may not be related to a specific injury recalled by the patient. It is often impossible to distinguish tears from rotator cuff tendinitis. Patients are middle-aged or older and complain of gradual and progressive pain which is worse at night. There is restricted active abduction and external rotation. Patients are often unable to hold the arm abducted and there is crepitus and pain on passive movement. Radiographs may show a non-specific sclerosis of the humeral head, degenerative joint disease at the acromioclavicular joint and osteophytes. These patients require analgesia and a supportive sling followed by early orthopaedic follow-up and physiotherapy. Although a number of specific tests of rotator cuff function can be used, these rarely allow the non-specialist to make an accurate anatomical diagnosis. Tendinitis or tear of the rotator cuff can be confirmed by ultrasound or magnetic resonance imaging.

The tendon of the long head of biceps traverses the bicipital groove anterior to the subacromial bursa. This tendon is best identified by palpating it in its groove as the patient rotates the humerus internally and externally. It may become inflamed and cause intense localized pain at the anterior aspect of the shoulder. Palpation of the tendon and resisted supination of the forearm will reproduce the pain. Analgesia, activity modification and rest will be required.

Calcific tendinitis is a condition that appears to be unrelated to chronic impingement and is thought to represent primary tendon degeneration. There is deposition of calcium hydroxyapatite crystals within one or more tendons of the rotator cuff (again most commonly supraspinatus). These crystals are eventually spontaneously reabsorbed and it is at

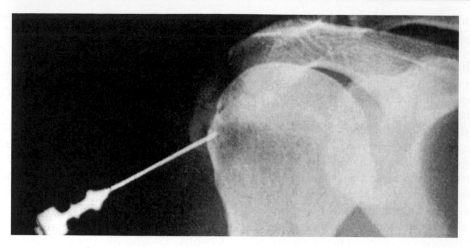

Figure 31.2: Radiograph of shoulder with calcium deposits visible within the rotator cuff. (Reproduced with permission from L. Solomon, D.J. Warwick and S. Nayagan (eds). *Apley's System of Orthopaedics and Fractures*, 8th edition, published by Arnold, London, 2001.)

this stage that the patient experiences sudden severe shoulder pain. Any movement causes pain and patients tend to hold their arm in a similar manner to those who have dislocated the shoulder. Radiographs reveal calcific deposits in the rotator cuff (Fig. 31.2). The pain, which is thought to be due to a relative increase in the pressure and volume within the tendon during reabsorption, lasts for 1–2 weeks. Patients require adequate analgesia and steroid injection if the pain fails to resolve.

Adhesive capsulitis is often referred to as a 'frozen shoulder'. Following injury, recurrent inflammation or prolonged immobilization (such as after a stroke), the shoulder joint capsule becomes thickened and contracted. Pain initially limits motion. This immobility allows additional inflammation, fibrosis and thickening of the capsule. The range of joint motion is thus further restricted. The aetiology of this condition is unclear but autoimmune mechanisms are implicated, given the strong association with diabetes and thyroid disease in these patients.

The patient complains of poorly localized pain and an insidious onset of stiffness. The shoulder is stiff on examination, with marked reduction of active and passive motion. Often, no specific cause is found and the condition improves slowly with physiotherapy and analgesia.

Osteoarthritis and rheumatoid arthritis commonly affect the acromioclavicular joint but osteoarthritis seldom involves the glenohumeral joint, unless there is a predisposing cause such as an old fracture. The glenohumeral joint is best palpated anteriorly by placing the thumb over the humeral head (just medial and inferior to the coracoid process) and asking the patient to rotate the humerus internally and externally. Pain localized to this region is indicative of glenohumeral pathology and merits plain radiography and specialist referral if symptoms do not settle with rest and analgesia.

THE PAINFUL ELBOW

The cause of elbow pain is often much more obvious than for pain in the shoulder or wrist. The most common causes of elbow pain are medial and lateral epicondylitis, olecranon bursitis, osteoarthritis and inflammatory arthritis. In medial epicondylitis, the insertion of the common flexor tendon is painful and inflamed (golfer's elbow). In lateral epicondylitis, the common extensor tendon is inflamed (tennis elbow). Both conditions may occur spontaneously or result from repetitive strain. They are often unrelated to either sporting activity. These patients require advice, rest and analgesia. Both conditions settle spontaneously with time, but occasionally become disabling and require follow-up and possibly corticosteroid injections or rarely surgery.

Tennis elbow: lateral epicondylitis
Golfer's elbow: medial epicondylitis.

Olecranon bursitis may occur as a result of infection of the bursa, spontaneously or following injury. Aspiration of the contents of the bursa may both be diagnostic and contribute to therapy. If the cause is thought to be infection, aspiration of the bursa and antibiotic therapy is required and flucloxacillin is the most appropriate choice until the results of a culture and sensitivity are available. More commonly, olecranon bursitis is a sterile, inflammatory process resulting from local minor trauma ('student's elbow'). In these cases avoidance of further injury or pressure to the area and anti-inflammatory medication will result in resolution. It is important always to be aware that olecranon bursitis may be the first manifestation of a polyarticular inflammatory arthropathy.

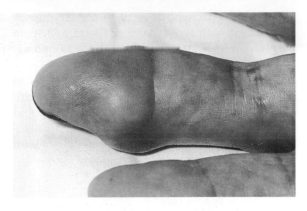

Figure 31.3: Gout in the hand.

PAIN IN THE WRIST, HAND AND FINGERS

Focal or unilateral, non-traumatic hand and finger joint pain may result from overuse, infection, reactive arthritis or crystal arthropathy. In contrast, bilateral hand and finger joint pain suggests osteoarthritis or a systemic inflammatory arthritis. The pattern of joint involvement is perhaps more useful in the hand than for any other body region. Osteoarthritis may manifest as distal interphalangeal (DIP) and proximal interphalangeal (PIP) joint pain with bony hypertrophy. This may result in the well-known Heberden's and Bouchard's nodes. In the acute phase these are inflamed and very tender. The nodules remain once the inflammation resolves but are no longer tender. Pain in the base of the thumb (first carpometacarpal joint) is also highly suggestive of osteoarthritis.

Rheumatoid arthritis tends to involve the PIP, metacarpophalangeal (MCP), intercarpal and carpometacarpal joints with pain, stiffness and synovial hypertrophy. The classic 'swan-neck' finger deformities and the ulnar deviation with volar subluxation at the MCP joints may be obvious. Psoriatic arthritis may also involve the DIP and PIP joints and the carpus with inflammatory pain, stiffness and synovitis. There may also be nail pitting or onycholysis. Gout commonly affects the small joints of the hand and will often be recognized by the patient. It can be difficult to differentiate gout from a septic arthritis (Fig. 31.3).

Pain over the dorsum of the forearm, hand and wrist may be due to an inflammatory extensor tendon tenosynovitis, possibly caused by overuse, infection, gout or inflammatory arthritis. The diagnosis of tenosynovitis may be suggested by local warmth and swelling and can be confirmed when pain is reproduced by maintaining the wrist in a fixed, neutral position and stretching the extensor tendons (by flexing the fingers). Focal wrist pain localized to the radial aspect may be caused by DeQuervain's tenovaginitis resulting from inflammation of the tendon sheaths of abductor pollicis longus or extensor pollicis brevis.

Extensor tenosynovitis and DeQuervain's tenovaginitis resulting from overuse are common causes of presentation to the emergency department. A history of excessive and unaccustomed activity is usually available. Classically, fine crepitus is palpable as the patient flexes and extends the digits. Treatment consists of rest, anti-inflammatory medication and splintage. In resistant cases later steroid injection or surgery may be required.

Carpal tunnel syndrome is another common cause of hand pain and results from compression of the median nerve within the carpal tunnel to produce paresthesiae in the thumb and the index, middle, and radial half of the ring fingers. There may also be atrophy of thenar musculature. Symptoms are classically present at night. Carpal tunnel syndrome is commonly associated with pregnancy, oedema, osteoarthritis, inflammatory arthritis and infiltrative disorders. The diagnosis is suggested by a positive Tinel's or Phalen's sign. With each test, paraesthesiae in a median nerve distribution is induced or increased by tapping the volar aspect of the wrist (Tinel's sign) or asking the patient to press the extensor surfaces of the two flexed wrists against each another (Phalen's test).

Some patients who present to the emergency department with wrist, hand or finger joint pain may have a small joint septic arthritis or an undiagnosed carpal, metacarpal or finger fracture. Any suggestion of infection in the hand should be taken seriously and a senior review sought. A low threshold for plain radiographs of the wrist, scaphoid and hand should be maintained. If a specific diagnosis cannot be made, conservative treatment with rest, activity modification, analgesia and out-patient or GP review will be required.

THE PAINFUL HIP

Diseases of the hip present with pain, stiffness, instability or deformity. Irritability in the hip is suggestive of acute inflammation and is manifest by acute pain and voluntary resistance to any movement (particularly internal rotation). Patients who complain of hip pain without any history of injury may have degenerative joint disease, trochanteric bursitis, iliopsoas bursitis or referred pain from the lumbosacral spine or knee. Septic arthritis and crystal arthropathy must always be considered with hip pain because as the joint is deep there will be little external evidence of inflammation. Assessments of injuries to the hip and problems associated with prosthetic hips are discussed in Chapter 26.

If the hip pain is localized to the buttock and radiates down the back or outside of the thigh then it is likely to represent referred pain from the lumbosacral spine. This results from degenerative arthritis of the lumbosacral spine with involvement of nerve roots between L2 and S1. The pain commonly follows a dermatomal distribution and is made worse by active movement and stretching of the nerve roots by straight leg raising. There may be neurological signs in the lower limbs and a history of back pain.

If the hip pain is localized laterally to the area overlying the trochanteric bursa then trochanteric bursitis may be the cause. Because of the depth of this bursa, swelling and warmth are usually absent although there will be tenderness directly over the greater trochanter. Ultrasound may be appropriate if there is suggestion of a septic bursitis. This will also allow the bursa to be drained.

Pain from the hip joint itself tends to be localized anteriorly over the inguinal ligament with radiation down the front and medial aspect of the thigh or along the groin. The commonest cause of true hip pain in adults is osteoarthritis, although any rheumatological condition that affects the hip, spine or sacroiliac joints may present with hip pain. Iliopsoas bursitis or a psoas abscess may mimic true hip joint pain. Pain associated with these conditions tends to worsen with extension of the hip. Patients therefore tend to flex and externally rotate the hip to reduce the pain from a distended bursa.

Hip function in all of these conditions is best assessed by observing the patient's gait, looking for deformity of the joint and assessing range of motion (Table 31.6). Patients with acute hip joint pathology tend to have an antalgic (pain-relieving) gait. Patients with an antalgic gait lean towards the painful side and take short steps. A useful screening test for hip irritability is to gently roll the leg as it lies extended on the bed. The patient will resist rolling the painful hip and may experience pain. The common deformities in hip pathology are flexion, adduction and external rotation; these can often only be revealed by measuring true and apparent leg lengths and performing Thomas's test.

True leg length is measured from the anterior superior iliac spine to the medial malleolus. Apparent leg length is measured from a central point such as the pubic symphysis to the medial malleolus. Apparent shortening indicates an adduction deformity. In Thomas's test, the patient is asked to lie on their back and flex the good hip and knee to bring the knee as close to the chest as possible. Flexion deformity in the diseased hip will be revealed if the patient is unable to maintain full extension of the hip. An alternative is to ask the patient to flex both hips and knees as far as they can and then ask them to lower the bad leg whilst the good side is being held. Adduction or flexion deformities are signs of chronic disease and,

Table 31.6: Range of movement at the hip

Movement	Normal
Flexion	125°
Extension	20°
Abduction	45°
Adduction	45°
Internal rotation	45°
External rotation	45°

together with the results of plain radiography, will often confirm degenerative joint disease.

Patients with chronic hip problems should be provided with adequate analgesia and walking aids if necessary. They should then be followed up by their GP. If there is any uncertainty as to whether an elderly patient may have fallen prior to the onset of pain, then a hip fracture should be excluded. It may be necessary to review the patient in the emergency department with repeat radiographs in these cases. Patients with acute bursitis should be treated conservatively once infection has been excluded. Those with referred pain should have the underlying condition assessed and, if possible, be referred for specialist advice.

Very occasionally, an elderly patient who can still walk, albeit with discomfort, will be found to have a fractured neck of femur (usually impacted).

> Always have a low threshold for X-raying painful hips in the elderly.

THE PAINFUL KNEE

There is a wide range of causes of knee pain. The knee is often affected by osteoarthritis and inflammatory, septic and crystal arthropathies. Bursitis, soft-tissue injuries, chronic knee pain syndromes and referred pain from the hip occur frequently. In addition, bone tumours and exostoses are also relatively common around the knee. Thus, evaluation of knee pain unrelated to injury can appear daunting. However, most conditions can be approached logically and the joint is easy to examine and investigate by aspiration and plain radiography.

The four cardinal symptoms of mechanical disruption of the knee are:

- giving way
- locking
- swelling
- pain.

Patients may present to the emergency department with a meniscal tear, articular cartilage or ligament injury which has arisen following an apparently minor stress some time previously. Thus, a full assessment of the integrity of the ligaments and menisci of the knee should be undertaken (see Chapter 26).

A common presentation is an acutely painful and swollen knee with no apparent cause. This may, rarely, be a septic arthritis but is more commonly a first presentation of reactive arthritis or crystal arthropathy. Less frequently, it may represent sudden onset of rheumatoid arthritis. In any case, the principles of history, examination and investigation discussed above apply.

With regard to intermittent exacerbations of chronic knee pain, the most common complaint is of non-specific anterior knee pain caused by malalignment, osteochondral injury, degenerative change or chondromalacia patellae. Other causes of pain apparently unrelated to injury are Osgood–Schlatter's disease, Sinding-Larsen–Johansen syndrome and patellar tendinitis. All of these improve with symptomatic management and physiotherapy.

Several forms of bursitis may also present as knee pain. The prepatellar bursa is superficial and is located over the inferior portion of the patella. The infrapatellar bursa is deeper and lies beneath the patellar ligament before its insertion on the tibial tubercle. The pes anserine bursa underlies the semimembranosus tendon and may become inflamed and painful owing to overuse or inflammation. Anserine bursitis manifests primarily as point tenderness inferior and medial to the patella (over the medial tibial plateau). In contrast to prepatellar and infrapatellar bursitis, swelling and erythema may not be present and this condition may easily be misdiagnosed.

PAIN IN THE ANKLE, FOOT AND TOES

The ankle is as equally susceptible to the inflammatory and non-inflammatory arthritides as other weight-bearing joints in the lower limb. Pain may also result from chronic sprain (recurrent injury in the past). There is often little evidence of acute injury on presentation but radiographs may reveal subluxation due to repeated lateral ligament injury and weakness. In most cases pain will settle with rest, analgesia and physiotherapy.

Pain in the joints of the foot may arise from collapse of the longitudinal arch (flat feet), collapse of the transverse arch (metatarsalgia), osteoarthritis of the mid-foot joints, stress fractures and plantar fasciitis. Most of these conditions are readily identifiable from the history, examination and plain radiography. Bone scans may be required to diagnose a stress fracture.

Plantar fasciitis is inflammation at the attachment of the plantar fascia to the medial calcaneal tubercle. It may be a manifestation of reactive arthritis. The patient complains of pain under the heel that is worse on standing after a period of rest but improves with walking. Firm pressure on the medial calcaneal tubercle reproduces the pain. Treatment involves provision of analgesia and a soft heel pad. Metatarsalgia is pain under the metatarsal heads (usually the second and third) following collapse of the transverse arch (often associated with obesity). The forefoot is broad and there are callosities beneath the metatarsals. Treatment involves analgesia and provision of a transverse arch and weight-supporting insole. Morton's metatarsalgia is due to a fibrous thickening of a digital nerve, usually between the third and fourth metatarsals. Chronic or repetitive trauma is thought to be responsible. Lateral pressure produces pain that may radiate to the toes. Diagnosis may only be confirmed by magnetic resonance imaging or surgical exploration.

Pain in the big toe is classically associated with gout. Otherwise, the toes can be involved in inflammatory and non-inflammatory arthritis in similar ways to the hands and fingers. Other conditions include hallux valgus (bunions), hallux rigidus (osteoarthritis of the metatarsophalangeal joint of the great toe), hammer toe and claw toes. These toe deformities may give rise to metatarsalgia and pain secondary to the formation of callosities.

The first metatarsal head is exposed with hallux valgus as the great toe drifts laterally. A bunion is then formed which contains a bursa and thickened skin. Hallux rigidus presents as stiffness and pain in the first metatarsophalangeal joint. Unlike gout, there is no evidence of acute inflammation and radiographs show osteoarthritic changes. A hammer toe is a fixed flexion deformity at the PIP joint. Pain often arises from the overlying callosity rather than the joint itself. Claw toes are toes with flexion deformities of both interphalangeal joints.

In this brief discussion of pain in the foot and toes, it should be clear that management of these conditions is largely outside the scope of the emergency department. Most patients should be referred back to their GP for further referral to podiatry or orthopaedic services. Treatment often requires specialist advice, physiotherapy and the creation of arch supports.

Septic arthritis, crystal arthropathies and reactive arthritis may all present as acute arthritis in the foot.

IMPORTANT CONDITIONS

Arguably the most important causes of joint pain presenting to the emergency department are septic arthritis, reactive arthritis, crystal arthropathies and degenerative joint disease. These are all considered in further detail below.

SEPTIC ARTHRITIS

An infected joint is an emergency. Articular cartilage can be destroyed within a relatively short period following bacterial proliferation and acute inflammation. While staphylococci, streptococci, *Haemophilus influenzae* and *Neisseria gonorrhoeae* are the most common causes of septic arthritis, mycobacteria, spirochaetes, fungi and viruses can also infect joints.

The commonest organism responsible for septic arthritis is *Staphylococcus aureus* but the clinical presentation is the same for all pyogenic organisms. They reach the joint by haematogenous spread, following a penetrating injury of the joint or rarely as a result of infection spreading from an adjacent focus of osteomyelitis. The result is a sudden acute arthritis with classic signs of inflammation.

The knee is most often affected by septic arthritis.

There may be an obvious focus of infection elsewhere in the body but it is normal to find no precipitant. There is an increased incidence of septic arthritis in patients with gout, rheumatoid arthritis and immunosuppression. It is important to realize that acute gout and septic arthritis may coexist. Intravenous drug users, immunocompromised individuals and patients with in-dwelling catheters for dialysis or parenteral medications are at increased risk of Gram-negative bacterial arthritis. This may occur in unusual joints such as the sacroiliac or sterno-clavicular joints.

The affected joint is generally clearly inflamed unless it is a deep-seated joint like the shoulder or hip. Movements at the joint are restricted and there is local tenderness. Ultrasound may be required to demonstrate (and aspirate) an effusion in deeper joints. Systemic upset with fever and rigors is common.

Aspiration of the suspected joint is the most important investigation and will be diagnostic. A full blood count and blood cultures should also be checked if the patient is unwell. Radiographs may be normal or show evidence of an effusion only (displacement of capsular fat planes). They may also reveal an underlying joint condition that may have predisposed the patient to infection.

Normal synovial fluid contains fewer than 180 white cells μl^{-1}. These are predominantly mononuclear cells. White cell counts averaging 100 000 μl^{-1} (range 25 000–250 000 μl^{-1}), with more than 90% neutrophils, are characteristic of acute bacterial infections. Crystal-induced, rheumatoid and other non-infectious inflammatory arthritides are usually associated with fewer than 30 000–50 000 white cells μl^{-1}. Counts of 10 000–30 000 white cells μl^{-1}, with 50–70% neutrophils and the remainder lymphocytes, are common in mycobacterial and fungal infections. Definitive diagnosis relies on identification of the bacteria on Gram-staining, isolation from cultures of synovial fluid and blood, or detection of microbial nucleic acids and proteins by polymerase chain reaction (PCR)-based assays and immunological techniques.

Once the diagnosis is made, the joint should be immobilized and antibiotics commenced. Blind therapy with intravenous benzyl penicillin and flucloxacillin should be started pending results of microscopy, Gram-staining and culture. Penicillin-allergic patients should have erythromycin. Infected joints should then be drained and, ideally, irrigated in the operating theatre. With effective treatment, resolution of symptoms occurs within a week.

REACTIVE ARTHRITIS

Reiter's syndrome consists of a triad of:

- seronegative arthritis
- non-specific urethritis
- conjunctivitis.

Two types are described, an arthritis which follows a gastrointestinal infection and an arthritis which follows a non-specific urethritis. Typical enteric infections that precipitate Reiter's syndrome are caused by *Shigella*, *Salmonella*, *Yersinia* and *Campylobacter* species. In both cases, an acute monoarthritis or oligoarthritis occurs within approximately 2 weeks of an enteric or venereal infection. The knees, ankles and feet are the most common sites and the arthritis is typically an asymmetrical mono- or oligoarthritis. In Reiter's syndrome there is an associated urethritis with mild dysuria and a sterile urethral discharge. Rarely, circinate balanitis (a rash around the glans of the penis) may be present. A third of patients have a mild bilateral conjunctivitis that resolves spontaneously. In very few patients the classic pustular rash and scaling of the skin of the soles of the feet and toes (keratoderma blenorrhagica) may be seen. Patients may not recognize symptoms associated with the urethritis and conjunctivitis unless specifically asked.

Reactive arthritis has all the same characteristics of Reiter's syndrome but without the associated conjunctivitis and urethritis. It is much more common than the classic triad of Reiter's syndrome and is the commonest cause of acute arthritis in young men.

The diagnosis of reactive arthritis and Reiter's syndrome is purely clinical. The acute arthritis may be very difficult to differentiate from septic arthritis or gout and the possibility of reactive arthritis may be suggested by the history alone. Acute-phase proteins will be elevated in the initial stages but other investigations are of little value. Synovial fluid analysis will reveal a sterile inflammatory fluid.

Once infection has been excluded, the patient should be referred to a rheumatologist for further management. This consists of resting the joint and providing non-steroidal anti-inflammatory drugs. Other anti-inflammatory agents and immunosuppressants may also be used. The acute arthritis resolves within a few weeks but many patients go on to develop recurrent synovitis and joint effusions.

CRYSTAL ARTHROPATHY

Several types of crystal can be deposited in joints and cause acute arthritis. Monosodium urate, calcium pyrophosphate, calcium hydroxyapatite and calcium oxalate can induce acute or chronic arthritis or periarthritis. In spite of differences in crystal morphology, chemistry and physical

Table 31.7: Causes of hyperuricaemia

Impaired excretion of uric acid:
   Idiopathic gout
   Chronic renal disease
   Drug therapy (thiazide diuretics)
   Hypertension
   Primary hyperparathyroidism
   Hypothyroidism
   Increased lactic acid production (alcohol, starvation)

Increased production of uric acid:
   Idiopathic gout
   Increased turnover of purines due to myeloproliferative and lymphoproliferative disorders
   Increased purine synthesis (due to inborn errors of metabolism)

properties, the clinical events that result from deposition and release of these microcrystals are usually indistinguishable. The type of crystal involved can only be identified by synovial fluid analysis. The generic term gout is often used to describe the whole group of crystal-induced arthropathies, although it refers specifically to monosodium urate crystal deposition. Pseudogout is used to describe the arthritis associated with calcium pyrophosphate crystals.

Gout is caused by hyperuricaemia secondary to overproduction or under-excretion of uric acid. A high dietary intake of purines can be an additional factor. Uric acid is the final step in the breakdown pathway of nucleoprotein and purines. The final two stages are the conversion of hypoxanthine to xanthine and of xanthine to uric acid. Both of these reactions are catalysed by the enzyme xanthine oxidase. Uric acid is then excreted by the kidneys. Most patients with idiopathic gout have increased uric acid production and a small degree of impaired renal excretion. There is, however, a wide range of causes of hyperuricaemia and these should be considered in all patients (Table 31.7). Asymptomatic hyperuricaemia is 10 times more common than gout.

Gout predominantly affects men and often begins in middle life. The classic acute episode begins in the early hours of the morning with severe pain in the big toe. Dietary or alcohol excess is often the immediate precipitant although drugs can also be to blame. Joints of the lower limb are most often involved and the attack is most commonly an acute monoarthritis. The joint is red, warm, swollen and tender. Examination of the synovial fluid and measurement of serum uric acid are the only useful investigations, although the differential diagnosis must always include infection, reactive and acute inflammatory arthritis. Following repeated attacks of gout there may be permanent deposition of urate in and around joints. When these gouty 'tophi' are present, the diagnosis is much easier.

Polarized-light microscopy of synovial fluid can identify most typical crystals, although more sophisticated techniques are required to confirm the presence of calcium hydroxyapatite. Monosodium urate crystals are long, needle-shaped, negatively birefringent and usually intracellular. Calcium pyrophosphate crystals are usually short, rhomboid-shaped and positively birefringent. Otherwise, the synovial fluid characteristics are non-specific and can be either inflammatory or non-inflammatory. It must always be recognized that the presence of crystals does not exclude the existence of an associated acute or, more rarely, chronic infection.

Serum uric acid will always be detectable during an episode of acute gout but it may not be abnormally high and there is a high incidence of false-positive and false-negative results.

A normal or high uric acid neither confirms nor excludes the diagnosis of acute gout.

A very low serum uric acid does, however, make the diagnosis of acute gout very unlikely. Acute attacks are treated with indomethacin or alternative non-steroidal anti-inflammatory drugs. Aspirin should not be used. Once the acute attack has settled, the patient should be advised to reduce uric acid levels and consult their GP if symptoms persist or recur. Uric acid levels can be reduced by weight loss, reduction in alcohol intake, withdrawal of drugs such as thiazide diuretics and avoidance of food and drinks containing high levels of purines (game and lager). In some cases, the patient will require admission to control pain, exclude other causes of acute arthritis and investigate the underlying cause. In the longer term, a xanthine oxidase inhibitor or a uricosuric agent can be prescribed.

Pseudogout generally affects older people, with an equal sex distribution. It produces an acute arthritis, which is similar to osteoarthritis and generally affects large, weight-bearing joints. The affected joint is painful, warm and swollen, with a large effusion. It is a more difficult condition to treat than acute gout but the principles are the same.

DEGENERATIVE JOINT DISEASE

This term is used to describe the chronic arthritic conditions that primarily affect the joints and are frequently seen in the emergency department. They include osteoarthritis and rheumatoid arthritis.

Osteoarthritis is the commonest type of arthritis. It is present in 20% of the population as a whole and in 50% of those aged over 60 years. It is primarily a disease of cartilage that becomes progressively eroded and thinned. Pain is typically in the knees, hips and hands and is made worse by activity. Pain therefore tends to be worse towards the end of the day and is relieved by rest. There is thickening of subchondral bone, so affected joints become characteristically swollen with hard, bony swellings as well as effusions. There is marked crepitus with movement. In the knee, varus and valgus joint deformities may be particularly troublesome as the disease progresses. Although osteoarthritis is characterized by joint inflammation, there is no systemic involvement and thus no systemic illness.

Radiographic changes with osteoarthritis are characteristic. There is narrowing of the joint space (owing to loss of cartilage) accompanied by formation of osteophytes at the margin of the joint. Sclerosis of the subchondral bone and formation of bone cysts may also occur (Fig. 31.4). There are no diagnostic markers for osteoarthritis and acute-phase proteins are generally not elevated.

Treatment involves analgesia with simple analgesics and non-steroidal anti-inflammatory drugs. Physiotherapy is effective in maintaining muscle power and knee and hip movement. An increasing number of patients eventually undergo prosthetic joint replacement.

RHEUMATOID ARTHRITIS (FIG. 31.5)

Rheumatoid arthritis is a common, chronic systemic disease that produces a symmetrical inflammatory polyarthritis with progressive joint destruction and disability. It affects about 2% of the population and can begin at any age. It most often starts in the

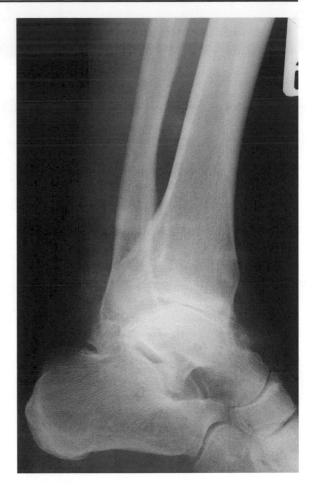

Figure 31.4: Radiographic changes of osteoarthritis.

30–40-year-old age group. It is an autoimmune disease, which has many extra-articular manifestations. It is, however, primarily a disease of the synovium. Synovial inflammation and proliferation account for much of the joint destruction.

Rheumatoid arthritis usually presents with the insidious onset of pain and stiffness in the small joints of the hands and feet. In 25% of cases it presents as arthritis of a single joint, such as the knee. An acute onset is sometimes seen in the elderly. Joint pain is worse on waking in the morning and is associated with marked stiffness that may take several hours to improve. Fatigue and general malaise are often associated with rheumatoid arthritis, as are a number of other non-articular conditions such as bursitis, tenosynovitis, anaemia and carpal tunnel syndrome.

Diagnosis relies initially on clinical features and the presence of rheumatoid skin nodules. These

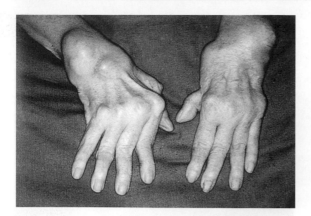

Figure 31.5: Clinical appearance of rheumatoid arthritis.

are seen in 20% of cases and are most often felt on the ulnar surface of the forearm. Radiographic abnormalities are also characteristic. There is loss of joint space and erosions on the articular surface of affected joints. Subluxation and destruction of joints may be seen. Serum tests for rheumatoid factor (an autoantibody) are positive in approximately 80% of patients and inflammatory synovial fluid can be aspirated from affected joints. Treatment involves specialist rheumatology input to protect joints, relieve symptoms, modify the disease process and manage the wide spectrum of complications.

FURTHER READING

Barkin, R., Rosen, P., Hockberger, R. *et al.* (Eds) (1998) *Emergency Medicine Concepts and Clinical Practice*, 4th Edn. Mosby, St Louis.

DERMATOLOGY

INTRODUCTION

Many patients present to emergency departments for assessment and treatment of a skin rash. As there are few genuine dermatological emergencies, these patients are generally given a low priority, an abbreviated consultation and referral back to their general practitioner (GP). It is, however, important that dermatological emergencies and presentations of serious systemic disease as a rash are identified and appropriately managed.

> Genuine dermatological emergencies are rare but important.

With these exceptions most patients can be safely discharged to their GP, who generally has more experience of the management of rashes. However, explanation, reassurance and, when applicable, symptomatic relief may be necessary.

This chapter covers the assessment of skin disease with particular reference to important factors in the history and examination. The immediate management of dermatological emergencies and other acute and common conditions that present to emergency departments, is also discussed. We have not provided black and white illustrations of rashes and the reader is referred to a suitable colour illustrated text (see Further Reading) to aid visual identification of specific rashes.

ASSESSMENT

As in most forms of diagnosis the history plays a pivotal role in the diagnosis of rashes (Table 32.1). Questions to elucidate the pattern and time course of evolution of the rash are followed by specific enquiry to search for causal factors. Many rashes that develop rapidly and therefore cause alarm to patients are related to allergy, and often to the use of a new type of medication or exposure to an environmental allergen. The association of the rash with systemic features such as nausea or vomiting is particularly important as it suggests the presence of systemic illness. This may, however, be a

Table 32.1: The dermatology history

How long have you had the rash, on which part of your body did it start and how has it spread and changed?
What other symptoms have accompanied the rash? Is it itchy?
Any allergen exposure (known allergies, new medications, unusual food, chemical exposure)?
Contact history – has anyone you know got a similar rash?
Travel history.
Past medical history of previous rashes, current or chronic other illness. Current medications.
Any family history of skin disease?

Table 32.2: A dermatological glossary

Erythema	Redness
Macule (macular)	Areas of altered skin colour not raised above the surface
Papule (papular)	An area of altered skin colour raised above the surface
Nodule (nodular)	Palpable lesion within the skin
Vesicle (vesicular)	A raised skin lesion containing fluid
Bulla (bullous)	A large vesicle
Circumscribed	Lesions are separate and well demarcated at their edges
Confluent	Lesions joining together to form larger continuous areas of rash
Scaling	Separation of flakes of skin from the surface
Crusting	Implies exudate (serous, purulent or blood) from the surface
Petechiae	Tiny collections of blood within the skin
Purpura	Larger collections of intracutaneous blood
Telangiectasia	Dilated but intact blood vessels

Table 32.3: Viral-induced skin rashes

Herpes zoster
Herpes simplex
Molluscum contagiosum
Erythema infectiosum
Hand, foot and mouth disease

VIRAL INFECTIONS (TABLE 32.3)

The commonest forms of rashes related to viral infections are the childhood exanthemata, chickenpox, measles and German measles. The chickenpox virus (varicella zoster) can also cause shingles, usually following reactivation of the virus, which remains dormant in the dorsal root ganglion for long periods. Severe and unremitting pain in the dermatome usually precedes appearance of the rash and therefore causes diagnostic difficulty. The commonest sites are the thoracic region and the ophthalmic division of the trigeminal nerve. Later eythema develops which is confined to the anatomical distribution of the dermatome and specifically does not cross the mid-line. This is followed by the appearance of vesicles which may become secondarily infected and crust. The lesions eventually heal over the course of a month.

Patients who develop infection in the ophthalmic division of the fifth cranial nerve are at risk of developing keratitis and corneal ulceration. They should be referred to an ophthalmologist for further management. In other cases a course of aciclovir will speed resolution of the illness and may reduce the risk of subsequent postherpetic neuralgia if given early. Those patients who are immunocompromised may develop more widespread infection and merit admission for treatment with intravenous aciclovir.

The herpes simplex viruses may cause a variety of illnesses. A systemic illness of pyrexia with headache may be accompanied by a widespread ulcerative gingivostomatitis that may leave the patient unwilling to take fluids and therefore dehydrated and requiring admission for rehydration. Following sexual transmission there may be an acute vulvovaginitis, and referral to a genitourinary medicine department should be made.

On occasions, a patient with established eczema develops secondary infection with the herpes simplex virus known as eczema herpeticum. The

trivial and self-limiting viral infection or a major life-threatening illness such as meningococcal septicaemia. Many skin diseases are recurrent, in which case there will be a past history of similar episodes, or relate to an existing systemic disease such as one of the connective tissue diseases.

The examination will largely consist of an attempt to describe accurately the nature and distribution of the rash. The accurate use of certain terms, especially if communicating with a specialist, is vital to achieving a correct diagnosis (Table 32.2).

SKIN INFECTIONS AND INFESTATIONS

A variety of viral, bacterial and fungal skin infections commonly present to emergency departments. The results of infestation of the skin are also frequently seen.

patient is usually systemically unwell with a widespread vesicular eruption. Treatment with aciclovir should be commenced urgently and in-patient treatment will be required.

Other virally induced skin conditions include molluscum contagiosum, which presents with a classic appearance of small shiny papules with central umbilication. It is most commonly seen in children and there is often a contact history. Untreated, it usually resolves over the course of several months leaving no scarring.

Fifth disease (erythema infectiosum) often occurs in epidemics in the spring in children. Marked erythema of the cheeks is accompanied by an upper body erythema that may be reticulate. The child is systemically well and no treatment is indicated. Hand, foot and mouth disease presents again mostly in children, with buccal ulceration and a vesicular eruption on the hands and feet. Again the child is systemically well and no treatment is indicated.

BACTERIAL INFECTIONS (TABLE 32.4)

The commonest micro-organisms responsible for bacterial skin infections are staphylococci and streptococci. Cellulitis is infection of the skin and subcutaneous tissue, usually by *Streptococcus pyogenes*. The classic clinical signs of infection, heat, erythema, swelling and tenderness are present with a varying degree of systemic illness. Signs of spreading infection, particularly lymphangitis, may also be seen. A search for a portal of entry for the infection must be made. This may reveal treatable causes such as athlete's foot. Underlying problems such as diabetes and neuropathy should also be considered. Treatment consists of rest, elevation and antibiotics. The most appropriate antibiotic is penicillin V, though more broad-spectrum antibiotics are commonly used. Admission for intravenous antibiotics is indicated where there is

significant systemic illness, failure to respond to oral antibiotics or where the patient is unable to manage their condition at home.

Erysipelas is also a streptococcal infection but usually involving the face and with a more acute onset and marked systemic illness. The erythematous area is circumscribed and indurated. Again treatment is with penicillin, but is often as an in-patient to allow parenteral administration.

A spectrum of infections caused by *Staphylococcus aureus* may occur. Folliculitis is infection of the hair follicles and responds to treatment with flucloxacillin. The infection may develop into furunculosis (boils) or even a carbuncle when multiple collections of pus have formed. In these cases treatment is by incision and drainage of the collection of pus. Antibiotics are usually not indicated. Infection in the nail fold may lead to the development of a paronychia where pus collects and may extend under the nail. Again treatment is adequate drainage of the pus, usually under a local anaesthetic ring block.

Impetigo is a virulent and contagious infection often occurring in outbreaks in schools. On examination in the early stages there is a collection of vesicles that break down, leaving a typically golden-coloured, encrusted area, often on the face. Bacteriological analysis usually demonstrates infection with either *Staphylococcus aureus* or a streptococcus. Treatment with oral penicillin and flucloxacillin should be accompanied by advice to reduce spread of infection.

Unusual infections of the skin include erysipeloid caused by *Erysipelothrix insidiosa*. This is an occupational disorder occurring in patients who handle infected meat or fish. It presents as a slowly enlarging, purple area with a raised edge. It responds rapidly to treatment with penicillin. In wounds sustained in or around fish tanks, infection with atypical mycobacteria may occur, causing fish-tank granulomata. These respond poorly to antibiotics and diagnosis is often only made after biopsy of the lesion.

FUNGAL INFECTIONS (TABLE 32.5)

Fungal infections of the skin not uncommonly present to emergency departments as a result of failure to respond to initial management from the GP. Tinea infections are caused by dermatophyte

Table 32.4: Bacterial-induced skin disease

Cellulitis
Erysipelas
Impetigo
Folliculitis, furunculosis, carbuncles and paronychia
Erysipeloid

Table 32.5: Fungal infections

| Tinea pedis, t. cruris, t. corporis, t. unguium |
| Candidiasis |

Table 32.6: Infestations

| Scabies |
| Pediculosis |
| Papular urticaria |

organisms and are suffixed by the anatomical location of the infection.

The commonest infection is tinea pedis or athlete's foot. On occasions patients present with this as the primary complaint. A macerated area of skin, usually in the web space between fourth and fifth toes, is diagnostic. More commonly, it is found either coincidentally during examination or as a portal of entry for a lower limb cellulitis. In either case it should be treated with a 2-week course of antifungal agents, which can be purchased without prescription from a chemist. General advice regarding regular hygiene may be necessary.

Tinea cruris (Dhobi itch) occurs in the skin folds of the groins as an irritant area of raised erythema with scaling. T. corporis has a similar appearance on the trunk, though on occasions as the lesion enlarges the central area of skin clears, leaving a target appearance. Both conditions are again simply treated with proprietary antifungal agents.

Fungal infection of the nails (T. unguium) will eventually produce a thickened, separated, yellow nail. Accurate diagnosis should be obtained by taking scrapings, as treatment involves a prolonged course of antifungal agents.

Infection with *Candida albicans* is most commonly recognized in the mouth as plaques of white material which leave a raw base when removed. Treatment is with nystatin or amphotericin. *Candida* may also superinfect areas of intertrigo, as in the groins, abdominal wall and inframammary areas. General advice regarding drying and hygiene in combination with a topical antifungal agent is usually effective. Infections involving the genitalia are dealt with in Chapter 18 but should prompt investigation for undiagnosed diabetes mellitus.

INFESTATIONS (TABLE 32.6)

Scabies is caused by infestation with the mite *Sarcoptes scabiei*. The female mites form burrows, usually in the web spaces of the hands or on the palmar surfaces of the wrists and extensor aspects of the elbows. As transmission of infection requires prolonged bodily contact, spread often occurs after sexual contact. Lesions on the genitalia are occasionally seen.

The condition presents with a gradual onset of itching, which becomes severe and intractable particularly in warm weather and when in bed. Any rash is usually as a result of scratching. On examination the burrows are usually visible as greyish tracks in the appropriate regions. The mite is sometimes visible within the burrow, which can be scraped open and its presence confirmed. Effective treatment with malathion or gamma benzene hexochloride is available, though clear instructions to treat all family members and sexual partners is needed.

Infestation with body lice (pediculosis) commonly affects the head, trunk or genitalia. The eggs of the lice are attached to the base of the hair follicles and are associated with itching. The lice are often seen around the genitalia. Secondary bacterial infection may occur. Treatment with malathion solutions should include treatment of contacts and be repeated after a week.

Papular urticaria presents as an irritant papule predominantly distributed on the limbs. It is a result of an allergic response to an insect bite and may be delayed in onset by several days. Treatment is symptomatic with antihistamines. Precautions to prevent further episodes may include disinfestation of house or pets.

DERMATOLOGICAL MANIFESTATIONS OF SYSTEMIC DISEASE

Many major systemic diseases may present with dermatological features. A list of these is provided in Table 32.7. Accounts of these are provided in the relevant sections of this text or in medical texts. One particularly worrying finding is that of purpura and a rapid assessment of the differential

Table 32.7: Systemic diseases with dermatological manifestations

Collagen vascular disorders and vasculitis:
  Systemic lupus erythematosus
  Scleroderma and systemic sclerosis
  Dermatomyositis
  Polyarteritis nodosa

Endocrine and metabolic disorders:
  Diabetes mellitus
  Thyroid disorders
  Hyperlipidaemia
  Vitamin deficiency

Infections:
  Human immunodeficiency virus infection
  Viral exanthemata
  Toxic shock syndrome
  Meningococcal septicaemia

Miscellaneous:
  Inflammatory bowel disease
  Sarcoidosis
  Liver disease
  Malignancy
  Arthropathies

Table 32.8: Differential diagnosis of purpura

Thrombocytopenia:
  Bone marrow replacement
  Drug induced
  Idiopathic

Coagulopathy:
  Congenital (e.g. haemophilia)
  Acquired (e.g. warfarin, liver disease)

Disorders of the vessel wall:
  Vasculitis (e.g. Henoch–Schönlein purpura)
  Emboli
  Fragility of vessel (steroid therapy)

diagnosis is necessary to allow initiation of definitive management (Table 32.8).

URTICARIA, ALLERGY AND DRUG REACTIONS

Patients with degrees of allergic reactions to a variety of substances may present to emergency departments. The degree of reaction may vary from

Table 32.9: Types of drug reactions

Exanthemata	Erythematous, maculo-papular and pruritic
Exfoliative	Red, scaly
Allergic vasculitis	Papules and nodules
Fixed drug eruptions	Erythematous areas the same site with each ingestion
Bullae	Large blistered lesions
Photosensitivity	Like sunburn in areas of light exposure

anaphylactic shock (see Chapter 16) to mild cutaneous manifestations. Often the provoking allergen may not be discovered. The skin eruption may consist only of erythema, although subcutaneous oedema may result in a pale papular central area. The lesions usually resolve within a few hours and will only recur if further exposure to the allergen occurs. Management consists of attempts to identify the allergen from the history and symptomatic treatment with antihistamines.

Angioedema is characterized by marked subcutaneous oedema occurring predominantly around the mouth or eyes. This may be life threatening if the swelling obstructs the airway.

With the increasing range of medications available to patients, either on prescription or without, drug reactions are an increasing cause of skin rashes. These may take a variety of forms (Table 32.9). Diagnosis is reliant on relating the onset of the rash to use of the medication. The disappearance of the rash on withdrawal of the medication adds evidence that the correct diagnosis was reached. Specific drugs may be associated with specific types of eruption.

REACTIVE ERYTHEMA

Erythema nodosum and erythema multiforme are poorly recognized but not uncommon. Erythema nodosum is diagnosed by the appearance of tender papules occurring predominantly in groups along the shins, thighs and extensor aspects of the upper limbs. Histologically, the lesions are areas of acute inflammation in the subcutaneous fat.

Table 32.10: Causes of erythema nodosum

Infective	Streptococci, tuberculosis, infectious mononucleosis, fungal
Drugs	Contraceptive pill
Idiopathic	
Sarcoidosis	
Inflammatory bowel disease	
Lymphoma	

Table 32.11: Causes of erythema multiforme

Infections	Viral (herpes simplex), bacterial (streptococcus) or fungal
Drugs	
Malignancy	
Pregnancy	
Idiopathic	

Table 32.12: Differential diagnosis of bullae

Infections	Herpes, varicella, impetigo
Drug eruptions	
Pemphigus	
Pemphigoid	

The underlying causes are listed in Table 32.10. Management consists of investigating the differential diagnosis, and a chest X-ray, anti-streptolysin-O titre and blood count are often performed. Symptomatic treatment includes use of an anti-inflammatory painkiller.

Erythema multiforme is initially seen as erythematous lesions first noticed on the extremities and then spreading proximally. Classically, the lesions later become pale centrally in which a further lesion appears giving the 'target' appearance. The main causes are listed in Table 32.11. In its most severe form, the Stevens–Johnson syndrome, there is widespread blistering and oral ulceration with systemic illness. Investigation involves defining the cause from the differential diagnosis and specific treatment of the cause. Patients with Stevens–Johnson syndrome require admission. Otherwise courses of oral steroids may shorten the course of the illness.

BULLAE

The differential diagnosis of bullous skin diseases is shown in Table 32.12. Many of these are dealt with elsewhere in this chapter. Pemphigoid and pemphigus are autoimmune skin disorders characterized by bullae. In pemphigus the bullae are intraepidermal and easily disrupted. In pemphigoid, the bullae are subepidermal and more durable. In both cases urgent dermatological advice and treatment are necessary.

Toxic epidermal necrolysis is a life-threatening condition usually resulting from a drug reaction. There is widespread loss of the epidermis associated with systemic illness. Management consists of withdrawal of the precipitating medication and management of the skin similar to a burn wound.

ECZEMA

This common skin condition is largely diagnosed and managed by GPs, though patients may attend the emergency department as an initial presentation or with complications of the established condition. The appearances are of a scaly erythema predominantly affecting the flexor creases. The patient often complains of intractable itching. In cases where the cause is an exogenous allergen, the distribution of the rash will match that of exposure.

In endogenous eczema the affected individual is usually a child with a positive family history for eczema and a past history of other atopic disorders such as asthma. The first line of treatment is emollients, and decisions regarding the use of other medications such as steroid creams should be left to the GP responsible for the patient's long-term management. Oral antibiotics are indicated where there is evidence of secondary bacterial infection.

In exogenous eczema, the patient should try to identify the allergen and avoid further contact. The allergen may be virtually any substance that the patient comes into contact with. Treatment of the presenting episode is otherwise as for endogenous eczema.

PSORIASIS

This is a chronic condition and the patient with established psoriasis will usually seek help from their GP rather than the emergency department. However, in certain circumstances the development of symptoms may be so acute that emergency treatment is indicated.

In erythrodermic psoriasis there is generalized erythema. This is often precipitated by changes in treatment or exposure to sunlight. Heat loss can result in hypothermia. The patient will require emergency management by a dermatologist. Pustular psoriasis presents as patches of scaling and erythema with superimposed pustules on the soles and palms. Systemic illness develops and in its generalized form admission is indicated. Guttate psoriasis presents acutely as multiple red scaly patches.

It often follows an acute streptococcal infection and clears after 4–6 weeks. Treatment with steroids or ultraviolet light may speed recovery.

FURTHER READING

Buxton, P. K. (1998) *ABC of Dermatology*. BMJ Publishing, London.

Fitzpatrick, T. Johnson, R. Wolff, K. and Suurmond, R. (2000) *Colour Atlas and Synopsis of Dermatology*. McGraw Hill, New York.

PART FIVE

OBSTETRICS AND GYNAECOLOGY

CHAPTER THIRTY THREE

OBSTETRIC AND GYNAECOLOGICAL EMERGENCIES

INTRODUCTION

It is common for women with gynaecological emergencies to present to the emergency department. The presenting complaint is generally either lower abdominal pain or abnormal vaginal bleeding. On occasions the conditions may be life threatening, requiring early surgical intervention to prevent mortality. Patients with problems in late pregnancy often present directly to obstetric units and are less commonly seen in emergency departments; however, the principles of dealing with obstetric emergencies, particularly in relation to trauma, are covered in the latter part of this chapter.

ASSESSMENT

Just as in other areas of clinical practice, accurate diagnosis in obstetric and gynaecological problems requires a complete although focused history and examination. In addition, investigations such as pregnancy testing and ultrasound scanning may be required in order to help decide on a working diagnosis.

Table 33.1: The gynaecology history

Vaginal bleeding	How long and how heavy?
Abdominal pain	How long, where and radiation?
Menstrual history	Normal cycle, last menstrual period?
Pregnancy	Result of pregnancy test. Contraception?
Vaginal discharge	Type?
Previous obstetric history	Expressed as P_{x+y} X number of pregnancies >24 weeks Y number of pregnancies <24 weeks

HISTORY

The history will initially focus on the presenting complaint although as a gynaecological diagnosis is considered, specific additional information will be required (Table 33.1).

EXAMINATION (TABLE 33.2)

As in other emergencies, initial consideration should be given to the airway, breathing and circulation.

Table 33.2: The gynaecology examination

Abdominal examination	
Inspection of the vulva	Bartholin's cyst, trauma
Speculum examination	Observe cervical os
	Take bacteriologiocal specimens
	Vaginal wall lacerations
Bimanual examination	Uterine and adnexal masses
	Local tenderness
	Cervical excitation (pain on moving the cervix)

Shock is a common presentation in conditions such as ectopic pregnancy and measures to control bleeding and initiate fluid resuscitation must be commenced immediately on recognition of the haemorrhage.

The examination of the gynaecological patient will then include an abdominal examination, with particular attention being paid to signs of pregnancy, including auscultation of the fetal heart after 12 weeks' gestation. Vaginal examination, including speculum and bimanual examination, may be necessary. It is, however, important to limit these examinations to circumstances where the findings will result in changes to decisions regarding investigation and management. There is no value in performing intimate examinations that will not alter the emergency department management and will need to be repeated by the gynaecologist.

Vaginal examination is contraindicated in suspected ectopic pregnancy and late pregnancy bleeding.

Emergency departments are uncomfortable places for patients to undergo vaginal examination. If this is necessary, the doctor must ensure that the examination takes place in a room where privacy can be ensured, interruptions avoided, and where the procedure cannot be overheard. A female chaperone should be present (for both male and female doctors) and the procedure should be explained prior to the examination taking place. The patient's legs and pelvis should be covered by a sheet as much as possible throughout the examination.

INVESTIGATIONS

A pregnancy test must be carried out on all females of potential child-bearing age (in other words from about 15 years, although pregnancy is possible before this, to patients in their late 40s). Most emergency departments are able to carry out sensitive near-patient pregnancy testing on urine samples with minimal delay. Urinalysis for signs of infection should also be performed.

The most useful imaging investigation is ultrasonography. This is usually carried out transabdominally but may be performed transvaginally where fine detail is required. Ultrasound is particularly useful in defining the position and viability of a pregnancy and in defining the nature of adnexal masses.

DIFFERENTIAL DIAGNOSIS

The common gynaecological diagnoses to be considered in the emergency department will now be considered individually.

ECTOPIC PREGNANCY

This is defined as a pregnancy that has implanted outside the uterine cavity. The commonest site of implantation is in the fallopian tube.

The diagnosis of ectopic pregnancy must be considered in all women of reproductive age with abdominal pain.

Ectopic pregnancy remains a cause of maternal death as a result of exsanguinating haemorrhage and occurs in up to 3% of all pregnancies.

Presentation

Ectopic pregnancy may present with abdominal pain, vaginal bleeding or collapse as a result of haemorrhage. There may be a previous history of ectopic pregnancy or other conditions that predispose to ectopic implantation, such as pelvic inflammatory disease or the use of an intrauterine contraceptive device.

The abdominal pain is usually of sudden onset, severe and localized to the right or left side of the lower abdomen.

Shoulder-tip pain is a classic though uncommon symptom of ectopic pregnancy.

The menstrual history is usually of 5–7 weeks' amenorrhoea and vaginal blood loss is present in most, although not all, cases.

Prior to rupture of the tubal pregnancy there is no haemodynamic abnormality although abdominal tenderness is usually found. Vaginal examination, if performed, may reveal tenderness in the right or left fornix and cervical excitation. Following rupture there are signs of hypovolaemic shock with more diffuse abdominal signs.

Management

If the diagnosis of unruptured tubal pregnancy is suspected, intravenous access must be obtained and samples sent for a baseline blood count and group and save. A pregnancy test is performed. If the pregnancy test is positive the patient will require an ultrasound scan to determine the location of the pregnancy.

Obtain senior help if you suspect a patient has an ectopic pregnancy.

The diagnosis of ruptured ectopic pregnancy is usually made on the basis of abdominal pain and shock in a patient with a positive pregnancy test. Arrangements must be made to get the patient to an operating theatre as rapidly as possible. Blood should be cross-matched and intravenous fluid resuscitation commenced through wide-bore cannulae.

Fluid resuscitation must not delay surgical intervention.

EARLY PREGNANCY LOSS

Spontaneous miscarriage is common, occurring in up to 40% of all pregnancies. Many women bleed

Table 33.3: Types of early pregnancy loss

Threatened miscarriage
Inevitable miscarriage
Incomplete miscarriage
Missed miscarriage
Septic miscarriage

in early pregnancy but subsequently deliver normal babies at full term. There is no treatment which will prevent miscarriage occurring and it is a distressing condition for the patient. It is also important to exclude other more serious conditions, such as ectopic pregnancy.

The term miscarriage is preferable to abortion in discussions with patients with early pregnancy loss.

Early pregnancy loss can be clinically divided into five categories (Table 33.3).

Presentation

The determination of the type of early pregnancy loss is predominantly based on the results of ultrasound examination. A number of clinical findings may, however, inform this decision.

In threatened miscarriage there is bleeding with a closed cervical os. The bleeding is usually light and pain may be minimal or absent. The prognosis for the pregnancy is good.

In inevitable and incomplete miscarriage there is heavier bleeding, often accompanied by abdominal pain with an open cervical os. In incomplete miscarriage products of conception are passed. If these are present in the cervical os they may produce a vagally mediated collapse. The products should be removed from the cervical os.

Missed miscarriage occurs when there is fetal death but the os remains closed, with retention of the products of conception. In septic miscarriage there is infection of the retained products resulting in purulent vaginal discharge and possibly septic shock.

Management

For patients who do not have excessive bleeding or pain, most hospitals will have an early pregnancy assessment unit which can provide further investigation and treatment, usually the following day.

Patients with profuse bleeding may require intravenous fluid therapy. Those with evidence of sepsis should have swabs and blood cultures taken and be admitted for intravenous antibiotic therapy.

It is important to consider at an early stage whether anti-D immunoglobulin therapy will be required to prevent rhesus iso-immunization. Guidelines are shown in Table 33.4.

OVARIAN CYST DISEASE

Ovarian cysts may present as an abdominal emergency as a result of the cyst undergoing torsion, rupture or haemorrhage.

Presentation

Lateralized lower abdominal pain is present which may be severe and intermittent. Rupture of the cyst will result in peritonism. The patient may have a previous history of ovarian cysts or be undergoing ovarian stimulation as a treatment for infertility. Abdominal examination will reveal tenderness although the cyst itself is rarely palpable. Bimanual examination will reveal adnexal tenderness and possibly a mass. Appendicitis, pelvic inflammatory disease and ectopic pregnancy should be considered as alternative diagnoses.

Investigations should include a pregnancy test. Definitive diagnosis is by ultrasound scan. Prior to this effective parenteral analgesia should be provided.

Management

The patient should be referred to a gynaecologist for possible surgical intervention.

Table 33.4: Guidelines for administration of anti-D immunoglobulin

Any rhesus-negative woman bleeding after 12 weeks of pregnancy
Any rhesus-negative woman:
  with an ectopic pregnancy
  with heavy bleeding or abdominal pain if gestation less than 12 weeks
  with inevitable, complete, septic or missed miscarriage at less than 12 weeks

PELVIC SEPSIS (TABLE 33.5)

Pelvic inflammatory disease arises as a result of ascending infection through the genital tract in sexually active women. It has potentially serious sequelae, particularly secondary infertility.

Presentation

The patient complains of lower abdominal pain with an offensive vaginal discharge. There may be symptoms and signs of sepsis, including pyrexia, flushing and tachycardia. Examination reveals lower abdominal tenderness with pain on cervical excitation.

Management

Bacteriological specimens should be taken whilst vaginal examination is being performed; these should include an endocervical swab for chlamydia. A pregnancy test, full blood count and blood cultures are also required. Treatment consists of antibiotic administration (Table 33.6).

Follow-up and contact tracing in a genitourinary medicine clinic must be arranged following detection of chlamydia infection.

Table 33.5: Types of pelvic sepsis

Pelvic inflammatory disease	Salpingitis
	Tubo-ovarian abscess
Infection of uterine contents	Retained products of conception

Table 33.6: Antibiotic treatment of pelvic sepsis

Type of infection	Treatment
Acute pelvic inflammatory disease	Metronidazole + doxycycline (or erythromycin) + cefotaxamine
Chlamydia	Doxycycline (or erythromycin)

OTHER COMMON GYNAECOLOGICAL PROBLEMS

BARTHOLIN'S CYST AND ABSCESS

The paired Bartholin's glands are situated in the posterior third of the vestibule and may become blocked, forming a cyst. This may subsequently become infected, resulting in an abscess. The patient complains of a unilateral painful labial swelling which may be recurrent and results in difficulty sitting. Examination reveals a tender, inflammed swelling in the labia.

If treated early the infection may resolve with oral amoxycillin. More commonly, formal incision and drainage is required and referral to the duty gynaecologist is therefore appropriate.

MENORRHAGIA

Excessive menstrual bleeding is a common problem and whilst it is more commonly dealt with in primary care and gynaecology out-patient departments, patients may present to the emergency department for assessment and treatment.

> Always check that the patient with menorrhagia is not also pregnant.

A history and examination are required to assess the severity of the bleeding and to check for serious underlying pathology. A blood count should be performed to identify the patient who is bleeding sufficiently to be anaemic and to require hospitalization. However, in most cases treatment to relieve the symptoms (Table 33.7) can be provided and the patient advised to see their general practitioner.

In general, mefenamic acid is particularly useful in patients with painful and heavy bleeding. Tranexamic acid is more effective in reducing menstrual blood loss. If in doubt advice should be sought from a senior doctor or the duty gynaecologist.

Table 33.7: Treatment of menorrhagia

Norethisterone
Combined oral contraceptive pill
Mefenamic acid
Tranexamic acid

EMERGENCY CONTRACEPTION

The availability of emergency contraceptive services varies and access to help can be difficult, particularly at weekends or out of normal working hours. As a result, patients may attend the emergency department seeking emergency contraception (Table 33.8). In general, these services should be provided by a doctor specifically trained in fertility control; however, hormonal postcoital contraception is more effective the earlier it is taken and doctors should therefore be familiar with the procedures for prescribing it safely. Departmental procedure regarding the provision of emergency contraception should always be followed.

In assessing the patient it is important to ascertain the date of the last menstrual period and the usual length of the cycle. The time of unprotected sexual intercourse should be documented. Contraindications to use of hormonal methods are established pregnancy, current focal migraine, jaundice or sickle-cell crisis as well as previous thromboembolic disease (combined hormone method only).

> Hormonal methods can be used up to 72 h after unprotected intercourse.

The combined hormone method was previously used with two pills taken immediately and a further two 12 h later. Although effective there was a significant incidence of nausea and vomiting which potentially rendered the treatment ineffective. If patients return having vomited after the medication, a further dose should be given after an antiemetic. More recently, the progestogen-only method has been found to be effective with a reduced incidence of side-effects. The preparation used is levonorgestrel, with two doses again taken 12 h apart. Patients should be provided with clear discharge instructions (Table 33.9) and their general practitioner should be informed.

The insertion of an intrauterine contraceptive device (IUCD) should be carried out by an

Table 33.8: Postcoital contraception

Progestogen-only method
Combined hormone method
Insertion of an intrauterine contraceptive device (IUCD)

Table 33.9: Instructions after using hormonal postcoital contraception

Take the first tablets as soon as possible and the second dose 12 h later
If you vomit after taking the tablets they should be considered to have been ineffective. Return to the emergency department
See your GP in 4 weeks to check the tablets have been effective and to discuss future contraception
Attend a genitourinary medicine clinic if you are worried you may have contracted a sexually transmitted disease

experienced practitioner, usually in a family planning clinic. It may be effective in preventing pregnancy up to 5 days after unprotected intercourse.

FOREIGN BODIES

The most common vaginal foreign bodies are lost tampons or condoms. Occasionally, something more exotic is retrieved. A careful speculum examination and removal of the item with sponge forceps is required. If tampons are left *in situ* for a prolonged period, toxic shock syndrome can result.

If a child presents with a possible vaginal foreign body, get senior help.

On occasions patients may present complaining of having 'lost' the threads of their IUCD. These are often found at speculum examination and the patient can then be reassured. If the device appears to have migrated, an abdominal X-ray and ultrasound may be helpful in locating it. In the meantime, alternative methods of contraception should be used.

POSTOPERATIVE PROBLEMS

When patients present with symptoms of pain and vaginal bleeding following childbirth or termination of pregnancy, the possibility of retained products of conception should be considered. More seriously, infection can occasionally develop. In general these

patients should be referred on to the duty gynaecologist for further management.

SEXUAL ASSAULT

Any allegation of sexual assault requires careful investigation in order to preserve and document evidence for use in any subsequent prosecution. If sexual assault is alleged, emergency department doctors should confine themselves to attending to any life-threatening injuries and summoning the police (with the patient's consent). An appropriate physical examination for forensic purposes should be carried out by a police surgeon.

OBSTETRICS

Most patients in the later stages of pregnancy will be dealt with in the delivery suite. However, a number of circumstances may lead to a presentation to the emergency department.

EMERGENCY NORMAL DELIVERY

Fortunately, there is normally time for a patient to be transferred to the delivery suite prior to delivery. However, on occasions labour is rapid (precipitate) and emergency department staff may be called on to perform the delivery. Often in large departments one of the nursing staff has had midwifery experience and will step forward. It is, however, worth revising the management of a normal delivery here.

Labour is diagnosed on the basis of painful uterine contractions that result in cervical dilatation. Rupture of the membranes may occur before onset of contractions or not until immediately prior to delivery. If delivery is thought to be imminent, help should be summoned from the obstetric team and the paediatricians.

The first stage of labour involves progressive cervical dilatation with descent of the baby's head. Following full cervical dilatation, contractions result in descent and rotation of the head. This stage is characterized by the overwhelming urge of the mother to push. The third stage is expulsion of the placenta and membranes.

Management

Help should be summoned. The abdomen should be examined and baseline vital signs recorded. The fetal heart rate should be assessed using a Pinard's stethoscope. If on examination of the perineum delivery is not imminent, the patient should be transferred to the delivery suite. If delivery is imminent, sterile procedures should be adopted. The left hand should apply pressure to slow the rate of delivery of the head and keep it flexed. As the head reaches the perineum the mother should be told to pant and not push. As the head is delivered it is allowed to extend. The neck should be checked for the presence of the cord and, if necessary, the cord should be pulled over the head or divided. The shoulders, followed by the rest of the baby, are then delivered and oxytocin and ergometrine administered intramuscularly to assist the third stage.

Delivery of the placenta and membranes should occur within 5 min of the end of the second stage. Gentle traction on the cord may be used and the placenta and membranes should be checked for completeness.

COMPLICATIONS OF PREGNANCY

This section deals with the commoner emergency presentations in late pregnancy.

Antepartum haemorrhage

This is defined as haemorrhage after the 20th week of pregnancy. The differential diagnosis is between abruption and placenta praevia.

Abruption is premature separation of the placenta and results in abdominal pain and vaginal bleeding. Depending on the degree of separation, the woman may go into labour or fetal death may occur. Placenta praevia occurs when the placenta is implanted in the lower segment of the uterus or over the internal cervical os. Haemorrhage may be profound and is usually painless. The patient may know that they have placenta praevia as a result of routine antenatal ultrasound scanning.

The priority in the emergency department is resuscitation with intravenous fluids and early obstetric consultation. If bleeding is profuse large volumes of blood should be cross-matched.

Table 33.10: Differential diagnosis of abdominal pain in pregnancy

Labour
Urinary tract infection
Ectopic pregnancy
Appendicitis
Ovarian cyst disease
Cholelithiasis
Abruption
Haemorrhage or infarction of a fibroid

Postpartum haemorrhage

Haemorrhage following delivery is predominantly caused by retained products of conception. Infection of the uterine cavity may also result in late bleeding. The immediate priorities are fluid resuscitation and involvement of the obstetric team. In profuse haemorrhage, oxytocin may be helpful in causing uterine contraction to reduce blood loss.

Abdominal pain in pregnancy

There are a large number of causes of abdominal pain in pregnancy (Table 33.10). These may be directly or indirectly related to the pregnancy or may be a coincidental occurrence.

Particularly in the late stages of pregnancy, the diagnosis may be more difficult to make clinically. Useful investigations include urine testing and ultrasound scanning. There should be a low threshold for referring these patients to the obstetric team.

Eclampsia and pre-eclampsia

Eclampsia is defined as maternal convulsions after the 20th week of pregnancy. It remains a cause of maternal and fetal mortality. Pre-eclampsia is characterized by two or more of:

- hypertension
- proteinuria
- oedema.

Eclamptic fits may be preceded by headache, tremor, hypertonicity and an altered mental state.

If an eclamptic fit occurs, oxygen should be administered and attempts made to abort the convulsions with intravenous diazepam and phenytoin. An experienced obstetrician and anaesthetist must be called urgently. The patient should be taken to the delivery suite since an emergency caesarean section will almost certainly be required.

Thrombo-embolic disease

Pregnancy results in a significant additional risk of deep venous thrombosis and pulmonary embolism, particularly in the last trimester. There should be a low threshold for investigating any patient with symptoms suggestive of these diagnoses.

TRAUMA IN PREGNANCY

Dealing with a pregnant traumatized patient presents a number of challenges. The way in which injury may affect pregnancy changes with the variations in anatomy and physiology as the pregnancy progresses. The initial assessment and management should follow the concepts of advanced trauma life support course.

> Good care for the mother will provide good care for the fetus.

Anatomical and physiological changes in pregnancy

In the first trimester the uterus is protected within the pelvis and injury is rare. In the second trimester the uterus rises out of the pelvis. The fetus is initially protected by the thick-walled uterus, although with time and thinning of the uterine wall fetal susceptibility to injury increases.

Maternal physiology changes during pregnancy with elevation of the blood volume and cardiac output and a raised respiratory rate. The blood pressure remains constant unless pre-eclampsia develops. During haemorrhage the blood supply to the placenta is reduced early on, making the fetus vulnerable to maternal hypovolaemia.

> The pregnant woman may lose 30% of her blood volume before signs of shock are detected.

Particularly relevant in the third trimester of pregnancy is the supine hypotension syndrome. The gravid uterus in the supine position lies on the inferior vena cava, resulting in reduced venous return to the heart, low cardiac output and maternal shock. Manual displacement of the uterus to the left or placing the patient in a lateral position (whilst protecting the spine if necessary) will alleviate the problem.

> Supine hypotension syndrome should be considered as a cause of shock in late pregnancy trauma.

Assessment

The primary survey assessment of the traumatized pregnant patient is exactly the same as for any adult. Optimum care of the mother results in the best care for the unborn child. In the secondary survey the abdomen should be examined and the fetal heart sounds checked. The fundal height should be assessed and compared with the known gestational age (Fig. 33.1). Visual examination of the vulva will reveal any vaginal bleeding. Initial investigations should include a group and crossmatch, coagulation studies and Kleihauer test. Any X-rays necessary for the management of the mother should be carried out regardless of concerns about irradiating the fetus.

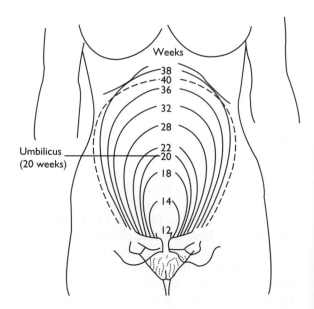

Figure 33.1: Fundal height and gestational age.

Management

Aggressive attempts should be made to correct hypoxia and hypovolaemia. Surgical techniques such as intercostal drainage and diagnostic peritoneal lavage may have to be modified to avoid the gravid uterus. Manual displacement of the uterus or turning the patient into a partially lateral position may be necessary for supine hypotension syndrome. Obstetricians should be called to help assess the patient, and in the rare event of a cardiac arrest, perimortem caesarean section should be considered. If the mother is rhesus-negative, anti-D immunoglobulin must be considered even after minor injury.

Specific injuries

Direct injury to the fetus may occur, although this is often the result of penetrating trauma and is rare in the UK. Injury to the uterus may result in abruption, with abdominal pain and tenderness and usually vaginal bleeding. Uterine rupture may also occur, resulting in fetal anatomy being easily palpable through the mother's abdomen. Injury to the uterus may also result in amniotic fluid embolism with disseminated intravascular coagulation, circulatory collapse and convulsions. All are associated with high fetal and maternal mortality. Early recognition of the injuries to mother and fetus and involvement of the obstetric team in trauma management offer the best chance of a successful outcome.

FURTHER READING

Stevens, L. and Kenny, H. (1996) *Emergencies in Obstetrics and Gynaecology.* Oxford University Press, London.

PSYCHIATRIC EMERGENCIES

PART SIX

PSYCHIATRIC EMERGENCIES

CHAPTER THIRTY FOUR

PSYCHIATRIC EMERGENCIES

- Introduction
- Assessment
- Referral to a psychiatrist

- Specific psychiatric emergencies
- Mental Health Act 1983 for England and Wales
- Further reading

INTRODUCTION

With the recent moves in the UK towards provision of care for psychiatric illness within the community, assessment and management of mental illness has become an increasingly common reason for attendance at or referral to an emergency department. Primary psychiatric problems account for 2.5% of emergency department attendances and 20% of patients suffer from a psychiatric disorder. As many patients previously managed in long-stay psychiatric hospitals have been discharged into the community they have reappeared in vulnerable groups who historically have relied on emergency departments for provision of routine healthcare. One in three homeless people suffers from psychiatric illness, most commonly schizophrenia and alcohol dependence.

It is important to recognize that serious physical illness may present with predominantly behavioural features. In addition, many psychiatric illnesses may initially present as a result of deliberate self-harm and require treatment prior to psychiatric assessment. The spectrum of conditions that may present to emergency departments is shown in Table 34.1.

ASSESSMENT

Just as in the management of patients with physical illness, the assessment of a patient with mental illness is reliant on a thorough history and examination. This may, however, be more difficult

Table 34.1: Common psychiatric conditions presenting to the emergency department

Acute confusional state
Unexplained physical symptoms
Self-harm
Psychosocial problems
Antisocial or violent behaviour
Alcohol and drug dependency
Anxiety states
Acute psychosis
Dementia

in the emergency department than in a ward or out-patient setting. Pressure of work often limits the most important resource for evaluating psychiatric problems – time.

The interview with the patient should be carried out in a quiet private room; however, the safety of the staff performing the assessment must also be considered. Fortunately, few patients with mental illness are dangerous and it is rare to have to use methods of physical or chemical restraint. A doctor interviewing a patient should, however, routinely position themselves in a room such that the patient would be unable to come between them and the door. The doctor, if alone, should always carry some form of personal alarm to alert other staff should they feel threatened.

Rarely, a patient is brought to the emergency department whose behaviour is potentially dangerous to them and those trying to assist. In this situation the minimum amount of physical restraint necessary to protect the patient and the staff from injury should be applied. In general, it is often possible to calm the patient and gradually remove the physical restraints. In some cases the patient's behaviour may make it necessary to use sedative drugs for the patient's own protection or that of the staff. However, this is a step that should not be taken lightly and will result in subsequent difficulty in assessing the patient's mental state.

HISTORY

A full psychiatric history is beyond the expertise and resources of most emergency departments. It is, however, important to gather sufficient information to rule out serious underlying physical illness and to allow a decision to be made on the need for referral or admission. Table 34.2 lists the items that are essential for a satisfactory assessment (Table 34.2).

Although most of this information is often obtained from the patient, valuable additional information may often be available from friends and relatives. The general practitioner and other healthcare workers such as community psychiatric nurses and social workers may also contribute to the assessment.

EXAMINATION

The physical examination of the patient is important in excluding a physical cause for their illness and should not be omitted. The mental state examination (Table 34.3) concerns information gathered by observation of the patient and by enquiring about unusual beliefs and experiences.

The patient's appearance gives many clues as to mental state. It is important to assess the patient's non-verbal behaviour, such as eye contact and expression, as this may offer valuable clues. There

may also be obvious signs of self-neglect from the patient's appearance, suggesting low self-esteem.

Behaviour and speech are typically altered in the major psychiatric illnesses. The speech of the hypomanic is pressured and their behaviour manifests an excess of energy and restlessness. In contrast, the severely depressed patient has limited speech and reduced energy.

Alterations in cognitive functions, such as disorientation and memory loss, are particularly important as they suggest the presence of underlying organic disease. Although severe mental illness, particularly when associated with alcohol abuse, may produce these features, extra care should be taken in carrying out a physical examination and further investigations may be indicated. It is important to assess the patient's orientation in time and place, short-term memory (recall of a name and address after 5 min), long-term memory (current affairs) and concentration (recite the months of the year backwards).

Delusions are beliefs that are 'unshared and unshakeable'. The patient may think that they have special powers or status and cannot be convinced otherwise.

The patient's emotions may vary from depression with suicidal ideation to euphoria. The emotions may be constant throughout the interview or swing markedly from one end of the spectrum to the other.

Hallucinations may be auditory or visual. Auditory hallucination described as outside the person's head are genuine, and in schizophrenia are often of voices criticizing the patient. Visual hallucinations are more typical of intoxication with drugs or withdrawal states.

REFERRAL TO A PSYCHIATRIST

Decisions regarding which patients require immediate referral to a psychiatrist should be based on a

Table 34.2: Components of psychiatric history

Presenting complaint
Past psychiatric history:
Previous admissions
Doctor's name
Diagnosis
Drugs:
Prescribed
Abused
Alcohol
Current relationships

Table 34.3: The mental state examination

Appearance
Behaviour and speech
Cognitive function
Delusions
Emotions
Hallucinations

number of key points. Following assessment of the patient's history, including past psychiatric history, and a mental state examination it is important to consider whether the patient may be a danger to him/herself or others. Although many patients express some degree of suicidal ideation not all are at significant risk of serious self-harm. It is, however, not the role of a junior doctor to make this judgement and all patients expressing suicidal ideas should be referred to a psychiatrist for assessment immediately.

> A psychiatrist should assess all patients expressing suicidal ideas.

Many patients with established psychiatric illness may present to emergency departments as a result of a crisis or deterioration in their condition. It is valuable to discuss these patients with their carers or relatives in order to assess the degree of support available to them in the community. Admission is often required to prevent further deterioration and re-establish compliance with therapy.

For patients with symptoms of mental illness who have not previously required contact with the psychiatric services, a decision regarding referral should be made on the basis of the severity of the patient's symptoms, whether there is evidence of self-neglect and on the patient's wishes. The family or carers' wishes should also be considered.

SPECIFIC PSYCHIATRIC EMERGENCIES

DELIBERATE SELF-HARM (DSH)

Patients choose to harm themselves in a number of ways. Most commonly in the UK this takes the form of the ingestion (or occasionally inhalation or injection) of drugs or chemicals. It is also common to encounter patients who inflict lacerations, particularly around their wrists or necks. Patients may also choose to harm themselves by jumping from a height or by setting fire to themselves. Despite this wide spectrum of self-injury it is important to remember that the duty of the doctor is not only to assess and treat the resultant poisoning or injury but also to detect underlying psychiatric illness and intervene to prevent recurrence.

The aim of the psychiatric assessment is therefore to quantify the suicidal intent by determining the reason for the episode of DSH and recognizing underlying psychiatric illness. Specifically, the doctor must identify patients at risk of further self-harm.

The suicidal intent is assessed by considering three key factors:

- the risk to which the person was exposed
- the actual injury sustained
- the likelihood that the patient meant to kill themselves.

A number of factors detected by taking a careful history and performing a mental state examination point to serious suicidal intent and risk of subsequent completed suicide (Table 34.4).

Completed suicide is associated with a number of features and these can therefore also be used as indicators of future risk in deliberate self-harm cases (Table 34.5). The greater the number of these

Table 34.4: Indicators of suicidal intent from assessment

Before (preparation):
  Act planned in advance
  Suicide note written
  Anticipated death (written a will)

During (circumstances):
  Patient alone at time of event
  Attempt timed so that intervention unlikely
  Precautions taken against discovery

After (afterwards):
  Did not seek help
  Stated wish to die
  Stated belief that act would have killed them
  Regrets that act failed

Table 34.5: Other factors associated with suicidal intent

Male sex
Age greater than 45 years
Divorced or single status
History of previous deliberate self-harm
Psychiatric illness – depressive disorders, alcohol or drug abuse, personality disorder
Social isolation
Unemployed
Any serious medical illness

factors present, the greater the risk of suicide. Overall, 10% of patients admitted after an overdose commit suicide within 10 years.

It is important to recognize that the motive for an act of deliberate self-harm may be one other than suicide. It is often an impulsive act undertaken as a 'cry for help' or as an attempt to influence others. The patient may also seek an escape from emotional distress or use the act to express anger directed at loved ones. In the absence of mental illness there is little evidence to suggest that psychiatric treatment will prevent repetition.

Acts of deliberate self-harm, however, predominantly occur in the setting of a depressive illness. Admission for the patient's protection will be necessary if the suicide risk is high and there is evidence of neglect. Biological features of depression, such as early morning wakening, poor appetite and weight loss, also suggest severe disease, which requires urgent treatment. Patients who have a lack of social support and evidence of failure of treatment in the community should also be referred for admission.

> Self-harm is not in itself a mental illness. The majority of people who self-harm have no psychiatric illness.

An objective technique for assessing suicidal risk is the 'sad person's' scale (Table 34.6). A score of less than 6 indicates that it may be safe to discharge the patient if appropriate support and follow-up are available. If the score is greater than 8, admission will probably be required. An intermediate score indicates formal psychiatric assessment.

Table 34.6: The 'sad person's' scale

- **S**ex male
- **A**ge <19 or >45
- **D**epression or hopelessness
- **P**revious DSH or psychiatric care
- **E**xcessive alcohol or drug use
- **R**ational thinking loss (psychosis, organic)
- **S**eparated, widowed, divorced
- **O**rganized or serious attempt
- **N**o social support
- **S**tated future intent (repeat or ambivalent)

<6 can consider discharge
6–8 probably requires psychiatric consultation
>8 probably requires admission

ACUTE PSYCHOSIS

Psychosis is a term that is poorly understood and often used inappropriately. The term implies a major mental illness in which the patient has lost contact with reality and their behaviour is no longer constrained by reasoning and morality. The patient has usually lost any insight into the abnormal nature of their beliefs and behaviour. It is characterized by hallucinations, delusions and thought disorder.

> Psychosis is characterized by hallucinations, delusions and thought disorder.

Psychotic symptoms may occur in a number of conditions (Table 34.7).

It is sometimes difficult to distinguish between drug-induced psychosis, the affective disorders (mania and depression) and schizophrenia.

Mania

Mania (or its less extreme form, hypomania) may occur as part of a manic–depressive illness (bipolar disorder) or as an isolated illness. The patient typically demonstrates insomnia without fatigue, with an increased appetite and libido and psychomotor acceleration. The patient has delusions, which are grandiose and expansive ideas regarding their self-importance. This often manifests itself as spending sprees way beyond their financial means.

Mental state examination reveals pressure of speech with a mood of euphoria, although the latter is often mixed with periods of anger and irritability. The patient's speech often shifts rapidly from one subject to another (flight of ideas) and there is an inability to concentrate on a subject, accompanied by loss of insight.

Table 34.7: Conditions presenting with symptoms of psychosis

Schizophrenia
Mania
Severe depression
Acute confusional states
Dementia
Drug-induced psychoses, including alcohol abuse

Admission is usually required in order to protect the patient from their own actions. As a result of the patient's lack of insight into their behaviour, voluntary admission is often refused.

Schizophrenia

Schizophrenia is a group of disorders which is classically subdivided into four types (Table 34.8).

In simple schizophrenia there is insidious social withdrawal and odd behaviour, although an absence of hallucinations and delusions. Paranoid schizophrenia is more florid, with systemized persecutory delusions and hallucinations. Mood and thought processes are reasonably well preserved so that the patient may appear normal until abnormal beliefs are uncovered. This disorder is more common with increasing age. The hebephrenic type manifests childish behaviour with prominent affective symptoms, disordered thought, delusions and hallucinations. This is commonest in adolescents and young adults. Catatonic schizophrenia initially presents with stupor or excitement, repetitive speech or actions (echolalia, echopraxia), autonomic obedience and perseveration. The acute syndrome manifests the positive symptoms, the chronic syndrome (dementia praecox) the negative ones.

Schizophrenia is often diagnosed on the presence of Schneider's first rank symptoms (Table 34.9).

The differential diagnosis of schizophrenia includes drug-induced psychosis (amphetamines and alcohol), temporal lobe epilepsy, dementia and affective disorders.

When assessing a patient with known schizophrenia it is important to attempt to establish a cause for their relapse. This may be iatrogenic (reduction or change in medication), non-compliance with medication, or an environmental or emotional crisis.

THE ACUTELY DISTURBED PATIENT

The behaviour of acutely disturbed patients is alarming and leads to relatives and bystanders seeking help urgently. This often results in the patient being brought to the emergency department by the ambulance service, police or their carers. These patients may manifest a wide variety of behavioural abnormalities and pose a risk to

Table 34.8: Types of schizophrenia

Simple
Paranoid
Hebephrenic
Catatonic

Table 34.9: Schneider's first rank symptoms of schizophrenia

Hallucinations:
Third-person auditory – two or more voices discussing or arguing about the patient
Running commentary
Thought echo – a voice speaking his thoughts simultaneously or just afterwards
Interference with thinking:
Thought insertion
Thought withdrawal
Thought broadcasting
Other symptoms:
Primary delusions (arising *de novo*)

Table 34.10: Differential diagnosis of the acutely disturbed patient

Alcohol or drug dependence
Prescribed drugs
Metabolic disturbance
Head injury
Schizophrenia
Mania
Personality disorders

themselves, their carers and healthcare staff. There is a wide range of potential causes (Table 34.10).

Most patients who present with disturbed, violent and abusive behaviour are not psychiatrically ill. The doctor should seek a physical cause for the patient's behaviour, such as hypoglycaemia, postictal state, drug intoxication or drug withdrawal. If no evidence of these conditions is found the behaviour may, rarely, be the result of a major psychiatric illness but is more commonly the result of a personality disorder.

Most violent patients are not psychiatrically ill.

The priority must be to ensure the safety of the patient and staff. In general, the use of drugs should be avoided and attempts made to calm the patient by talking to them and listening to their complaints.

Management

In the first instance it is vital to try to engage the patient by providing a calm and reassuring environment in which provocation is avoided. This will allow the patient to be assessed and the differential diagnosis to be considered. A senior and experienced doctor should be involved in the management of all acutely disturbed patients.

The matter of consent to treatment is complex. If a patient has a disorder such that they are unable to comprehend and retain information, particularly in respect of the consequences of accepting or refusing treatment, they may be judged incompetent to consent or refuse. In such a case treatment may continue in line with accepted medical practice.

Physical restraint and sedative medication may, however, be necessary to protect the patient and the carers from injury. Restraint should be to the minimal degree and should be provided by personnel trained in safe control and restraint techniques.

> Physical and chemical restraint should be a last resort if there is no other way of protecting the patient and attendants from injury.

If sedation is unavoidable haloperidol is better than chlorpromazine as it is less sedating, causes less postural hypotension and has fewer anticholinergic side-effects. It does, however, cause more extra-pyramidal side-effects. Up to 30 mg may be given intramuscularly. If further sedation is required, lorazepam 4 mg intravenously is the drug of choice. The patient must be closely monitored. Patients presenting to emergency departments are much more likely to have an organic aetiology to their psychiatric symptoms and should be investigated accordingly. Specific psychiatric assessment and treatment may also be required.

ORGANIC DISORDERS

Acute organic disorder (delirium)

This is usually characterized by an acute onset with marked cognitive impairment, including changes

Table 34.11: Causes of an acute confusional state

Alcohol and drugs:
  Intoxication or withdrawal
Metabolic:
  Uraemia
  Electrolyte imbalance (hyponatraemia, hypercalcaemia)
  Cardiac or respiratory failure
  Hepatic failure
  Acute intermittent porphyria
  Systemic lupus erythematosus (SLE)
Endocrine causes:
  Thyroid disorders
  Hypoglycaemia
Infective causes:
  Intracranial infection
  Systemic infection
Other intracranial causes:
  Space-occupying lesion
  Raised intracranial pressure
  Head injury
  Epilepsy
Vitamin deficiency:
  Wernicke's encephalopathy

in the level of consciousness and a fluctuating course. A wide range of conditions may cause delirium (Table 34.11).

Typical features of an acute confusional state include impairment of consciousness with disorientation in time and place and poor concentration. The patient often has no insight into their illness and there may be visual hallucinations and misinterpretations and tactile hallucinations. These are classically demonstrated by the visual and tactile hallucinations of the patient in delirium tremens. Mood is often labile and the thought processes slow and muddled.

> Alcohol withdrawal and drug abuse are probably the commonest causes of delirium seen in emergency department practice.

The management of the acutely disturbed patient should involve determination of the underlying cause and specific measures relevant to that cause. This may be straightforward (glucose for hypoglycaemia) but is usually more complex.

The patient should be managed in a well-lit room and the familiar faces of relatives may help provide reassurance to the patient. Fluid and electrolyte abnormalities should be corrected. If drugs are considered necessary to aid management they should be prescribed with consideration to the patient's underlying illness. Haloperidol may be indicated to calm the patient and benzodiazepines to sedate. Chlordiazepoxide is particularly useful in alcohol withdrawal states. In hepatic failure haloperidol may precipitate coma and benzodiazepines are therefore preferred, despite their sedating effects.

Alcohol excess and withdrawal

Emergency departments commonly see the effects of both acute alcohol intoxication and long-term alcohol dependence. Although the effects of alcohol use may be obvious in the case of an acutely intoxicated or withdrawing patient, the role of alcohol may be much less obvious. It is of course now widely recognized that a large proportion of road traffic accidents are the result of intoxication. There is also a wide range of traumatic and medical morbidity, which is the direct or indirect result of alcohol abuse. The long-term use of alcohol may result in a varying degree of symptoms when alcohol is withdrawn, or in symptoms related to nutritional deficiency.

Following withdrawal of alcohol after a prolonged period of abuse, the patient may experience tremor, agitation, nausea, retching and sweating. Perceptual distortions and, on occasions, convulsions may also occur.

> Delirium tremens is a life-threatening medical emergency.

Delirium tremens, the fully developed withdrawal syndrome, is a life-threatening emergency. It is characterized by clouding of consciousness with disorientation in time and place. Visual hallucinations and delusions occur on a background of agitation and restlessness. There is prolonged insomnia, with truncal ataxia and autonomic overactivity.

Malnutrition commonly occurs in patients who are dependent on alcohol, since their energy and financial resources are directed at ensuring a supply of alcohol to the exclusion of a proper diet. Sustained lack of thiamine may produce Wernicke's

Table 34.12: Features of Wernicke's encephalopathy

Ophthalmoplegia
Nystagmus
Clouding of consciousness with memory disturbance
Ataxia
Peripheral neuropathy

Table 34.13: Features of Korsakoff's psychosis

Impairment of recent memory
Confabulation
Retrograde amnesia
Disorientation
Euphoria or apathy
Lack of insight
Ataxia

encephalopathy, the features of which are shown in Table 34.12.

Similarly, Korsakoff's psychosis may occur, the features of which are shown in Table 34.13.

The management of alcohol withdrawal consists of the use of drugs to reduce the distressing physical symptoms (typically chlormethiazole or chlordiazepoxide) and the provision of vitamin supplements to provide thiamine. It is important that this treatment is properly supervised and the doctor should refer the patient to the local agency responsible for providing this service and subsequent follow-up.

In delirium tremens, in-patient treatment may be required to provide rehydration, glucose should the patient develop hypoglycaemia, and anticonvulsants if withdrawal fits occur.

BORDERLINE PSYCHIATRIC CONDITIONS RELEVANT TO EMERGENCY DEPARTMENT PRACTICE

Repeat attenders

A small number of patients are responsible for a disproportionately large number of attendances. Usually they have one of two underlying problems, a chronic psychiatric illness or somatization. Patients with chronic psychiatric illness often do not register with a general practitioner and use the emergency department as a source of primary healthcare. While the department is not an appropriate place to deal with their healthcare needs, it is appropriate to try to place the patient in contact with appropriate services. Referral to a community psychiatric nurse or social worker can often lead to a reduction in the patient's use of the emergency department.

Somatization describes a number of patients who describe symptoms in the absence of sufficient underlying cause. It is assumed that there is some form of psychological gain for the patient. Once again, an active strategy of intervention through community psychiatric services may result in a reduction in the patient's demands and attendances.

Factitious disorders

Patients with Munchausen's syndrome seek medical attention by simulating physical illness. Many will submit to an extraordinary amount of investigation and treatment, including surgery. Most departments will have access to a list of patients who are thought to have this condition. If this condition is suspected, serious illness must be excluded and a senior doctor involved in decisions regarding further management.

Another group of patients will attempt to obtain drugs such as opiates by simulating illness (classically ureteric colic). These patients often demand opiates for their symptoms and fail to respond to the administration of other drugs which would normally be effective (e.g. diclofenac for ureteric colic). Further investigation will often reveal that the patient is using an assumed name and address and may be known to other departments in the region. Again a senior doctor should be involved in the management of the patient.

SIDE-EFFECTS OF PSYCHIATRIC MEDICATION

Drugs used in psychiatric practice may have a narrow therapeutic window and it is not uncommon for patients to present with side-effects of their medication. It is important to recognize these and provide appropriate treatment.

The major tranquillizers

These cause side-effects which are predominantly due to central blockade of dopamine receptors. Acute dystonia usually occurs shortly after starting treatment and may also be seen as a side-effect of related drugs used for other conditions (e.g. metoclopramide as an antiemetic). Typical features are oculogyric crisis (involuntary eye movements), torticollis and opisthotonus (involuntary arching of the back.). To the inexperienced clinician this condition appears bizarre and it is not uncommon for a diagnosis of 'hysteria' to be made. However, treatment with the anticholinergic procyclidine rapidly resolves this condition.

In the long term, a pseudoparkinson's syndrome with extrapyramidal features of rigidity, akinesia and pill-rolling tremor is often seen, and treatment consists of dose reduction and anticholinergics.

Neuroleptic malignant syndrome is a life-threatening emergency characterized by hyperpyrexia with autonomic instability and severe muscular rigidity. It occurs as an idiosyncratic reaction to antidopaminergic drugs and is often precipitated by intercurrent infection or dehydration. The mortality may be up to 20%. Treatment is with rehydration and cooling. Patients often require paralysis and ventilation. Bromocriptine and dantrolene have been successfully used.

Antidepressants

Monoamine oxidase inhibitor (MAOI) antidepressants are now rarely used owing to the high incidence of serious side-effects. However, a small number of patients are still prescribed these drugs for conditions resistant to conventional therapies. The tyramine reaction is caused by the inhibition of peripheral metabolism of tyramine by MAOIs. Tyramine-rich foods may therefore produce a hypertensive crisis.

The tricyclic antidepressants are effective but often produce side-effects and are dangerous in overdose (see Chapter 15). Anticholinergic features of dry mouth, blurred vision, constipation and urinary retention may occur. Arrythmias and heart block may also occur, particularly in patients with pre-existing heart disease.

The more modern selective serotonin re-uptake inhibitors (SSRIs) have a much improved safety profile and are relatively safe even in overdose. They may, however, cause nausea, vomiting and headache.

Lithium

Lithium is an effective therapy used predominantly in bipolar affective disorder. There is, however, only a narrow range of therapeutic serum levels, above which significant and occasionally life-threatening toxicity may occur. Lithium toxicity causes fine tremor, polyuria, polydipsia, sleepiness, nausea and diarrhoea. Levels above $1.5\,mmol\,l^{-1}$ cause central nervous system manifestations of ataxia, dysarthria and drowsiness. Levels greater than $2\,mmol\,l^{-1}$ cause impairment of consciousness and seizures. Toxicity is often precipitated by dehydration or by concomitant administration of a diuretic or anti-inflammatory drug (NSAID).

Treatment should involve rehydration and osmotic diuretics. With severe toxicity haemodialysis may be necessary.

Anxiolytics

Although these drugs are relatively safe, overuse can cause falls in the elderly. Sudden withdrawal may produce a severe reaction, with mood changes, nightmares and perceptual disturbances, especially skin sensitivity.

MENTAL HEALTH ACT 1983 FOR ENGLAND AND WALES

Any actions necessary to preserve life or prevent serious injury or illness can and should be taken without the patient's consent if the patient is deemed to be unable to understand the nature and seriousness of their condition and the treatment required. Such actions are not covered by the Mental Health Act but are lawful under common law. Detention under the Mental Health Act does not necessarily mean that a patient is incompetent to consent to or refuse treatment.

Treatment of mental illness, including admission to hospital, should be voluntary other than in a minority of circumstances dictated by the Mental Health Act. The act allows for compulsory admission and detention when the patient suffers from a mental disorder of a nature and degree that warrant hospital detention for assessment or treatment in the interests of their own health or safety or for the protection of others.

The following are not regarded as mental disorders and are therefore excluded from the Mental Health Act:

- alcohol or drug dependence
- promiscuity or immoral conduct
- sexual deviancy.

> There is no specific part of the Act designed for use in the emergency department.

The Act grants (under Section 12) specific powers to approved doctors. These are usually senior psychiatrists and police surgeons. Such doctors are usually referred to as Section 12 approved. The preferred option is always voluntary admission; failing this, a Section 2 is the next best choice. In exceptional circumstances (i.e. non-availability of a Section 12-approved doctor), a Section 4 may be completed.

SECTION 2

This is an order for compulsory admission. Detention is for assessment or assessment followed by treatment. It requires a medical recommendation by two doctors, one of whom is Section 12 approved; the other has previous knowledge of the patient (usually the GP). The application is made by the patient's nearest relative or an approved social worker. The duration of the Section is 28 days.

SECTION 4

This is an emergency order for the compulsory detention of a patient. It should only be used where there is insufficient time to obtain the opinion of a Section 12-approved doctor who could then complete a Section 2. This is normally converted to a Section 2 as soon as possible. It requires a medical recommendation by one doctor who must have examined the patient within the last 24 h. The doctor need not be Section 12 approved.

Application is made by the patient's nearest relative or an approved social worker. The duration of the Section is 72 h.

Variations in these orders occur in Scotland and Northern Ireland. The Mental Health Act (Scotland) describes a Section 24 order (similar to the English Section 4) and a Section 26 which is equivalent to the English Section 2. In Northern Ireland compulsory admission for assessment of mental illness requires application by the nearest relative or an approved social worker. Three doctors are required to sign the order, which lasts for 7 days.

If a patient who is felt to be mentally ill and is likely to be a danger to themselves or others leaves the emergency department the police should be informed. They can detain the patient under Section 136 of the Act and return the patient to a place of safety for further assessment.

FURTHER READING

Merson, S. and Baldwin, D. (1996) *Psychiatric Emergencies*. Oxford Handbooks in Emergency Medicine. Oxford University Press, Oxford.

ENVIRONMENTAL

EMERGENCIES

CHAPTER THIRTY FIVE

ENVIRONMENTAL EMERGENCIES

- Introduction
- Heat illness
- Cold injuries
- Chemical incidents
- Radiation illness
- High-altitude sickness

- Diving emergencies
- Near drowning
- Electrocution (including lightning strike)
- Venomous snake bites
- Further reading

INTRODUCTION

This chapter considers the assessment and management of a variety of conditions presenting to the emergency department as a result of accidental or deliberate exposure to dangers in the patient's environment. The following subjects are covered:

- heat illness
- cold injury
- chemical incidents
- radiation illness
- high-altitude sickness
- diving emergencies
- near drowning
- electrocution (including lightning strike)
- snake bites.

HEAT ILLNESS

Although the climate in the UK makes it unusual to see patients with heat illness, it is important that it is recognized and treated appropriately. Heat illness may be contributed to by a number of factors other than the environmental temperature. These include strenuous exercise, age and pre-existing illness.

Heat illness may be divided into minor and major. The major heat illnesses comprise heat exhaustion and heat stroke. These may be regarded as being part of a continuous spectrum of heat illness, with progression from heat exhaustion to heat stroke occurring if the provoking conditions persist.

MINOR HEAT ILLNESS

Minor heat illness may manifest as heat cramps in muscles. This appears to be related to salt deficiency and advice to supplement food with salt and avoid excessive sweating will usually lead to resolution. Heat syncope occurs as a result of the opening of cutaneous vascular beds in response to heat, and tends to occur in the elderly and others with diminished cardiovascular reserve. General advice to maintain adequate fluid intake and avoid prolonged periods of standing is usually all that is required.

HEAT EXHAUSTION

This occurs as a result of volume depletion when loss through sweating exceeds fluid intake. It is most commonly, seen in those undertaking vigorous exercise, such as long-distance running in hot weather. Over a more prolonged period salt depletion can also occur if there is insufficient dietary intake to replace salt losses in sweat.

Presentation

The early symptoms are non-specific, with lethargy and headache. As the condition progresses there is dizziness, vertigo and syncope. Examination will reveal postural hypotension and tachycardia but the core temperature remains normal.

Management

In mild cases oral rehydration and rest in a cool environment will be sufficient. In more severe cases intravenous fluid therapy with normal saline will produce rapid recovery. The volumes of fluid administered should be titrated to produce restoration of normal pulse and blood pressure. In more complex cases, particularly in patients with significant pre-existing illness, the serum electrolytes should be checked and the patient admitted for a period of observation.

HEAT STROKE

Heat stroke is a result of a failure of the body's homoeostatic mechanisms for temperature regulation. There is marked elevation of the core temperature and evidence of multi-organ failure.

> Heat stroke is a life-threatening emergency.

Presentation

Heat stroke is characterized by marked elevation of body temperature and evidence of central nervous system dysfunction, with a confusional state, seizures and coma. The skin is characteristically hot and dry and absence of sweating is common, although not universal. Coagulation failure and hepatorenal failure are common.

Management

The most important initial measures are to secure the airway and ensure oxygen delivery. Cooling must be initiated by removing clothing and commencing more active measures to rapidly decrease body temperature, including immersion in cold water or tepid sponging under fans. The core temperature must be continuously monitored. Intravenous fluids are required but their administration must be carefully monitored as pulmonary oedema may occur. If excessive shivering is preventing

rapid cooling, chlorpromazine will be of benefit. The patient will require further treatment on an intensive care unit.

COLD INJURIES

Cold may be considered as resulting in either local injury such as frostbite, or systemic as in hypothermia.

LOCAL HYPOTHERMIA

Frostnip

This is the mildest form of cold injury, characterized by reversibility, pallor, pain and numbness.

Frostbite

Historically, frostbite has been not only a military problem, but also a problem in high-altitude climbers and the homeless. Frostbite can be classified into superficial and deep injuries. Superficial injuries are characterized by hyperaemia, oedema, clear vesicle formation and partial-thickness skin involvement. Deep injuries are characterized by haemorrhagic vesicles, full-thickness skin involvement and, in extreme cases, gangrene and bone destruction (Fig. 35.1).

Non-freezing injury

This type of injury results from chronic exposure to wet and cold conditions. At first the limb is cold,

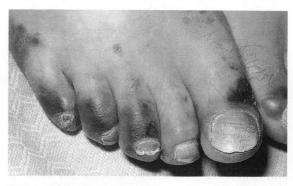

Figure 35.1: Severe frostbite.

but in 1–2 days it becomes painful and hyper-aemic, with blistering and ulceration. A classic example of non-freezing injury is trench foot.

Management of cold injuries

This includes warm blankets and hot drinks as general warming measures. The affected limb is rewarmed by immersing it in warm water (40–42°C) for 20–30 min. Analgesics are necessary as this process is very painful. Other modalities of treatment for frostbite include institution of oral and topical antiprostaglandin therapy to limit the release of inflammatory mediators. Antibiotics may be indicated when the skin barrier is broken. Surgical debridement should be postponed until a clear demarcation has occurred.

SYSTEMIC HYPOTHERMIA

Hypothermia is defined as a core temperature of less than 35°C.

Hypothermia may occur primarily, predominantly as a result of accidents and exposure to low temperature. Alternatively it may occur secondarily to a disease process, which it then complicates, contributing to the subsequent mortality and morbidity. Measurement of the core temperature allows definition of severity (Table 35.1).

Hypothermia is characterized by depression of the cardiovascular and central nervous systems.

The elderly, children and trauma patients are particularly susceptible to hypothermia and therefore extra care is required when these patients present to the emergency department. Elderly patients have impaired ability to increase heat production and a decreased vasoconstrictor response. Children

Table 35.1: Classification of hypothermia

	Temperature (°C)
Mild	32–35
Moderate	30–32
Severe	<30

have an increased surface area to body mass ratio as well as low energy sources. The typical clinical signs are given in Table 35.2 and are correlated to the degree of hypothermia. A low-reading thermometer is required and a temperature reading should be taken from a central site such as the rectum.

Investigations

A full baseline assessment should be undertaken. Hypothermic patients may manifest a number of abnormalities (Table 35.3 and Fig. 35.2).

Management of hypothermia

Initial priority must be given to securing a patent airway and providing oxygen. The core temperature should be assessed with a central low-reading thermometer. Many treatments, including defibrillation, are ineffective when the core temperature is less than 30°C. The patient in hypothermic cardiac arrest should therefore be rewarmed with continuing cardiac massage and ventilation until a core

Table 35.2: Symptoms and signs of hypothermia

Mild:
  Lethargy
  Confusion
  Shivering
  Ataxia
Moderate:
  Hypotonicity
  Bradycardia and hypotension
Severe:
  Coma
  Arrhythmias
  Pupils fixed and dilated
  Pulselessness

Table 35.3: Abnormalities on investigation of a hypothermic patient

- High haematocrit due to cold diuresis and dehydration
- Hyperkalaemia (poor prognosis)
- Coagulopathy
- High amylase
- ECG J wave and arrhythmias (see Fig. 35.2)

HYPOTHERMIA

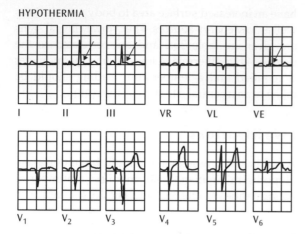

Figure 35.2: ECG showing J waves in hypothermia.

temperature of 30°C is reached before defibrillation is attempted. There is some evidence that bretylium is effective in profoundly hypothermic patients.

Rewarming is started by the removal of cold or wet clothing and insulation of the casualty in a warm environment (passive rewarming). Active external rewarming involves exposing the patient to exogenous heat sources such as heating blankets. Active internal rewarming techniques are indicated in patients with severe hypothermia. These include the following:

- ventilation with warm humidified oxygen
- intravenous warm fluids
- gastric, bladder, peritoneal or pleural lavage with warm fluid
- blood rewarming by cardiopulmonary bypass or haemodialysis.

In general, patients who are conscious with cardiac output and who improve with simple external rewarming methods do not require aggressive treatment. Invasive active internal rewarming should be used in profoundly hypothermic patients, including those with no cardiac output.

For those with previous good health, the prognosis is good and recovery is usually complete. In those with significant co-morbidity the mortality rate may be above 50%. Many patients will develop multiple organ failure and will require treatment on an intensive care unit.

Over the years there has been much debate regarding the determination of death in hypothermia. A well-known adage is that *'a patient is not dead until they are warm and dead'*. Profound hypothermia

may mimic death with the absence of any cardiorespiratory activity, yet aggressive resuscitation and rewarming (particularly in cold-water drowning) may produce a neurologically intact survivor. However, there are patients in whom it is impossible to restore body temperature. The decision regarding when to discontinue resuscitation in a hypothermic patient should therefore be made by a senior doctor.

> Decisions to discontinue resuscitation of hypothermic patients should only be made by experienced clinicians.

CHEMICAL INCIDENTS

A chemical incident is *'an unforeseen event leading to an acute exposure of two or more individuals to any non-radioactive substance resulting in illness or a potentially toxic threat to health'* or *'two or more individuals suffering from a similar illness which might be due to such an event'*.

Examples of chemical incidents include fires or explosions in a chemical plant or chemical spills causing water pollution. Patients may present having been exposed to a wide range of substances of varying toxicity.

> Do not become a further victim of the incident yourself.

MANAGEMENT

The rescuers' safety is the first priority. On site, the police, together with other emergency services, will always attempt to contain the chemical hazard. Rescue teams are allowed to approach casualties only once the scene is declared safe.

There are three triage categories for chemically contaminated casualties:

- resuscitation required during decontamination
- treatment may be delayed until after decontamination
- minor injuries may walk unaided to an ambulant decontamination facility.

Decontamination starts by identifying contaminated 'dirty' areas and uncontaminated 'clean' areas. Decontamination prior to transfer to hospital is desirable but may not always occur. Decontamination of casualties is the responsibility of the ambulance service, who are able to provide portable cold water decontamination facilities.

Resuscitation is provided according to established guidelines. Treatment for such victims includes removal of contaminated clothing. This will remove 70–80% of the contamination. The same principles apply to the emergency department. Advice on identified specific chemicals can be sought from the National Poisons Unit. Relevant biological samples are collected to confirm exposure and the dose received. Other injuries are also treated.

RADIATION ILLNESS

Accidents producing life-threatening radiation exposure are very rare. Protection from external contamination is best achieved with protective clothing. There should be no eating, drinking or smoking in areas considered to be contaminated in order to prevent internal contamination. Moreover, in situations where there is a risk of release of radioactive iodine, a large dose of stable iodine should be administered by mouth before or shortly afterwards in order to saturate the thyroid gland and increase excretion of the radioactive form. This should lessen the risk of thyroid cancer.

Human factors, such as lack of elementary safety rules and inadequate training, play a major role in most of the accidents occurring in industry. Preplanning is essential and may minimize the severity and the deterioration of the situation.

MANAGEMENT

Patients with whole-body irradiation should have their radiation dose assessed. Vomiting within 2 h is suggestive of significant irradiation. Patients should be transferred to a specialized unit. Antiemetics such as ondansetron can be very helpful. Where there has been local irradiation, skin erythema may develop which may subsequently proceed to vesiculation.

Pain, infection and malignant change are long-term complications. External contamination is dealt with by clothing disposal and soap and water decontamination. Radiation monitoring should be carried out after each attempt. Specialist advice should always be sought. In cases of internal contamination the aim of the treatment is to reduce absorption and enhance elimination.

HIGH-ALTITUDE SICKNESS

The higher the altitude, the lower the partial pressure of oxygen and therefore the greater the hypoxia experienced. Hyperventilation results in respiratory alkalosis. Hypoxia causes the pulmonary vessels to constrict and the pulmonary artery pressure to rise. At a later stage, red blood cell production increases to enhance the oxygen-carrying capacity of the blood. Acute mountain sickness, high-altitude pulmonary oedema and high-altitude cerebral oedema are all caused primarily by hypoxia and the associated circulatory changes.

ACUTE MOUNTAIN SICKNESS

Acute mountain sickness develops within the first 24 h after a high ascent. This will not be seen in mountain ascents within the UK. The commonest symptom is headache and this is classically frontal or bitemporal and throbbing in nature. Other manifestations include shortness of breath, insomnia, anorexia, nausea, vomiting, dizziness and fatigue. These symptoms usually resolve after a few days at levels below 3050 m but can take weeks at higher altitudes. If acute mountain sickness is left untreated this may lead to pulmonary or cerebral oedema.

Prevention includes slow ascent to allow for acclimatization as well as taking acetazolamide where indicated. Acetazolamide has been shown to reduce the incidence and severity of acute mountain sickness. It is a carbonic anhydrase inhibitor that causes metabolic acidosis by enhancing the renal excretion of bicarbonate ions. The resultant acidosis stimulates ventilation and therefore the rate and depth of breathing. Moreover it causes diuresis, which reduces peripheral oedema.

HIGH-ALTITUDE PULMONARY OEDEMA

This is due to non-uniform, hypoxic pulmonary vasoconstriction. The result is over-perfusion of the remaining patent vessels with transmission of the high pulmonary artery pressure to capillaries. Dilatation of the capillaries and high flow results in capillary injury, with leakage into the alveoli. It is a non-cardiogenic pulmonary oedema that leads to shortness of breath, cough and haemoptysis as well as fatigue. Signs include tachypnoea, tachycardia, an altered mental state and pulmonary crepitations. The chest X-ray may show pulmonary oedema.

High-altitude pulmonary oedema is treated using oxygen, nifedipine, hyperbaric oxygen, or simply by transferring the patient to a lower altitude. Some studies have shown that frusemide may be of some benefit.

HIGH-ALTITUDE CEREBRAL OEDEMA

The blood–brain barrier is believed to be altered in high-altitude cerebral oedema, causing an increase in the cerebral blood flow. Symptoms include headache, insomnia, nausea and vomiting, as well as cranial nerve palsies, paralysis and seizures. Treatment in these cases involves descent to low altitude, oxygen, dexamethasone and hyperbaric oxygen.

DIVING EMERGENCIES

Medical emergencies related to diving can be divided into:

- decompression sickness
- barotrauma
- arterial gas embolism.

DECOMPRESSION SICKNESS

For the diver, every 10 m of submersion below sea level increases the surrounding pressure by one atmosphere. This causes more nitrogen to dissolve in the tissues (Henry's law). Decompression sickness – the 'bends' or Caisson's disease – results as gas bubbles form in the tissues if the diver ascends

Table 35.4: Types of decompression sickness

| Type I | Affecting skin, lymphatics, musculoskeletal areas |
| Type II | Neurological changes |

Table 35.5: Symptoms by area affected in decompression sickness

Joint	Joint pain, dysaesthesia
Cutaneous	Subcutaneous emphysema, pruritus, rash
Pulmonary	Cough, shortness of breath, chest pain, cyanosis, hypotension, shock, death
Neurological	Any neurological event, low back pain, paraesthesia, paralysis, bladder dysfunction

too rapidly. If enough time is given during the return to the surface nitrogen can be eliminated and decompression sickness prevented.

Decompression sickness presents within an hour of ascent and symptoms are the result of:

- mechanical obstruction of the vascular system
- activation of complement and inflammatory mediators
- bubbles in the tissues causing distension.

The types of symptoms are classified in Table 35.4.

Categorizing decompression sickness by anatomical distribution is more relevant to clinical practice (Table 35.5).

Any symptoms in a diver following a dive should be considered to be the result of decompression sickness until proved otherwise.

The gold-standard treatment is hyperbaric oxygen therapy. The sooner this is commenced the better the prognosis, and doctors should know the location and contact details of the nearest hyperbaric centre. Treatment will also include oxygen and isotonic fluid resuscitation.

BAROTRAUMA

Boyle's law states that the volume of a given mass of gas is inversely proportional to the pressure in that environment. Therefore the expansion and contraction of gas in the natural air cavities of the body, as a diver ascends or descends, can cause damage to the surrounding structures (barotrauma).

Barotrauma of descent

MIDDLE EAR SQUEEZE
During a dive the surrounding pressure increases and in effect the volume of any body cavity decreases. In the middle ear, pressure outside the tympanic membrane increases and the middle ear cavity is squeezed. If the pressure on either side of the membrane is not equalized the tympanic membrane will be damaged or ruptured. Resulting haemorrhage can cause pain, hearing loss and vertigo. If the membrane perforates, the pain resolves but the rest of the symptoms persist, along with vomiting. If the membrane is intact most patients recover within a few weeks. If it has ruptured then antibiotics are prescribed and ENT involvement is mandatory.

INNER EAR BAROTRAUMA
This involves rupture of the round or oval windows. Symptoms include vertigo, tinnitus, nystagmus, ataxia and sensorineural hearing loss. Treatment includes bed rest with the head of the bed elevated, as well as an appointment with an ENT surgeon. The patient should not fly or dive unless instructed by an ENT specialist.

SINUS SQUEEZE
This occurs when the sinuses are blocked and the pressure is not equalized. This causes haemorrhage, mucosal congestion and pain over the affected sinus as well as bloody nasal discharge. Management includes nasal decongestants.

Barotrauma of ascent

PULMONARY BAROTRAUMA
As the diver ascends to the surface, air in the lungs expands. If the air is not exhaled during the period of ascent the alveoli overinflate and can rupture. Overdistension of the alveoli often presents with haemoptysis but not necessarily with chest pain. If there is rupture of the alveoli the end result is pneumomediastinum, or pneumothorax. The patient presents with chest pain and, on examination, subcutaneous emphysema as well as decreased

breath sounds are present. A chest X-ray is often diagnostic. In the former case oxygen along with observation may be the only treatment required. In the latter case treatment depends on the size of the pneumothorax. Divers with pre-existing small lung cysts or end-expiratory flow limitation may be at risk of pulmonary barotrauma. Pulmonary barotrauma is second only to drowning as a cause of death in divers.

ARTERIAL GAS EMBOLISM

This condition is a true medical emergency since pulmonary veins can be injured and alveolar gas enter the systemic circulation, causing embolism. Symptoms include loss of consciousness, confusion, seizures, hemiparesis and other neurological disturbances. An elevated serum creatine kinase level may be a marker for arterial gas embolism, as well as a predictor of outcome. Management includes oxygen, intravenous fluids and hyperbaric oxygen. Expert advice should always be sought.

NEAR DROWNING

Near drowning is survival after submersion (Table 35.6). Death from drowning is most commonly caused by aspiration of liquid but can also be caused by asphyxia secondary to laryngospasm (so called dry drowning). If death is not immediate from hypoxia there is intrapulmonary shunting, decreased lung compliance, ventilation/perfusion mismatch and further hypoxia, leading to cerebral ischaemia, cardiac arrhythmias and multi-organ failure.

Aspiration of water often causes non-cardiogenic pulmonary oedema, which presents as adult

Table 35.6: Factors associated with near drowning

Inability to swim
Hypothermia
Drugs or alcohol
Trauma
Seizures
Myocardial infarctions
Cerebrovascular accidents
Non-accidental injury

respiratory distress syndrome (ARDS). A chest radiograph may be normal at first but later on will show evidence of pulmonary oedema. The patient may deteriorate after a few hours (secondary drowning). This is due to influx of proteins and fluid into the alveoli as a result of loss of surfactant and leaky respiratory membrane due to acidosis and hypoxia. Near-drowning patients must always be observed in hospital, no matter how well they seem at the time of their emergency department attendance.

TREATMENT

Immediate resuscitation is essential in the prehospital setting. Care must be taken to protect the cervical spine in cases of suspected injury, particularly where the patient has dived into shallow water. In these cases the airway should be opened by using a jaw thrust rather than head tilt. Oxygen (100%) should be administered to all patients. Apnoeic patients or those with decreased respiratory effort require bag and mask ventilation or endotracheal intubation. Asystole and ventricular fibrillation require cardiopulmonary resuscitation. Sinus bradycardia, atrial fibrillation and junctional rhythms are commonly seen after hypothermia but require no immediate management.

In the hospital setting, the patient is reassessed and resuscitation continues. Blood should be sent off for baseline investigations and large-bore intravenous lines inserted. The patient's arterial blood gases and temperature must be monitored. Positive end-expiratory pressure ventilation may be needed as this will reduce the degree of intrapulmonary shunting, decrease the ventilation/perfusion mismatch and improve the functional residual capacity and hence the oxygenation of the blood. Bronchodilators can improve bronchospasm in near drowning. Hypothermia should be corrected appropriately and any other injuries treated.

Asymptomatic patients can be discharged after 6–8 h if their observations, chest radiograph and arterial blood gases are normal. Most near-drowning victims will require at least 24 h of observation.

PREVENTION

Approximately 25% of victims of near drowning presenting to the emergency department will die and another 6% will develop neurological sequelae. Prevention is therefore crucial. Community education in basic life-support is vital, as immediate cardiopulmonary resuscitation before the arrival of paramedical personnel is associated with a significantly better outcome in terms of prevention of death or severe anoxic encephalopathy. Moreover, adequate adult supervision and properly fenced swimming pools are essential.

ELECTROCUTION (INCLUDING LIGHTNING STRIKE)

Over 90% of deaths due to electrocution result from generated electricity and half are due to contact with low voltages (less than 1000 V). There are approximately 200 electricity-related fatalities in the UK each year. There are essentially four categories of electrical injury:

- domestic
- industrial
- railway related
- lightning strike.

There are two forms of electrical current, direct and alternating, of which alternating current, for example in the ordinary domestic supply, is the most dangerous. Alternating current, in which the flow of electrons switches from positive to negative at a frequency of 50 Hz, is more likely to induce ventricular fibrillation than is direct current. In the industrial environment, direct current is more likely to be the cause of electrical injury. Railway-related injuries may be either alternating current (AC) or direct current (DC). Many lines are electrified on a 25 000 V overhead system; others use a 750 V third rail, although the London Underground uses a system based on a 630 V fourth rail.

Deaths from lightning strike are uncommon in the UK with, on average, four fatalities occurring each year. The majority of lightning victims were struck whilst working or indulging in recreational activities in rural rather than urban areas. Thus victims include farm workers, walkers and golfers. The voltage of lightning varies from a few million volts to 2×10^{12} V and usually averages $10–30 \times 10^{6}$ V.

Injuries due to burns may be classified as follows:

- flash burns
- arc burns

- direct (contact) burns
- cardiac effects
- other injuries (neurological and ophthalmic)
- secondary injuries (due to inhalation, blast, falls, muscular spasm and ignition of clothing).

Flash burns occur when the energy of an electric shock (including lightning strike) passes over the surface of the body. The resultant burns tend to be superficial and involve exposed areas.

Arc burns result from a source short-circuiting through the air to a victim. They are associated with very high temperatures and the victim may be thrown by the energy of the shock, resulting in secondary injuries. Partial- or full-thickness burns may result, which will be more severe if the clothing ignites.

Direct (contact) burns result from current flowing through the body. The degree of tissue damage is proportional to the current flow and its duration. Direct current characteristically produces a small entrance and a much larger exit wound. These are full-thickness burns.

Tissue damage is usually more extensive than the visible burn. Current follows the line of least resistance. Dry skin has a high resistance, followed by bone, muscle, blood vessel and nerve. The higher the resistance, the greater the resulting damage.

> Tissue damage due to electric shock is usually more extensive than the visible burn.

In some respects, severe electrical injury is similar to crush injury since it can result in muscle breakdown, with release of myoglobin and the potential for cardiac arrhythmias, renal failure and electrolyte disturbance. Severe muscle oedema may result in compartment syndrome.

Alternating current tends to result in ventricular fibrillation whereas lightning results in a massive shock producing asystole and respiratory arrest. Arrhythmias are more common with shocks that pass through the chest rather than involving a single limb.

The neurological effects of electric shocks include loss of consciousness (in up to 50% of victims of high-voltage injury), headaches, peripheral neuropathy, transient paralysis and mood disturbances. Delayed neuropathy in high-voltage injury is well described. A number of ophthalmological effects have been described, including delayed cataract formation, glaucoma, retinal injuries, iritis and injuries to the cornea.

Secondary injuries include fractures and dislocations from electricity-induced muscle spasm, injuries due to being thrown or falling from a height, burns from the ignition of clothing, inhalational burns and blast injuries to the lungs and elsewhere.

LIGHTNING STRIKE

Clothing may ignite or, in the case of lightning, be blasted off the body by the vaporization of sweat or rain; the same mechanism may result in tympanic rupture. Flashover burns result in a characteristic fern-like appearance which typically resolves in 24 h.

A depressed conscious level may result from secondary head injury, cardiac arrest or the direct effects of the strike. Confusion and amnesia lasting for several days is common. Coolness and mottling of the limbs may result from arterial spasm that resolves in a matter of hours. Limb paralysis is common but generally resolves over a few days. A wide variety of ophthalmic problems, most notably cataract, may occur. Temporary deafness is common and tympanic rupture occurs in more than half of victims. Secondary injury should always be excluded and any patient with evidence of arrhythmia or ECG changes will require continuous ECG monitoring. All victims of lightning strike must be admitted for observation.

MANAGEMENT

Asymptomatic patients from, usually domestic, low-voltage incidents can be allowed home as long as they have a normal ECG, normal urinalysis and no evidence of any injury requiring specialist treatment. Review after a couple of days is recommended. All patients with high-voltage injuries, ECG abnormalities or myoglobinuria must be admitted. Superficial burns are treated in the conventional manner; however, it is important to remember that the tissue damage may be disproportionate to the superficial appearance of the burn wound and an approach to these injuries of extreme caution is recommended. Unless deeper damage can be absolutely excluded, all electrical burns should be reviewed before discharge by a senior doctor, and if there is any doubt as to the nature of the wound they should be referred for a specialist opinion.

VENOMOUS SNAKE BITES

Snake bite envenomation in tropical areas affects an estimated 1 million people each year according to the World Health Organization. Estimated annual mortality is between 30 000 and 50 000 people. Worldwide, only about 10% of the 3000 species of snake are venomous. In the UK the adder is the only native venomous snake; however, it is increasingly common to see exotic animals being kept as pets, and bites from these may present to UK departments.

One common family of venomous snake is the Crotalidae or pit-vipers (rattlesnakes, moccasins). Other snake families include Elapidae (cobras, kraits) and Hydrophydae (sea snakes). Fifty to seventy-five per cent of snake bites result in envenomation. Since even a dead snake can envenomate a handler they should all be treated with great respect.

EFFECTS

Venom consists of proteins that are cytotoxic, neurotoxic and haemotoxic. The first symptom is pain around the puncture site that increases over the next few hours. Swelling and oedema progress rapidly to involve the whole extremity. With pit-viper bites there is also erythema, ecchymosis and coagulation defects. With coral snake bites there is less oedema and the pain can develop after a few hours. Moreover, neurological effects are more prominent with the latter and include ptosis, dysphagia, dysarthria, loss of deep tendon reflexes and respiratory depression. Patients can also develop cardiac and kidney failure. Compartment syndrome is rare.

TREATMENT

There is no evidence that suction or the use of a tourniquet proximal to the wound site will affect the outcome. In addition, the use of ice can cause thermal injuries and circulatory compromise. A splint can be used in order to limit movement and avoid spread of venom. It can also decrease the pain. Marking the border of advancing oedema with a pen every 15 min is recommended.

The patient should be observed for at least 6–12 h. Intravenous access should be gained and blood sent off for full blood count, electrolytes, coagulation studies and group and save. In addition, the patient should be placed on a cardiac monitor and urine sent for analysis. The main treatment is antivenom therapy. Antivenoms are hyperimmune sera collected from animals immunized with venom. The antibodies contained in the serum bind and inactivate venom components. This offers a specific treatment that can significantly reduce the injury and symptoms of the envenomation. The main adverse effect encountered when using antivenoms is anaphylaxis, which may be life threatening. Preparations to treat anaphylaxis must be made before initiating antivenom therapy. Blood tests are then repeated. The swollen limb is elevated and tetanus toxoid booster is given as necessary. Finally, broad-spectrum antibiotics are usually given. Standard antitetanus immunoglobulin should be administered to non-immune patients.

FURTHER READING

Steedman, D.J. (1994) *Environmental Emergencies*. Oxford Handbooks in Emergency Medicine. Oxford University Press, Oxford.

PART EIGHT

OPHTHALMOLOGY, ENT AND DENTAL CARE EMERGENCIES

OPHTHALMOLOGY

INTRODUCTION

Most emergency department medical staff have little ophthalmic training yet eye emergencies represent a significant proportion of a department's workload. As in other areas of medical practice, early and accurate diagnosis requires only the skill to take an accurate history and perform a simple ophthalmic examination. In most cases further examination is not required. While most eye complaints in an emergency department are relatively trivial and self-limiting, a few are time dependent and require early intervention to preserve visual function. It is important to recognize those conditions that require further specialist management and refer them appropriately to an ophthalmologist.

HISTORY

The history should be brief yet define the presenting symptom, its duration, severity and location. Associated symptoms, past medical and ophthalmic history and the current use of eye and other medications should be documented. The presenting symptom for an eye complaint will usually be one of those listed in Table 36.1.

Trauma to the eye may be blunt or penetrating and may occur in isolation or in association with more significant injuries, which should take precedence. A history of injury from a high-velocity foreign body should raise the suspicion of a penetrating injury with intraocular foreign body.

Visual loss may occur with or without pain. The loss may be partial or complete. Determine whether the visual impairment is unilateral or bilateral and the time scale of onset. Also take a wider medical history to elicit previous symptoms of diabetes mellitus, cerebrovascular disease or demyelination.

An acute red eye may occur in association with pain and visual disturbance. The diagnosis may be obvious if the onset of symptoms can be related to a specific incident such as a chemical splash, but often no cause can be easily identified. Document the length of symptoms and rapidity of onset. If any discharge occurs note the type (serous or purulent).

Table 36.1: Common presenting complaints

Eye presenting complaints:
Trauma
Visual loss or disturbance
Acute red eye
Periocular infection
Contact lens problems

Table 36.2: Components of an eye examination

Ophthalmic examination:
Visual acuity
Inspection of conjunctival sac
Fluorescein
Anterior chamber
Pupil
Funduscopy

Periocular infection involves the structures of the lids and the lacrimal system and is usually minor, but on occasions may become life threatening by involvement of the central nervous system.

Contact lens problems are seen with increasing frequency. It is important to determine the type of lens used (hard, soft or gas permeable) and the duration of use. Problems are often associated with prolonged use, poor lens hygiene and allergy to cleaning solutions.

OPHTHALMIC EXAMINATION (TABLE 36.2)

A satisfactory ophthalmic examination can be performed with a minimum of equipment. If a slit lamp is available the doctor should learn how to use it correctly, but it is often not an essential component of the assessment of patients in emergency departments.

VISUAL ACUITY

Recording of visual acuity is a mandatory component of the examination of any patient with an eye complaint. It assesses visual function and there may be significant medico-legal consequences if it is not recorded. Patients who normally use glasses should wear these for testing.

If the patient's glasses are unavailable, use of a pinhole will provide an acceptable substitute. A Snellen chart (Fig. 36.1) is usually used and is read at either 6 m (or 3 m for a half-size chart) with one eye covered. The visual acuity is recorded as a fraction, with 6 as the numerator and the number of the lowest line read as the denominator. 6/6 indicates

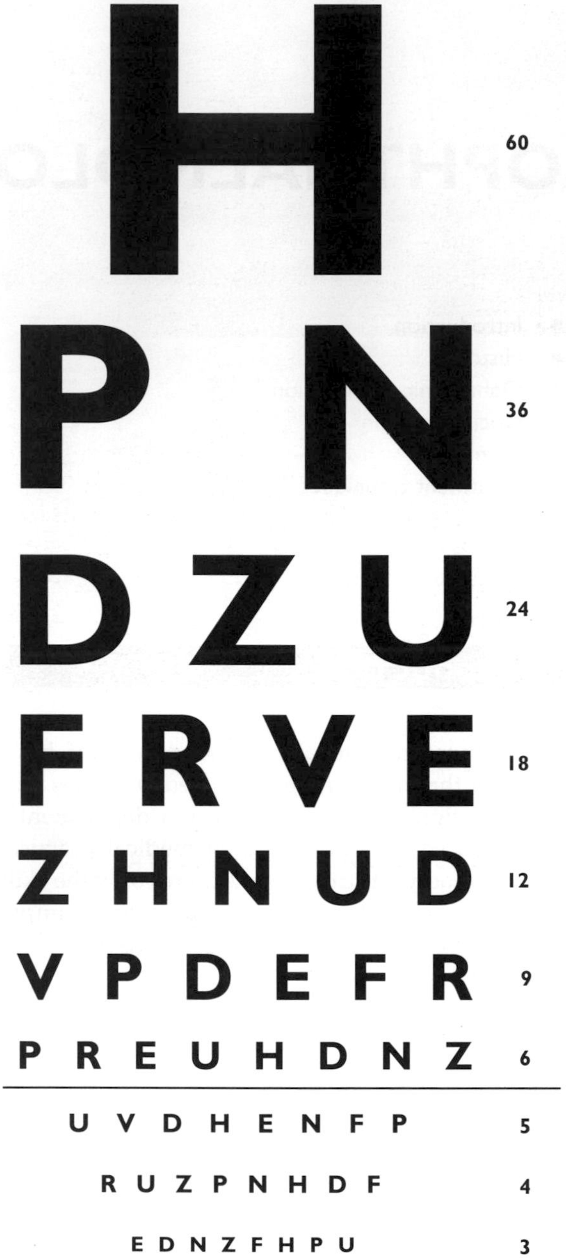

Figure 36.1: Snellen chart.

normal vision, 6/12 reduced acuity and 6/4 better than average vision.

If the patient is unable to read the largest letter on the Snellen chart, they can be assessed on their ability to count fingers at a distance of 1 m. If they are again unsuccessful, their ability to differentiate light from dark can be tested.

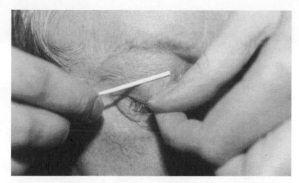

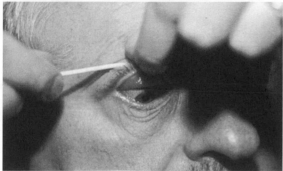

Figure 36.2: Eversion of the upper lid to inspect the subtarsal area.

INSPECTION OF CONJUNCTIVAL SAC

A thorough search for foreign body involves visualizing the whole conjunctival sac and the subtarsal area by everting the tarsal plate (Fig. 36.2). Also note the degree of conjunctival injection and whether this is localized or generalized.

FLUORESCEIN STAINING

Fluorescein selectively stains areas of the cornea where there is epithelial loss. Uptake is typically seen in a corneal abrasion or ulcer. View the cornea under a cobalt blue light to define the areas of staining.

ANTERIOR CHAMBER

The anterior chamber should be clear. Inspect it visually and with an ophthalmoscope. Any cloudiness of the aqueous humour suggests the presence of either blood or inflammatory cells.

PUPIL

The pupil should be symmetrical and react briskly to light. Assymetry or poor reaction as a new clinical finding is significant whether you are dealing with trauma or an inflammatory process.

FUNDUSCOPY

This is important in any condition where there is disturbance of vision. Full assessment of the posterior chamber requires a slit-lamp and a trained ophthalmologist.

SLIT-LAMP EXAMINATION

The slit lamp provides a magnified and well-illuminated image of the eye. Conditions that would pass unnoticed on conventional examination, such as small foreign bodies and the flare of the inflammatory cells in the aqueous humour of anterior uveitis, are detected by use of the slit lamp. It also facilitates the accurate and atraumatic removal of corneal foreign bodies. Correct use of the instrument does require training and experience, and junior doctors should be aware of when to refer the patient to an ophthalmologist for slit-lamp examination rather than spend time learning the technique.

The measurement of intraocular pressure is usually carried out with an applanation tonometer and slit lamp but is not often available in an emergency department. Although a rough assessment of the pressure can be made by digital palpation, the patient should be referred for a formal ophthalmic assessment if there is any suspicion of glaucoma.

DOCUMENTATION

As in other areas of emergency work it is important to accurately yet concisely document the history, examination and treatment (Fig. 36.3).

Use of diagrams is often helpful to describe the position of foreign bodies or the pattern of fluorescein staining.

JOHNSON 1035

24-hour h/o right eye pain and photophobia

No trauma. Known ank. spond. 4 y

No previous episodes

O/E VA R 6/12 L 6/4

Circumcorneal inj. No FB

Fluor. NAD

AC ?flare

Pupil small no reaction

PC poor view

Imp Iritis

Ref Eyes (1040) – to clinic

GJ

Figure 36.3: Example of documentation of an ophthalmic complaint.

FORMULARY

LOCAL ANAESTHETICS

A variety of local anaesthetics are available in single-use dispensers. Amethocaine and lignocaine are the most commonly used and one or two drops will anaesthetize the conjunctiva in 3 min. Proxymetacaine has the advantage of rapid onset and brief duration of action. Anaesthetized eyes should be covered with an eye pad as the blink reflex is lost.

Local anaesthetic eye drops should not be given to the patient as a method of analgesia. With repeated use, wound healing is inhibited.

ANTIBIOTICS

Antibiotics are available as drops or ointment. Drops need to be used every 2–3 h whereas ointment is usually only applied three times a day. Chloramphenicol is the most commonly used drug, with fucidic acid often prescribed as a second line.

FLUORESCEIN

This is available either as drops or on strips, which should be dampened before application to the eye. Areas where the corneal epithelium has been lost will stain selectively under a cobalt blue light.

MYDRIATICS

It may be necessary to dilate the pupil, either to examine the posterior chamber or for pain relief in corneal abrasion or arc eye. The mydriatics differ in their duration of action, a short-acting drug such as tropicamide (3 h) being used to assist funduscopy, whereas a longer-acting one such as cyclopentolate or homatropine (up to 24 h) can be used for pain relief. Owing to its prolonged duration of action in the eye (up to 7 days), atropine must not be used in emergency departments.

Mydriatics are contraindicated in glaucoma.

STEROIDS

The use of steroid drops or ointments is potentially disastrous in an eye with an undiagnosed dendritic ulcer. They should not therefore be prescribed by emergency department doctors and the patient should be referred to an ophthalmologist.

Never prescribe steroid preparations for eyes in the emergency department.

TREATMENT TECHNIQUES

DROP AND OINTMENT INSTILLATION

The lower eyelid should be everted and the patient asked to look up with the head extended. A single drop is placed into the eye, which is then gently closed. Ointments are similarly inserted within the lower eyelid. Patients should be warned that the ointment will blur their vision temporarily and they should not drive for 30 min. Excess ointment may be removed with a tissue whilst the eye is held firmly closed.

CONTACT LENS REMOVAL

Contact lenses must be removed prior to examination and in an unconscious patient the eyes should be checked to ensure that lenses are not *in situ*. The lens may migrate up into the superior conjunctival sac and be difficult to find. Removal of soft lenses is usually best accomplished by pinching them between finger and thumb. Hard lenses may be particularly difficult to remove after they have been left in an excessive length of time. Lubricating the eye with saline may be necessary, but if this is unsuccessful a suction cup designed for this purpose can be used.

IRRIGATION

This can be an important measure in flushing out chemical irritants or foreign bodies. Saline (0.9%) is the most common and convenient fluid as a drip bag with giving set can be used. This procedure is often unpleasant for the patient and the use of local anaesthetic prior to irrigation is recommended.

EYE PATCHING

The application of an eye pad is most commonly used to protect the eye when the protective blink reflex has been removed by use of local anaesthetic. Though previously used in the treatment of corneal abrasion, this is no longer recommended.

A pad is folded in half across its long axis and is then placed with the folded edge under the supra-orbital ridge. A second pad is placed on top in line with the orbit and taped in place.

Patients wearing an eye patch should be instructed not to drive.

EYE INJURIES (TABLE 36.3)

FOREIGN BODIES

Identification of a foreign body requires a careful visual assessment of the conjunctival sac and

Table 36.3: Types of eye injury

Eye injuries:
Foreign bodies
Corneal abrasion
Ultraviolet keratitis (arc eye)
Blunt injury
Penetrating injury
Chemical burns

cornea, including eversion of the tarsal plate (see Fig. 36.2). Local anaesthetic is usually required to allow removal of the foreign body, which is often easily accomplished with a cotton-wool bud. When the foreign body is embedded on the surface of the cornea the tip of a hypodermic needle may be used to aid removal, but in order to minimize trauma to the cornea this may be better performed under a slit lamp, especially when the foreign body is deeply imbedded.

Metallic foreign bodies may leave a rust deposit on the surface of the cornea, which requires removal. This is often accomplished more easily after a period of 24 h during which the eye is treated with chloramphenicol ointment, so the patient can usually be referred to an eye clinic.

When the patient gives a history of a high-speed metallic foreign body it is important to be aware of the possibility of an intraocular foreign body and to arrange an X-ray (Table 36.4).

CORNEAL ABRASION

This results from direct injury to the cornea with a variable depth of injury to the corneal epithelium. The patient complains of pain and often foreign body sensation, with watering of the eye (epiphora). In severe cases blepharospasm results in inability to open the eye for examination. Instillation of anaesthetic drops may be necessary.

Staining of the cornea with fluorescein reveals the site and size of the abrasion. Treatment involves the use of prophylactic antibiotics. An eye pad should be used for 4 h if anaesthetic drops were used but is not otherwise required. If pain is severe a mydriatic such as homatropine may be helpful. The patient should be told to expect resolution in 24–48 h but to return if symptoms fail to settle. On occasions, spontaneous recurrence of the abrasion may occur at a later date following initial healing.

Table 36.4: Case history of a missed penetrating foreign body

Case history
A man presents to the emergency department complaining of foreign body sensation in the right eye. The onset occurred while he was using a hammer and chisel to cut stone. Visual acuity in the right eye is 6/9 but no foreign body is visible. A small area of haemorrhage was visible on the sclera but examination was otherwise normal. He was discharged with an eye pad and chloramphenicol ointment. He returns 48 h later with an inflamed eye with visual acuity of 6/60. An X-ray of the orbit shows an intraocular metal fragment. He is admitted, but as a result of endophthalmitis subsequently has to have the eye removed.

ULTRAVIOLET KERATITIS (ARC EYE)

The patient typically presents some hours after exposure to ultraviolet light, such as from an arc welder or a sun lamp. They complain of pain and epiphora. Examination reveals an injected eye and on fluorescein staining superficial pitting of the surface of the cornea may be seen. The condition is self-limiting and almost always resolves in 24–48 h. Treatment is largely symptomatic with eye pads, mydriatics and oral analgesics. Local anaesthetics provide temporary symptomatic relief but repeated instillation is not recommended.

BLUNT INJURY

Any structure in the eye may be injured by blunt force. Assessment is often difficult as periorbital swelling may obscure significant injury to the eye.

Injuries to the cornea have already been discussed. Bleeding into the anterior chamber of the eye produces hyphaema. If the patient has been sitting still in an upright position prior to examination, this will easily be seen as a fluid level with blood in the lower part of the chamber (Fig. 36.4). However, if the patient has been lying flat, the anterior chamber will merely look hazy.

Blunt injury may produce traumatic mydriasis in which the pupil is dilated and paralysed. This may be the cause of some concern in the patient who has sustained a significant head injury, and investigations should be initiated to exclude an intracranial mass lesion. Any reduction in visual acuity suggests injuries to the iris, lens, vitreous or retina and will require urgent specialist assessment.

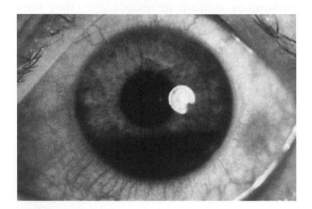

Figure 36.4: A hyphaema.

PENETRATING INJURY

Early recognition and repair is vital if ocular function is to be preserved. The history usually provides an important clue to the correct diagnosis, though the actual site of penetration may not be obvious. In many cases prolapse of the iris through the wound may cause obvious irregularity of the pupil (Fig. 36.5). The eye should be protected against further injury with an eye shield. Antibiotic and tetanus prophylaxis must be provided and the patient referred to the ophthalmologist.

CHEMICAL BURNS

A large variety of chemicals may be splashed into the eye. Fortunately, most of these are harmless. Alkali burns to the cornea, however, can cause significant permanent visual impairment. These most

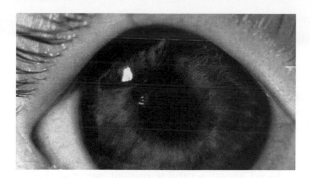

Figure 36.5: Penetrating injury with iris prolapse.

commonly occur from drain and oven cleaners and concrete and plaster. The mainstay of treatment is early and continuous irrigation of the eye with large volumes of saline, and this should not be delayed by attempts to identify the substance involved. Any particulate matter should be identified by careful inspection of the whole eye and removed.

After completion of irrigation, the cornea should be stained with fluorescein. If there is any corneal injury the patient should be referred to the ophthalmologist.

VISUAL LOSS

Acute deterioration in visual acuity (Table 36.5) in an uninflamed eye implies significant disease in the posterior chamber or optic nerve and requires prompt referral.

VITREOUS HAEMORRHAGE

Although most commonly associated with diabetes this condition may occur spontaneously. The examination finding of loss of the red reflex and inability to visualize the retina should suggest this diagnosis.

RETINAL DETACHMENT

This may occur in relation to trauma or in a diabetic patient but also occurs spontaneously. The patient complains of visual disturbance, with flashing lights or floaters, or the appearance of a veil over

Table 36.5: Differential diagnosis of acute visual loss

Causes of visual loss:
Vitreous haemorrhage
Retinal detachment
Central retinal artery occlusion
Central retinal vein occlusion
Optic neuritis

the affected eye. The lesion may be demonstrated by ophthalmoscopy but a full ophthalmic assessment is necessary to exclude the diagnosis. Treatment is surgical.

CENTRAL RETINAL ARTERY OCCLUSION

This typically presents with sudden and painless loss of vision. If a branch artery only is occluded there may be a field defect rather than complete visual loss. The occlusion is usually embolic from a carotid atheromatous plaque. The retina usually appears pale through the ophthalmoscope. Always consider the possibility of temporal arteritis as a cause, especially if there is a history of preceding headaches and lethargy. Prompt treatment with steroids may save the unaffected eye. Otherwise massage of the globe may on occasions break up the embolus. The prognosis is otherwise poor, as the retina tolerates ischaemia poorly.

CENTRAL RETINAL VEIN OCCLUSION

The onset of symptoms following venous occlusion is more gradual. Again thrombosis of a branch vein will lead to a field defect. Ophthalmoscopy will reveal an engorged retina with haemorrhages. Spontaneous resolution may occur but treatment is generally ineffective. Long-term follow-up is necessary to detect and treat the complications of secondary glaucoma and neo-vascularization.

THE ACUTE RED EYE

The acute red eye has a large number of potential causes (Table 36.6). Assessment requires a careful history to establish whether trauma has occurred or if there is a possibility of a foreign body. In the absence of these factors one of the atraumatic causes of red eye is likely (Table 36.6). In some cases a preceding general medical problem may be related to the development of red eye. A thorough examination will usually result in an accurate diagnosis (Table 36.7), though further assessment with a slit lamp by an ophthalmologist may be necessary to define the cause.

CONJUNCTIVITIS

The most common diagnosis in acute red eye is conjunctivitis. This may be viral, chlamydial or bacterial. The condition is usually bilateral and caution must be applied to the use of this diagnosis in unilateral red eye, though involvement of the second eye may be delayed in onset.

> Be cautious about diagnosing conjunctivitis in unilateral red eye.

Viral conjunctivitis presents with an inflamed eye and the patient often complains of a foreign body sensation. There is generalized injection of the eye and there may be symptoms of an associated systemic viral illness. Although most conjunctivitis is viral, treatment with topical antibiotics is usually used as clinical differentiation from bacterial infection is difficult.

A highly contagious form, epidemic keratoconjunctivitis, is caused by an adenovirus. The conjunctival inflammation is follicular, initially uniocular, and is associated with tender enlargement of the preauricular lymph nodes. Photophobia and reduced visual acuity, if present, suggest corneal involvement. This condition is self-limiting but may take several weeks to resolve. Precautions taken by staff and patients to avoid spread should include use of separate towels and advice to stay away from work until resolution occurs. Treatment is with topical antibiotic ointment to prevent secondary infection.

Chlamydial infection most commonly occurs after use of swimming pools or jacuzzis that have been poorly maintained. Transmission from genital infection may also occur. Again, clinically the appearances are similar to those of other types of conjunctivitis but, if suspected, treatment with oral tetracyclines should be considered.

Bacterial conjunctivitis is a result of infection by skin commensals such as *Staphylococcus aureus* or *Streptococcus pneumoniae*. Discharge is often purulent but sometimes serous. Treatment is empirical with topical antibiotics for 5 days. Lack of response by 48 h should prompt re-evaluation and, if necessary, change of antibiotics.

ALLERGY

The appearances of conjunctival oedema (chemosis) as a result of allergy are characteristic, with itching and boggy translucent swelling. A large

Table 36.6: Causes of atraumatic acute red eye

Conjunctivitis
Allergy
Subconjunctival haemorrhage
Episcleritis
Scleritis
Keratitis
Anterior uveitis
Acute glaucoma
Herpes zoster infection
Orbital cellulitis

Table 36.7: Examination findings in acute red eye

	Conjunctivitis	Keratitis	Anterior uveitis	Acute glaucoma
Visual acuity	Normal	Reduced	Reduced	Poor
Pain	Mild	Moderate	Moderate	Severe
Photophobia	None	Mild	Severe	Mild
Injection	Generalized	Circumcorneal	Circumcorneal	Generalized
Pupil	Normal	Normal	Constricted	Oval
Cornea	Normal	Cloudy	Normal	Oedematous
Anterior chamber	Normal	Normal	Flare	Shallow
Ocular pressure	Normal	Normal	Normal	High

number of airborne allergens can be the cause, as well as substances inserted into the eye such as medications. The rather dramatic appearances will usually resolve spontaneously on removal from the provoking substance. The prescription of further medication in this situation often only causes a further allergic response.

SUBCONJUNCTIVAL HAEMORRHAGE

When this occurs spontaneously in the absence of trauma, the patient requires only reassurance that this benign condition will resolve without treatment.

EPISCLERITIS

This usually presents as a localized inflamed nodule on the sclera. It is often recurrent and responds to the use of local steroids, though an ophthalmic opinion should precede the prescription of this medication.

SCLERITIS

Pain is more intense and deep-seated than in conjunctivitis. The eye is often tender to palpation. This condition is often symptomatic of a collagen disease and requires treatment with systemic steroids.

KERATITIS

Inflammation of the cornea results in an acutely painful, watering red eye. The injection is around the cornea (circumcorneal) rather than generalized and there is often punctate uptake of fluorescein on the cornea or, more rarely, a discrete ulcer that is characteristically dendritic in shape in herpes simplex infection. The patient should be referred for further assessment. Treatment is likely to include the use of a mydriatic to relieve pain and prophylactic antibiotics or aciclovir in the case of a dendritic ulcer.

ANTERIOR UVEITIS

Inflammation of the iris (iritis) or ciliary body (cyclitis) presents with an acutely inflamed eye with reduced visual acuity and photophobia. Recurrences are common. On examination, injection is circumcorneal and a flare in the anterior chamber may be seen, though often this is only visible under a slit lamp. The pupil is often small and may be assymetrical as a result of adhesions to the surface of the lens.

There is often an associated systemic illness such as ankylosing spondylitis or reactive arthritis. Referral to an ophthalmologist is required and treatment consists of a mydriatic to dilate the pupil to prevent adhesions and steroids.

ACUTE GLAUCOMA

Acute glaucoma classically presents with the sudden onset of severe pain that may be felt by the patient to be generalized rather than localized to the affected eye. Vomiting and collapse are common associated symptoms and glaucoma may be misdiagnosed as a neurological emergency. Visual acuity is often markedly reduced and the cornea is oedematous and appears cloudy, with conjunctival injection (Fig. 36.6). The pupil is characteristically a vertical oval shape and is unresponsive. The eye feels hard on palpation.

This is a genuine emergency and prompt treatment will preserve visual function. As intraocular pressure approaches systolic blood pressure the retina becomes ischaemic and permanent injury results. Initial treatment is medical, with miotics and acetazolamide. If intraocular pressure remains elevated a peripheral iridectomy is necessary. Urgent referral is essential.

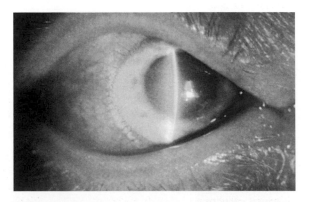

Figure 36.6: Appearance of acute glaucoma.

HERPES ZOSTER OPHTHALMICUS

In herpes zoster ophthalmicus, pain characteristically precedes the development of clinical signs. The pain and rash are limited to the fifth nerve distribution and ocular complications occur in approximately half of the cases, with ophthalmic division involvement. This may vary from conjunctivitis to panophthalmitis. Treatment with aciclovir orally and topically, topical antibiotics to prevent secondary infection, and occasionally steroids may be used.

PERIOCULAR INFECTIONS (TABLE 36.8)

BLEPHARITIS

Blepharitis is characterized by erythema, which is maximal on the eyelids. There is usually infection in either the follicles or the meibomian glands. Treatment in the first instance is with topical antibiotic ointment, though the response to treatment may be slow and the condition may recur. On occasions an underlying dermatological condition requires treatment.

STYE (HORDEOLUM)

This is a suppurative infection of the lash follicles or their associated glands that usually progresses to abscess formation and spontaneous discharge of pus. Again treatment is with topical antibiotic ointment, though resolution will occur with or without treatment.

MEIBOMIAN CYST

Infection of one of the meibomian glands results in a tender inflamed lesion, usually visible on the tarsal plate. Treatment initially is with topical antibiotic ointment, though referral to an eye clinic for curettage of the cyst is necessary if the cyst is large and fails to resolve.

DACROCYSTITIS

Infection of the lacrimal sac results in a painful, inflamed swelling below the medial canthus. Pressure over the lacrimal sac may produce pus at the punctum. The causal organism is usually *Staphylococcus aureus* and antibiotic therapy should be systemic.

ORBITAL CELLULITIS

Infection has usually spread from adjacent structures such as the sinuses or teeth or from a wound. There is local injection and swelling, with proptosis and painful restricted eye movement. There is usually systemic disturbance with fever. Urgent treatment with intravenous and topical antibiotics is required, as well as identification and treatment of the primary infection site. Prompt treatment will prevent serious complications such as meningitis, optic nerve compression and cavernous sinus thrombosis.

CONTACT LENS PROBLEMS

A number of ophthalmological problems occur which are specific to the use of contact lenses. Failure to comply with instructions regarding length of use and cleaning results in an increased incidence of the following complications. All patients who experience problems as a result of contact lens wear should be reassessed by either an ophthalmologist or an optician prior to resuming use of the lens.

CORNEAL HYPOXIA

Corneal oxygenation occurs through the corneal surface. This process is impaired when a lens is *in situ*, although many soft lenses are gas permeable. Corneal hypoxia results in superficial ulceration and the symptoms of painful red eye with photophobia are often delayed in onset until after the

Table 36.8: Causes of periocular infection

Blepharitis
Stye
Meibomian cyst
Dacrocystitis
Orbital cellulitis

lens has been removed. The treatment is to stop use of the lens and prescribe prophylactic antibiotics. Mydriatics may provide symptomatic relief when symptoms are severe. More severe cases should be followed up in the eye clinic.

KERATOCONJUNCTIVITIS

As with any prosthesis, the presence of a contact lens predisposes to infection. The infection usually resolves rapidly with removal of the lens and the use of topical antibiotics. Infection of a corneal ulcer is a potentially sight-threatening condition as a result of corneal scarring and the patient should be referred for immediate ophthalmic assessment.

MECHANICAL INJURY

The use of damaged or unclean lenses may lead to abrasion of the corneal surface. Again symptoms will resolve once the lens and the foreign material is removed.

FURTHER READING

Chawla, H.B. (1993) *Ophthalmology*, 2nd Edn. Churchill Livingstone, London.

Okhravi, N. (1996) *Primary Eye Care*. Butterworth-Heinemann, Oxford.

CHAPTER THIRTY SEVEN

EAR, NOSE AND THROAT

- Introduction
- Ear problems
- Nasal problems

- Throat conditions
- Further reading

INTRODUCTION

The majority of emergency department doctors have received no formal training in ear, nose and throat (ENT) conditions. Optimal management is therefore hampered by this and by inadequate conditions and equipment. Most ENT conditions are straightforward and easy to manage if appropriate attention is paid to the history and examination. However, if there is any possibility of significant pathology, junior doctors should have a low threshold for specialist referral.

EAR PROBLEMS

ASSESSMENT AND EXAMINATION

Symptoms

It is important to establish the predominant complaint and whether it affects one or both ears. Table 37.1 illustrates the important points in the history taking.

Table 37.1: Taking a history in ear problems

Hearing loss – onset and rate of progression
Otalgia (pain in the ear)
Otorrhoea (discharge from the external auditory meatus)
Tinnitus
Loss of balance
Noise exposure

In addition any history of nasal obstruction or discharge, recent ototoxic medication (such as the aminoglycosides) and any family history of hearing loss should be sought.

Signs

It is important to examine the ear in good lighting with adequate equipment. The largest auroscope speculum available which will fit the ear canal should be used in order to examine the tympanic membrane properly. The pinna should be pulled backwards and upwards (backwards and downwards in children), and scars crusting and weeping sought on the pinna and especially around the external auditory meatus. The ear canal should be inspected before, and as the speculum is inserted, as in acute otitis externa this will be very sore. Finally, the tympanic membrane is examined.

Auditory testing

By talking to the patient in a quiet room the clinician will soon appreciate their hearing ability. Tuning-fork tests can be used to distinguish between conductive and sensorineural hearing loss but are less reliable in children. Conductive deafness results from mechanical obstruction of the sound waves in the outer or middle ear. Sensorineural deafness results from defective function of the cochlea or of the auditory nerve.

Two tuning-fork tests are usually employed using a 512-Hz fork. The fork is sounded by striking the tines against the elbow.

Rinne test

This test compares air conduction (hearing via the ear canal and middle ear) with bone conduction (direct transmission to the inner ear via the mastoid process). The tuning-fork is struck and held in front of the patient's ear. It is then firmly placed on the mastoid process and the patient asked to state which position of the tuning-fork was louder. If the fork is heard better in front of the patient's ear this is Rinne positive, indicating that the sound can be heard better by air conduction than by bone conduction. A Rinne-negative result occurs with disease in the external or middle ear, producing a conductive deafness. In this instance the fork is louder when applied to the mastoid. A false Rinne-negative result occurs in cases of severe unilateral sensorineural loss, and care should be taken to remember this.

Weber test

The Weber test is more sensitive than the Rinne test. The tuning-fork is placed on the forehead and the sound waves are transmitted to both ears via the skull. The patient is asked whether the sound is heard centrally or is referred to one or both ears. If the sound is heard centrally the patient has either normal bilateral hearing or bilateral sensorineural hearing loss. A conductive deafness in one ear causes the sound to be heard on that side (the deafer ear). A sensorineural deafness causes the sound to be heard on the opposite side (the better ear).

EAR INFECTIONS

Acute otitis externa

Inflammation of the ear canal may be due to trauma from the use of cotton buds or secondary to eczematous ear canal skin. Symptoms range from mild irritation to severe pain, and movement of the pinna at its root or pressure on the tragus will exacerbate the condition. The most common infective agents are *Staphylococcus, Pseudomonas* and fungi.

Examination of the ear will reveal a red and tender canal with a thin discharge that should be sent for culture. Hearing loss occurs as a result of oedema of the canal and accumulation of debris.

Treatment consists of gentle removal of the ear canal debris and application of antibiotic and steroid drops, ointment or spray. A dressing can be inserted into the ear canal for 48 h and this will expand when the drops are applied. Prolonged use of the medication should be avoided in order to prevent secondary fungal otitis with organisms such as *Aspergillus*. Hydrocortisone cream (1%) will reduce itching after the infection has been controlled.

Furunculosis

Infection of a hair follicle in the ear canal may produce severe pain, slight deafness and pyrexia. Drainage, antibiotics and analgesia are required. A short course of flucloxacillin is usually appropriate.

Infections of the pinna

These may follow severe otitis externa or trauma such as ear piercing. In perichondritis, the infected cartilage produces a swollen, red and tender pinna with spreading oedema on to the face. This is rare. Any precipitating cause must be removed, with incision and drainage as necessary. Systemic antibiotics are required. The patient should be referred to an ENT clinic for follow-up.

Infected earrings in small children are the most common source of infection of the pinna, usually due to the ulceration of a small 'butterfly' through the soft skin of the posterior of the pinna. Removal of both parts of each earring is necessary, with appropriate advice to the parents about not reinserting the earrings until the child is older. A short course of flucloxacillin or a similar antibiotic should be given. The cartilage is not usually involved; if such involvement is suspected, referral to the ENT department is indicated.

Acute otitis media

Inflammation of the middle ear cavity is a common condition that occurs frequently in children and may be bilateral. It usually follows an upper respiratory infection that ascends the eustachian tube to reach the middle ear. Inflammatory exudate in the middle ear and oedema of the eustachian tube preventing drainage produce increasing pressure and severe pain.

The ears must always be examined in a child with a pyrexia of unknown course.

On examination the patient is generally unwell with pyrexia. The eardrum will initially bulge, but subsequent rupture produces release of pus and relief of pain.

Treatment consists of analgesia and broad-spectrum antibiotics. The usual organisms producing acute otitis media are *Haemophilus influenzae* and streptococci. Nasal decongestants may help to unblock the nose.

Acute mastoiditis

Inflammation of the mastoid lining may occur if acute otitis media is inadequately treated medically. It is usually seen in young children and produces severe pain, pyrexia and tachycardia. On examination there will be swelling and redness behind the ear and the pinna will be pushed down and out. The tympanic membrane will be either perforated or red and bulging. Treatment involves systemic antibiotics, which should be prolonged to ensure healing.

Acute labyrinthitis

Inflammation of the labyrinth may follow acute or chronic ear disease. The patient will complain of giddiness and loss of balance, associated with nausea and vomiting. On examination there is marked sensorineural hearing loss and the patient will be lying still with the affected ear uppermost. Treatment with high-dose systemic antibiotics is essential but surgical drainage may be required.

PINNA HAEMATOMA

Blunt trauma to the ear may result in a subperichondrial haematoma of the pinna, which strips the cartilage from the perichondrium. Failure to recognize and treat this may result in marked deformity (cauliflower ear). On examination the whole of the pinna is swollen and the outline of the cartilage is lost. Drainage of the haematoma is essential using a wide-bore needle. A pressure dressing applied for 24 h should prevent further accumulation of the haematoma but re-examination of the ear may suggest that re-aspiration is necessary. If blood clot has already formed and aspiration is impossible then surgical drainage through a skin flap and a course

of antibiotics are indicated. ENT referral is almost always appropriate.

Lacerations of the pinna should be managed by repair under sterile conditions: simple superficial lacerations can be sutured in the emergency department but lacerations involving cartilage or where there is significant cosmetic damage should be referred to an ENT or plastic surgeon.

Occasionally, complete avulsion of the pinna may occur. In these circumstances the pinna should be preserved and reattached, although the outcome is unpredictable. Human bites to the pinna can become infected, and perichondritis may be prevented by dressing the wound and prescribing a course of antibiotics, with delayed review and repair at 2 days in the ENT clinic.

FOREIGN BODIES

Children often put small objects such as beads into their ears and this may go unnoticed. Otalgia or otorrhoea may be the presenting complaint. Clumsy attempts at ear cleaning by adults may also result in foreign bodies, such as cotton wool, becoming lodged in the ear canal. Visualization of some foreign bodies can be difficult if not impossible, depending on their anatomical location.

Removal of the foreign body requires good lighting and the correct instruments. Crocodile forceps (Fig. 37.1) are most useful. Clumsy attempts with inadequate equipment must be avoided: the patient should be referred to ENT. In children it may be necessary to remove the object under general anaesthesia. Many can be removed using

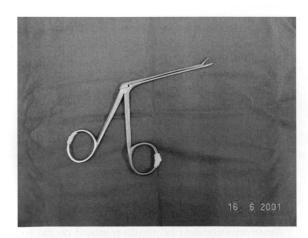

Figure 37.1: Crocodile forceps.

crocodile forceps, although round smooth bodies cannot be grasped properly. However, a blunt hook inserted behind a round object is a useful alternative. Syringing is ideal for most foreign bodies except vegetable material such as rice that may swell and impact in the ear. Insects can cause tinnitus and should be killed using olive oil or spirit before syringing. Suction is another useful method for removing most foreign material.

PERFORATED TYMPANIC MEMBRANE

Injury to the tympanic membrane can occur following direct or indirect trauma. Direct trauma can follow attempts to clean the ear using buds and other instruments or by syringing. Inadequate care in removing a foreign body may also cause perforation. Indirect trauma can result from a slap or from a blast injury.

The patient will complain of transient pain at the time of rupture, deafness and tinnitus. On examination the patient will have conductive deafness, bleeding from the ear, and possibly a clot in the canal. A tear will be seen in the tympanic membrane.

Treatment is conservative. The ear should not be cleaned out nor should drops be inserted. Antibiotics are necessary if the trauma was direct. The patient should be reviewed in the ENT clinic until the hearing returns to normal, the tear usually healing quickly.

VERTIGO

Balance relies upon inputs from the ears, eyes, joint proprioception sensors and signals from the cerebellum into the vestibular system. If the equilibrium is disturbed dizziness or vertigo results.

Vertigo is a subjective sensation of movement, usually rotatory in nature, which is worse in the dark. The patient should be questioned regarding the first attack, in particular the mode of onset and duration. Any alteration in hearing or relationship to activity must be recorded. Tinnitus may be an associated symptom and the condition may be worse in the dark or when the eyes are closed. A medical history may reveal anxiety, cardiovascular disease or the use of antihypertensive or aminoglycoside medication. Alcohol consumption should be noted.

Examination includes assessment of the cranial nerves and cerebellar function. The tympanic membranes are examined for middle ear disease and the eyes tested for nystagmus (an objective sign of vertigo). Romberg's test, in which the patient is asked to stand and then close their eyes, may produce swaying or falling if there is loss of joint proprioception or vestibular disturbance. The causes of tinnitus are listed in Tables 37.2 and 37.3.

Benign paroxysmal positional vertigo

Benign paroxysmal positional vertigo may follow an upper respiratory tract infection or head injury and occurs on turning the head, especially in bed. The episode lasts for a few seconds and is episodic. In the majority of cases it settles spontaneously.

Menière's disease

Menière's disease affects young to middle-aged adults and attacks occur in clusters. The patient

Table 37.2: Otological causes of vertigo

Middle ear disease:
Otitis media with effusion
Acute otitis media
Chronic suppurative otitis media
Trauma:
Temporal bone fracture
Otological surgery (stapedectomy)
Benign paroxysmal positional vertigo
Menière's disease
Labyrinthitis
Ototoxic drugs (aminoglycosides)

Table 37.3: Non-otological causes of vertigo

Cervical spondylosis
Migraine
Transient ischaemic attacks
Head injury (without temporal bone fracture)
Epilepsy
Ageing (poor eyesight, impaired proprioception, cerebral ischaemia)
Cardiovascular disease (postural hypotension, arrhythmia)
Drugs (alcohol, antihypertensives, vestibular sedatives)

complains of vertigo, hearing loss, tinnitus and a feeling of fullness in the ear. An acute episode of vertigo should be managed symptomatically, with reassurance and bed-rest. Vestibular sedatives may be required and nausea and vomiting should be controlled. Betahistine or metoclopramide are effective. ENT referral for formal assessment and follow-up is indicated.

Labyrinthitis

Bacterial labyrinthitis has been discussed above. Viral labyrinthitis presents with acute vertigo, nausea and vomiting. Treatment is symptomatic.

Differential diagnosis will include the non-otological causes of vertigo in which the patient complains of lightheadedness or unsteadiness. Many of these patients will have cardiovascular or neurological disease and should be referred appropriately.

NASAL PROBLEMS

ASSESSMENT AND EXAMINATION

Symptoms

The features of nasal conditions are listed in Table 37.4.

Common causes of nasal obstruction include septal deflection, adenoidal hypertrophy, neoplasia, allergic and infective rhinitis, nasal polyps and vasomotor rhinitis.

Signs

A thorough examination of the nose is important and again good lighting is necessary. The nose should be examined externally, first looking for any deformity that may suggest either a recent or chronic injury. Recurrent injury to the nose may be indicated by scarring or saddle deformity and the nasal septum may be deflected into one of the nostrils.

The Thudicum's speculum (Fig. 37.2) is useful for internal examination of the anterior nose.

The anterior septum and inferior turbinates are easily seen – the latter often being mistaken for a nasal polyp. The nasal airway of each nostril is assessed by obstructing each in turn.

FOREIGN BODIES

Most commonly seen in children, many objects have been found up small noses. Although the patient may not complain or admit to inserting a foreign body into their nose, the most frequent sign is a unilateral nasal discharge that is foul smelling. There may be infection around the nasal vestibule extending to the upper lip.

In a co-operative child the object may be easily visualized and removed using forceps or a blunt, hooked probe. General anaesthetic may, however, be the only alternative, particularly if there is any danger of the child inhaling the object.

An adult complaining of nasal obstruction and foul-smelling discharge may on examination have a rhinolith, a foreign body surrounded by layers of calcium. There is often a history of previous nasal packing for epistaxis. The rhinolith is preferably

Table 37.4: Nasal symptoms

Nasal obstruction
Nasal discharge
Sneezing
Facial pain
Otological:
Otalgia
Hearing loss
Disorders of smell:
Anosmia (loss of smell)
Cacosmia (unpleasant smell)
Halitosis

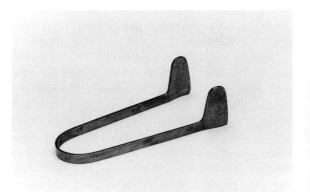

Figure 37.2: Thudicum's speculum.

removed in one piece, by an ENT surgeon, although this is often impossible owing to the size.

NASAL INJURY

Injury to the nose is considered in detail in Chapter 21.

EPISTAXIS

Epistaxis is a common presenting complaint in all ages. A single episode that has stopped requires no further treatment and the patient can be reassured, discharged and advised to return if it restarts. The patient should be shown how to control epistaxis by pressure between thumb and finger *over the soft part of the nose* (Fig. 37.3). Ongoing epistaxis may be treated by the insertion of expanding foam packs into both nostrils (Fig. 37.4): if this is effective in

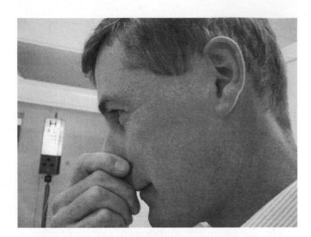

Figure 37.3: Controlling epistaxis.

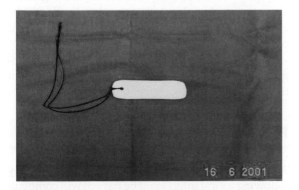

Figure 37.4: Merocel® foam packs.

controlling bleeding, review and removal of the packs by an ENT surgeon within 24 h is appropriate. Persistent minor epistaxis should be referred to ENT for cautery. Major epistaxis which cannot be controlled should be referred to the ENT surgeons for admission and cautery or packing.

THROAT CONDITIONS

EXAMINATION AND ASSESSMENT

Symptoms

The throat may be divided into the pharynx and the larynx and the symptoms will vary according to the region affected. The pharynx is further considered as three parts, each with its own symptoms. These are given in Table 37.5.

Signs

The neck should be examined systematically to include all the areas from the clavicles to the mandible. Standing behind a seated patient, the examiner should feel both sides of the neck at the same time, commencing at the clavicles and

Table 37.5: Symptoms of throat conditions

Nasopharynx:
    Nasal obstruction with discharge (mucopurulent or bloody)
    Deafness
    Adenoidal speech

Oropharynx:
    Dysphagia
    Articulation
    Airway obstruction

Hypopharynx:
    Dysphagia
    Regurgitation
    Dysphonia
    Airway obstruction

Larynx:
    Voice alteration
    Respiratory difficulties
    Pain
    Otalgia
    Aspiration of solids and liquids

palpating upwards along the anterior border of the sternomastoid muscle to the mandible. The areas between the posterior border of the muscle and the trapezius muscle should also be examined. Any lumps should be noted. The submandibular, submental and parotid regions should be palpated in turn.

An intraoral examination follows systematically, commencing at the lips and noting the tongue, sublingual, buccal and gingival mucosal surfaces. The hard and soft palate should be visualized. An intraoral examination requires a good light and ideally a mirror, care being taken to view all mucosal surfaces. The pharynx can be seen directly using a tongue depressor and mirror. Use of a flexible fibreoptic scope introduced via the nose allows visualization of the nose, nasopharynx, oropharynx, hypopharynx and larynx, and referral to ENT for a formal examination may be necessary.

FOREIGN BODIES

Children and adults may swallow or inhale foreign bodies, either accidentally or deliberately. The object may lodge anywhere in the pharynx or the upper airway and may scratch or tear the mucosa. Very occasionally, foreign bodies may cause perforation, abscess or mediastinitis, with fatal consequences.

A good history should be taken, including the nature of the foreign body and the time of ingestion. There may be a history of sudden onset of coughing, wheezing or stridor in a previously healthy child. Alternatively, a chest infection may develop. Examination of the patient may reveal the foreign body stuck in the tonsils or valleculae (especially fish bones). The mucosa may be torn, suggesting that the foreign body has passed on, rather than being stuck in the throat. A plain radiograph of the neck (lateral view) may reveal the object, although some fish bones and plastics are radiolucent (Fig. 37.5).

Any patient who is convinced that they have a foreign body stuck in their throat (unless the history is inconsistent) should be referred to ENT for laryngoscopy, even if the neck X-ray is normal.

Inhalation of a foreign body may be suggested by the history. Examination may show unilateral wheezing, poor chest movement or reduced breath sounds. A chest X-ray in expiration may demonstrate the foreign body or show distal

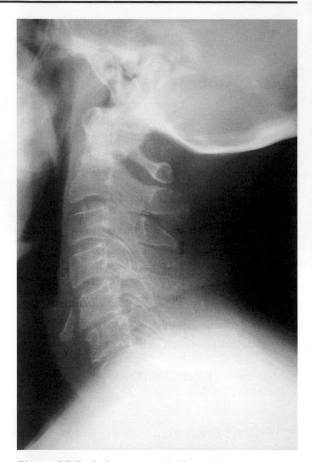

Figure 37.5: Soft-tissue neck X-ray showing a foreign body.

hyperinflation, infection and collapse, although these are usually late signs.

If the airway is compromised, a sharp blow to the back may dislodge the object. Alternatively, the Heimlich manoeuvre can be employed (Chapter 12). It may be necessary to secure the airway prior to removal of the object under general anaesthetic. An object that is visualized can be grasped with forceps and removed. Care should be taken not to tear the mucosa.

Patients with objects impacted in the oesophagus should be referred for endoscopic removal of the foreign body.

PHARYNGITIS

Acute pharyngitis is a common condition usually following a viral infection. The patient will complain of pain and difficulty swallowing, together with malaise. On examination the mucosa will be red and swollen. Symptomatic treatment including fluids and analgesia is usually all that is required. Antibiotics should not routinely be prescribed.

Chronic pharyngitis produces a persistent soreness of the throat and a complaint of dryness. On examination the mucosa is red with nodular lymph node enlargement on the posterior pharyngeal wall. Treatment is aimed at removing predisposing factors such as smoking and excessive spirit drinking. There should always be a high index of suspicion for malignancy in any patient with a chronic sore throat.

TONSILLITIS

Tonsillitis is an acute illness associated with severe sore throat and difficulty swallowing. The majority of cases are viral. Most patients can be managed without admission, with aspirin gargles, compound analgesia and antibiotics such as ampicillin. Dehydrated patients with severe systemic symptoms should be admitted.

QUINSY (PERITONSILLAR ABSCESS)

In this condition pus forms outside the capsule of the tonsil. The abscess occurs as a complication of acute tonsillitis and is more common in adults. The patient complains of a severe unilateral sore throat and dysphagia. The patient may also complain of malaise, difficulty in opening the mouth (trismus) and otalgia. On examination, the patient may be dribbling saliva owing to difficulty in swallowing and the voice may have a 'hot potato' quality. Cervical lymphadenopathy may be found on the affected side. The trismus may be so marked as to make intraoral examination difficult. However, on inspection there is a unilateral tonsillar inflammation causing deviation of the uvula.

In the early stages of cellulitis a systemic antibiotic (penicillin) is appropriate. An abscess must be drained.

STRIDOR

Stridor is noisy breathing resulting from an upper airway obstruction. Children have narrower

Table 37.6: Causes of stridor

Neonates:
  Congenital tumours, cysts
  Webs
  Laryngomalacia
  Subglottic stenosis
Children:
  Acute laryngotracheobronchitis (croup)
  Epiglottitis
  Acute laryngitis
  Foreign body
  Retropharyngeal abscess
  Respiratory papillomata
Adults:
  Laryngeal neoplasia
  Laryngeal trauma
  Acute laryngitis
  Epiglottitis

airways and softer cartilage that collapses more easily than adults and are at greater risk from upper airway obstruction.

The differential diagnosis of stridor is given in Table 37.6.

Stridor in neonates is unlikely to present to an emergency department. Immediate anaesthetic referral is appropriate.

EPIGLOTTITIS

This condition, which affects children in the 3–7-year age group, requires urgent management owing to the short interval between the onset of stridor and respiratory obstruction. Epiglottitis is characterized by marked swelling of the supraglottic larynx and pyrexia. The patient, if old enough, may complain of a sore throat and be mouth breathing and dribbling.

No attempt should be made to examine the throat of a child with suspected acute epiglottitis as this may precipitate complete airway obstruction. For the same reason an oxygen mask should not be applied, although gentle wafting of oxygen from a mask by the child's parent may be helpful. The child should be kept as calm as possible, usually in the upright position as leaning forward improves airway opening, and an opinion sought urgently from a senior ENT surgeon. The presence of an experienced anaesthetist is essential. The majority of these cases can be managed by endotracheal

Table 37.7: Croup and epiglottitis

	Croup	Epiglottitis
Onset	Gradual – preceding coryza	Rapid
Drooling	Absent	Present – unable to swallow
Cough	Barking	Minimal
Respiratory distress	Variable	Severe – stridor
Pyrexia	Low grade	Marked
Appearance	Unwell	Toxic

intubation rather than a surgical airway, but neither of these procedures should be attempted by the inexperienced.

LARYNGOTRACHEOBRONCHITIS (CROUP)

This viral infection (caused by parainfluenza or respiratory syncytial viruses) affects children aged between 6 months and 3 years. The patient is unwell with a barking cough. Initially there is inspiratory stridor due to mucosal swelling in the subglottis with thick secretions. An expiratory component may develop in advanced cases as respiratory obstruction increases.

Management with humidified and warmed air will loosen the secretions but intubation or tracheostomy may be required in a small number of cases.

The symptoms and signs of croup and acute epiglottitis are compared in Table 37.7.

ACUTE LARYNGITIS

Inflammation of the vocal cords may follow a respiratory infection or be secondary to tobacco, spirits or overuse of the voice. The patient may complain of hoarseness or discomfort in the throat.

Treatment is symptomatic, avoiding predisposing factors. Oedema of the subglottis in children may require intubation or tracheostomy.

LARYNGEAL TRAUMA

Any patient with a history of trauma to the neck may have direct injury to the larynx. The patient may complain of alteration of the voice or dyspnoea. On examination there may be neck bruising or swelling with surgical emphysema. Patients at risk of cervical spine injury must have a full examination of the neck with appropriate immobilization (Chapter 22), and it should be remembered that a well-fitting collar may conceal relevant signs. Intubation or tracheostomy may be necessary, although difficult if the continuity of the airway is disrupted. Surgical airway may also be difficult if the normal anatomy is deranged. Severe laryngeal injuries are fortunately rare, resulting from such mechanisms as wires stretched across roads or direct blows resulting from impacts with fences. In severe cases, the patient will be severely distressed and cyanosed and urgent senior anaesthetic assistance will be required.

FURTHER READING

Bull, P.D. (1996) *Diseases of the Ear, Nose and Throat*, 8th Edn. Blackwell Science, Oxford.

DENTAL PROBLEMS

INTRODUCTION

The most common dental emergencies presenting to an emergency department are toothache, infection and trauma. The commonest of these is toothache. Wherever possible, patients who ring the department seeking advice regarding a problem that is obviously dental in origin should be advised to seek advice from their own general dental practitioner in the first instance.

ANATOMY

The nomenclature of the permanent dentition is given in Figure 38.1.

TOOTHACHE

The most common causes of toothache are pulpitis, periapical periodontitis and dental abscess. Toothache may also result from 'dry socket' following dental extraction.

PULPITIS

Pulpitis (inflammation of the tooth pulp) is the commonest cause of dental pain and is the most likely cause following the destruction of a tooth by caries (decay). Pulpitis may be acute or chronic. The causes of pulpitis are given in Table 38.1.

It is important to take a careful history from the patient. The only symptom of pulpitis is pain and

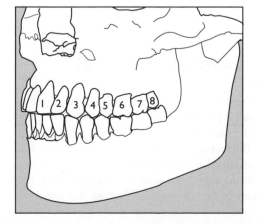

1 Central ⎫
2 Lateral ⎬ incisor
3 Canine

4 First ⎫
5 Second ⎬ premolar

6 First ⎫
7 Second ⎬ molar
8 Third* ⎭

• The corresponding teeth of the upper and lower jaws have similar names.
* The third molar tooth is sometimes called the wisdom tooth.

Figure 38.1: Nomenclature for permanent dentition.

Table 38.1: Causes of pulpitis

Dental caries
Fracture of tooth

Dental treatment:
  Traumatic exposure of nerve
  Chemical irritation from filling materials
  Over-heating of tooth

this may be poorly localized. In the early stages the tooth is hypersensitive to hot and cold and this will cause a stabbing pain, which stops when the stimulus is removed. As the inflammation progresses the pain becomes more persistent and will occur spontaneously. The patient may then give a history of being kept awake at night because of it. The pain becomes increasingly severe and is usually described as sharp and stabbing in nature. Analgesics are of little value.

Chronic pulpitis may develop without symptoms. It often occurs under a large carious lesion in a tooth. There may be occasional episodes of dull pain following hot or cold stimuli, or the pain may arise spontaneously.

Pulpitis may be poorly localized in the jaw and the patient may not be able to point to the tooth. Occasionally, all the teeth on the affected side of the jaw may feel painful, or the pain may be referred to the ear.

Examination of the patient with adequate lighting is essential. The patient will be able to point to the affected side and the examiner should look at all the teeth on that side. Usually there will be an obvious carious lesion on one of the teeth and the pain can be elicited by applying a hot or cold stimulus to the tooth (ethyl chloride on a pledget of wool gives a good cold stimulus).

Radiographic examination of the tooth (periapical X-ray) will be required and may reveal caries hidden below a filling, but this should be performed by the patient's general dental practitioner.

Treatment of pulpitis involves either extraction or preservation of the tooth. If the tooth is to be saved the cause of the pulpitis must be removed and root treatment commenced. For this reason, the appropriate emergency department treatment is referral to a dental practitioner. A non-steroidal anti-inflammatory drug will ease the pain.

PERIAPICAL PERIODONTITIS

Inflammation of the periodontal membrane around the apex of the tooth may follow death of the pulp. It is due to spreading infection from the pulp and will usually remain localized at the apex of the tooth.

A patient with acute periapical periodontitis will often give a history of pain due to initial pulpitis. However, as the inflammation develops, exudate enters the tissues around the apex of the tooth causing it to be extruded slightly in the socket. As a result the patient complains of increasing pain on biting on the tooth. The tooth becomes increasingly painful to touch and the pain becomes throbbing in nature. Hot and cold stimuli have no effect.

The patient may give a history of increasing pain as described above which is suddenly relieved and is often accompanied by a foul taste in the mouth. This usually occurs 24–48 h after the onset of symptoms and represents discharge of pus through the overlying bone and gingiva or from around the tooth.

Examination of the patient may reveal some ipsilateral cervical lymphadenopathy. Intraorally, there may be some redness of the gum overlying the root of the tooth. The gum may also feel slightly swollen and there may be signs of a discharging sinus. The tooth will be clearly identified by the patient and will be tender to touch. It may be slightly extruded from the socket and mobile.

Treatment is aimed at either removing the tooth or preservation. Extraction will relieve the pain but conservation of the tooth is preferable. The patient should be directed to a general dental practitioner.

DENTAL ABSCESS (FIG. 38.2)

Prompt treatment of acute periapical periodontitis will usually prevent the development of a periapical (dental) abscess. Persistence of infection around the periapical area of a tooth can lead to direct spread of pus into the surrounding tissues. The point at which an abscess emerges from the jaw depends on the relationship of the involved

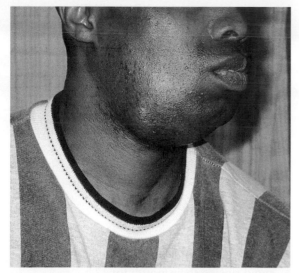

(a)

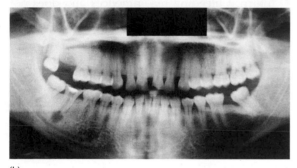

(b)

Figure 38.2: A dental abscess.

root and the thickness of the cortical bone. The facial muscles attached to the upper and lower jaws are important in providing planes along which pus can spread before it emerges into the mouth or on to the face.

A patient may complain of pain due to acute periapical periodontitis preceding the onset of swelling. The swelling may appear inside the mouth or on the face, depending on the tooth that is involved.

Many patients may present with pyrexia and may be generally unwell. In addition, they may not have eaten or drunk because of the trismus. These patients may require admission for fluid replacement and systemic antibiotics.

The patient should be commenced on suitable antibiotic therapy, for example benzyl penicillin and metronidazole, and given adequate analgesia such as a non-steroidal anti-inflammatory drug or

a compound analgesic. Subsequent treatment by the patient's dentist is aimed at extracting the offending tooth and draining the abscess.

DRY SOCKET

'Dry socket' occurs following dental extraction and is characterized by an acutely painful tooth socket that contains bare bone and blood clot. Analgesia and saline mouthwashes should be prescribed together with penicillin or erythromycin. Referral to a dentist is necessary for definitive management.

LUDWIG'S ANGINA

This is a rare but life-threatening spreading infection, usually from a lower molar tooth. A hard, non-fluctuant swelling develops in the floor of the mouth and gradually increases in size. The tongue is forced upwards against the palate as the swelling spreads to the opposite side. Eventually both sublingual and submandibular spaces become involved. This condition must be treated immediately with high-dose systemic antibiotics and drainage of all the spaces. The airway should be managed by intubation or tracheostomy. Urgent referral to a maxillofacial surgeon is therefore necessary.

SINUS FORMATION

Occasionally, a patient may present complaining of a discharging sinus on the chin (Fig. 38.3). The patient often gives a history of recurrent discharge and crusting from the lesion for 1–2 years. The discharge may have been treated by antibiotics on previous occasions. The most common cause of the sinus is as a complication of periapical periodontitis. On examination intraorally the patient may have a discoloured and non-vital lower incisor. Radiographs will confirm a chronic infection related to the apex of the tooth. The patient should be referred for removal of the dead pulp. Treatment is aimed at preservation of the tooth.

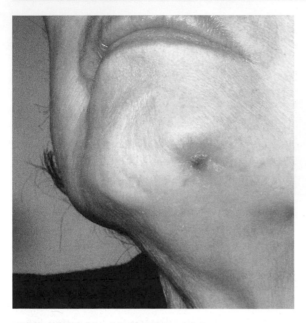

Figure 38.3: Dental sinus formation.

POST-EXTRACTION BLEEDING

Patients presenting in the emergency department with a history of bleeding from their mouth following a dental extraction are usually upset and agitated. They should be managed in a quiet and efficient manner. A careful history should determine when the extraction took place, how many teeth were extracted and when the bleeding commenced. The following are causes of post-extraction bleeding:

- alveolar bone trauma
- soft tissue trauma
- bleeding disorder
- anticoagulant therapy
- infection
- failure to follow postoperative instructions.

The patient should be examined in a good light and preferably with an assistant to suck away any blood. The socket should be carefully examined and signs of trauma to the bony socket wall or soft tissue noted.

Treatment is usually carried out under local anaesthetic. If, however, there is a possibility that the patient has a previously undiagnosed bleeding diathesis or is taking anticoagulants and that the International Normalized Ratio (INR) was not at the appropriate level prior to the extraction, then the patient should be admitted.

The patient should be reassured and seated in a suitable chair with good lighting. The bleeding can sometimes be stopped just by asking the patient to bite on a piece of gauze that has been placed over the socket. The patient should sit quietly for 30 min before being re-examined. Bleeding is most likely to stop with this treatment if the patient had previously ignored the postoperative instructions. Failure to control the bleeding is an indication for referral.

Once the bleeding has stopped, the patient should be advised to:

- rest for 12 hours
- avoid drinking hot fluids for 12 hours
- avoid rinsing their mouth for 12 hours
- return if bleeding recommences and does not stop by biting on gauze.

LACERATIONS TO INTRAORAL SOFT TISSUES

The soft tissues of the mouth are well perfused and bleed profusely when cut. This may be accompanied by marked swelling which may compromise the airway (Chapter 21). The history will reveal the mechanism of injury and there may be associated bony tissue damage. Dog bites can produce severe lacerations around the mouth, particularly in children, and usually these should be treated under general anaesthetic.

A careful examination of the patient must be carried out in good light with an assistant to suck away the blood. The lacerations may be covered firmly with gauze and this may be all that is required to stop the bleeding. Suturing of the wound is performed under local anaesthetic as above. Each tissue plane should be closed. Deep tissues are closed using 3/0 reabsorbable suture material. Intraoral mucosa may be closed using 3/0 reabsorbable material. Lacerations within the mouth which are less than 1 cm long can usually be managed without suturing as the mouth is an area of rapid healing. Attempting to suture small lacerations within children's mouths is almost impossible without a general anaesthetic, and sutures tend to work free owing to the constant attention of a small tongue. Full-thickness lacerations of the lips should be sutured. The commonest cause of such lacerations is a fall resulting in the teeth being pushed through the lower lip. Damage to the teeth must therefore also be excluded.

Lacerations involving the vermilion border and skin of the lip must be carefully closed, and complex lacerations are usually best referred to a plastic or maxillofacial surgeon. Minor lacerations may be managed by careful suturing with fine non-absorbable sutures (for example 6/0 prolene or nylon) but the vermillion border must be carefully approximated in order to avoid a cosmetically unacceptable 'step'.

Foreign bodies penetrating the intraoral tissues should usually be left *in situ* until they can be removed in controlled circumstances under general anaesthetic. If they are causing airway obstruction they may be removed.

INJURY TO THE TEETH

Teeth may be *avulsed* (completely lost from the socket) (Fig. 38.4), *extruded* (partially lost from the socket), *intruded* into the socket or *subluxed* (displaced in a forward, backward or sideways direction). A good history will give the mechanism of injury and the likely damage to the tooth.

Injuries to the tooth may be confined to the enamel, the enamel and dentine, or extend to involve the pulp. A tooth with a fractured crown and an associated soft-tissue injury to the lip may suggest that there is a buried fragment that must be looked for. A soft-tissue radiograph should therefore be considered. An apparently intact tooth may have a fractured root below the gum margin or there may be a longitudinal fracture.

Parents or school-teachers may contact an emergency department if a child has avulsed a tooth. This is usually a front tooth. The adult must not touch the root surface if possible, but hold the tooth by the crown. No attempt should be made to clean the tooth as this may damage the root surface.

The immediate management is to reinsert the tooth into the socket and ask the child to hold it in place until they reach the emergency department (Fig. 38.5). Alternatively the tooth can be carried with the patient in a container of milk. The child should

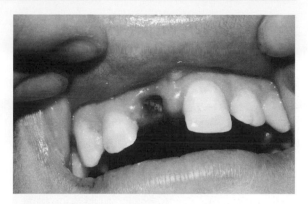

Figure 38.4: Avulsed teeth.

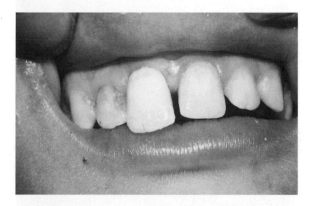

Figure 38.5: Avulsed tooth replaced in socket.

not hold the tooth in the buccal sulcus, as has been advised in the past, because of the danger of inhalation, particularly in patients with a head injury.

The patient may complain of pain from the involved teeth, that pieces of the teeth seem to be missing or that there are loose fillings. They may also report that the teeth do not appear to be meeting in the usual bite or that they are mobile. If a tooth has been completely avulsed the patient may have the tooth (preferably in a container of milk, but more usually wrapped in tissue paper). Alternatively, the tooth may be lost.

On examination, all missing and mobile teeth should be noted. Missing and loose fillings must also be noted. A radiograph may show fractured teeth below the gum margin (Fig. 38.6) and may also reveal an associated bony injury. It is essential that a chest X-ray be taken if an avulsed tooth or fragment has been lost. An inhaled tooth may cause respiratory obstruction or become a source of infection.

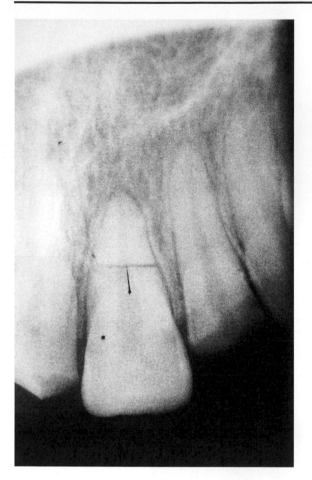

Figure 38.6: Fractured tooth revealed on an X-ray.

The treatment aim is to preserve the teeth. Fractured teeth involving the pulp may be reimplanted by a dentist and referral is therefore appropriate.

A completely avulsed tooth can be reimplanted into the socket. Under local anaesthetic the socket is gently irrigated with saline solution to remove any blood clot. The tooth can then be inserted into the socket (the correct position can be assessed by looking at the teeth in the opposite side of the mouth). There are a number of different ways to hold the tooth in place temporarily, depending on what equipment is available. A piece of aluminium X-ray foil can be cut to size and held over the tooth with dental cement. Alternatively the tooth can be splinted with a piece of wire (paper clip) and dental cement. Mobile and extruded teeth can also be splinted in this way. All these procedures should be carried out by a dentist or maxillofacial surgeon.

Children may have teeth at different stages of development and this will affect treatment. Adult teeth should be managed as above. Deciduous teeth are not usually reimplanted because they will be shed at a later date. A mobile deciduous tooth should be removed. Intruded or extruded deciduous teeth can be left, although the parents will need reassurance. Rarely the adult tooth developing in the bone beneath a deciduous tooth may be damaged, particularly with intrusion injuries. Parents should be warned about this possibility.

Antibiotics and tetanus cover are essential, especially if the tooth was avulsed. Penicillin or metronidazole will cover most intraoral organisms.

FURTHER READING

Hawkesford, J. and Banks, J. (1994) *Maxillofacial and Dental Emergencies*. Oxford Handbooks in Emergency Medicine. Oxford University Press, Oxford.

PAEDIATRICS

PAEDIATRIC TRAUMA

INTRODUCTION

This chapter covers major and minor trauma in children. Non-accidental injury in children is also discussed. Major trauma in children is thankfully rare. Having said this, trauma is the leading cause of death in childhood. An emergency department seeing 35 000 children a year would expect to see a severely injured child every couple of weeks. Dealing with traumatized children is distressing for patients, parents and staff. Appropriate management reduces morbidity, mortality and the distress for all involved. Although the approach to major trauma is the same in any age group, the patterns of injury are different in children and management of these cases differs significantly.

Trauma is the leading cause of childhood death.

MECHANISM OF INJURY

Children, by their nature, are prone to different injuries. Falls and road traffic accidents, either as pedestrians struck by a vehicle or as occupants of cars, are the main causes of trauma deaths in childhood. Drowning and burns are relatively common in small children. Car bumpers that would strike the knee of an adult will cause life-threatening injuries to the abdomen and chest in a small child. Children also travel in a different area of a car and are restrained in different ways. For instance, the use of lap belts has resulted in a pattern of injury characterized by abdominal contusions, hollow visceral injury, mesenteric avulsion and lumbar vertebral fractures. Burns are common in children, most commonly with children who pull on kettle or iron flexes but more seriously in house fires. In addition, children's skin is significantly less resistant to thermal injury. Penetrating trauma in children is rare in northern Europe and is usually the result of a fall on to an object.

ANATOMICAL AND PHYSIOLOGICAL DIFFERENCES

The priorities in resuscitating a severely injured child are the same as in an adult. The airway must be secured with control of the cervical spine, breathing must be assessed and assisted if necessary, and circulatory abnormalities must be identified and treated, initially by fluid therapy. A thorough secondary survey identifies other injuries requiring further management. However, children have certain anatomical and physiological differences that influence their response to trauma and dictate differences in management. It is vital that an effort is made to estimate the weight and height of the

Paediatric resuscitation chart

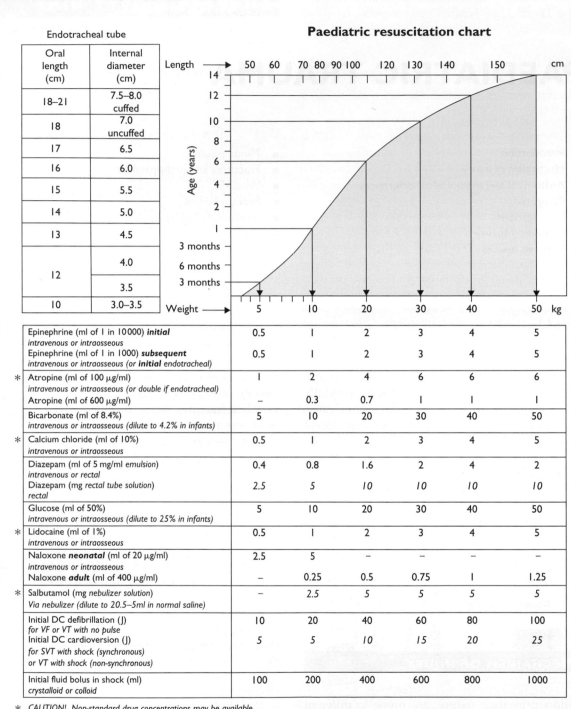

Endotracheal tube

Oral length (cm)	Internal diameter (cm)
18–21	7.5–8.0 cuffed
18	7.0 uncuffed
17	6.5
16	6.0
15	5.5
14	5.0
13	4.5
12	4.0
12	3.5
10	3.0–3.5

Length → 50 60 70 80 90 100 120 130 140 150 cm
Age (years): 14 12 10 8 6 4 2 1 — 3 months 6 months 3 months
Weight → 5 10 20 30 40 50 kg

	5	10	20	30	40	50
Epinephrine (ml of 1 in 10000) **initial** intravenous or intraosseous	0.5	1	2	3	4	5
Epinephrine (ml of 1 in 1000) **subsequent** intravenous or intraosseous (or **initial** endotracheal)	0.5	1	2	3	4	5
* Atropine (ml of 100 µg/ml) intravenous or intraosseous (or double if endotracheal)	1	2	4	6	6	6
Atropine (ml of 600 µg/ml)	–	0.3	0.7	1	1	1
Bicarbonate (ml of 8.4%) intravenous or intraosseous (dilute to 4.2% in infants)	5	10	20	30	40	50
* Calcium chloride (ml of 10%) intravenous or intraosseous	0.5	1	2	3	4	5
Diazepam (ml of 5 mg/ml emulsion) intravenous or rectal	0.4	0.8	1.6	2	4	2
Diazepam (mg rectal tube solution) rectal	2.5	5	10	10	10	10
Glucose (ml of 50%) intravenous or intraosseous (dilute to 25% in infants)	5	10	20	30	40	50
* Lidocaine (ml of 1%) intravenous or intraosseous	0.5	1	2	3	4	5
Naloxone **neonatal** (ml of 20 µg/ml) intravenous or intraosseous	2.5	5	–	–	–	–
Naloxone **adult** (ml of 400 µg/ml)	–	0.25	0.5	0.75	1	1.25
* Salbutamol (mg nebulizer solution) Via nebulizer (dilute to 20.5–5ml in normal saline)	–	2.5	5	5	5	5
Initial DC defibrillation (J) for VF or VT with no pulse	10	20	40	60	80	100
Initial DC cardioversion (J) for SVT with shock (synchronous) or VT with shock (non-synchronous)	5	5	10	15	20	25
Initial fluid bolus in shock (ml) crystalloid or colloid	100	200	400	600	800	1000

* CAUTION! Non-standard drug concentrations may be available
Use **Atropine** 100 µg/ml or prepare by diluting 1 mg to 10 ml or 600 mg to 6 ml in normal saline
Note that 1 ml of **Calcium chloride** 10% is equivalent to 3 ml of **Calcium gluconate** 10%
Use **Lignocaine** (without adrenaline) 1% or give twice the volume of 0.5%. Give half the volume of 2% or dilute appropriately
Salbutamol may also be given by slow intravenous injection (5 µg/kg, but beware of the different concentrations available (e.g. 50 and 100 µg/ml)

Figure 39.1: The Oakley chart.

child and the Oakley chart (Fig. 39.1) and Broselow tape (Fig. 39.2) are useful in this respect.

AIRWAY

The differences between adult and child airways are shown below:

- Infants are obligate nose breathers until 6 months of age.
- Children have relatively large heads on small bodies (the ideal position for intubation is with the head flat on the bed, not on a pillow).
- The mandible is less developed.
- A small oral cavity with a large tongue.
- Milk teeth are often loose and an aspiration hazard.
- Tonsils are relatively larger and more vascular.
- The epiglottis and the arytenoid folds are relatively larger.
- The larynx is higher (C3–4) than in the adult (C5–6).

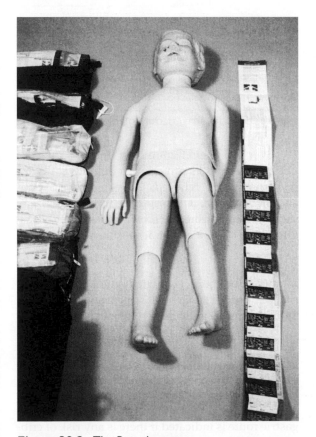

Figure 39.2: The Broselow tape.

- The trachea is shorter: in the newborn 4–5 cm, at 18 months 7–8 cm.
- The soft tissues of the mouth are more prone to injury.

These anatomical differences mean that airway protection is practised differently.

Basic airway care

FACE-MASKS
When using a face-mask, care must be taken to make sure that the supporting fingers do not press in the submental triangle. This causes posterior displacement of the tongue and subsequent airway obstruction. The correct position of the supporting fingers is along the margin of the mandible.

ASSISTED VENTILATION
Bag inflation must be gentle. Pressures greater than $20 \, cm \, H_2O$ cause gastric distension and an increased risk of aspiration.

GUEDEL (OROPHARYNGEAL) AIRWAYS
The correct size can be selected by placing the airway on the side of the child's head. An adequate airway runs between the incisors and the tragus of the ear. These should be inserted 'the right way up'. Rotating the airway can traumatize the soft tissues at the back of the mouth and cause bleeding and airway obstruction.

Advanced airway management

Children desaturate quickly. It is important to administer high-flow oxygen and adequate basic airway management before intubation. The pulse oximeter is a useful adjunct in assessing oxygenation, but because of the sigmoid-shaped oxygen disassociation curve, large falls in PaO_2 may occur despite relatively normal saturation readings.

> Children die of hypoxia, not failure of intubation.

> Do not attempt endotracheal intubation in children without administering high-flow oxygen and adequate basic airway support.

Table 39.1: Endotracheal tube sizes in children

Age	Internal diameter in mm
0–3 months	3.0
3–12 months	3.5
2 years	4.0
3	4.0
4	4.5
5	5.0
6	5.5

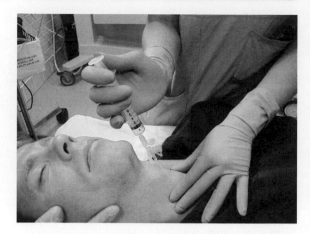

Figure 39.3: Needle cricothyroidotomy.

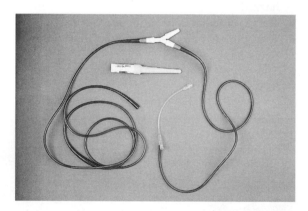

Figure 39.4: Needle cricothyroidotomy apparatus.

TRACHEAL INTUBATION

A straight-bladed (MacGill) laryngoscope is more suitable in children under 12 months of age. This is designed to pick up the epiglottis, not sit in the vallecula like a MacIntosh laryngoscope blade. Older children require the standard curved MacIntosh laryngoscope, with allowance for size. Table 39.1 shows the endotracheal tube size appropriate for children under 6 years old.

Alternatively, the internal diameter of a tracheal tube in millimetres for a child over 6 years old can be calculated by the formula:

Diameter = Age/4 + 4

Tracheal tubes should be uncuffed to allow a small air leak. (Pressure on the glottis causes oedema and stridor at extubation and for up to 8 hours afterwards.)

NEEDLE CRICOTHYROIDOTOMY (FIGS 39.3 AND 39.4)

Surgical cricothyroidotomy is contraindicated in children less than 12 years old as damage to the cricoid cartilage can result in damage to the only circumferential support to the airway. Needle cricothyroidotomy is indicated when intubation has failed and there is an overwhelming need to provide the airway. A 14 gauge intravenous cannula is attached to a syringe. The cricothyroid membrane is pierced at 45°, with the needle pointing caudally. When air is aspirated, the cannula is advanced into the trachea. The needle is withdrawn, a 5 ml syringe, with the plunger removed, is connected to the external end of the cannula. A cuffed 6 mm endotracheal tube should then be placed in the syringe, and the cuff inflated. This apparatus can then be connected to the oxygen supply. This technique only buys time and should not be regarded as providing a definitive airway. Hypoxia can be relieved, but expiration is poor and hypercarbia will result. A definitive airway should be established as soon as possible either by intubation or by formal tracheostomy.

VENTILATION

Infants should be ventilated at 40 breaths per minute, older children at 20 breaths per minute. Tidal volumes should be between 7 and 10 ml kg^{-1}.

GASTRIC DECOMPRESSION

Distressed children swallow air and trauma impairs gastric emptying. A full stomach impairs respiration and is a significant aspiration hazard. Early nasogastric intubation is recommended. The orogastric route is indicated if there is any risk of cribriform plate damage.

Table 39.2: Vital signs in children

Age (years)	Respiratory rate (breaths min^{-1})	Heart rate (beats min^{-1})	Systolic blood pressure (mmHg)
2–5	25–30	95–140	80–90
5–12	20–25	80–120	90–110

Table 39.3: Chest drain sizes in children

Age	Chest drain size
6–12 months	12–18
1–3 years	14–20
4–7 years	14–24
8–11 years	16–30

BREATHING

Assessment can be difficult in a distressed, crying child. Children's normal vital signs vary with age (Table 39.2).

Children's chest walls are much more compliant and the absence of rib fractures does not exclude serious intrathoracic injury. Conversely, the presence of rib fractures in a child merits greater suspicion of life-threatening injuries. The mediastinum of children is more mobile and consequently more vulnerable to blunt trauma.

The assessment and management of thoracic injuries in children is broadly similar to that in adults. Intercostal drainage requires smaller tubes (Table 39.3).

CIRCULATION

The diagnosis of shock in children is clinical. Children can tolerate substantial fluid losses while maintaining a relatively normal blood pressure and pulse and have a greater physiological reserve than adults. Assessment of circulation should pay particular attention to the mental state, the respiratory rate and the capillary refill time (normal capillary refill is less than 2 s). It is vital to aim to identify and control significant sites of haemorrhage in the primary survey. A classification of haemorrhagic shock is shown in Table 39.4; however, its divisions are artifici and not all children will demonstrate the classic signs of shock. All authorities agree that repeated observation is vital, ideally by the same doctor.

The diagnosis of hypovolaemia in children is clinical.

The child's normal blood pressure can be estimated by using the formula below:

Systolic blood pressure = $80 + (2 \times$ the age of the child).

Fluid resuscitation

Crystalloid is the usual first line of intravenous fluid resuscitation – 20 ml kg^{-1} should be infused as rapidly as access will allow (20 ml kg^{-1} corresponds to 25% of the patient's circulating volume). Reassessment of the circulation should follow. Persisting evidence of circulatory instability necessitates a further 20 ml kg^{-1} bolus; 10 ml kg^{-1} of blood should then be transfused if necessary. Any shocked child should be assessed by a surgeon to determine the source and management of any haemorrhage.

The large surface area of a child relative to its body weight increases the risk of iatrogenic hypothermia. Hypothermia impairs coagulation and strenous efforts should be made to keep the child warm. Warm fluids should be given if possible, and the child should be covered with blankets when not being examined. Children differ from adults in that they can more readily become hypovolaemic from scalp lacerations.

Vascular access and intraosseous infusion

Children are significantly more difficult to cannulate than adults, even when well-perfused, relaxed and warm. Femoral lines are useful, but require experience. In children under 6 years old, intraosseous cannulation of the proximal tibia just below the tibial tuberosity provides an interim site of vascular access. An effort should be made to direct the needle away from the epiphysis since this can

Table 39.4: Classification of shock

	Class 1	Class 2	Class 3	Class 4
% Blood volume loss	< 15	15–30	30–40	> 40
Capillary refill	Normal	Prolonged	Very prolonged	Very prolonged
Skin	Normal	Cold and clammy	Cold and pale	Cold and pale
Respiratory rate	Normal	Increased	Increased	Increased
Mental state	Normal	Irritable	Lethargic	Comatose
Heart rate	Slight increase	Tachycardia	Tachycardia	Bradycardia
Blood pressure	Normal	Normal	Reduced	Very reduced

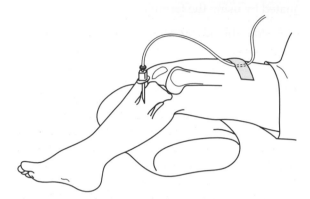

Figure 39.5: An intraosseous needle being inserted.

interfere with subsequent growth. An intraosseous needle should be placed when two attempts at venous cannulation have failed (Fig. 39.5). Aspiration of bone marrow confirms placement. Bone marrow can be used for subsequent cross-matching; however, rapid infusion of fluid requires manual pressure with a syringe.

ANALGESIA

Morphine ($0.1 \, \mathrm{mg \, kg^{-1}}$) is the analgesic of choice in the traumatized child. There is no place for intramuscular injection in potentially shocked patients. The dose should be given intravenously and titrated to achieve adequate analgesia. This has benefits beyond the relief of pain: cardiovascular physiology is improved, the patient will be more co-operative and physical signs may become easier to elicit. Regional anaesthesia may be used, for instance femoral nerve blocks for fractured femoral shafts. A mixture of lignocaine and marcain provides longer analgesia than lignocaine alone (see Chapter 8).

INVESTIGATIONS

Radiographs of the chest and pelvis should be obtained early in the severely injured child. Blood should be sent for cross-match, a full blood count and biochemistry. An amylase is useful if pancreatic trauma is suspected.

SECONDARY SURVEY

An ordered systematic head-to-toe examination follows the primary survey. The aim is to detect every injury, no matter how trivial, in order to allow appropriate treatment.

REGIONAL INJURIES

This section considers the effects of major trauma on regions of the body and subsequent management.

HEAD INJURIES

Assessment of conscious level in children requires use of a modified Glasgow Coma Scale (Table 39.5). Diffuse cerebral injury is commoner than in adults and focal injuries such as extradural haematoma rare. In the infant, lax sutures and the open fontanelle allow significant cerebral swelling and haematoma to be accommodated before intracranial pressure rises.

A short neurological examination should include:

■ inspection of the pupils
■ visual examination of the face and scalp

Table 39.5: Glasgow Coma Scale in children under 4 years old

Eyes:	
4	Opens spontaneously
3	React to speech
2	React to pain
1	No response
Motor:	
6	Spontaneous or obeys verbal command
5	Localizes to pain
4	Withdraws to pain
3	Abnormal flexion to pain
2	Extension to pain
1	No response
Verbal:	
5	Smiles, orientated to sounds, follows objects and interacts
	Crying and interacts
4	Consolable
3	Inconsistently consolable, moans
2	Inconsolable and irritable
1	No response

- palpation of the anterior fontanelle
- inspection of the ears for blood
- movement of the limbs and reflexes.

The anterior fontanelle, when open, provides a simple guide to intracranial pressure. A bulging fontanelle in an infant that is not crying implies significantly raised intracranial pressure.

Head injuries are classified as severe if the Glasgow Coma Scale (GCS) is 8 or less, moderate if 9 to 12 and mild if 13 or above. The term 'minor head injury' is unsatisfactory and its use should be discouraged.

Severe head injury

Severe head injury is the main cause of death in traumatized children. Management in the emergency department aims to reduce secondary brain injury by prevention of hypoxia, hypoperfusion and raised intracranial pressure. Clumsy intubation may cause coughing and raise intracranial pressure.

Hypovolaemia should be treated aggressively. It is safe to give fluid therapy as any effect on brain swelling is offset by the benefit of correcting hypovolaemia. Only in small infants can intracranial bleeding cause hypovolaemia. An alternative source

of bleeding should therefore be sought prior to attributing shock to intracranial bleeding. Seizures are common, and should be controlled with diazepam. Continuing seizures need treatment with a phenytoin infusion. All severe paediatric head injuries must be discussed with the neurosurgeons and a plan of investigation and management agreed. Generally, prognosis in children with severe head injury is better than in adults.

Moderate and mild head injuries

The aim is to detect a small group of children who may initially appear to have sustained a minor injury but who subsequently deteriorate as a result of cerebral swelling or intracranial haematoma. As in all aspects of trauma the mechanism of injury is important. An estimate of the forces involved should be made and noted. The child's parent should be questioned about behavioural changes as they will often notice subtle changes. Skull radiographs are commonly performed, though their role in head injury assessment is controversial. A child can have significant brain damage without a skull fracture, and a child with a skull fracture may do very well with minimal treatment. Skull X-rays are of greatest use in assessing a child with a head injury who is likely to be discharged. A child with no skull fracture and normal conscious level is highly unlikely to deteriorate at home. In a child with a reduced conscious level following a head injury, the appropriate investigation is a CT scan of the head and skull X-rays only delay diagnosis.

Interpretation of skull radiographs can be difficult, with a high incidence of both false positives and false negatives. In particular, distinguishing between fractures and vascular lines can be difficult for junior staff. Skull fractures are usually lucent and rarely branch. White sclerotic lines may indicate a depressed skull fracture. Where any uncertainty exists, the advice of a senior colleague should be sought (Fig. 39.6).

Admission of head injuries

The guidelines are shown below; these are not intended to replace clinical judgement but to provide advice and guidance:

- confusion or any other depression of the level of consciousness at the time of examination

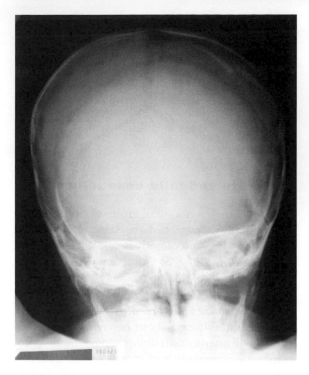

Figure 39.6: A skull X-ray showing a depressed skull fracture.

(if under 5 years old, at any time following the injury)

- neurological symptoms or signs (headache or vomiting more than twice)
- skull fracture on radiograph or clinical evidence of a base of skull fracture, including cerebrospinal fluid rhinorrhoea/otorrhoea
- difficulty in assessing the patient (e.g. suspected drugs, alcohol, non-accidental injury, epilepsy)
- other medical conditions (e.g. coagulation disorders)
- patient's social conditions or lack of a responsible adult or relative.

Post-traumatic amnesia of less than 2 min or transient loss of consciousness with full recovery are not necessarily indications for admission. Patients sent home should be accompanied by a responsible adult who should receive written advice to return immediately if there is any deterioration (Fig. 39.7).

Increasing use of CT scans allows early detection of significant intracranial lesions and therefore reduced morbidity and mortality. Potential indications for head CT include confusion (GCS less than 13–14) or worse, persisting after initial assessment and resuscitation. Fully conscious children with a skull fracture or following a first fit should also undergo a head CT scan. However, do not send an unstable patient to the CT scanner. Resuscitating an unstable child in a cramped, unfamiliar room is difficult and dangerous.

Discussion with local neurosurgeons should occur for patients with coma continuing after resuscitation, deterioration in level of consciousness or progressive neurological deficits, and open injury or depressed fractures. Following a CT in the receiving hospital the neurosurgeons should be contacted regarding any child with an abnormality on CT, or when the CT is normal but the patient's progress is considered unsatisfactory.

Analgesia, antiemetics and antibiotics for head injuries

MAJOR HEAD INJURIES

There is concern that giving opiate analgesia to severely head-injured children may impair their respiratory drive and conscious level. There are also concerns that opiate-related pupillary constriction may mask a dilating pupil. On the other hand, appropriate and effective analgesia is a priority in trauma, not only for relief of pain but for the beneficial effects on cardiovascular physiology and subsequent intracranial pressure.

Vomiting should be controlled since it raises intracranial pressure and presents risks to the airway. An antiemetic and a gastric tube may be required. Patients with open skull fractures should have their tetanus status checked. Prophylactic antibiotic administration should be discussed with local neurosurgeons.

MODERATE AND MILD HEAD INJURIES

Paracetomol is a suitable first-line analgesic in these patients. Any children discharged with a head injury should receive (or their parents should receive) written instructions and this should be documented in the notes.

CERVICAL SPINE

Severely traumatized children should be assumed to have a cervical cord injury until a decision is made by senior medical staff that the spine is normal. This usually requires normal radiographs and clinical

Do

✓ rest completely at home for at least 24 hours
✓ take the painkillers suggested by the doctor

Do not, for at least 24 hours

✗ drive or operate machinery
✗ garden, shop or carry out DIY
✗ drink alcohol
✗ take a bath unsupervised

Do not

✗ play contact sports, eg, football, rugby for 3 weeks
✗ return to sport or occupation that involves balance or heights, eg. gymnastics, window cleaner, for 1 week

Please retain this card for future reference

Head Injury

This advice must be given to patients and the accompanying adult.

You have had a head injury. You have had a thorough examination and are now considered fit to be discharged. Some people who have had a minor head injury later develop problems, which occasionally can be serious. **If you experience any of the following, please contact your nearest Accident & Emergency department.**

● Persistent headache that does not improve with simple painkillers, eg, paracetamol
● Vomit more than twice
● Develop double vision
● Develop slurred speech

If the accompanying adult notices any of the following please return to your nearest Accident & Emergency department or contact us on 01773 874803.

● Increasing drowsiness
● Abnormal or unusual behaviour
● Fitting
● Slurred speech

Hospitals **NHS**
NHS Trust

ADVICE SHEET

HEAD INJURY

ACCIDENT & EMERGENCY DEPARTMENT

Figure 39.7: A head injury advice card.

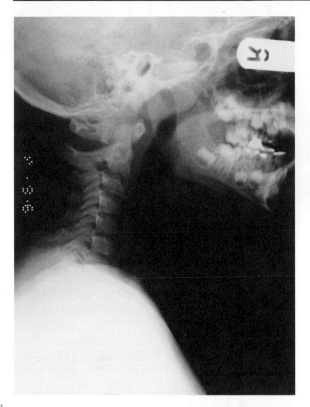

Figure 39.8: A child's cervical spine X-ray. Note the pseudosubluxation at C2–C3.

examination of an alert patient. If a child is ventilated and sedated, this may not occur for days and immobilization should be maintained. The relatively large mass of a child's head on a poorly developed neck makes injury relatively more likely. Spinal cord injury without radiographic abnormality (SCI-WORA) may occur due to the flexibility of the child's spine. Fifty per cent of children with serious spinal cord injury have normal initial radiographs.

Whilst the airway is being established, an assistant should provide manual in-line immobilization. Subsequently, the child's head and torso must be immobilized with a semi-rigid cervical collar, sandbags and tape. If the child is unco-operative and moving, the best option is to immobilize the neck with a collar alone.

Radiographs of the neck are often difficult to interpret. There is a high false-positive rate. Pseudo-subluxation of C2 on C3 occurs in a third of children under 7 years of age (Fig. 39.8). Pseudosubluxation of C3 on C4 also occurs, but less frequently. The thickness of the prevertebral tissues varies with respiration and this can give the appearance of a

prevertebral haematoma. Growth plates can also have the appearance of a fracture.

Clinical examination when cervical trauma is suspected should include:

- neurological assessment of the limbs
- assessment of the pattern of breathing (cord damage above the intercostal nerves leads to pure diaphragmatic breathing)
- palpation of the abdomen for a distended bladder (if present it should be catheterized)
- a log roll should be performed, looking for bruising and palpable steps in the vertebral column
- assessment of anal tone.

ABDOMEN

The management of blunt abdominal trauma in children differs from that in adults. Children have less protection than adults; the abdominal wall is thinner, and compliant ribs protect the upper abdomen less. Bladder rupture is more common in children since the bladder is intra-abdominal rather than pelvic.

Assessment

A traumatized, frightened child is a difficult historian. Efforts should be made to make the child pain free. It is important to consider the mechanism of injury and how this could have affected the abdomen.

The abdomen should be inspected for distension, bruising and lacerations. Gentle palpation may indicate areas of tenderness, guarding and rebound. Clumsy and painful examination makes further assessment difficult, since the child will associate further examinations with pain. This will make distinction between voluntary and involuntary guarding difficult. Adequate analgesia improves the sensitivity and specificity of examination of the abdomen: there is no 'masking' of signs. Distressed children swallow air and fill their stomachs, making assessment of guarding and distension difficult. Gastric drainage is recommended. The femoral pulsations should be palpated, absence or asymmetry suggesting major arterial damage. A rectal examination is rarely indicated in children and vaginal examination almost never.

Regular reassessment is vital.

The presence of haematuria should be sought in all children with trauma to the abdomen. Frank haematuria should be investigated with an intravenous pyelogram. A non-functioning kidney mandates urgent exploration. With lesser degrees of haematuria a conservative approach is justified, with follow-up and later investigation if haematuria is persistent. (The exception is when penetrating trauma causes any degree of haematuria; these cases must be investigated with an intravenous pyelogram.) The external urethral meatus should be examined for the presence of blood that suggests urethral injury. A retrograde urethrogram may be necessary in boys. Girls, with shorter urethras, are unlikely to damage their lower urinary tract.

Investigations

A full blood count is of limited value. A raised amylase is suggestive of pancreatic damage. Other non-invasive tests are extremely useful, in particular CT scanning, which is both sensitive and specific for abdominal injury. Ultrasound is good at detecting fluid in the peritoneal cavity and injury to the solid organs, but is less good at detecting bowel injuries, and has an early high false-negative rate.

There is good evidence that solid organ injuries (liver, spleen and kidney) can be managed conservatively. However, the decision not to operate on a traumatized abdomen is surgical and should only be undertaken if the following conditions can be met:

- a surgical opinion is readily available
- the child can remain haemodynamically stable with less than $40\,ml\,kg^{-1}$ of fluid being tranfused
- there is no evidence of hollow viscus injury
- close observation of the child's vital signs is available.

Diagnostic peritoneal lavage is rarely useful in children since a positive result does not invariably indicate laparotomy. Lavage also renders the peritoneum irritable for up to 48 h. Penetrating wounds usually need exploration. Haemodynamically unstable children, where the source of bleeding is presumed to be in the abdomen, require laparotomy.

LIMBS

The adage that the word limbs is a mnemonic for 'Last In My Basic Survey' holds some truth.

Extremity trauma is rarely immediately life threatening; however, appropriate and early assessment and treatment are important for many injuries to the extremities. A supracondylar fracture of the humerus with brachial artery injury is a limb-threatening injury. Actively bleeding wounds should be covered with a sterile pad, compressed and elevated.

All limbs should be examined gently for tenderness, bruising and deformity. Distal pulses should be sought and, if possible, distal neurological function should be assessed. An absent pulse below an injury requires urgent management. Open fractures should be photographed with a Polaroid camera, and then covered with a sterile dressing. This dressing should remain in place until the patient is in the operating theatre. Prophylactic antibiotics should be given, though the choice of drug varies.

MINOR TRAUMA

Minor trauma is only minor in that it is not immediately life threatening. Minor trauma is certainly not minor to the child or parents. Parental anxiety is transmitted to all but the youngest children. Acknowledging their concerns can make a consultation run much more smoothly. One out of every four attenders at emergency departments is under 16 years of age; the majority of these attendances are for injuries. Accurate diagnosis and early management are important to avoid complications.

Assessment of a child with an injury follows similar principles to assessment in adults, namely, history and mechanism of injury, examination, special tests and management.

HISTORY

It is helpful to ask the child about the problem in terms that they can understand. In children under 5 years of age some useful information may be gained, but the accompanying adult will probably provide most of the history. In older children, their history may be all that is required. It is important to find out whether the accompanying adult witnessed the injury. A history of an injury is not complete until the interviewing doctor can visualize the mechanism of injury. Unfortunately, the history may not be fully available or be interpreted wrongly by the parents. A common example is a limping child that the parents assume must be due to trauma: there are many non-traumatic causes of limp.

The relationship of the accompanying adult to the child should be documented, even if it seems unimportant at the time. It becomes very important if non-accidental injury is later suspected. A brief past medical history, medication and allergy list should be taken. Multiple fractures suggest non-accidental injury. Immunizations should be enquired about, particularly tetanus status. Do not assume that all children are automatically immunized.

EXAMINATION

This needs to be done in an opportunistic, non-threatening manner. Young children may be distressed by the strange environment, the injury, and sometimes the doctor. Some children may be so upset that they refuse examination. Demonstrating an examination on a soft toy can be helpful. Asking the child to perform part of the examination can also be useful, for instance pulling the lower eyelid down in eye injuries. More than any area of medicine, inspection and careful observation is the most useful part of the examination.

If lower limb injuries are suspected, watch the child walking or crawling. A child that will crawl happily but adamantly refuses to walk implies a problem below the knee. If knee pain is complained of and the knee appears normal, consider a hip injury. If an upper limb injury is suspected, asking the child to pick up a toy with the injured arm is useful. Leave invasive parts of the examination until the end.

FRACTURES AND ORTHOPAEDIC PROBLEMS IN CHILDHOOD

Children's fractures heal much more quickly than those in adults. For instance, a femoral shaft fracture will usually unite in 1 week in an infant, 1 month in a 1-year-old, 2 months in a 10-year-old, compared to 3 months in an adult. Growing bone has good capacity to correct angulation, this

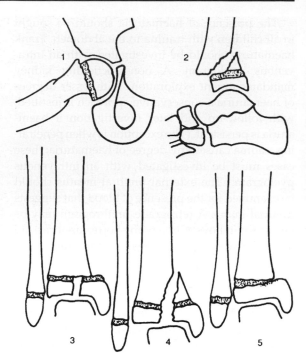

Figure 39.9: The Salter–Harris classification of fractures.

remodelling occurring along the lines of stress. Remodelling is greatest near the epiphyseal plate and in younger children. Remodelling, however, does not correct rotational deformity: reduction is necessary for this.

Fractures near growth plates are important because of the risk of subsequent growth deformity. They are also common, since this is the weakest part of the bone. The Salter–Harris classification (Fig. 39.9) is a way of categorizing these injuries.

- *Type 1.* A separation through the epiphyseal plate. This usually occurs in infants but also occurs in adolescents as a slipped femoral epiphysis. This will only be visible radiologically if displaced.
- *Type 2.* A fracture through the metaphysis and epiphyseal plate. This is the commonest and usually has a benign course.
- *Type 3.* An intra-articular fracture of the epiphysis and epiphyseal plate. This is rare but important, since accurate reduction is necessary to restore the joint surface.
- *Type 4.* Splitting of the metaphysis and the epiphysis. If this is displaced it needs open reduction, since it can interfere with both joint function and growth.

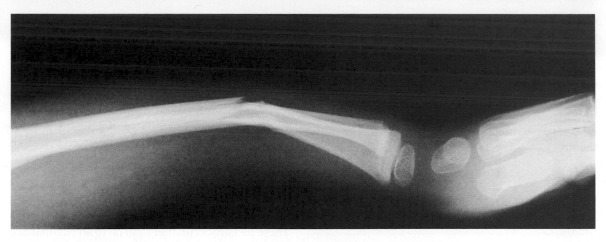

Figure 39.10: Greenstick fracture.

- *Type 5*. Crushed epiphyseal plate. This is difficult to identify, but has important consequences as growth can arrest.

Salter–Harris types 1 and 2 have a good prognosis; types 3, 4 and 5 have a poor prognosis for subsequent growth. All displaced epiphyseal injuries should be referred to the orthpaedic surgeons for reduction.

GREENSTICK FRACTURES (FIG. 39.10)

These are fractures in children where the cortex of bone is incompletely broken. On one side of the injury the cortex is broken, on the other side it is intact or slightly buckled. Rarely, greenstick fractures can have significant deformity and angulation that requires manipulation.

TORUS FRACTURES

Torus or buckle fractures are small disruptions in the cortex. The significance of these injuries is the pain they cause. Plaster casts are often applied to immobilize these for analgesia.

SPRAINS

These are relatively less common in children than in adults, since ligaments are more likely to avulse

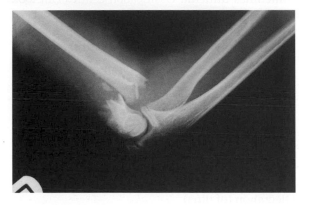

Figure 39.11: A supracondylar fracture of the humerus.

flakes of bone than to tear. A higher index of suspicion and liberal radiographs are necessary if fractures are not to be missed.

FRACTURES AND SOFT-TISSUE INJURIES SPECIFIC TO CHILDREN

Elbow (Fig. 39.11)

Supracondylar fractures of the humerus are one of the commonest fractures in childhood, usually occurring in the 6–9-year-old age group. The usual mechanism of injury is a fall on to the hand. These fractures have a high risk of brachial artery injury and subsequent forearm ischaemia and development of Volkman's ischaemic contracture. The earliest sign of compromised arterial flow is pain on passive extension of the fingers. Later, pallor, pulselessness and paraesthesiae appear. Paralysis is usually a sign of irreversible damage.

Undisplaced supracondylar fractures require only a collar and cuff and follow-up in fracture clinic. Displaced fractures may require manipulation, whilst those with vascular compromise need immediate reduction and fixation in an operating theatre.

OSSIFICATION CENTRES AND THE CONDYLAR FRACTURES

Interpreting radiographs of children's elbows is sometimes difficult. Ossification centres can look like fractures. The large amount of radiolucent cartilage in the developing elbow means that significant injuries can result in only slight radiological abnormalities.

The acronym CRITOL indicates the order in which ossification centres become visible on a radiograph:

Capitellum (of humerus)
Radial head
Internal (or medial) epicondyle
Trochlea (of humerus)
Olecranon (of ulna)
Lateral epicondyle.

The age at which ossification occurs is unimportant: what is important is the sequence. In particular, the medial epicondyle ossifies before the trochlea. If the medial epicondyle is not visible and the trochlear ossification centre is, then there is a high chance that the medial epicondyle has been avulsed into the elbow joint (Fig. 39.12)

Medial epicondylar fractures

A fall on to an outstretched hand causes the wrist flexors to avulse the medial epicondyle at its insertion. There is a high risk of ulnar nerve damage and this should be actively sought. There is an association with lateral dislocation of the elbow. Radiological signs can be subtle. Significant displacement merits reduction; undisplaced avulsions can be treated with a collar and cuff.

Fractures of the neck of the radius

These usually occur after a fall on to an outstretched hand – the radius is pushed against the capitellum. The neck is the most likely fracture site in children whereas in adults the head of the radius fractures more often. Characteristic findings are of minimal swelling, and pain on pronation and supination of the forearm. The radiograph shows a transverse line proximal to the growth plate. The degree of tilt of the radial head must be assessed. Angulation of greater than 15° implies that reduction is necessary.

Pulled elbow

This commonly occurs in children under 5 years of age who have sustained a traction injury to their extended arm. The parents complain that the child will not use the affected arm, which is usually held in extension. The injury is a partial dislocation of the head of the radius out of the poorly formed annular ligament. If the history is clear, then it is reasonable to attempt reduction without a radiograph. Flexion and supination of the elbow with a thumb pressed on the radial head usually produces an audible 'click'. The child will initially cry,

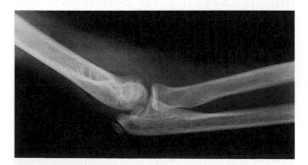
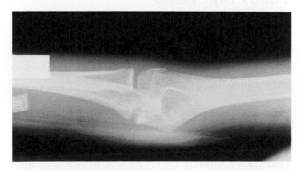

Figure 39.12: Major displacement of the medial epicondyle below the trochlea.

but should start using its arm within the hour. The parents should be advised to bring the child back if it is not using the arm in 24h. The parents should be advised not to lift the child by its hand until after the age of 5 years, since pulled elbows are frequently recurrent. Long-term sequelae are very rare indeed. Without reduction, most pulled elbows relocate themselves over a couple of days. Early relocation reduces the pain that a child suffers.

Slipped femoral epiphysis (Fig. 39.13)

This is separation of the femoral epiphysis and is an example of a Salter–Harris type 1 epiphyseal injury. The epiphysis slips downwards and backwards, sometimes chronically, but often there is a history of trauma. It occurs most commonly in obese adolescent boys and is practically unheard of in children under 8 years of age. It is frequently bilateral.

The child may present with a painful groin, a limp, or even a painful knee. Physical examination reveals an externally rotated leg that is 1–2 cm shorter than the normal side. Standard anteroposterior radiographs may be normal, or have very slight radiological abnormalities. A lateral radiograph is much more sensitive. When looking at the radiograph, draw an imaginary line along the superior surface of the neck of the femur (Trethowan's line). In the normal hip this line should pass through the epiphysis. When the epiphysis has slipped, the line passes superior to the epiphysis. When the

diagnosis is confirmed these children should be referred to an orthopaedic surgeon without delay for treatment. Untreated, there is a risk of coxa vara and avascular necrosis. Other non-traumatic disorders of hip pain are discussed in the section on the limping child.

Toddler's fracture

This is a spiral fracture of the tibia that is usually caused by twisting on a fixed foot. The force required is surprisingly small. The injury is often not recollected, though the parents notice that the child was walking normally but now prefers to crawl. Initial radiographs are often normal and the fracture may not become apparent for up to 10 days. These injuries do not invariably require placing in a cast though a cast provides good analgesia.

Fractures specific to non-accidental injury are discussed in that section.

WOUNDS

The principles of wound management in childhood are the same as in adults (Chapter 5). Adequate wound toilet and optimal opposition ensure the best results. Adequate wound toilet is unlikely unless there is adequate anaesthesia.

Use of tissue glue and adhesive wound tapes in children reduces the need for suturing and the inevitable distress that surrounds this procedure.

(a)

(b)

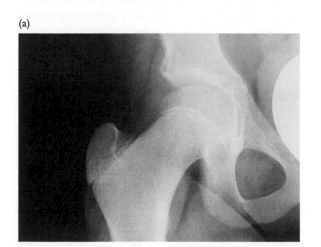
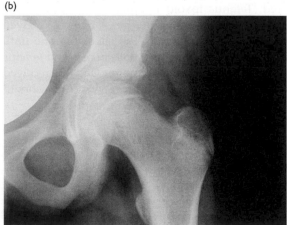

Figure 39.13: X-ray of slipped femoral epiphysis. (a) Normal; (b) abnormal.

However, suturing remains the gold-standard method of closing gaping wounds. In children, sedation often with oral or nasal midazolam may make the procedure less traumatic for the child, its parents and the clinicians. It is vital to have an experienced nurse to help restrain the child: wrapping the child in a blanket is sometimes useful. Extensive lacerations should, however, be sutured and explored under general anaesthesia.

The choice of suture material will depend on the site and extent of the wound. Scalp lacerations are best closed with absorbable sutures, since finding and removing the stitches can be difficult. Absorbable sutures are also preferred for repair of nail-bed lacerations. Non-absorbable sutures should be used on the face. Early removal reduces the risk of cross-hatched marks forming across the wound: 3–4 days is usually adequate, especially for facial wounds.

The maximum safe dose of lignocaine for subcutaneous injection is $3\,mg\,kg^{-1}$. One per cent lignocaine solution contains 10 mg of lignocaine ml^{-1}. If adrenaline is combined with lignocaine, the maximum safe dose is 7 mg of lignocaine kg^{-1}. Lignocaine with adrenaline is very useful in profusely bleeding wounds, but potentially dangerous in end-artery territories such as digits, the pinna and the penis.

Do not exceed the maximum safe dose of lignocaine.

TETANUS PROPHYLAXIS

Do not assume that children are adequately immunized. Tetanus toxoid is administered to children at 2, 3 and 4 months of age. A booster is given at 5 years. This renders the child immune until 15 years old. A child who has not received tetanus immunizations almost certainly has not received diphtheria and polio immunizations. These should also be administered in a non-immune child.

FACIAL LACERATIONS AND TRAUMA

Trauma to a child's face is often a particularly distressing experience for parents and children. The majority of wounds do not need suturing and can be closed relatively painlessly, with good cosmetic results. There are, however, a number of situations where specialist input may be necessary:

- The vermilion border of the lip needs meticulous opposition. A malopposed vermilion border will heal with unsightly scars. These wounds are best repaired by plastic or maxillofacial surgeons, depending on availability.
- The eyelids contain the lacrimal apparatus. Any laceration involving the margin of the eyelid must be sutured by an ophthalmologist in theatre, usually using a microscope to ensure accurate apposition.
- Extensive lacerations should be sutured under a general anaesthetic.
- Heavily contaminated lacerations such as dog bites require aggressive surgical debridement and are often best treated under a general anaesthetic.
- Where the child is too unco-operative to allow adequate wound toilet and suturing, exploration and suturing under a general anaesthetic may be necessary.
- Where there is any doubt about the integrity of the underlying structures, such as the facial nerve. These cases should be formally explored by surgeons.

Lacerations to the inside of the mouth are common. Common mechanisms of injury include falling while sucking a pen (in which palatal damage may occur), falling with the tongue between the teeth, and self-inflicted bites. Injuries to the hard palate should be explored under general anaesthesia. Fortunately, healing within the mouth is excellent and many initially alarming injuries heal well with conservative management. It is important to consider the possibility of non-accidental injury in these cases.

Injuries to teeth are common. Loose teeth are more likely to fall out and children fall over more. Out of hospital, a traumatically avulsed tooth should be washed gently in tap water and then transported in milk. The tooth should be reimplanted into the socket as soon as possible and within 6 hours. The prognosis is improved if the delicate blood vessels and nerves at the proximal end of the tooth are handled as little as possible. Traumatically avulsed milk teeth are still worth implanting since they guide further development. The duty maxillofacial surgeon should be contacted. Teeth can also remain in their sockets after injury but be displaced and point backwards or forwards. These should be repositioned, usually by the duty dentist.

FOREIGN BODIES

Children are naturally curious, and will place foreign bodies in all sorts of orifices. It is important to try to found out what the foreign body is, and in particular whether it is corrosive (a bleach tablet) and whether it is organic or not.

EARS

All sorts of matter finds its way in to children's ears. Occasionally, a child will have a foreign body in both ears. There are a number of ways of removing these, though you may only get one chance! A hook is better than forceps since the latter may drive the foreign body further into the ear. Syringing the ear is useful, but contraindicated if the foreign body is organic as it may become softer and less easy to remove. Some foreign bodies will be too difficult to remove in the emergency department and may even have to be removed under a general anaesthetic. Children with these should be referred to the next ENT clinic.

NOSE

These may present acutely, when witnessed. Later presentation is with a unilateral foul discharge from the nostril. Ask the child to occlude the open nostril and blow out: this may dislodge the object. If the object is visible, then hooking it may be appropriate. Suction with a large bladder syringe may be useful. If these measures fail then the child will need to be referred to the duty ENT surgeon. There is more urgency in these cases since aspiration and airway obstruction, though uncommon, can occur.

INHALED FOREIGN BODIES

A description of the management of inhaled foreign bodies is given in Chapter 40 (p. 491).

SWALLOWED FOREIGN BODIES

These are common. The history should aim to answer the following questions:

- Is the foreign body a poison, for instance a mercury battery or a bleach tablet?
- Is the foreign body actually in the airway?
- Is the foreign body causing any gastrointestinal symptoms such as dysphagia, abdominal pain or constipation? Sharp foreign bodies usually cause no more problems than blunt ones.
- Is the foreign body likely to be radio-opaque?

An algorithm for swallowed coins is shown in Figue 39.14.

Button batteries need to be taken seriously, since they are a potential poison. Neuropsychiatric symptoms and an acute corrosive gastroenteritis may result. A management protocol is shown in Figure 39.15.

Ingestion of bleach tablets is an emergency. The bleach causes ulceration in the oesophagus and may result in stricture formation. Any child who has ingested bleach must be admitted and endoscoped and have copious lavage of the oesophagus.

NON-ACCIDENTAL INJURY

An abused child is one that is treated in a way that is regarded as unacceptable by the present culture. Different cultures treat children in different ways. Every year in England about 100 children die from abuse. Thousands of children are placed on the Child Protection Register. Diagnosis and management are often difficult. This section aims to help in the diagnosis and initial management of child abuse. Child abuse takes many forms. The forms that may present to emergency departments are listed below:

- non-accidental injury, usually a direct assault
- neglect. The normal protection provided for a child is lacking and accidents occur as a result
- Munchausen by proxy. The mother or carer invents false illnesses in the child in order to obtain medical attention
- emotional abuse
- sexual abuse.

Non-accidental injury and neglect are the most likely forms to present to emergency departments.

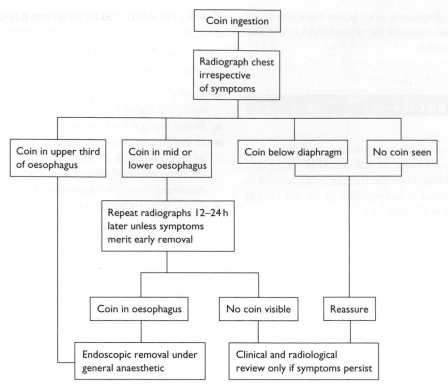

Figure 39.14: Protocol for swallowed coins.

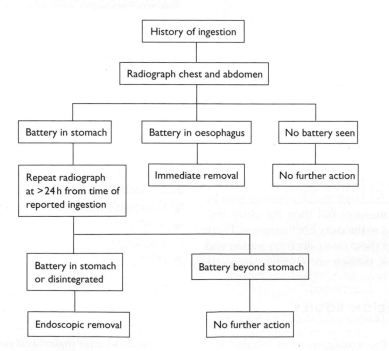

Figure 39.15: Protocol for swallowed batteries.

Although the range of presentations is extremely varied, there are a number of suggestive, common features in the history that should be looked for There are also a number of characteristic physical findings that should suggest non-accidental injury.

HISTORY

None of the following features is diagnostic, but they should raise suspicion of child abuse:

- Delay in seeking medical help.
- Providing an inconsistent or inappropriate history (2-month-old babies do not crawl and fall).
- A very vague or history of minor trauma which is out of keeping with the observed injuries (this is increasingly suspicious if the story changes).
- Multiple attendances at the emergency department, or at other nearby departments.
- The interaction of the child and the parent should be observed, though abused, distressed children will still look for support from their carer. Normal parents are concerned with the child first; abusing parents may be more concerned with their own problems.
- The parents may become hostile, abusive and behave in an inappropriate manner.
- The child may give an account of abuse: in this case, the actual words should be recorded verbatim.

It is vital to record from whom the history is taken: just stating 'history from parent' is inadequate. The child's development should be assessed (Table 39.6). and the family composition noted. A past medical history should be taken and the child's height and weight should be recorded on a centile chart.

Table 39.6: Developmental milestones

2 months	Smiles
4 months	Rolls over
6 months	Resists taking toy from grasp
	Bears some weight on legs
12 months	Just stands, walks and can make a pincer grip
18 months	Walks backwards
	Throwing objects on to the floor and drooling is abnormal
24 months	Can kick a ball

RISK FACTORS FOR NON-ACCIDENTAL INJURY

There are various factors that make child abuse more likely, though abuse occurs in all sections of society.
Parent factors include:

- age under 30
- single parent
- lack of extended, available family
- adverse social circumstances, such as unemployment
- stepfather
- criminal record
- abuse of parent as a child.

Child factors include:

- first born
- unwanted
- prolonged neonatal illness (a long stay in an incubator interferes with parental bonding)
- chronic illness.

EXAMINATION

There are a number of injuries that are virtually diagnostic of non-accidental injury. Injuries that arise from neglect are often indistinguishable from simple accidents and the history is the main pointer. No single feature should be taken in isolation. Where there are visual signs these should be photographed.

The following physical findings are suggestive of non-accidental injury.

Skin

Burns are a common non-accidental injury. Children's skin is more prone to burn injury (above 60°C a child's skin will burn four times as quickly as an adult's).

- Cigarette burns.
- Hot water burns to both feet result from dipping into hot water. There may also be burns to the buttocks, with no burns on the rest of the lower limb. This pattern results from the child lifting its legs up to withdraw in pain.
- 'Doughnut' sparing of the buttocks results when a child is forced into a hot bath. The 'hole

Table 39.7: The age of bruises

Colour of a bruise	Probable age of a bruise
Red or purple	Less than 24h old
Purple or blue	12–48h
Brown	48–72h
Yellow or green	More than 72h

in the doughnut' results from being pressed on to the cooler floor of the bath.

- Children touch hot objects with the palm of the hand: injuries to the dorsum of the hand are more suspicious.

Bruising should be looked for and described with respect to colour and distribution. Beware of trying to date a bruise too accurately (Table 39.7):

- Finger-tip bruises result from gripping the child forcibly, either on the torso, on the face or around the neck.
- Lash marks. A central white area is surrounded by bruising. This occurs because blood is forced from the point of impact to the surrounding tissue, where it tears capillaries.
- Bites. Cats and dogs cause semicircular bites, adults cause straight bites.

Eyes

RETINOSCHISIS

Shaking causes the vitreous humour to move in the eyeball. This can separate the retinal layers causing a dome-shaped cavity that may have a blood level. Shaking causes retinal tears; these may be caused by other diseases, including acute hypertension, fulminant meningitis and endocarditis. Normal birth also causes retinal haemorrhages but these resolve by 2 weeks.

Mouth

Shaking can cause the frenulum of the tongue to tear. Aggressive feeding with a bottle causes bleeding to the mouth. Simple falls can also tear the frenulum.

Fractures

- Multiple fractures in various stages of healing are highly suspicious, as is a single fracture with multiple bruises.

Table 39.8: The age of fractures. (Adapted from Kleinman, P.K. (1987) *Diagnostic Imaging of Child Abuse.* Williams and Wilkins, Baltimore)

Radiographic sign	Age of fracture
Resolution of soft tissue swelling	4–10 days
Periosteal new bone formation	10–14 days
Loss of fracture line definition	14–21 days
Soft callus	14–21 days
Hard callus	21–42 days

- Metaphyseal and epiphyseal fractures. The usual sites are at the knee, wrist, elbow and ankle. Shaking of the infant causes twisting and pulling injuries at the ends of long bones; fragments of bone are torn off.
- Rib fractures are highly suggestive of non-accidental injury, particularly if they are healing at the time of presentation, or multiple.

It is important to attempt to date the fracture from its radiographic appearance (Table 39.8).

Brain

Non-accidental injury characteristically causes two types of head injury. Shaking injuries cause diffuse axonal injury and subdural haematomas, while impacts from punches or throwing the child result in fractures. Subdural haematomas in children are almost invariably the result of violent shaking. They may occur after birth trauma, but do not become chronic. The diagnosis may be suspected clinically when a child presents with irritability, vomiting and a reduced level of consciousness. Retinal haemorrhages should be looked for carefully. Fractures have a different nature from those arising from simple accidents. Multiple fractures of different ages are highly suspicious. Fractures of the occiput are particularly suspicious, as are fractures wider than 5mm.

POISONING

Non-accidental injury need not be traumatic, poisoning being well described. The symptoms and signs will depend on the poison ingested. Salt poisoning, due to high intake and fluid restriction, is relatively common and should be suspected when the child has hypernatraemia and a high urinary

Table 39.9: Munchausen by proxy

False symptom or signs	Explanation
Seizures, apnoea attacks	Smothering, suffocation
Haematuria	Tampered sample (often by a vaginal tampon)
Fever	Tampered thermometer Repeated vaccination
Diarrhoea	Laxative abuse

sodium content. The child will present with thirst and irritability, followed by seizures.

MUNCHAUSEN BY PROXY

This is a rare disorder in which the parent or carer invents illness in the child in order to obtain medical attention. The form most likely to present to emergency departments is of fabricated illness. Some examples are shown in Table 39.9.

EMOTIONAL ABUSE

This term refers to the persistent verbal abuse of a child by criticism and ridicule. This form of child abuse is unlikely to be the sole cause of attendances at emergency departments. Children who do not receive affection and encouragement suffer in many ways. There is general developmental delay, with poor growth, poor immune function and poor social interaction with peers.

GENITAL INJURIES AND SEXUAL ABUSE

It is uncommon for this to present to emergency departments. It is inappropriate for staff to examine children who may have been sexually abused, unless the injury is so severe as to require immediate, life-saving treatment.

It is important to be able to recognize when these children need further help (see below). This help is usually provided by the police surgeon and a consultant paediatrician.

Possible presentations of child sexual abuse include:

- teenage pregnancy

- altered behaviour, for example truancy, deliberate self-harm or inappropriate sexuality
- prepubertal vaginal bleeding or discharge
- proven sexual transmitted disease
- anal trauma.

DISEASES WHICH MAY MIMIC CHILD ABUSE

Occasionally, a child may present with signs suggestive of child abuse that are actually caused by underlying disease:

- Breech deliveries can cause fractures of the clavicle and humerus. These fractures invariably have callus formation by 2 weeks of age.
- Prematurity causes a form of rickets, predisposing to fractures.
- Osteogenesis imperfecta. Abnormal collagen allows bone to break with minimal trauma. Blue sclera, deafness, skin fragility, dental abnormalities and a positive family history should be looked for.
- Copper deficiency predisposes to pathological fractures.
- Many haematological disorders, such as Henoch–Schönlein purpura, leukaemia, idiopathic thrombocytopenia, and haemophilia can produce bruising. A full blood count, platelet count and coagulation screen are often indicated when a child presents with unexplained bruising.
- Burns. Impetigo may be mistaken for a contact burn.

MANAGEMENT OF CHILD ABUSE IN EMERGENCY DEPARTMENTS

Every child that attends an emergency department should have a careful history and a thorough examination documented. Aim to record as much information as possible, and as accurately as possible. It is inappropriate for staff to attempt to manage suspected child abuse without adequate support from senior paediatricians and social workers. It is vital that doctors in the emergency department feel able to draw on the expertise of these specialists. It is also important that staff do not approach the parents in a confrontational manner. Angry parents can be extremely difficult to deal with later. The parents should be told that their child is being referred for a further opinion. They must not be misled or lied to, since this will create problems for everyone involved. The roles of emergency department staff in the management of child abuse are outlined below:

- Identify suspected abuse and refer to the paediatrician for an opinion. Some children will be referred and the diagnosis subsequently refuted. This is preferable to 'missing' cases. This also illustrates why a non-confrontational approach is important.
- Provide appropriate initial treatment for physical injuries, such as burns or fractures.

Emergency Protection Orders

Occasionally, parents may refuse to see a paediatrician and remove their child from hospital. If necessary, an Emergency Protection Order can be sought. This allows the court to '*Detain the child in a place of safety if there is reasonable cause to believe his or her proper development is being avoidably prevented or neglected or his or her health is being avoidably impaired or neglected or he or she is being mistreated*'. An Emergency Protection Order lasts for up to 8 days. The duty social worker will usually make an application to the court of behalf of the local authority.

Emergency department staff should also be fully aware of safeguards in the emergency department and use them:

- The 'at-risk register' comprises a list of children in the area who are felt to be at increased risk of abuse. Staff should have easy access to their local register.
- The number of times that a child has attended a department should be clearly visible on the record.

- A dedicated social worker or health visitor should work in the emergency department. He or she should have close contact with the paediatric ward, the community paediatricians, social workers in the community, child's family doctor and health visitors.
- A letter to the child's family doctor should follow every attendance at the department, with the diagnosis clearly stated.
- New medical and nursing staff should be taught when to suspect child abuse.

SUMMARY

Children are not miniature adults but are subject to a whole spectrum of different injuries, to which they behave in physiologically different ways. The whole approach to the multiply injured child is therefore different while maintaining the same basic objectives. Trauma that is not life threatening is different in children: in presentation, pathology and management. They are also subject to the phenomenon of child abuse, where a multidisciplinary approach is important.

FURTHER READING

Advanced Life Support Group. (1997) *Advanced Paediatric Life Support*. BMJ, London.

Meadow, R. (1993) *ABC of Child Abuse*. BMJ, London.

Milner, A. and Hull, D. (1992) *Hospital Paediatrics*. Churchill Livingstone.

Morton, R. and Philips, B. (1996) *Accidents and Emergencies in Children*. Oxford University Press, Oxford.

CHAPTER FORTY

THE SICK CHILD

- Introduction
- Cardiac arrest
- Neonatal resuscitation
- What to do after a cardiac arrest
- Recognizing the ill child
- The breathless or wheezy child
- Shocked children
- The unconscious child
- Convulsing children
- The hot and feverish child

- The poisoned child
- The vomiting child
- Acute diarrhoea
- Abdominal pain in childhood
- Rectal bleeding
- Diabetic emergencies
- Anaphylaxis
- Drowning and near drowning
- Further reading

INTRODUCTION

The majority of children who present to emergency departments have relatively minor injuries and illnesses. It is important that the minority with life-threatening illnesses are identified early and treated promptly. Children have different physiology and anatomy from adults and respond to disease in different ways.

CARDIAC ARREST

Cardiac arrest in childhood is uncommon and has different causes from those in the adult. Primary cardiac arrest is rare. Cardiac arrest usually occurs as a result of respiratory or circulatory failure. This suggests that if the primary cause of the cardiac arrest can be treated adequately then many arrests might be prevented.

Neonatal deaths are those that occur in the first month of life. Since the vast majority of these occur in hospital and are managed by paediatricians, they are not discussed further.

'Cot death' refers to deaths that occur from the first month to 1 year of age. Some of these are due

to previously unrecognized disease. In others, no cause is ever found even after post-mortem examination and these are referred to as deaths from the 'sudden infant death syndrome' (SIDS).

After 1 year of age, trauma is the commonest cause of death until adulthood. Further advice on the management of major trauma in childhood can be found in Chapter 39.

PREPARATION PRIOR TO RECEIVING A CARDIAC ARREST

Staff

There must be adequate staff numbers, while avoiding overcrowding. A doctor competent in airway management must take control of the airway. He or she will require a skilled assistant. Another staff member provides chest compressions. One staff member provides vascular access and is responsible for administering intravenous drugs. The most senior doctor should act as team leader and it is preferable that the team leader stands back and directs and monitors the resuscitation. It is very helpful if someone documents events as they proceed. If there are sufficient staff to explain what is happening, there is no reason why the parents cannot be present during the resuscitation, but adequate care and supervision are essential.

Environment and equipment

Ideally, children should be resuscitated in a separate area from the adult resuscitation area. There must be adequate space. There should be an available method of estimating the child's weight quickly: a Broselow tape (see Fig. 39.2) which relates weight to height is ideal and provides information on equipment sizes and drug doses. A simple set of marks along the trolley can provide the same information. The formula below is also useful for determining the weight of children between 1 and 10 years old:

Weight (kg) = 2 (Age + 4).

A clock should be started when the child arrives. Whatever equipment is available, staff must ensure that they are familiar with its use.

BASIC LIFE SUPPORT IN CHILDREN

Though the objective of adequate perfusion with oxygenated blood is the same as for adults, the means by which this is achieved is very different. This reflects the different anatomy of the child. The initial assessment and initiation of basic life support for children is shown in Table 40.1. All emergency department doctors should receive formal training in paediatric basic life support.

> Basic life support for children requires different techniques.

In hospital environments help is usually readily available and the paediatric cardiac arrest team should be called immediately. In the unusual situation of a cardiac arrest occurring where it is necessary to leave the patient to get help, basic life support should be performed for at least 1 min before leaving to call for help. This differs from adults and reflects the fact that hypoxia is the commonest cause of cardiac arrest in children.

> 1 min of cardiopulmonary resuscitation (CPR) must be administered before leaving the child to get help.

Table 40.1: Initial assessment and management of paediatric cardiac arrest

> Check awareness (Are you all right?)
> Airway opening manoeuvres
> Look, Listen, Feel for breathing
> 5 breaths
> Check carotid pulse
> Start cardiopulmonary resuscitation (CPR)
> 20 × 5:1 CPR cycles

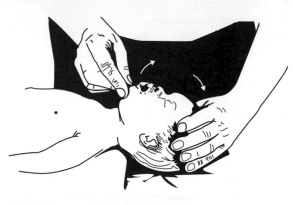

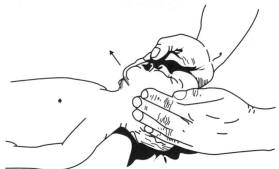

Figure 40.1: Opening an infant and child airway.

Shaking a child gently by the shoulders and talking is a good way to assess consciousness. If trauma is a possibility, the cervical spine should be immobilized by placing one hand on the forehead and shaking the arm.

Airway and breathing

The airway in infants is opened by performing a chin lift while keeping the head in a neutral position (Fig. 40.1). Older children's airways are opened by lifting the chin with the head in a 'sniffing' position.

The adequacy of the airway is assessed by:

- Looking for chest movements
- Listening for breath sounds
- Feeling for breath.

This should take no longer than 10 s. Because hypoxia is the commonest cause of cardiac arrest in children, five initial rescue breaths should be given. If there are no airway adjuncts available, mouth-to-mouth respiration should be started. In smaller children this may entail mouth-to-mouth and nose respiration. Whatever technique is used, the adequacy of ventilation should be assessed by observing chest movements.

Circulation

The carotid artery should be palpated for 10 s although in infants it is easier to palpate the brachial or femoral arteries. Cardiac compressions should be started if the pulse is absent. In infants, a pulse of 60 or less is assumed to be inadequate and cardiac massage should be initiated at or below this rate.

TECHNIQUES OF CARDIAC COMPRESSION

For infants (under 1 year old) an imaginary line is drawn between the nipples and the sternum compressed one finger breadth below this line. The sternum should move one third of the depth of the child's chest. This can be achieved by the two-finger technique or the hand-encircling technique (Fig. 40.2). The hand-encircling technique requires the thumbs to be placed on the sternum.

For small children (under 8 years old) the sternum should be compressed one finger breadth above the xiphisternum using the heel of one hand, and for older children the sternum should be compressed two finger breadths above the xiphisternum using interlocked hands. The compression rate should be at least 100 per minute.

ADVANCED LIFE SUPPORT

Advanced life support aims to provide further interventions in cardiac arrest in order to restore cardiac output. These skills are harder to learn, require equipment and drugs, and are therefore not widely taught to the public. It is important that there is

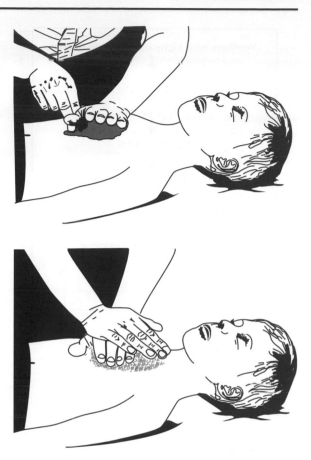

Figure 40.2: Technique of cardiac compression for older children.

adequate basic life support in progress before and while these are performed. ECG electrodes should be placed on the patient as soon as possible and the rhythm should be identified promptly.

> Always look for underlying pathology causing cardiac arrest.

Asystole

This is the commonest presenting rhythm in paediatric cardiac arrests (Fig. 40.3), since bradycardia is the normal response to hypoxia. The absence of any electrical activity and a gently undulating baseline usually confirm the diagnosis. A completely straight line suggests that a lead has become disconnected. The gain should be increased and the selected lead changed if there is any doubt about the diagnosis. If dehydration or vascular insufficiency is the cause of the cardiac

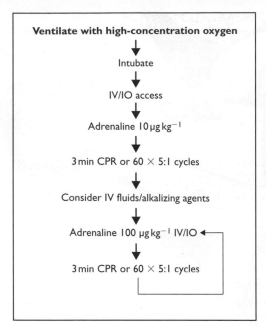

Figure 40.3: Management of asystole.

arrest, intravenous fluids should be administered at $20\,ml/kg^{-1}$. Alkalizing agents and atropine are of unproven benefit. The management of asystole is summarized in Fig. 40.3.

Ventricular fibrillation

Although this is the commonest arrythmia of cardiac arrest in adults, it is much less common in children. In children it is usually caused by hypothermia, tricyclic poisoning, and in those with cardiac disease (usually congenital). An algorithm for the management of ventricular fibrillation in children is given in Figure 40.4.

PULSELESS ELECTRICAL ACTIVITY

Otherwise known as electromechanical dissociation (EMD), pulseless electrical activity (Fig. 40.5) is usually the result of hypovolaemia. Tension pneumothorax and cardiac tamponade are possible causes when there is trauma. Pulmonary emboli are rare in children. Calcium chloride should be given if electrolyte disturbances are thought to have caused the cardiac arrest.

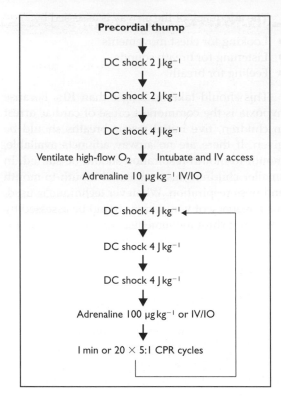

Figure 40.4: Management of ventricular fibrillation.

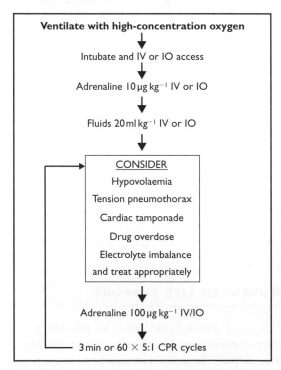

Figure 40.5: Management of pulseless electrical activity in children.

NEONATAL RESUSCITATION

Cardiorespiratory arrest in neonates is fortunately extremely rare in emergency departments but unexpected deliveries do occur in the department or are brought in from close by. Any neonate with apnoea or a pulse of less than 60 requires aggressive resuscitation. Urgent expert assistance should be sought.

Apnoeic newborn infants are likely to breathe with some stimulation, and suction to the nares and mouth together with oxygen by mask may be effective. After 1 min, ventilation with a bag and appropriate mask should be commenced. If the baby remains apnoeic, intubation may be necessary. Chest compressions may be required if there is bradycardia.

Endotracheal intubation in the newborn (3 mm tube, 2.5 mm in premature infants) must be preceded by pre-oxygenation except in suspected meconium aspiration. If meconium aspiration has occurred, intubation should be followed by direct suction on the endotracheal tube which is simultaneously withdrawn. The procedure can then be repeated with a clean tube.

Newborns with bradycardia of less than 60 b.p.m. that is not clearly improving with ventilation require external cardiac compressions. The method of chest compression has already been described and a compression-to-ventilation rate of 3:1 should be used. The chest should be depressed by 2 cm at a rate of 120 compressions per minute.

If the baby remains bradycardic (less than 60 b.p.m.) after 1 min of chest compressions, adrenaline $10 \mu g \, kg^{-1}$ should be given intravenously. Further doses should be given every 3–5 min during CPR. Consideration should also be given to the administration of sodium bicarbonate $1 \, mmol \, kg^{-1}$ ($2 \, ml \, kg^{-1}$ of 4.2% solution) intravenously. Hypovolaemic cardiac arrest is treated with intravenous fluids ($20 \, ml \, kg^{-1}$) and hypoglycaemia must be excluded or treated.

AIRWAY

There are a variety of airway adjuncts available to assist in paediatric advanced life support. A description of paediatric airway and circulatory management is provided in Chapter 39.

DEFIBRILLATION

A normal adult defibrillator is used with paediatric paddles of an appropriate size. An appropriate energy level must be selectable. An infant requires paddles 4.5 cm in diameter; a small child requires 8-cm diameter paddles.

WHAT TO DO AFTER A CARDIAC ARREST

OUTCOME SUCCESSFUL

The return of spontaneous output moves the management from cardiac arrest to resuscitation of a seriously ill child. The aim of interventions is to improve oxygenation and perfusion while treating the underlying cause of the cardiac arrest.

Following cardiac arrest the child should be closely monitored (Table 40.2). A series of investigations should also be performed (Table 40.3).

Oxygenation should be improved so that oxygen saturations are above 95%. Most children will have an impaired conscious level, and a period of intubation and ventilation to optimize oxygenation is beneficial.

Table 40.2: Post-arrest monitoring

Pulse oximetry
ECG
Blood pressure (initially non-invasive)
Rectal temperature
Urine output: consider urinary catheter
Consider central venous pressure (CVP)
End-tidal CO_2

Table 40.3: Post-cardiac arrest investigations

Arterial blood gases
Bedside and formal laboratory glucose
Chest radiograph
Urea and electrolytes
Haemoglobin and haematocrit
Group and save serum
12-lead ECG
Coagulation screen

Metabolic acidosis following cardiac arrest should be corrected by optimizing ventilation and perfusion.

Perfusion may be impaired because of hypovolaemia or poor cardiac function. Poor cardiac function may result from underlying cardiac disease, but is more likely to result from acidosis and electrolyte disturbance. The best initial treatment of post-arrest acidosis is adequate oxygenation and perfusion. The circulation should be optimized with volume expansion or inotropic support. This usually requires central venous access. Hypothermia and hypoglycaemia are common following cardiac arrest. These problems should be anticipated and avoided. The child should be monitored and observed in an intensive care unit.

The parents will be extremely upset and the most senior team member should find time to explain what has happened to their child. An explanation of all the interventions that have been performed should be given. Unfortunately, some children who have been successfully resuscitated die later and over-optimistic prognoses should be avoided. These deaths may be due to the underlying cause or to the physiological insult of a cardiac arrest.

OUTCOME UNSUCCESSFUL

It is reasonable to stop resuscitation after 30 min if there has been no sign of a spontaneous circulation or cerebral activity. Hypothermic children should be resuscitated until their core temperature is above 32°C. Prolonged resuscitation is also necessary following overdose of cerebral depressant drugs. The decision to stop CPR should be made by the most senior doctor on the team with the agreement of all involved.

Following an unsuccessful resuscitation the child should be examined for bruising, rashes and dehydration. The paediatric team should be involved and, in the case of suspected SIDS, local policies should be followed in taking samples for further investigation. If the cause of death is clearly fulminant meningococcal septicaemia, local infection-control physicians should be informed and disease prophylaxis should be given to all family members. The general practitioner, health visitor and coroner should also be informed. Follow-up with a consultant paediatrician should

be arranged in a few weeks, to discuss the causes of the death.

The most senior doctor available should inform the parents. It is important that this is done with sensitivity, tact and sympathy. A nurse should accompany the doctor. A separate room should be available for breaking bad news. The doctor should also try and ascertain some history from the parents. This should be done gently and may take some time. The relatives should be encouraged to see and hold their child. This will have enormous significance later on and aid the bereavement process. The parents should also be told that the coroner and police will be informed. It should be emphasized that this is routine in all cases, and does not suggest blame.

RECOGNIZING THE ILL CHILD

One of the most important functions of emergency staff is the prompt recognition of seriously ill children. The identification of sick children who need further investigation is a skill that takes experience to acquire. However, an appreciation of normality and recognition of deviation from this is helpful.

General observation should begin from the moment the doctor sees the child. It is essential to observe the affect of the child: are they interested, interactive and playing? Can you make them smile?

Ill children are usually miserable and uninterested.

AIRWAY AND BREATHING

Respiratory rate is a sensitive marker for respiratory distress and should be recorded in all potentially ill children. The normal value varies with age (Table 40.4).

Table 40.4: Normal values for respiratory rate by age

Age (years)	Respiratory rate (breaths min^{-1})
<1	30–40
2–5	25–30
5–12	20–25
>12	15–20

Recession of the subcostal, intercostal or sternal regions indicates increased respiratory effort. Older children have less compliant chest walls and so recession, when seen, is progressively more significant. The use of the sternocleidomastoid muscles indicates respiratory distress, and can cause head bobbing in infants. Stridor is an inspiratory noise that implies upper airway obstruction. Wheeze is an expiratory noise implying lower airway obstruction. Grunting usually occurs in infants and indicates severe respiratory distress. Flaring of the alar nasi is also seen in infants with respiratory distress.

Pulse oximetry is a useful and simple investigation, although significant decreases in arterial oxygenation may not cause significant desaturations, because of the sigmoid-shaped relationship between oxygen saturation and oxygen tension. Cyanosis, bradycardia and confusion are all very late signs of respiratory failure and are preterminal. Rapid action is necessary to prevent cardiac arrest.

CIRCULATION

Heart rate increases in response to hypoperfusion. It also increases when there is pain and anxiety. In the late (preterminal) stages of hypoperfusion a bradycardia may appear. Again normal pulse rate varies with age (Table 40.5).

The volume of a pulse is important in assessing shock. Hypoperfusion causes a decline in the volume of a pulse. An absent peripheral pulse and a weak central pulse are signs of significant hypoperfusion. Capillary refill time is a useful indicator of peripheral perfusion and is obtained by pressing on a warm digit for 5 s. It is prolonged if the skin does not return to a normal colour in 2 s.

Hypotension is a late sign of hypoperfusion. An estimate of expected blood pressure can be made by using the formula below:

$$\text{Systolic blood pressure} = 80 + (\text{Age in years} \times 2).$$

Table 40.5: Normal pulse rate by age

Age (years)	Heart rate (beats min^{-1})
<1	110–160
2–5	95–140
5–12	80–120
>12	60–100

NEUROLOGICAL ASSESSMENT

The AVPU system is very quick and easy to use:

A ALERT
V responds to Voice
P responds to Pain
U UNRESPONSIVE.

Pulling frontal hair is an appropriate painful stimulus. Children in deep coma may assume a decorticate (flexed arms, extended legs) or even a decerebrate posture (extended arms, extended legs). The size, symmetry and reactivity of the pupils should be recorded. Reflexes and tone should be assessed, particularly for asymmetry.

THE BREATHLESS OR WHEEZY CHILD

There are many causes of respiratory distress in children. Usually a characteristic pattern allows the diagnosis to be made. The causes that are likely to present to emergency departments are listed in Table 40.6.

This list is not comprehensive. There are many other causes of respiratory distress in children, for instance cystic fibrosis and congenital malformations. These tend to have a more protracted course and usually present to the patient's general practitioner or to the paediatricians. However, familiarity

Table 40.6: Causes of breathlessness by age group

	Age
Upper airway:	
Acute laryngeotracheitis (croup)	6 months to 5 years
Pseudomembranous croup (bacterial tracheitis)	6 months to 5 years
Epiglottitis	2–3 years
Retropharyngeal abscess	6 months to 3 years
Inhaled foreign body	Any age
Lower airway:	
Acute viral bronchiolitis	Under 1 year
Asthma	From 12 months
Pertussis (whooping cough)	6 months on
Inhaled foreign body	Any age
Pneumonia	Any age
Acute bronchitis	Any age

with the above conditions will ensure that the majority of breathless children in emergency departments are managed appropriately.

UPPER RESPIRATORY TRACT DISORDERS

Croup (acute laryngotracheobronchitis)

This is a common viral infection of the upper airway. It occurs in children from 6 months to 5 years old. It usually presents 1–2 days after the onset of an upper respiratory tract infection. The symptoms are worse at night, or when the child is upset. The voice is hoarse and there is a characteristic cough which sounds like a barking seal. These children are usually systematically well and may not have a pyrexia. A coarse inspiratory stridor is usually heard. Upsetting the child makes their symptoms worse.

The diagnosis is mainly clinical although recording oxygen saturations is useful. Normal saturations may be present with severe croup, but low saturations indicate increased severity. Lateral neck radiographs are usually normal, although a narrowed subglottic airway may be seen. These should not be taken routinely.

The illness is usually benign and self-limiting. Admission is not always necessary. A child with croup can usually be sent home safely if there is no stridor at rest, no sternal or subcostal recessions, and the child is well saturated on pulse oximetry. The parents should be willing and able to provide care and have the ability to return to hospital promptly. Parents of children sent home should be advised to keep the child warm. It is useful to expose the child to steam. This can be achieved by turning on the hot taps in the bathroom.

Children who do not fulfil the above criteria need admission. The reason for admission is to provide close observation for those children who may require intubation. While observation needs to be close, the child should be upset as little as possible. If the child is clearly unwell and requires intubation, 1 ml of 1 in 1000 adrenaline mixed with 4 ml of normal saline can be given by a nebulizer while arrangements are made for intubation. This only 'buys time', as symptoms usually recur within 20 min.

Bacterial tracheitis

This is an uncommon, but potentially life-threatening condition. There is a bacterial infection of the trachea, usually by *Staphylococcus aureus*. The child has usually had a fever for a couple of days and presents with a croupy cough. Signs of upper airway obstruction are progressive. Laryngoscopy at the time of intubation usually confirms the diagnosis. A normal epiglottis is seen and the trachea is full of pus-like secretions. Intubation is invariably required. Flucloxacillin and amoxycillin therapy is usually appropriate.

Acute epiglottitis

This is rare and should become even less common with the introduction of the *Haemophilus influenzae* vaccine given at 1 year. However, it is important that knowledge exceeds experience, since prompt recognition and treatment saves children's lives. *Haemophilus influenzae* type B (HIB) causes a rapid swelling of the epiglottis and pharynx. Upper airway obstruction occurs rapidly, with subsequent hypoxia and death. Children are usually 2–3 years old, although adults can also be affected. The child's parents will state that the child has become unwell very rapidly. The child will be toxic, with a fever in excess of 39.0°C, look anxious and sit very still with his or her head forward. Drooling occurs because the child does not want to swallow. A low, soft stridor is heard and there is often an added expiratory noise. Cough is not usually a feature.

Senior staff from the emergency department, paediatrics and anaesthesia should be summoned immediately, along with a surgeon skilled in performing tracheostomy. It is essential not to interfere with the child any more than is strictly necessary. The child should be left sitting with his or her mother. Laryngoscopy to visualize the epiglottis must not be attempted, since this may well provoke complete laryngeal obstruction. Providing oxygen by a face-mask may only increase the child's anxiety and should not be forced. Nebulized drugs may provoke coughing and should be avoided. The child requires endotracheal intubation, usually after a gas induction. The anaesthetist usually confirms the diagnosis at laryngoscopy. The surgeon is there to provide an emergency tracheostomy should airway obstruction occur. Once the airway is secure the child needs an intravenous line and antibiotics.

> Summon senior staff immediately for the child with acute epiglottitis.

Retropharyngeal abscess

This is another uncommon but life-threatening infection of the upper respiratory tract and is usually caused by β-haemolytic streptococcus. Children from the age of 6 months to 3 years are usually affected. The usual story is of 2–3 days of coryza. Feeding difficulties emerge before respiratory problems. The child looks ill, may assume an opisthotonic posture, is toxic, drooling, and has inspiratory stridor. A pharyngeal mass may be visible with a torch and a tongue depressor. A lateral neck radiograph shows widening of the retropharyngeal space and air/fluid levels may be seen. Treatment is with intravenous antibiotics (usually benzyl penicillin) and possible incision and drainage. Drainage should be performed with a secured airway since aspiration of the pus can cause a pneumonia. If there is any doubt about the diagnosis or epiglottitis is suspected then the treatment of acute epiglottitis should be instituted.

Inhaled foreign bodies

These are another cause of upper airway obstruction. Suspicion should be high when there are signs of acute upper airway obstruction with no systemic illness. (see section on foreign bodies.) A child with 'croup' who has not got better over a week may well have a tracheal foreign body.

LOWER RESPIRATORY TRACT DISORDERS

Acute viral bronchiolitis

This tends to occur in epidemics over winter. It usually affects children under the age of 12 months and is usually caused by respiratory syncytial virus (RSV). The illness begins with an upper respiratory tract infection, but over a couple of days the child becomes progressively more short of breath and wheezy. There may be problems feeding and

Table 40.7: Features of severe and life-threatening asthma

Features of severe asthma in children:
  Too breathless to feed or talk
  Recession or use of accessory muscles
  Respiratory rate > 50 breaths per minute
  Peak flow $< 50\%$ expected or best

Features of life-threatening asthma in children:
  Depressed conscious level/agitation
  Exhaustion
  Poor respiratory drive
  Oxygen saturation $< 85\%$ on air
  Cyanosis
  Silent chest
  Peak flow $< 33\%$ expected or best

signs of respiratory distress. Fine inspiratory crackles and expiratory wheeze may be heard on auscultation. Pulse oximetry shows reduced oxygen saturation; arterial blood gases (if done) show hypoxia and normocarbia. A chest radiograph may show hyperinflated lungs and peribronchiolar thickening. Areas of consolidation suggest an alternative diagnosis of pneumonia.

If the child is alert, playing well, has no problem feeding and has no signs of respiratory distress, then admission to hospital is probably not necessary. Arrangements for further review by the patient's family doctor are necessary if the child is discharged. Children who are admitted should receive oxygen as the mainstay of their treatment. Intubation is occasionally necessary.

Asthma

This is very common in children. It is, however, unusual in children who are under 1 year old. Despite being common, there are still a number of deaths every year among children. The diagnosis of an acute attack is not usually difficult, although bronchiolitis, an inhaled foreign body and croup can produce similar clinical features. Assessing a young child with an asthma attack is more difficult than in an adult.

Certain features may be obtained in the history and examination which should suggest that an asthma attack is severe or life threatening (Table 40.7). The presence of any of these should prompt aggressive management. Increased use of

Table 40.8: Expected peak flow rates by age

Age	Mean length (cm)	Expected peak flow (l min^{-1})
6	110	150
8	120	200
10	130	250
12	150	350
14	160	400

bronchodilators with reduced effect at home indicates worsening asthma. It is important to note that severity of wheeze and cough do not correlate with the severity of the disease.

Children under 5 years old and severely dyspnoeic children cannot reliably perform peak flow measurements. Children over 5 years should have at least two attempts and their best effort should be recorded. The result is dependent on the child's height. The formula below gives a rough guide to working out the expected peak flow for children longer than 110 cm:

Peak expiratory flow rate (PEFR) = 150 + 5 × (length of child in cm − 110).

Example: A child of 160 cm has an expected PEFR of 150 + 5 × (160 − 110) = 400.

Actual peak flows should be recorded as a percentage of the expected (Table 40.8).

The child should dealt with in a calm manner. Staff anxiety will be transmitted to the parent and then the child; this often makes the asthma worse. High-flow rate oxygen should be administered in all cases. There is little indication for routine chest radiographs. Chest radiographs should be reserved for first presentations, where genuine doubt exists about the diagnosis and where there is good reason to suspect a pneumothorax or a chest infection (chest pain, abnormal physical findings.) Arterial blood gases are not very useful, and are distressing for children. Pulse oximetry gives similar information non-invasively, but the initial assessment of asthma remains dependant on clinical skills. The algorithm shown in Figure 40.6 is widely used.

Children with mild asthma who are discharged should receive some form of follow-up. Inhaler technique should be checked in all children and their parents prior to discharge. Parents who bring

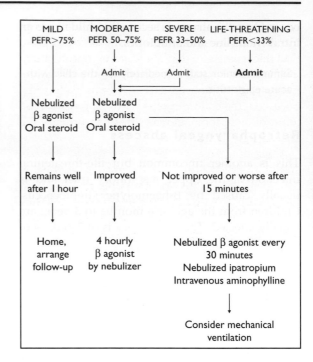

Figure 40.6: Asthma management algorithm.

their children to emergency departments at night with worsening asthma are often exceptionally worried: a cautious approach is recommended in these children and there should be a very low threshold for seeking admission.

Pertussis (whooping cough)

This is still seen despite vaccination programmes, as uptake of the vaccine has been suboptimal owing to misinformed concerns about safety. Vaccination does not provide complete protection and the disease should still be considered in a fully immunized child. The disease is caused by *Bordetella pertussis.* The illness is commoner in those over 3 years old, and more severe in those under 1 year. The child usually presents with coryzal symptoms, and develops a paroxysmal cough with an inspiratory whoop. A bout of coughing terminates with vomiting. The coughing bouts may be so violent as to induce intracranial and subconjunctival haemorrhages. Secondary bacterial infections can occur anywhere in the respiratory tract. Bronchiectasis is a late complication in a few children.

The illness has a characteristically prolonged course and most children are symptomatic for 4–8 weeks. Cases lasting up to a year are well recognized. The chest radiograph shows some bronchial wall thickening and may show some consolidation.

If the diagnosis is suspected, a swab should be taken from the pharynx. This is only likely to be positive if the child presents within 2 weeks of the onset of symptoms. Paired titres can provide the answer in equivocal cases.

Whooping cough is a notifiable disease. Antibiotics such as amoxycillin are of questionable benefit, although they are often prescribed early in the disease. Cough suppressants are of no value. Children under 6 months of age should be admitted to hospital, since good nursing care reduces complications. Older children probably do not need to come into hospital provided the parents are able to cope. A child with whooping cough is a considerable strain for their parents.

Inhaled foreign body

This important differential should be considered in the diagnosis of most cases of childhood respiratory disease. These cases constitute an emergency, since an inhaled foreign body is potentially life threatening and the majority occur in children under 5 years of age. A significant proportion present with no suggestive history. Peanuts, seeds and pieces of toys are commonly recovered. The most usual history is of an episode of choking and stridor, which resolves, the child then developing wheeze, or even pneumonia, a few days later. The diagnosis should also be considered in any child with croup who is not getting better after a few days.

The symptoms and signs will depend on the site of the obstruction. Stridor implies a foreign body in a main stem bronchus, the trachea, the oesophagus or the larynx. Unilateral wheeze implies that the foreign body is in the lower airways. The commonest site of obstruction is in the right main bronchus. Initial radiographs may be normal, although increased lung volume on the side of the obstruction may be seen, since a foreign body in the bronchus causes air trapping on expiration. Bilateral decubitus films show failure of the affected side to 'collapse down' when the affected side is inferior. Collapse distant to the obstruction may also be seen. Bronchoscopy is necessary and can be technically difficult in small airways.

Table 40.9: Causative organisms of pneumonia by age

Under 1 year	Streptococcus pneumoniae
	Staphylococcus
	Escherichia coli
	Chlamydia
Over 1 year	Streptococcus pneumoniae
	Mycoplasma

Secondary complications are common: pneumonitis is especially associated with aspirated peanuts.

Pneumonia

This remains common in younger children although the causative organisms vary with age (Table 40.9).

The onset of symptoms is usually acute, with coughing following coryzal symptoms. The child may also describe extrathoracic symptoms: for instance, lower lobe involvement can cause abdominal pain and upper lobe consolidation can cause neck stiffness. The child is usually febrile, tachypnoeic, and may have grunting respiration. Percussion reveals areas of dullness. Auscultation may reveal areas of bronchial breathing, although this may be difficult to demonstrate in small chests. A radiograph will show areas of consolidation, confirming the diagnosis.

Blood and sputum cultures should be taken. The patient may well need intravenous hydration if feeding has been a problem. If oxygen saturations are at all compromised supplemental oxygen should be administered. Broad-spectrum antibiotics and anti-staphylococcal antibiotics should be given to children under 1 year old. Gentamicin and flucloxacillin is a popular combination. Older children, where the cause is usually *Streptococcus pneumoniae*, can be treated with amoxycillin and erythromycin.

Acute bronchitis

This is common in children and is caused by a variety of viruses. It presents with a dry cough that becomes productive after a couple of days. There may be mild systemic upset, and a few scattered wheezes and crackles may be heard. There are no radiographic changes. Treatment, other than reassurance, is unnecessary since the child

Table 40.10: Causes of shock

Hypovolaemia:
    Haemorrhage
    Diarrhoea and vomiting
    Burns
    Peritonitis
    Diabetic ketoacidosis
Maldistributive:
    Sepsis
    Anaphylaxis
Obstructive:
    Tension pneumothorax
    Haemopneumothorax

Table 40.11: Causes of pupillary abnormalities

Small reactive pupils:
    Opiate poisoning
    Metabolic disorders
    Medullary lesions
Fixed mid-size pupils:
    Mid-brain lesion
Fixed dilated pupils:
    'Ecstasy' ingestion
    Hypothermia
    Barbiturates
    Hypoxia
    Tricyclic ingestion
Unilateral dilated pupil:
    Tentorial herniation
    Rapidly expanding ipsilateral intracranial lesion

recovers over approximately 1 week. Cough suppressants do not provide much relief.

SHOCKED CHILDREN

Shock is a clinical syndrome that results from inadequate tissue oxygenation. The commoner causes are listed in Table 40.10.

RESUSCITATION OF THE SHOCKED CHILD

Assessment of the shocked child should identify the signs described in the section on recognition of the sick child. It is also important to look at the fullness of the neck veins. Full neck veins in the presence of shock suggest a tension pneumothorax or primary cardiac cause of shock and indicate the need for a different approach. High-flow oxygen should be given in all cases and urgent intravenous or intraosseous access should be established. Blood or bone marrow aspirate should be taken for cross-match. A fluid bolus of $20\,\mathrm{ml\,kg}^{-1}$ of crystalloid should be given as quickly as possible. The child should then be reassessed to see if there has been a clinical improvement. Failure to improve indicates another $20\,\mathrm{ml\,kg}^{-1}$ bolus of crystalloid. The child should then be reassessed and an attempt made to find the underlying cause. Blood ($10\,\mathrm{ml\,kg}^{-1}$) may need to be given at this point. Cross-matching blood takes about an hour; however, type-specific blood is available much more quickly and O-negative blood can be obtained almost immediately.

A bedside glucose should be taken since hypoglycaemia can mimic many of the symptoms and signs of shock. Conversely, shock can cause hypoglycaemia in children.

THE UNCONSCIOUS CHILD

The initial priorities in coma are airway protection, breathing, and circulatory assessment and management. The next priority is a methodical assessment of the depth of the coma and a mini-neurological examination. A Glasgow Coma Scale (GCS) of less than 9 is an indication for intubation and ventilation, provided the child is clearly not postictal. The GCS has been adapted for use in children under the age of 4 years (Table 39.5). The reliability and sensitivity are improved by repeated observation by the same person. The pupils should also be examined (Table 40.11).

The presence or absence of neck stiffness (never stress the neck if there is any possibility of trauma) and the presence or absence of lateralizing signs should be sought. A doll's eye reflex is said to be absent when the eyes move with the child's head, or move randomly, when the head is rotated. The normal response is for the eyes to move away from the direction the head is rotated. Abnormality indicates brainstem dysfunction. A bedside glucose

Table 40.12: Causes of paediatric coma

Infections:
  Bacterial meningitis
  Encephalitis
Traumatic:
  Head injury
  Hypovolaemia
Hypoxia:
  Ischaemia following respiratory or circulatory
    failure
  Drowning
Metabolic:
  Hypoglycaemia
  Diabetic ketoacidosis
  Liver or renal failure
  Hyperammonaemia
  Porphyria
Poisoning:
  Opiates
  Ethanol
  Tricyclic antidepressants
  Benzodiazepines
  Barbiturates
  Iron
Neurological:
  Postictal
  Epileptic
  Vascular events

Table 40.13: Signs suggestive of raised intracranial pressure

Abnormal posture, either decerebrate or
  decorticate
Abnormal respiratory pattern
Unequal pupillary size and reactivity
Abnormal doll's eye reflexes
Papilloedema
Slow pulse, high blood pressure and abnormal
  respiration (Cushing's triad)

Table 40.14: Initial management of raised intracranial pressure

Raise the head of the bed to 30°
Ensure a neutral neck position
Ask an anaesthetist to intubate and ventilate the
  patient
Mannitol 0.5 g kg^{-1} should be given, and the
  bladder should be catheterized
Arrange an urgent CT scan of the head
Arrange a prompt expert opinion from a
  neurologist or neurosurgeon

RAISED INTRACRANIAL PRESSURE

In an unconscious child, where there is doubt about the cause of the coma, an attempt should be made to see if there is evidence of raised intracranial pressure. Unfortunately, all the clinical signs in Table 40.13 occur late. Confusion can occur with children who are postictal, although the history is usually helpful. Raised intracranial pressure usually results from head injuries, meningoencephalitis and hypoxia. Space-occupying lesions cause a slower rise in intracranial pressure and usually present less urgently.

If the diagnosis is suspected, it is vital to get expert help. General supportive measures should also be instituted (Table 40.14).

CONVULSING CHILDREN

Children often attend emergency departments with convulsions, although the convulsion may have stopped by the time the patient arrives at the department. Status epilepticus occurs when fitting

should be recorded. The child should be exposed and any rashes should be looked for. The head should be carefully examined for bruises and lacerations indicating trauma. The temperature should be measured and intravenous access should be established. The causes of paediatric coma are given in Table 40.12.

The treatment of the coma will depend on the underlying cause. Hypoglycaemia (capillary blood sugar less than 4 mmol l^{-1}) may be the underlying cause of the coma or a reflection of depleted liver glycogen stores from a severe physiological insult. Regardless of the cause of the hypoglycaemia, blood should be taken for a formal laboratory assay and 2 ml kg^{-1} of 25% dextrose should be infused. If there is any doubt about excluding meningitis or encephalitis as the cause of the coma, treatment with cefotaxime 100 mg kg^{-1} and aciclovir should be instituted. Blood cultures should be taken at this time.

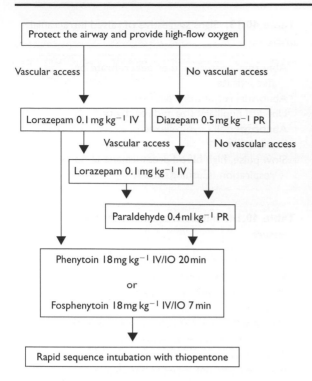

Figure 40.7: Management of status epilepticus.

does not stop, or there is incomplete recovery between fits for more than 20 min. Management is outlined in Figure 40.7.

Status epilepticus is a life-threatening emergency.

This protocol is designed for children over 1 month of age. If intravenous access is established immediately, two doses of lorazepam should be given 10 min apart, followed by phenytoin. Rectal paraldehyde is given whilst the phenytoin is being prepared. If intravenous access is not achieved, rectal diaezepam is given followed 5 min later by paraldehyde then, 10 min later, phenytoin. If intravenous access is established within 5 min of the administration of rectal diazepam, the intravenous pathway is followed from the second dose of lorazepam. If the child is already on oral phenytoin, the third step should be phenobarbitone ($15 \, mg \, kg^{-1}$).

Phenobarbitone with or without a benzodiazepine is most commonly used in children under 1 month of age pending definitive guidelines.

While the child is being stabilized as above, an attempt should be made to find the underlying cause (Table 40.15). An attempt should also be

Table 40.15: Common causes of status epilepticus

Febrile convulsions
Bacterial meningitis
Acute cerebral trauma
Idiopathic epilepsy
Sudden reduction in anti-epileptic medication in known epileptic
Poisoning, tricyclic antidepressants and carbamazepine

Table 40.16: Initial investigations in status epilepticus

Bedside glucose and formal laboratory glucose
Urea and electrolytes
Calcium and phosphate
Magnesium
Arterial blood gases
Full blood count

made to find out whether any injuries have occurred as a result of the fit. This requires a thorough history and examination and a few simple investigations (Table 40.16). It is important to remember that a paralysed child can continue to fit, and suffer adverse consequences as a result.

A fit that is uncontrolled for more than 1 h carries a substantial risk of neurological damage.

FEBRILE CONVULSIONS

Febrile convulsions are the commonest form of seizure in childhood. They are also a source of great alarm to parents, who will often seek urgent medical help. The current and generally accepted definition is a generalized seizure occurring between the age of 3 months and 5 years in a previously healthy and developmentally normal child in association with a fever, but without evidence of intracranial infection or defined cause. The fit will usually have stopped by the time the child presents to the emergency department. If the fit is ongoing, treatment should be instituted at once. The initial treatment of a febrile convulsion is no different from the emergency treatment of other seizures.

There are two main questions to be answered. First, is this a febrile convulsion, and second, what is the cause of the fever? It is essential to establish how long the fit lasted, although parental panic makes accurate time keeping unlikely. A complicated febrile convulsion is one that lasts 15 min or more, is focal, followed by a neurological deficit, or has repeated seizures within the same illness.

A family history of febrile convulsions is often obtained and febrile convulsions are recurrent in a third of children. The causes of febrile convulsions are not very different from those of simple fevers in children. The most frequent causes are upper respiratory tract infections, otitis media and tonsillitis.

Children with epilepsy are more likely to suffer fits when they have an intercurrent illness. This may be related to vomiting prophylactic medication or effects on the seizure threshold. Meningitis, encephalitis and septicaemia are important differential diagnoses. These occasionally present with convulsions.

The parents of a fitting child are often very upset and will require appropriate explanation and reassurance. They should be told that their child does not have epilepsy or a life-threatening disease. The prognosis is usually excellent. Measures to reduce the fever should be instituted, although whether this reduces further convulsions is debatable. Paracetamol should be given and tepid sponging and a fan may be useful.

In the UK children are usually admitted to hospital, although the need for this is again debatable. Children under 18 months usually receive a lumbar puncture to exclude meningitis; older children are usually observed.

THE HOT AND FEVERISH CHILD

The definition of what constitutes a fever is controversial, and there seems to be little agreement among authorities. For practical purposes, a fever is said to be present if the:

- rectal or tympanic temperature is greater than 38.3°C (if there is active ear inflammation the temperature taken here will be spuriously high)
- oral temperature is greater than 37.8°C
- axillary temperature is greater than 37.0°C.

Young children are frequently brought to emergency departments with fevers and the complaint of being 'generally unwell'. Happily, the majority of these children have minor self-limiting illness.

In a minority of cases the fever is a feature of a severe, life-threatening illness. Every child with a fever should therefore be assessed carefully and systematically. The term 'pyrexia of unknown origin' is defined as a fever that persists for more than a week, and in which routine investigations reveal no cause. The term is widely and wrongly used to describe children with acute fevers in which no cause is immediately apparent.

HISTORY AND EXAMINATION

The age of the child is important. Children under 3 months old are notoriously difficult to assess (no social smile, limited interaction) and a cautious approach is recommended.

Infants are difficult to assess and there should be a low threshold for admission for observation.

Children under the age of 2 years, but older than 3 months, are easier to evaluate since their interaction is developing. A smiling, playful and interactive child is probably not seriously unwell. Signs of meningism such as Kernig's and Brudzinski's signs may not appear in children under 2 years old. Older children become progressively easier to assess.

The history should cover the presenting complaint. How long has the child been unwell; how unwell is the child? Clues to the state of the child should include:

- feeding: less than half the usual feed in the preceding 24 h is a worrying symptom
- abnormal cries or high-pitched moans
- abnormally quiet or listless
- fewer than four wet nappies in the preceding 24 h.

It is also important to ask about other family members and to try to find localizing symptoms. Fever of any cause leads to vasodilatation, which in turn causes headache. Distinguishing benign headaches from those of meningitis may be very difficult. Urinary tract infections localize poorly and may only be picked up by culture of the urine. Ear infections also localize poorly in young children, although abnormal head movements may provide a clue.

In examining a child, particular attention should be paid to rashes, the throat and the ears

Table 40.17: Common causes of childhood fever

Otitis media
Pharyngitis and tonsillitis
Coryza
Bronchiolitis
Gastroenteritis
Urinary tract infections
Viral exanthemata:
    Measles
    Mumps
    Rubella
    Fifth disease
    Roseola infantum
    Chicken pox

Table 40.18: Significant rarer causes of fever

Meningitis
Septicaemia
Bacterial pneumonia
Appendicitis
Septic arthritis
Osteomyelitis
Epiglottitis
Retropharyngeal abscess

and to signs of meningism. Blood tests are often not necessary although urine dip-stick and culture is very useful and should be performed whenever a child has an unexplained fever. A chest radiograph is not routinely indicated unless the child is breathless or has suggestive signs.

TREATMENT

Fever in itself is not dangerous, and may be beneficial for the immune response. Apart from febrile convulsions, there are no complications of fever. However, children seem much more comfortable when their fever is reduced. Paracetamol is widely given for this and is very effective. Tepid sponging and fans are also widely used but hypothermia must be avoided.

The commonest (Table 40.17) and 'important not to miss' (Table 40.18) causes of childhood fevers are listed below. These lists are not comprehensive, since many diseases can cause fevers.

Gastroenteritis and bronchiolitis are dealt with in more detail elsewhere in this chapter.

OTITIS MEDIA

This is usually caused by a haemolytic streptococcus, *Staphylococcus aureus* or *Haemophilus influenzae*. The child will present with earache that is often severe and may wake the child from sleep. There may be a history of a preceding upper respiratory tract infection. The child or parent may volunteer that the pain lessened after noting some discharge in the ear canal, which implies that the tympanic membrane has burst. Younger children may not localize symptoms to the ear. They may only present with fever, vomiting and generally off colour, the diagnosis becoming clear after examining the ears. Examination may reveal a yellow tympanic membrane (indicating pus) and dilated vessels over the surface of the drum; later the drum becomes red. Otitis externa is uncommon in children, and is usually secondary to an underlying otitis media.

Oral amoxycillin for 10 days, with paracetamol and pseudoephedrine (a systemic decongestant), usually effects a cure. Chronic discharge implies a complication, such as acute mastoiditis, which should be referred to an ear, nose and throat surgeon.

PHARYNGITIS AND TONSILLITIS

These are considered together, since they represent opposing ends of a spectrum of disease. The majority of cases are caused by viruses. Only rarely are these conditions caused by group A beta-haemolytic streptococci. Presentation is usually with a fever and a sore throat, although earache is also common. An exudate occurs with both viral and bacterial infections. Antibiotics should probably not be administered since the majority of cases are viral in origin.

CORYZA

The common cold causes fever in children and should be suspected where multiple family members are affected. Parents should not receive antibiotics for their children. They should be advised that cold remedies are unlikely to do much good and that the disease can last up to 2 weeks. Fluids and paracetamol provide symptomatic relief.

URINARY TRACT INFECTIONS

These are commoner in girls than boys except in the neonatal period. Neonates and infants localize symptoms very poorly to the urinary tract and fever may be absent in younger children. The symptoms of frequency and dysuria are irrelevant in younger children. Normal bowel flora cause most infections, particularly *E. coli*. Diagnosis can only be made by culture of properly collected urine. Urine dip-stick may be normal even with pronounced infection; conversely, haematuria and proteinuria only indicate the need for further investigation.

Methods of urine collection

Prior to collection the genital area should be cleaned with normal saline. A mid-stream urine collection indicates infection if a single growth of greater than 100 000 bacteria ml^{-1} occurs. Less than 10 000 bacteria indicates sterile urine; a mixed growth implies contamination.

Suprapubic aspiration is safe and effective. It is indicated in children who are under 2 years old and who have not voided urine for 1 h. A syringe is connected to a 23 gauge needle, this is passed vertically just above the symphysis pubis. Constant aspiration is performed. Any growth indicates infection and the need for treatment.

Children with urinary tract infections are usually treated with trimethoprim or amoxycillin, but local advice should be followed. Although many children with urinary tract infections are not unwell, they must be investigated for urinary tract abnormalities. It is for this reason that most children are referred from the emergency department to paediatricians.

VIRAL EXANTHEMS

These diseases are less common in the UK since widespread vaccination was introduced. Cases are

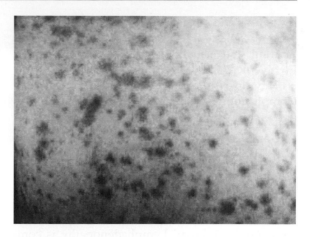

Figure 40.8: The rash of measles.

still seen, and it is important to be able to recognize them. In particular, measles, mumps, rubella and scarlet fever are notifiable diseases. If a case is seen then a report should be sent to the Communicable Disease Surveillance Centre.

Measles (Fig. 40.8)

A fever is the earliest sign. A runny nose and sore throat follow, with a hacking cough, and bilateral conjunctivitis develops. Koplik's spots, small white lesions on the buccal mucosa, develop before the rash. The rash develops 2–3 days after the onset of symptoms, is maculopapular and involves the whole body. The rash heals by desquamation. The child will be unwell for about a week.

The diagnosis is usually made clinically. Since most cases are self-limiting and highly contagious, children do not usually require admission. However, measles can be devastating if there is any immunosuppression. In these cases expert advice should be obtained.

Secondary bacterial infections are common, the middle ear being the commonest target, and amoxycillin usually covers the infecting agents. Encephalitis affects one in 1000 children with measles and should be suspected when there is a reduced level of consciousness and neurological findings.

Mumps

Initially there is a fever. The parotid glands swell and are tender on mastication. Bitter fluids stimulate the glands and also cause pain. The child is listless, with myalgia and a headache. The illness is self-limiting and usually lasts 7–10 days. Gonadal involvement is rare in children.

The disease requires no specific treatment. Complications are rare, but include pancreatitis and orchitis.

Rubella

A macular rash is the commonest early sign of rubella. This starts on the face and spreads to involve the trunk and limbs. Systemic upset is less common in children. Lymphadenopathy is common, particularly at the postauricular lymph node. The illness is self-limiting and usually requires no active treatment.

Arthritis is common and self-limiting, particularly in girls. There are devastating effects on fetal development and it is important to ascertain whether the mother of an affected child is pregnant. The fetus is most vulnerable in the first trimester. If there is good reason to suspect the mother to be pregnant, blood should be taken from the mother for IgM antibodies to rubella and the mother should receive an appointment to see an obstetrician in 10 days. Rising titres indicate infection, often subclinical, and a termination of pregnancy may be offered. A previous history of rubella exposure does not, unfortunately, carry lifelong immunity.

Fifth disease (slapped cheeks syndrome, erythema infectiosum)

This occurs in epidemics and presents with fever, malaise and arthralgia. There is a characteristic rash over the cheeks and a reticular rash on the limbs. In most children it is of little significance, but in children with abnormal red blood cell production (hereditary spherocytosis and sickle cell disease), the illness can cause a profound anaemia and transfusion may be necessary.

Exanthema subitum (roseola infantum, fourth disease)

This is caused by human herpes virus 6 and affects children from the age of 6–18 months. A high fever, irritability and runny nose precede the development

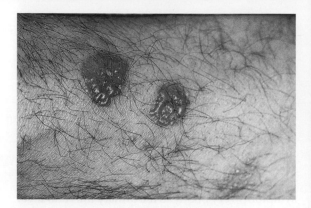

Figure 40.9: Rash of varicella infection.

of a macular rash. The fever resolves at the time the rash appears and this is characteristic. Complete recovery is the rule, and complications almost never occur.

Chicken pox (varicella)

The fever precedes the rash by a couple of days. The small red spots rapidly become fluid-filled vesicles. The vesicles are surrounded by a small area of erythema and are intensely itchy. Crusting subsequently develops (Fig. 40.9).

Children are usually well with chicken pox and scratching can be reduced by calamine lotion. Scratching increases the risk of secondary infection, usually staphylococcal, and of scarring. Cutting fingernails short is also helpful. Encephalitis occurs once in 1000 cases and is particularly associated with cerebellar signs. Most cases resolve well.

Chicken pox pneumonia is uncommon in children. If the diagnosis is suspected in an immuno-compromised patient, the child should be admitted for intravenous aciclovir.

BACTERIAL MENINGITIS AND MENINGOCAEMIA

Meningitis is an important cause of death in children. Around 2000 cases are reported annually in the UK in children, of whom 200 die.

Meningitis is caused by a variety of organisms. Neonates are susceptible to different organisms from older children (*E. coli*, *Listeria monocytogenes*,

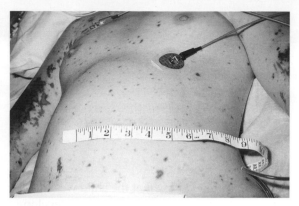

Figure 40.10: Rash of meningococcal septicaemia.

Table 40.19: Symptoms of meningococcal infection

Headache
Persistent vomiting
Abnormal high-pitched cry
Myalgia
Seizures
Abdominal pain

Table 40.20: Signs of meningococcal infection

Meningeal:
Stiff neck (the child can not kiss their knee)
Photophobia
Kernig's sign (resistance on extending the knee with the hip fully flexed)
Brudzinski's sign (flexing the neck causes the hips to flex)
Toxic:
Purpuric rash, though initially this may be even urticarial
Fever
Shock
Raised intracranial pressure
Focal neurological deficits
Seizures
Tachycardia

group B haemolytic streptococci). Outside the neonatal period, *Neisseria meningitidis, Streptococcus pneumoniae* and *Haemophilus influenzae* are the commonest causes of disease. The introduction of a vaccine has reduced the incidence of *Haemophilus influenzae* meningitis. Streptococcal disease is often associated with respiratory tract infections, skull fractures and neural tube defects.

Neisseria meningitidis is the most feared of the organisms causing meningitis. It can also cause a form of septic shock, meningococcal septicaemia, with a classic rash (Fig. 40.10). Meningococcal meningitis and septicaemia are not different conditions but extremes of a spectrum caused by one illness. Either can occur separately; a normal lumbar puncture can be obtained in the presence of meningococcal septicaemia.

A high index of suspicion should be maintained (Tables 40.19 and 40.20). The younger a child is the more non-specific the presenting symptoms may be and the more difficult signs may be to elicit. In particular, children under 4 years do not present with the classic symptoms and signs.

> Young children do not manifest the classic symptoms and signs of meningococcal infection.

Tragically, early symptoms and signs of meningococcal disease are often overlooked by parents and doctors alike until the diagnosis becomes obvious. Because it is a rare disease and trivial viral infections are exceptionally common this is not surprising. The risk of missing the disease is minimized by always undressing a febrile child and having a careful look for the rash and signs of poor tissue perfusion, such as prolonged capillary refill and tachycardia.

Senior emergency and paediatric staff must be involved early. Blind treatment with parenteral antibiotics should be instituted as soon as the diagnosis is suspected. Benzyl penicillin ($50\,\text{mg}\,\text{kg}^{-1}$) should be given by slow intravenous injection (there is a risk of convulsions with fast injections) together with $100\,\text{mg}\,\text{kg}^{-1}$ of cefotaxime. If intravenous access proves impossible, then the drugs should be given intramuscularly. If there is good reason to suspect penicillin allergy, intravenous erythromycin and cefotaxime should be used.

If there is any evidence of poor perfusion, intravenous fluids $20\,\text{ml}\,\text{kg}^{-1}$ should be given as a bolus and the child reasssessed. Blind treatment with dexamethasone ($0.15\,\text{mg}\,\text{kg}^{-1}$) has been shown to improve outcome in cases of *Haemophilus influenzae* meningitis, although this is now less common as a cause of meningitis. If there is rapid neurological deterioration and evidence of raised intracranial pressure (falling conscious level and a full fontanelle) the child should be nursed head-up at 30° and receive intravenous mannitol. The child should then be ventilated and transferred to a paediatric intensive care unit.

Lumbar punctures are potentially dangerous in acute meningitis and do not alter management of the acute resuscitation. Useful information about the causative organism can be obtained by blood cultures and a throat swab. Polymerase chain reaction (PCR) is also being used to detect organisms in doubtful cases. A clotting screen is useful since disseminated intravascular coagulation is common. CT scanning should only be performed if the child is well enough, when it is useful to demonstrate raised intracranial pressure and subdural effusions.

Many cases of meningitis appear to be suboptimally managed. Confusion with other diagnoses is common, resulting in delayed antibiotic treatment. If the cause of a small child's febrile illness is not clear, admission or observation are usually warranted. Shock is often underestimated and inadequately treated.

THE POISONED CHILD

Accidental poisoning is common in young children, who are naturally curious. Older children may deliberately take poisons or overdoses. Rarely, children can be poisoned as a form of abuse and in these cases the history may be misleading. The majority of accidental poisonings are preventable by simple safety measures and parent education. The poisons taken by children differ from those taken by adults and the management of childhood poisoning differs from that in adults.

The emergency department doctor can be confronted by an extremely wide range of potential poisons. It is unrealistic to expect a detailed knowledge of each poison. If there is any doubt, advice should be sought from a poisons unit or the Toxbase service. As full a history as possible should be given. The advice that these units give errs on the side of caution. Assessment of these children is similar to that of adults (Table 40.21).

Most poisoned children do not have abnormal physical findings on initial examination. However, a full examination must be performed and the findings documented. It is very useful for the

Table 40.21: Paediatric poisoning history

When was the poison taken?
How much was taken?
Were any other drugs taken?
Has there been any vomiting?
Is there any past medical history?
If the overdose is deliberate, attempt to find out why this happened

receiving team to know that the child was initially clinically normal should complications develop.

There are general and specific measures in treating poisoned children. Gastric lavage is rarely indicated in children (but see below). The diameter of the tube that can be passed into a child's stomach is too small to retrieve most swallowed tablets. Induced vomiting with ipecacuanha has been demonstrated to have no benefit. Activated charcoal is widely prescribed. It does reduce the absorption of most drugs, but certainly not all. A poisons centre should be contacted for advice.

Gastric emptying is rarely indicated for poisoned children.

It is appropriate to have some in-depth knowledge about the commoner childhood poisons.

IRON

This causes gastric haemorrhage, which may be severe. Later, iron disrupts cellular metabolism and causes third-space pooling. Shock occurs from hypovolaemia and lactic acidosis results. Late complications include small bowel scarring causing obstruction.

A child who has been asymptomatic for 8 h and is normal on physical examination can usually be sent home. Symptoms of abdominal pain, melaena, vomiting and haematemesis should be sought. If any of these symptoms are found, desferrioxamine ($30\,\mathrm{mg\,kg^{-1}}$) should be given intramuscularly as soon as possible. An abdominal radiograph will show the radio-opaque tablets and may confirm the diagnosis in doubtful cases. Unfortunately, a normal radiograph does not exclude the diagnosis. Gastric lavage may be necessary and $10\,\mathrm{g}$ of desferrioxamine should be left in the stomach. An intravenous desferrioxamine infusion should be started. Intravenous fluids should be started if there is any evidence of hypoperfusion. Blood should be taken for serum iron, although treatment should be based on symptoms and not levels. Assays of iron are extremely unreliable in acute poisoning.

CAUSTIC SODA

This is used as a cleaning agent. It is commonly used in dishwasher powders and tablets. It is important because even small amounts have the ability to cause oesophageal strictures. Children should be given as much milk as they can drink. Gastric lavage and forced vomiting are contraindicated, since this can compound the oesophageal damage. The child should be referred to the surgeons, since oesophagoscopy is usually necessary.

THE VOMITING CHILD

Children are commonly brought to emergency departments with vomiting. There are a number of questions that the doctor should attempt to answer while assessing the child:

- What do the parents mean by vomiting? A detailed description of the vomitus and its frequency is important.
- Is the vomiting bile stained? (Bile-stained vomiting is rarely benign in origin.)
- Is the cause of the vomiting intra-abdominal or extra-abdominal?
- Is there a self-limiting condition present, such as gastro-oesophageal reflux, or a potentially fatal condition, such as appendicitis?

The list given in Table 40.22 shows some of the conditions that may initially present with vomiting. This list is far from comprehensive but illustrates the difficulty in reaching an early, accurate diagnosis. If a young child has unexplained, persistent vomiting it is sensible to admit the child until the symptoms have resolved or the diagnosis evolves.

The extra-abdominal causes are not discussed further here.

Table 40.22: Causes of vomiting

Extra-abdominal:
  Hydrocephalus
  Subdural haematoma
  Renal failure
  Congenital adrenal hyperplasia
  Addison's disease
  Diabetic ketoacidosis

Intra-abdominal:
  Gastroenteritis
  Simple possetting
  Urinary tract infections
  Gastro-oesophageal reflux
  Appendicitis
  Intussusception
  Pyloric stenosis
  Malrotation with or without volvulus
  Strangulated inguinal hernia
  Iron overdose

GASTROENTERITIS

This is extremely common in children. In the less developed world it is a major cause of childhood death. The illness is usually caused by viruses in infants, especially rotavirus. Older children often have a bacterial infection such as *Shigella*, *Campylobacter* or *E. coli*. The vomiting often begins before the diarrhoea and a coryzal illness often accompanies the illness. There is often colicky abdominal pain and febrile convulsions may occur as there is usually a rapid rise in body temperature. There are a number of instances where a more cautious approach to management and admission is justified (Table 40.23).

The diagnosis is usually clear cut and infants are at most risk. The degree of dehydration should be estimated. Weighing infants is useful, especially if the child's weight before the illness is known. Table 40.24 gives a good guide to assessing the hydration of a child and is in wide clinical use.

If a child has any signs of moderate or severe dehydration, they should be admitted to hospital. In contrast to adults, who are often placed on an intravenous infusion, the purpose of admitting children is to provide close observation and regular feeding. Children with losses of up to 10% of their body weight can be successfully managed by oral rehydration therapy.

Table 40.23: Factors indicating admission in the vomiting child

Dehydration
Children under 1 month of age
Immunodeficent children
Major organ disease
Symptoms lasting more than 10 days
Vomiting without diarrhoea suggests an alternative diagnosis

Table 40.24: Clinical indices for estimating degree of dehydration

Mild dehydration:
   5% body weight loss
   Prolonged capillary refill time (>2 s)
   Thirsty, alert, irritable, restless
   Increased respiratory rate

Moderate dehydration:
   6–9% body weight loss
   Thirsty, lethargic, irritable
   Tachycardia, normal blood pressure
   Sunken fontanelles and eyes
   Pinched skin retracts slowly

Severe dehydration:
   More than 10% body weight lost
   Drowsy, comatose, cold, sweaty
   Tachycardia, feeble pulse, blood pressure may fall

Losses of greater than 15% are usually fatal

The fluid replaced should ideally be isotonic. Colas, apple juices, sports beverages and chicken soups are unsuitable. Oral rehydration mixtures are good, but many babies find them unpalatable. Breast-feeding should continue during the illness whenever possible. Even if there is extensive vomiting, some milk will be absorbed. The provision of maternal antibodies is also helpful. Nasogastric feeding is occasionally necessary.

Children who are severely dehydrated, with losses of greater than 10%, require urgent intravenous resuscitation. An initial bolus of $20\,ml\,kg^{-1}$ (of the child's expected premorbid weight) should be given and the child reassessed. A further bolus of $20\,ml\,kg^{-1}$ may be necessary. The commonest mistake is not to give enough fluid.

SIMPLE POSSETTING

This is often a worrying symptom for new mothers. The baby is systemically well but has small-volume milky vomits between feeds. The baby will grow out of this, although giving thicker feeds and feeding with the child in a more upright position may help.

GASTRO-OESOPHAGEAL REFLUX

This is also common in childhood and is characterized by large-volume vomits with neck posturing between feeds. It may be so severe as to cause failure to thrive, iron-deficiency anaemia and aspiration pneumonia. If the diagnosis is suspected the child should be referred to an out-patient clinic.

APPENDICITIS

This is the commonest childhood surgical emergency. The diagnosis is often less straightforward than in adults. It should be considered in all children with vomiting, abdominal pain, fever, irritability and anorexia. A child who tells you that he or she is hungry and can happily list all his or her favourite foods almost certainly does not have appendicitis. Mesenteric adenitis and urinary tract infections are common differential diagnoses. The presence of pyuria or the features of upper respiratory tract infection does not exclude appendicitis.

INTUSSUSCEPTION

This usually occurs in children from 6 to 9 months old. A segment of bowel 'auto telescopes' distally. The waves of peristalsis propel this segment of bowel on and an obstruction occurs. The baby presents with vomiting, intermittent pain and crying, and the passage of blood-stained stools. The stools have been described in the past as looking like redcurrant jelly. A sausage-shaped mass may be palpated in the right upper quadrant.

Fever and peritonism indicate that urgent operative involvement is necessary as a result of strangulation.

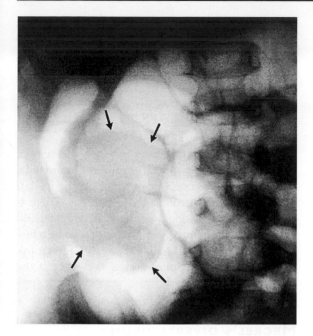

Figure 40.11: Abdominal X-ray of a child with intussusception.

An abdominal radiograph shows small bowel obstruction, absent gas in the ascending colon and a characteristic gas shadow at the apex of the intussusception (Fig. 40.11). These children require an urgent nasogastric tube to relieve vomiting. They should be referred to the surgical team. Unwell children require a laparotomy; other children can be managed by gas insufflation by a radiologist.

PYLORIC STENOSIS

This usually presents in babies in the first 6 weeks of life. The pyloric canal narrows, for reasons that are not clear. This causes an obstruction and spectacular projectile vomiting. The vomiting is never bile-stained since the obstruction is high. The child is usually hungry and diarrhoea does not occur. A mass may be felt in the epigastrium, and peristalsis may be visible. An ultrasound scan after a test feed is useful in doubtful cases. These children should be resuscitated with fluids before operation, since prolonged vomiting causes hypochloraemic alkalosis. A Ramstedt's pyloroplasty is curative.

MALROTATION AND VOLVULUS

This is rare but important, since prompt treatment prevents the mid-gut becoming gangrenous. It usually presents within the first year of life. Bilious vomiting with constant abdominal pain and streaks of blood in the stool is the commonest presentation. The abdomen may or may not be distended. A radiograph shows small bowel obstruction and a loop of bowel may be seen between the liver and the diaphragm. These children require a nasogastric tube, intravenous fluids and operative intervention.

INCARCERATED INGUINAL HERNIA

These occur in children, usually in the first year of life. The diagnosis is usually straightforward provided the possibility is considered. The hernial orifices should be examined in every child with poor feeding and vomiting. The majority of these cases can be gently reduced manually. A small proportion will require an emergency operation.

ACUTE DIARRHOEA

Breast-fed children normally pass liquid faeces. The commonest cause of diarrhoea is gastroenteritis. Assessment should aim to determine the state of hydration of the child. Other causes of diarrhoea are usually chronic, such as coeliac disease, and should be investigated on an out-patient basis.

ABDOMINAL PAIN IN CHILDHOOD

There are many causes of abdominal pain in childhood. Assessment should answer the following questions:

- Is the source of the pain in the abdomen or elsewhere?
- Is the child acutely unwell?
- Is there a surgical or medical cause for the pain?

A differential diagnosis is shown in Table 40.25.

INFANTILE COLIC

This occurs in children in the first few weeks of life. The cause is unknown. The parents are alarmed by a child who has sudden episodes of screaming, flexing the hips and distress. These episodes are not accompanied by vomiting, diarrhoea or constitutional upset. The child gains weight normally. The condition has a benign, self-limiting outcome.

MESENTERIC ADENITIS

The importance of this disorder is its similarity in presentation to appendicitis. Following a viral infection swollen, reactive lymph nodes cause right iliac fossa pain. A pyrexia is common. Palpable lymph nodes elsewhere suggest the diagnosis. The distinction from appendicitis is very difficult and a period of observation is recommended. Appendectomy may be necessary in doubtful cases.

LOWER LOBAR PNEUMONIA

This is a well-recognized cause of abdominal pain in children. Involvement of the lower lobes causes pain to be referred to the abdomen. A cough and

Table 40.25: Causes of abdominal pain in a child

Surgical:
Appendicitis
Intussusception
Volvulus
Torsion of the testes
Meckel's diverticulum
Medical:
Mesenteric adenitis
Urinary tract infection
Lower lobar pneumonia
Meningococcal septicaemia
Henoch–Schönlein purpura
Diabetic ketoacidosis
Sickle cell disease
Miscellaneous:
Constipation
Infantile colic
Munchausen's by proxy

shortness of breath are usually present, but this information may not be volunteered. Signs may be slight although a chest radiograph confirms the diagnosis.

TORSION OF THE TESTIS

This most commonly occurs between the ages of 15 and 30 years; however, it can occur at any age. The boy usually complains of pain in the ipsilateral iliac fossa, or around the umbilicus. There is usually extreme testicular tenderness and the child may walk with a limp. Vomiting may also be a feature. Epididymo-orchitis is rare in this age group. Urgent urological exploration is necessary if the testis is not to be lost.

MECKEL'S DIVERTICULUM

Meckel's diverticulitis can result in symptoms and signs identical to those of appendicitis. The diagnosis is usually made at operation. Bleeding can also occur from the diverticulum and usually occurs in children under 2 years of age.

HENOCH–SCHÖNLEIN PURPURA

This is a type III hypersensitivity reaction that occurs after an upper respiratory tract infection. A petechial or purpuric rash is characteristically seen over the lower limbs and the buttocks. There is arthralgia, and variable abdominal pain. Haematuria should be sought. The disease is usually benign, but a minority develop chronic renal failure and so these children should be followed up. The main differential diagnosis is meningococcal disease. If there is any doubt about the diagnosis, the child should be treated for meningitis until the diagnosis can be refuted.

RECTAL BLEEDING

This is a source of great alarm to many parents. Assessment should aim to identify children who need resuscitation, and make a provisional diagnosis. The causes are different from those in adults (Table 40.26). Although most cases result from constipation, the importance of the other diagnoses means that referral is usually warranted.

DIABETIC EMERGENCIES

DIABETIC KETOACIDOSIS (DKA)

This is common in childhood, either as a primary presenting event of diabetes mellitus or as a consequence of poor diabetic control. The clinical features (Table 40.27) are not very different from those of the adult. The diagnosis is not hard to make provided the possibility is considered. Liberal use of bedside glucose sticks is recommended.

A high blood glucose and ketones in the urine usually confirm clinical suspicion. The principles of management do not differ from adult practice:

- The child's airway should be protected by lying the child in the recovery position. The airway is potentially compromised by a reduced conscious level and vomiting. A nasogastric tube should be considered to decompress the stomach.
- Intravenous hydration. The child should be weighed and vascular access should be

Table 40.26: Causes of rectal bleeding in a child

Constipation
Meckel's diverticulum
Intussusception
Necrotizing enterocolitis (in neonates only)
Gastroenteritis (particularly *Campylobacter*)
Inflammatory bowel disease
Iron poisoning

Table 40.27: Clinical features of diabetic ketoacidosis

Vomiting
Drowsiness
Polyuria
Polydipsia
Breathlessness
Weight loss
Abdominal pain

established. Normal saline is the initial fluid of choice.

- Short-acting insulin should be given through an infusion pump. Intravenous boluses should be avoided.
- Underlying causes, such as an infection, should be sought.
- Urine output should be monitored, possibly by using a urinary catheter.

Most hospitals have local protocols for calculating fluid requirements and these should be followed. Table 40.28 is a useful guide in the absence of clear guidelines.

The degree of dehydration should be estimated clinically (see Table 40.24) and the fluid deficit calculated. The sum of the maintenance fluid and the fluid deficit is the fluid requirement. A third of the fluid requirement should be given in the first 4 h (Table 40.29).

HYPOGLYCAEMIA

Hypoglycaemia is usually the result of over-treatment of diabetes. As described in the section on coma, $2 \, \text{ml} \, \text{kg}^{-1}$ of 25% dextrose should be infused intravenously. If vascular access is impossible, glucagon 0.5–1 mg intramuscularly should be given. Once the acute episode of hypoglcaemia has resolved, an attempt should be made to find the cause of the event.

ANAPHYLAXIS

Anaphylaxis is an increasing problem in the allergy-prone western world. Anaphylaxis implies an IgE-mediated hypersensitivity reaction, whereas anaphylactoid reactions do not require hypersensitivity but are otherwise similar. In clinical practice, the distinction is of little relevance during the acute resuscitative phase.

The diagnosis is often less easy to make in children (Table 40.30) than in adults since children may not as readily exhibit classic clinical features. There is usually a rapid onset following exposure to an allergen. Peanuts, penicillins and insect stings are common culprits. Occasionally, a delay of a couple hours between exposure and

Table 40.28: Calculated maintenance fluid requirements for a child with diabetic ketoacidosis

Body weight	Fluid requirement day^{-1}	Fluid requirement h^{-1}
First 10 kg	100 ml kg^{-1}	4 ml kg^{-1}
Second 10 kg	50 ml kg^{-1}	2 ml kg^{-1}
Subsequent kg	20 ml kg^{-1}	1 ml kg^{-1}

Table 40.29: Worked example of fluid requirements in diabetic ketoacidosis

A child normally weighing 12 kg in diabetic ketoacidosis is 5% dehydrated.	
The maintenance fluid requirement is	$1000 + 100 = 1100$ ml day^{-1}
The fluid deficit is	$12000 \times 0.05 = 600$ ml
The fluid requirement is	1700 ml day^{-1}
In the first 4 h	560 ml should be given

Table 40.30: Clinical features of anaphylaxis

Angio-oedema
Urticaria
Stridor
Dyspnoea
Hypotension
Asthma
Rhinitis
Conjunctivitis
Abdominal pain
Vomiting
Diarrhoea
Agitation

Table 40.31: Management of anaphylactic shock

Discontinue causative agent (e.g. drug/blood)
Open and maintain airway
Give oxygen 100% via Hudson mask
If bronchoconstriction occurs give salbutamol 5 mg nebulized in oxygen
Obtain intravenous access
Titrate intravenous adrenaline 0.5–1 mg aliquots of 1/10 000 solution response to life-threatening symptoms
If IV access not available give 0.5 mg adrenaline IM
Repeat IM adrenaline if intravenous access not obtained and there is no clinical improvement
Give an antihistamine, e.g. chlorpheniramine 10 mg slow injection
Give intravenous fluid to correct hypotension
Administer steroids (hydrocortisone 200 mg IV)
Admit for observation

Beware of biphasic reactions: observe closely

the onset of symptoms makes the diagnosis difficult. A biphasic reaction is uncommon but well described.

Treatment of anaphylaxis should be commenced when there is a compatible history of severe allergic-type reaction with respiratory difficulty, with or without hypotension. Local protocols should be followed. Table 40.31 gives an outline of the management. Senior assistance is essential.

After initial resuscitation and stabilization, the patient should be admitted and observed for a biphasic reaction. Ten millilitres of clotted blood should be drawn within 6 h of an attack for mast-cell tryptase levels. Further assessment by an immunologist is recommended.

DROWNING AND NEAR DROWNING

Drowning is tragically common. Ponds and swimming pools mix poorly with unsupervised toddlers. Forty per cent of drownings occur in those under 4 years old. 'Dry drowning' occurs when laryngeal spasm and glottic closure prevent water aspiration but cause profound hypoxaemia. Fresh- and salt-water aspiration removes surfactant from the lung, resulting in atelectasis and stiff non-compliant lungs. Involuntary swallowing of large volumes of water can cause gastric dilatation and aspiration. The distinction between fresh- and saltwater drowning is of limited clinical significance, despite the different pathological changes.

MANAGEMENT

The history should take into account the length and mechanism of the immersion, and the possibility of coexistent trauma such as a spinal fracture or head injury. In older children the possibility of drug and alcohol intoxication should be considered. If the child is pulseless, standard CPR should be instituted as described earlier in the chapter. The prognosis of cardiac arrest following drowning is poor, although case reports suggest complete recovery is possible following a prolonged immersion in cold water. If a pulse is present, urgent assessment of the conscious level and temperature is required. Hypothermia is often associated and may be protective.

Unconscious patients usually require intubation of the airway with intermittent positive-pressure ventilation. A bronchoscopy is required if aspiration and soiling of the airway is considered possible. The stomach should be decompressed with a nasogastric tube. Hypothermia should be treated aggressively if present, and anticipated if absent.

Conscious patients require treatment with high-flow oxygen through a non-rebreathing bag. The presence of cough, wheeze or dyspnoea implies aspiration. A chest X-ray may show pulmonary oedema or perihilar infiltrates. Arterial blood gases are not always necessary, but may demonstrate hypoxaemia.

Children who are admitted in an unconscious state after a submersion usually do well. Most children who are admitted unconscious with reactive pupils recover fully. A third of children with fixed dilated pupils also recover fully. Neurological deficits are common in those who have fixed dilated pupils at 6 h.

FURTHER READING

Advanced Life Support Group (2000) *Advanced Paediatric Life Support*. BMJ, London.
Strange, G., Schafermayer, R., Lelyveld, S. *et al.* (1995) *Pediatric Emergency Medicine. A Comprehensive Study Guide*. Mcgraw Hill, New York.

PART TEN

PRE-HOSPITAL CARE

IMMEDIATE CARE

INTRODUCTION

Immediate care, defined as the provision of skilled medical help in the prehospital setting, is currently provided by a variety of organizations in the UK. These range from general practice-based schemes, particularly in rural areas, to designated teams from emergency departments. In many centres where there is no dedicated emergency team, individual staff members are asked to respond to prehospital incidents on an *ad hoc* basis.

The first national organization of immediate care practitioners was created in 1977 with the formation of the British Association for Immediate Care (BASICS). This association became the centre of integration of the various immediate care schemes in operation with the local ambulance services. In 1995 the Royal College of Surgeons of Edinburgh founded the Faculty of Pre-hospital Care with the aim of setting and maintaining standards of practice in immediate care. This is achieved by the promotion of education, teaching and research in immediate care, and there are several courses offered by the Faculty for paramedics, nurses and doctors.

IMMEDIATE CARE PROVIDERS

The provision of immediate care requires doctors who are trained and proficient in assessing and treating patients in the prehospital environment. Conditions are very different from an emergency department and patients are often treated in cold, damp and noisy conditions with poor access to the patient and little light. The hospital doctor should not therefore expect to be able to easily translate the skills used in a hospital environment to the roadside. The immediate care provider should also be adequately equipped and understand the roles of the other emergency services and work as a team with them.

Training and qualifications in immediate care are now provided by the Faculty of Pre-hospital Care and BASICS. Any doctor considering taking on the role of immediate care practitioner should also spend time working with experienced colleagues prior to practising on their own. The immediate care provider will also require a close working relationship with the local ambulance service and should acquire adequate protection against claims for medical negligence.

As in other emergencies the prioritized assessment and management of the airway, breathing and circulation is the cornerstone of clinical method. Clinical technique, however, often has to be modified to take account of the environment. The ability to undertake procedures in the field should also not delay transport of the patient to hospital, particularly when the patient has a time-critical injury requiring definitive care at a hospital.

Although the provision of immediate care by doctors is part of the formal system of prehospital care in many European countries, the National Health Service relies on ambulance service paramedics to provide advanced early interventions to its patients.

THE UNITED KINGDOM AMBULANCE SERVICE

Since 1974 there has been a move to make the ambulance service an integral part of the National Health Service (NHS). Currently, the service is responsible for delivering emergency and elective prehospital patient care and transportation. Ambulance services organized as NHS Trusts have their own administrative hierarchy that arranges contracts for the provision of services with local health authorities and other acute care trusts. The ambulance service has in recent years rapidly developed from a simple first aid and transport service to a sophisticated medical system that is an essential link in the chain of survival for many of the most sick and severely injured patients (Fig. 41.1).

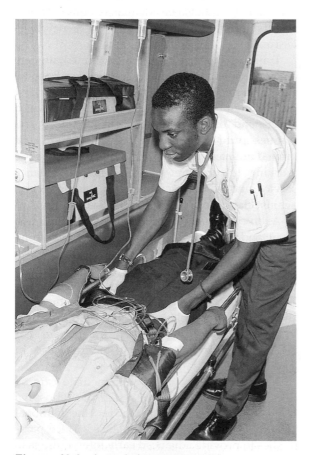

Figure 41.1: An ambulance paramedic.

TRAINING

The national training standards for ambulance personnel are set by the Institute of Health Care Development (IHCD). The basic award of ambulance technician can be achieved after the 6-week ambulance aid course, a 2-week driving skills course, an examination and a 12-month continuous assessment arrangement in the 'work-place'. The course covers the relevant basic sciences, the teaching of skills to lift and move patients, splinting and immobilization techniques, and basic life support and defibrillation. In addition, it may include the teaching of the therapeutic administration of oxygen, nebulized salbutamol, Entonox, glucagon, and the emergency management of conditions such as myocardial infarction, poisoning, eye injuries, childbirth and civil and major incident procedures.

Following this, ambulance technicians are eligible for the 8-week paramedic training course, followed again by a continuous assessment period. The paramedic course places emphasis on advanced airway and circulatory access skills, as well as cardiac rhythm recognition and a broader knowledge of therapeutic administration of drugs. Compulsory continuous education schemes exist and further optional training is available, such as the Pre-hospital Trauma Life Support, the Pre-hospital Paediatric Life Support and Advanced Life Support. Direct entry to training to paramedic level and 3-year university courses have recently become available which provide a greater core knowledge along with the skills necessary for recognition by the IHCD as a paramedic.

The relatively short period of formal training received by paramedics has dictated that they have relatively little clinical freedom and work largely to rigid protocols in assessing and treating patients. Despite this there are a large number of paramedics who have a vast experience of the prehospital environment and whose skills in treating patients in difficult conditions far outstrip their paper qualifications.

PARAMEDICS AND TECHNICIANS

The introduction of the paramedics in the UK was dictated by political necessity rather than scientific evidence, and has sparked controversy as to the enhanced effectiveness of paramedics compared to ambulance technicians. The advocates for paramedics argue that their introduction has converted the ambulance service to a more structured and professional service and is the first step to accountability in the service provision. In addition, it promoted the more active involvement and participation of physicians in the clinical supervision of the service. Critics would argue, with scientific evidence, that there was has been no significant change in survival of patients suffering a cardiac arrest when comparing resuscitation performed by paramedics and technicians. There is also little objective evidence that paramedics improve survival rates in trauma. It has been suggested, however, that the advanced airway skills of paramedics would make no difference to the outcome of the patients who are able to tolerate an endotracheal tube (with no anaesthetic) due to their abysmal initial prognosis. Paramedics are not yet allowed to use anaesthetic drugs and hence are unable to treat the patient who may still benefit from intubation and ventilation at the scene, such as severe isolated head injury cases and the multiply injured.

Furthermore, it has been widely reported that establishing intravenous access to begin fluid therapy at the scene (rather than in transit to the hospital) can prolong scene time significantly. The short transfer to hospital times in most UK practice (as opposed to the Australian and US experience), with the consequent small amount of fluid that can be infused, compromises any advantage by delaying the transfer to the hospital.

STANDARDS

The aim of the ideal ambulance system is to achieve the best clinical outcome, with the fastest response time, with the best patient satisfaction at the least cost. The achievement of such 'high-performance' systems is being aided by the introduction of computerized despatch and communication systems and the provision of first-aid advice by phone to the public by the ambulance control centre until the arrival of the ambulance vehicle at the scene. In 1996 the Steering Group on Ambulance Performance Standards published proposals to improve performance standards by linking them with patients' clinical needs. The proposed standards

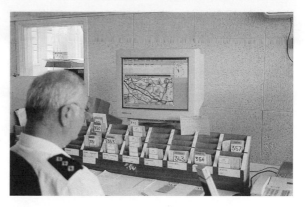

Figure 41.2: A modern ambulance control centre.

allow for triaging of calls and attendance at high-priority calls within 8 min.

DISPATCH

Until recently the role of the ambulance dispatcher was merely to send an emergency ambulance as rapidly as possible to every 999 call. Modern despatch systems incorporate vehicle tracking so that the control centre staff know the position of each available ambulance. They also recognize that different road and traffic conditions mean that the ambulance nearest to a call may not always be the one that can reach the scene first. Predictive software also allows the dispatchers to position available ambulances away from stations to provide the most rapid responses to calls (Fig. 41.2).

The modern ambulance dispatcher now uses a structured series of questions to determine the severity of the patient's illness or injury prior to the ambulance arriving. The dispatcher can also provide first-aid advice, such as instruction in basic life support and assisting childbirth. Calls are categorized as either A (immediate life threat), B or C (standard). In the future, instead of responding to each 999 call with a blue lights and sirens ambulance, alternative responses, such as redirection of calls to other agencies and transport of patients to general practice centres, may be used.

EQUIPMENT

In terms of equipment, the emergency ambulance is usually equipped with a single, centrally located

Table 41.1: Drugs commonly carried by ambulances

Adrenaline
Atropine
Lignocaine
Nalbuphine or tramadol (synthetic opioids)
Aspirin
Sublingual nitrates
Salbutamol
Glucagon
Naloxone
Diazepam (rectal or IV)

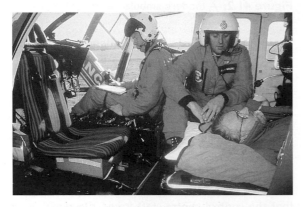

Figure 41.3: An air ambulance.

self-loading trolley, suction apparatus, mechanical ventilator, cardiac monitor and defibrillator units, traction splints and long spinal boards. A list of drugs used by paramedics is given in Table 41.1, though these do vary from service to service.

AIR AMBULANCES (FIG. 41.3)

Air ambulance operation, with the exception of the Scottish Ambulance Service and HEMS in London, lacks central government funding and hence has resulted in poor geographic organization of the facility. In addition, there are as yet no clear indications for aeromedical evacuation. The logical indication for use of a helicopter is of course clinical urgency, but other reasons, such as access to the incident and transport distance to be covered, can be equally important.

Most areas of the UK are now covered by air ambulance services, although these are financed predominantly through commercial sponsorship and charity. They are staffed mainly by paramedics and attend a variety of medical and trauma emergencies. Helicopters are also often used for inter-hospital transfer over longer distances.

The HEMS (London) service based at the Royal London Hospital is unique in carrying a doctor and exclusively attending trauma. The doctors are able to provide advanced airway interventions at the accident scene with the aid of anaesthetic drugs. They are also able to perform surgical procedures such as chest drainage and exercise a greater degree of clinical freedom in treating the patient and determining the receiving hospital. Despite this, independent evaluation of the service has failed to show any overall improvement in survival for its patients.

THE HOSPITAL TEAM

Most emergency departments will despatch a medical team to the scene of an incident at the request of the ambulance service. This may occur in a major incident (see Chapter 42) or when a patient is trapped at the site of the accident and cannot be rapidly removed to hospital. Each department should have in place procedures to allow rapid identification of appropriate team members (usually an experienced doctor and nurse) and rapid access to appropriate equipment. Whilst time as a member of a prehospital team is good experience for a junior doctor, they should always work under the supervision of a trained and experienced senior.

All staff attending a prehospital incident must have appropriate personal protective equipment (PPE). This includes comfortable waterproof fluorescent clothing with protective footwear, a helmet with eye protection and gloves. The hospital team must be sufficiently equipped to allow it to function separately from the other services at the incident. Personal lighting and communications equipment should be carried. The medical equipment taken may vary with the type of incident that is being attended. Most mobilizations of hospital teams are to trapped victims of road traffic accidents. A list of equipment the team should carry is shown in Table 41.2.

The team will usually be transported to the site of the incident by the ambulance service. On arrival at the scene of an incident the team should report to the senior officers of the police, fire or

Table 41.2: Equipment for hospital mobile
medical team

Airway equipment, including simple and
   endotracheal airways
Surgical airway equipment
Self-inflating bag/valve mask with reservoir
Chest drain set
Intravenous cannulae and fluids
Splintage for limbs and spine
Drugs, including opiates and ketamine
Monitoring – ECG, blood pressure, oximetry

ambulance services and check that it is safe to approach the patients. The team must be constantly aware of the dangers to themselves at the sites of incidents such as road traffic accidents, and follow the advice of the other emergency services. The best care can be provided only with proper training of the immediate care personnel, adequate mobile equipment and exemplary co-operation and communication between the emergency services. The prehospital care personnel should receive training in a structured approach to assessing patients. There are courses such as Pre-Hospital Emergency Care, Pre-Hospital Trauma Life Support and Advanced Trauma Life Support (ATLS) which emphasize these principles.

Scene safety – ensure that you do not become another victim.

As in a hospital environment, the initial assessment and treatment should be a primary survey of airway, breathing and circulation. The ability of the doctor to perform these may, however, be limited by reduced access to the patient, the often dark and wet conditions, and the noise of equipment being used by the other emergency services. The doctor should be able to determine the severity and the time criticality of the patient's injuries in order to decide with the other emergency services the best way to treat and evacuate the patient.

The predominant therapeutic role of the doctor with the entrapped patient is in providing effective analgesia in order to allow the fire service to rapidly extricate the patient in a controlled manner. The use of high doses of intravenous opiates may produce respiratory depressant effects and consequent hypoxia. Ketamine is an excellent drug in these circumstances but it should only be used by those familiar with it. In low doses it provides profound analgesia with little cardiovascular or respiratory depression. Titrated intravenous injection is recommended. Rarely, invasive procedures such as a surgical airway or chest drainage may be required.

Rarely, specialized doctors may be required at the scene of an accident, specifically an anaesthetist to undertake drug-assisted intubation, or a surgeon to perform an amputation of a trapped and non-viable limb to allow extrication and evacuation of the patient.

FURTHER READING

Greaves, I. and Porter, K. (Eds) (1999). *Pre-hospital Medicine*. Arnold, London.

CHAPTER FORTY TWO

MAJOR INCIDENTS

- Introduction
- Definition of a major incident
- Classification of major incidents
- Declaring a major incident
- The hospital response
- Planning and equipment
- Command and control
- Triage
- Treatment
- Dealing with the dead
- Admissions
- Urgent surgery
- Staffing

- Dealing with relatives
- Communications
- Dealing with the media
- Police liaison
- Mobile medical teams
- The scene of a major incident
- Emergency services organization at the scene
- Command and control
- The role of the emergency services
- Debriefing
- Training
- Further reading

INTRODUCTION

In today's complex society there are many potential causes of a major incident, and most emergency departments will have within their area sites where there has been recognized to be a particular risk of such an incident, for example an industrial site or sports stadium. Nevertheless, with the current rapid increase in motor transport and the rise in urban terrorism, every major road or city centre now has the potential to be the site of a major incident (Table 42.1).

DEFINITION OF A MAJOR INCIDENT

A major incident cannot be defined simply in terms of the number of people killed or injured. It is important that the ability of the emergency services to cope with the incident is taken into account. Fifty casualties from a motorway pile-up may have little effect on emergency departments if distributed around the hospitals of a major city.

Table 42.1: Types of major incident

Terrorism
Transport incidents
Industrial accidents
Sporting/mass gathering incidents
Natural disasters

The effect would be completely different if they were all taken to the local district hospital of a small market town 45 km from other health service facilities. The standard definition of a major incident, therefore, is:

> 'any emergency that requires the implementation of special arrangements by one or more of the emergency services, the National Health Service, or the local authority'.

It will be obvious, therefore, that what constitutes a major incident for one of the emergency services may not be a major incident for the National Health Service. For example, the plane crash at Lockerbie in 1988, which was associated with the wide dispersal of many bodies but few injured victims, represented a major incident for the forensic, body collection and

Table 42.2: Recent UK major incidents

Date	Place	Incident	Dead	Injured
11 May 1985	Bradford, England	Football stadium fire	55	200
9 September 1987	M4 motorway, England	Multiple vehicle accident	4	74
12 December 1988	Clapham Junction, England	Rail collision	34	115
21 December 1988	Lockerbie, Scotland	Aircraft explosion	270	
8 January 1989	Kegworth, England	Aircraft explosion	47	79
15 April 1989	Sheffield, England	Crowd crush, Hillsborough stadium	96	200
13 March 1996	Dunblane, Scotland	Shooting	17	
15 June 1996	Manchester, England	IRA bombing	0	220
19 September 1997	Paddington, England	Rail collision	7	>150
15 August 1998	Omagh, N. Ireland	Bombing	29	220
28 February 2001	Great Heck, England	Rail collision	10	56

crash investigation agencies, but did not seriously disrupt local healthcare provision. Similarly, a major warehouse fire may be a major incident only for the fire service, and a bus crash will have its main effect on the local emergency departments. The majority of major incidents, however, will involve more than one of the emergency services. A list of recent UK major incidents is given in Table 42.2.

CLASSIFICATION OF MAJOR INCIDENTS

Major incidents are usually classified into:

- compensated or uncompensated
- simple or compound.

When an incident can be effectively managed by mobilizing extra resources that are readily available, for example extra vehicles from the local and neighbouring ambulance services, military personnel and the local authorities, it is said to be compensated. The majority of incidents in the UK and the developed world, for example the Omagh bombing, are of this type. When the response to a major incident remains inadequate even after all the available resources have been mobilized, the incident is described as uncompensated.

When an incident is of sufficient magnitude to disrupt the structure of the society in which it has occurred, the incident is said to be compound. In a compound incident, communications, hospitals and other organizations required for an appropriate response to the incident are themselves disrupted and the ordered structure of society itself may descend into chaos. Such incidents usually result from natural phenomena such as hurricanes, floods and tidal waves. The fact that the majority of areas prone to such occurrences are in desperately poor parts of the world means that only too often preparation and planning for future problems are underdeveloped and mechanisms for dealing with them inadequate. The terms catastrophe and disaster are best reserved for these incidents. When the infrastructure of society remains intact, an incident can be described as simple.

This chapter describes the management of the hospital response to simple compensated incidents and the organization of the emergency services at the scene of an incident itself.

DECLARING A MAJOR INCIDENT (FIG. 42.1)

Members of staff of an emergency department will be informed of a major incident by the hospital switchboard or, if there is a direct radio or telephone link, by ambulance control. The language used in declaring a major incident is formalized. If an incident has already occurred, and it is felt that the implementation of emergency planning by the hospital is necessary, the phrase:

'major incident declared'

is used. In some circumstances, it may be appropriate to acquire further information before declaring

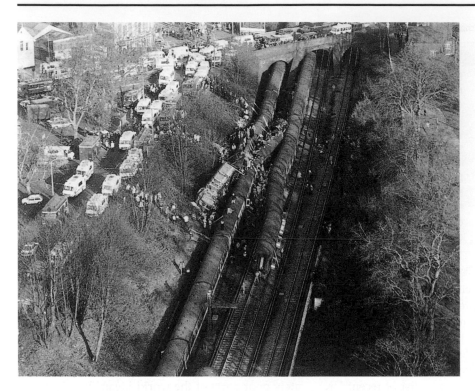

Figure 42.1: A simple uncompensated disaster. (Reproduced from *Investigation into the Clapham Junction Railway Accident*, Department of Transport, by permission of the Metropolitan Police Service.)

a major incident. Examples might include warnings of possible impending terrorist atrocities or assessment by the emergency services of the scene of a multiple-vehicle road traffic accident. Implementation of a hospital major incident plan will seriously disrupt the normal running of a hospital, and some caution should properly be exercised in declaring a major incident. However, it is usually appropriate to declare a major incident if in any doubt, as belated attempts to organize a response once patients are arriving in large numbers are very much less likely to be effective. If the declaration of an established major incident is imminent or likely, the phrase:

'major incident standby'

can be used.

THE HOSPITAL RESPONSE

Hospitals designated as 'primary receiving hospitals' are those deemed to be able to play a role in the reception of any casualty from a major local incident. It is essential, therefore, that all hospitals have a written, comprehensive major incident plan designed to ensure that an optimal response can be mounted. It is hardly necessary to say that all members of staff must be familiar with the outline of this plan and with their specific role in it. Unfortunately, it seems that too many people work on the principle that major incidents only happen to someone else, and studies suggest that many staff members remain sadly ignorant regarding their role should the unimaginable happen.

Specific details of individual major incident plans will depend very much on local factors (Fig. 42.2). It is possible, for example, that the presence in the area of a major airport, chemical plant or military establishment will make one particular type of incident more likely. This will affect the plan, although it must be flexible enough to deal with any possible type of incident. Other factors will include the numbers of available personnel, the layout of the hospital, and the need to send personnel to the scene of the incident.

The hospital response can be divided into the following key areas:

- planning and equipment
- command and control

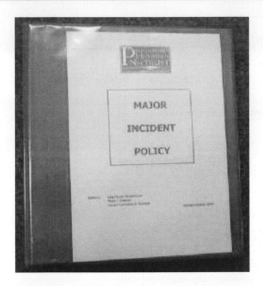

Figure 42.2: A hospital major incident plan.

- triage
- treatment
- dealing with the dead
- admissions
- urgent surgery
- staffing
- dealing with relatives
- communications
- police liaison
- dealing with the media
- mobile medical teams
- debriefing.

PLANNING AND EQUIPMENT

The preparation of a hospital major incident plan is a complex and time-consuming task, involving liaison with all the departments and professional groups within the hospital as well as the local emergency services and voluntary agencies. The majority of major incident plans now use an action card system. Each member of staff registers their availability to help in the incident response and collects an action card detailing their roles and responsibilities. Action cards simplify the response to a major incident as staff members need only know where to collect them; they also allow the development of a coherent integrated plan within which each individual staff member is clearly aware of their role. Correct distribution of tasks

between action cards allows a logical crescendo response as more staff become available (Fig. 42.3).

Once an effective major incident plan has been developed, it is essential that regular major incident practices are held. These are usually either table-top (or paper) exercises or full practice exercises. Table-top exercises, which are cheaper and easier to organize and do not disrupt the routine functions of the hospital, are important in streamlining and developing an efficient major incident plan. Full-scale practices, with staff being called in and simulated casualties, are expensive and can be disruptive and are therefore usually held at weekends. They are an essential component, however, of effective major incident preparedness and, better than anything else, give staff an impression of what 'the real thing' might be like. It is an important responsibility of those tasked with major incident planning to ensure that there is an ongoing programme of major incident response education for staff which also forms part of staff induction days.

It is also essential that any equipment that is likely to be needed for an appropriate major incident response is available, correctly located and 'in date'. This equipment is likely to include triage cards, documentation packs, resuscitation equipment and signage.

COMMAND AND CONTROL

Although the precise command structure will vary from hospital to hospital, all plans will have a number of features in common. The overall response is controlled by the medical co-ordinator, who is usually a consultant. The medical co-ordinator works closely with the triage officer, the senior nursing officer and the duty senior manager. In addition, there will be close liaison with the ambulance service, the police (and especially their documentation team) and the strategic (or gold) control for the incident (see below).

TRIAGE

The key to a successful hospital major incident response is effective and efficient triage. It is inevitable, particularly in the early stages of a major

```
┌─────────────────────────────────────────────────────────────────┐
│     Action Card 57-                                               │
│                                                                   │
│                    Medical Secretary Emergency                   │
│                                                                   │
│   Major Incident Declared                                        │
│                                                                   │
│      • Your role is to support the control team and record events within the control area │
│                                                                   │
│                                                                   │
│      Responsibilities:                                           │
│                                                                   │
│           Primary: To document the Major Incident Report         │
│                                                                   │
│      Action:                                                     │
│                                                                   │
│      1. Attend briefings and record events                      │
│      2. Collate Log Sheets                                       │
│      3. Liaise with Emergency Consultant                         │
│                                                                   │
│                                                                   │
│      NOTE: REMEMBER DURING A MAJOR INCIDENT ALL PATIENTS WILL BE  │
│   IDENTIFIED USING A MAJAX NUMBER, PLEASE USE THIS NUMBER WHEN    │
│              UNDERTAKING RELATED PROCEDURES                       │
│   ALL STAFF MUST WEAR ID BADGES TO GAIN ACCESS TO ANY AREA        │
│                                          Revised 10.04.00        │
└─────────────────────────────────────────────────────────────────┘
```

Figure 42.3: A hospital action card.

incident response, that the number of patients will exceed the availability of the staff and resources required to treat them. Triage ensures that those patients with immediately life-threatening injuries (Priority 1 or P1 patients) receive treatment first, followed by P2 (urgent) patients. In the initial response, P3 (delayed) patients, often referred to as 'the walking wounded', will be directed to an area where they can be carefully observed whilst waiting for treatment. Once the hospital response is fully established, medical and nursing staff will be able to manage patients from all these groups simultaneously. P1 patients will be labelled, directed to and treated in the emergency department resuscitation room and 'major side'. P2 patients will be directed to either the emergency department or a similar suitable area, and P3 patients to an area where they do not compromise the management of more severely injured patients but where full medical and nursing supervision is possible and from where transfer is practical should they deteriorate. Triage categories (T) are listed in Table 42.3.

Triage is carried out according to the triage sort (Table 42.4) and is usually performed by a senior member of the emergency department staff, such as the duty consultant.

Once each patient has been triaged, it is essential that they are clearly labelled with a triage category.

Table 42.3: Triage (T) categories

'P'	'T'	Description	Colour
1	1	Immediate	Red
2	2	Urgent	Yellow
3	3	Delayed	Green
	4	Expectant	Blue
Dead	Dead	Dead	White

There are a number of commercially available triage cards and the majority of patients will arrive at hospital with one already applied at the scene of the incident. Depending on the type of card, this can be changed to show the updated triage category or replaced with a new card. Probably the most effective triage card is the Cambridge Cruciform Triage Card (Fig. 42.4). Each limb of the card is colour coded and labelled with a particular triage category and the card can be folded so that the appropriate category lies uppermost before the card is placed in its bag. In addition, the inside of the triage card contains the information necessary to calculate the patient's triage category using the triage sort.

It must be remembered that a patient's triage category can change and constant vigilance is therefore required in order to ensure that patients do not deteriorate unnoticed. Similarly, a patient's

Table 42.4: The triage sort

	Measured value	Score
Respiratory rate	10–29	4
	>29	3
	6–9	2
	1–5	1
	0	0
Systolic blood pressure	>90	4
	76–89	3
	50–75	2
	1–49	1
	0	0
Glasgow Coma Scale (GCS)	13–15	4
	9–12	3
	6–8	2
	4–5	1
	3	0

Respiratory score + BP score + GCS score	Triage category
1–10	T1
11	T2
>12	T3
0	Dead

triage category will (it is to be hoped) improve following treatment.

TREATMENT

The patient treatment areas, as described above, will be clearly specified in the plan. Detailed action cards will indicate which areas individual staff are to work in. In general, those with the greatest experience of working with the acutely sick and injured will be allocated to the P1 and P2 areas. Senior surgeons and anaesthetists will determine patient priorities for transfer to theatre and the intensive care unit.

DEALING WITH THE DEAD

Dead patients will be labelled as such at the triage point. In general, if there are large numbers of dead at the scene, they will be held there prior to transfer to a temporary mortuary. The hospital should only have to deal with those who die after arrival at hospital or *en route*. Bodies should be placed in a secure area. If this can be locked, the continuous presence of a police officer is not necessary; if this is not possible, a police officer must remain with the bodies at all times in order to ensure that they are not tampered with, or that the possibility of this happening is eliminated so that evidence cannot subsequently be challenged. The numbers of fatalities will only be released in official information bulletins and should never be discussed informally with anyone. The identities of the deceased will only be released once the next of kin have been informed.

ADMISSIONS

During the hospital response to a major incident, it is likely that large numbers of casualties will require admission to hospital for treatment or observation. As a consequence of this, special plans are needed. A specific admissions ward is usually designated in the major incident plan. This ward, ideally, will have good access to the emergency department and operating theatres, and will not normally contain high-dependency patients who are difficult to move at short notice. For example, an ear, nose and throat (ENT) ward is likely to be more appropriate than a colorectal surgery ward.

In addition to the designation of an admissions ward, an accurate bed state must be maintained. Patients from the acute admissions ward must be either transferred to different wards or, if possible, discharged. Patients awaiting surgery should be discharged and their operations postponed. Other patients fit enough for or already awaiting discharge should be sent home. All routine admissions will be cancelled. It must be remembered that the effects of the incident do not stop when the response is formally stood down. It is likely that there will in most cases be a backlog of surgery and shortage of intensive care and other acute beds that will affect the hospital's routine function for several weeks.

The management of hospital beds and discharges is usually the responsibility of the duty

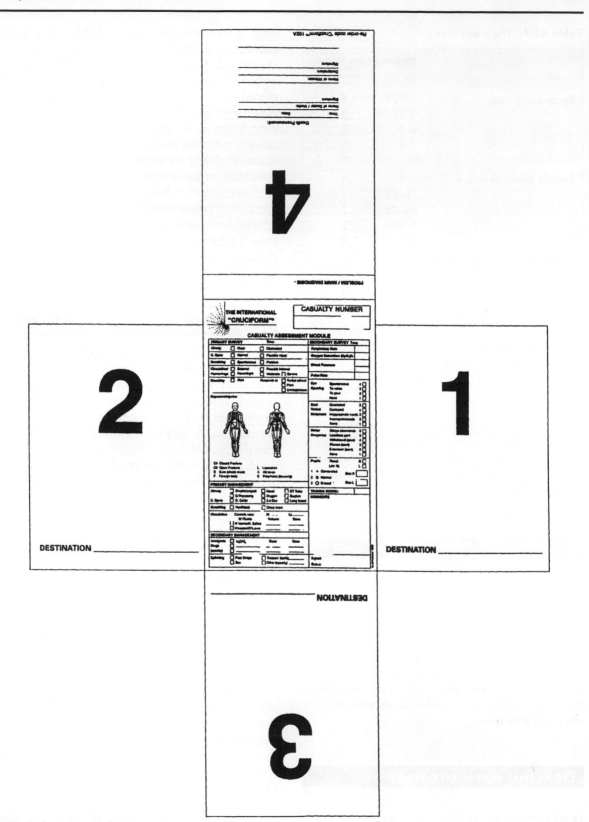

Figure 42.4: The Cambridge Cruciform Triage Card.

Figure 42.4: Continued.

senior hospital manager, often based on information gathered by bed managers or specialty nursing officers.

URGENT SURGERY

As discussed above, a major incident is likely to produce large numbers of patients who might require urgent surgery. In addition, many patients will subsequently require reconstructive surgery. During the initial phases of the incident, a senior orthopaedic surgeon, general surgeon and intensivist must be available to assess and prioritize patients for surgery.

STAFFING

During the response to a major incident, key hospital staff are usually informed by the hospital switchboard. These staff will include on-call consultants and other medical staff, the duty manager, senior nurses, and the senior clerical officer, porter and operating department assistant as well as the duty pharmacist and other technical support staff. Once these staff have been called, a cascade system operates so that each of these personnel calls in others. Staff are called in by role (e.g. duty pharmacist) rather than by name, and all lists of contact numbers must be regularly revised and up to date. In some departments, staff call other staff members in by ringing them from home before leaving for the hospital. In addition to the call-out system, other staff will come to the hospital having heard of the incident on national or local television or radio.

If the response to an incident is likely to be prolonged, it is the responsibility of managers and heads of department to ensure that adequate staffing levels can be maintained beyond the initial surge of enthusiasm. This may mean sending staff home, or asking them not to come in, so that they can form a second 'shift' of responders. In addition, those working nights should not be disturbed since they are likely to be best used on the next night shift.

Staff who cannot prove their identity will not be admitted: wear your ID badge!

DEALING WITH RELATIVES

Inevitably, the hospital will become a focus for relatives wishing to rejoin victims of the incident or simply seeking information. It is essential, therefore, that an area is established for this. This area needs to be comfortable, warm and distinct from the treatment areas, although not too far from them. In addition, the police will need facilities for gathering and collating information, and refreshments should be provided. Input from social workers, chaplains and nurses will assist relatives in coming to terms with bad news.

COMMUNICATIONS

Where possible, communications within the hospital will take place using normal mechanisms such as bleeps and internal telephones. For this reason, it is essential that lines are not blocked by staff making unnecessary calls. Telephones with direct access to outside the hospital should be used for calling in staff, in order to avoid swamping the hospital switchboard. The most appropriate communication method for staff members who are likely to be moving around the hospital but need ready access to other personnel is usually a radio system, and porters' radios can usually be utilized.

Once a major incident has been declared, the police will issue to the press a telephone number for the public to use when seeking or offering information. Enquiries made to individual staff members or to the hospital switchboard should be politely but firmly deflected.

DEALING WITH THE MEDIA

Any major incident will generate huge media interest. The pressure on journalists to achieve a 'scoop' is enormous. The key to success in dealing with journalists is to release sufficient information to ensure that they are for the most part satisfied, but to release it in a controlled manner in order to avoid speculation. The most appropriate method, therefore, is to provide regular bulletins, at which a pre-agreed statement is read by one individual who is responsible for media liaison. Speculation, particularly regarding who might be responsible for the incident, or death rates, must be avoided. Off-the-record statements by staff members only lead to confusion. In particular, information regarding the dead should only be released by the media liaison officer once the next of kin have been informed.

Once the response to the incident has reached a 'stable' phase, it is usually appropriate for representatives of the media to be given the opportunity to interview members of staff or victims. These interviewees should be carefully selected, and in the case of staff members, some agreement of the subjects to be discussed reached.

It is no longer appropriate to treat the press as an irritation best ignored. The public has some right to know what is happening, and it is the media's responsibility to inform them. Appropriate release in a controlled manner of sufficient information will satisfy the legitimate media and go a long way to preventing unacceptable intrusion. When journalists do behave in an inappropriate manner, the police should remove them.

POLICE LIAISON

The police service will despatch to the hospital a documentation team that will work closely with the hospital and liaise with the staff manning the telephone numbers released to the general public. The role of the police documentation team is to build up a complete picture of all those involved in the incident, whether missing, injured, dead or unharmed. Once this information is collated, relatives can be informed.

It should always be remembered that a major incident is the scene of a crime until proved otherwise. Inevitably, an enquiry into the cause of the incident will follow. The police have responsibility for all the forensic aspects of the incident. As a consequence, personal clothing and belongings should be carefully removed, bagged and labelled with the patient's identification. If this is done, evidence that might subsequently prove vital to the police enquiry will not be lost. Clothes should be cut distant from holes made by penetrating objects.

MOBILE MEDICAL TEAMS

Depending on the local policy, it may be part of the major incident plan that the hospital sends personnel to the scene. It is essential, however, that despatch of personnel does not denude the hospital of staff and reduce the effectiveness of the hospital response. The hospital may send either a medical incident officer, whose role is explained below, or a mobile medical team or mobile surgical team. Whichever is sent, they must be properly clothed, experienced and trained for the task (Fig. 42.5).

Mobile medical teams either work together with individual patients or are split up under the direction of the medical incident officer and work in the casualty clearing station or elsewhere on the site. It is now accepted that mobile surgical teams should be called out to deal with a specific surgical problem, such as a patient requiring an amputation for extrication, and then returned to

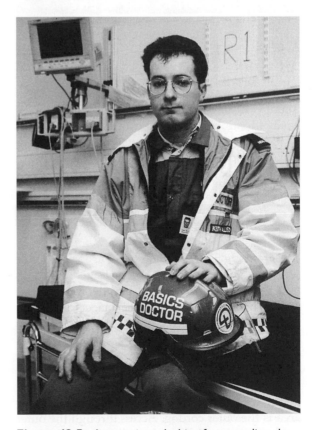

Figure 42.5: Appropriate clothing for attending the scene of an incident.

the hospital. With modern extrication equipment, the necessity for on-site surgical intervention is much less than in earlier years. A mobile medical team usually consists of two doctors and two nurses; a mobile surgical team of a surgeon, an anaesthetist and two nurses, or a nurse and an operating department assistant.

THE SCENE OF A MAJOR INCIDENT

It is possible that members of the hospital staff will be despatched to assist at the scene of a major incident. It is therefore important to be aware of the structure of the health and emergency services' response to a major incident.

EMERGENCY SERVICES ORGANIZATION AT THE SCENE

The first emergency services vehicle at the scene of an incident becomes the control unit and continues in this role until a dedicated vehicle arrives. The rotating beacon of this vehicle (and any subsequent control vehicle) remains lit so that it can be easily identified. Having shown appropriate proof of identity, and passed through the cordon, medical staff report to the control unit.

COMMAND AND CONTROL

The immediate area containing the incident (the wreckage in a plane crash, the damaged buildings and victims in a bombing) is called the bronze area. This is also termed the operational area. Surrounding the bronze area is the inner cordon (Fig. 42.6).

The area outside the bronze area is the silver or tactical area. This area contains the casualty clearing station and other components of the emergency services' response. Surrounding the silver area is the outer cordon. Access through the outer cordon is controlled by the police and only those who can prove their identity and need to pass through the cordon will be allowed to do so.

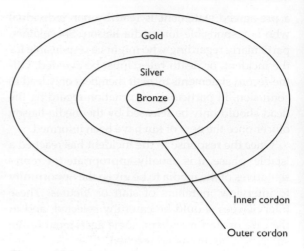

Figure 42.6: Areas and cordons.

In response to a major incident, a gold control or strategic control will also be established some distance from the scene, usually in a purpose-built control centre. This control is staffed by senior officers of all the emergency services, together with representatives of local authorities and government agencies where necessary. Among its responsibilities are liaison with adjoining services and national bodies.

Each emergency service at the scene of the incident is under the command of a commander, who will be clearly identifiable by means of a chequered tabard. The police commander, fire commander, ambulance commander and medical commander together constitute silver control and are in overall command of the incident at the scene. The ambulance and medical commanders work very much as a team. The commanders at the scene report to gold control.

Within the bronze area there will be a senior officer from each of the emergency services. These are the forward commanders (e.g. the forward ambulance commander). The forward medical commander is in charge of the medical response within this area. These officers report to silver control. (There has recently been a change in terminology and the term 'commander' has replaced 'incident officer'. The *forward fire incident officer*, for example, is now known as the *forward fire commander*. The old terminology is, however, still widely used.)

The ambulance service will establish a casualty clearing station within the silver area (Fig. 42.8).

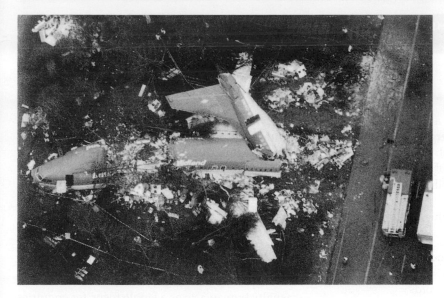

Figure 42.7: The bronze area – Kegworth. (Reproduced from *Report on the Accident to Boeing 737-400 G-0BME near Kegworth, Leicestershire on 8 January 1989*, Department of Transport. Crown copyright material is reproduced with the permission of the Controller of HMSO and the Queen's Printer for Scotland.)

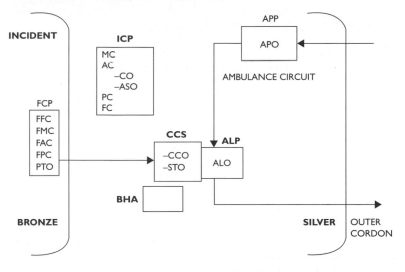

FCP	Forward control point	
FFC	Forward fire commander	
FMC	Forward medical commander	
FAC	Forward ambulance commander	
FPC	Forward police commander	
PTO	Primary triage officer	
ICP	Incident control point	
MC	Medical commander	
AC	Ambulance commander	
CO	Communications office	
ASO	Ambulance safety officer	
PC	Police commander	
FC	Fire commander	

CCS	Casualty clearing station
CCO	Casualty clearing officer
STO	Secondary triage officer
ALP	Ambulance loading point
ALO	Ambulance loading officer
APP	Ambulance parking point
APO	Ambulance parking officer
BHA	Body holding area

Figure 42.8: Organization of on-scene major incident response – schematic.

This is the main location for on-scene casualty treatment. Victims brought to the casualty clearing station from the bronze area will be retriaged and assigned to patient categories for treatment or evacuation. Mobile medical teams or their members may be assigned to work forward or tasked to treat patients in the casualty clearing station.

THE ROLE OF THE EMERGENCY SERVICES

THE POLICE

On arriving at the scene of a major incident, the police, like any of the emergency services, will assess the scene and establish a control point. The police are in overall control of the scene of a major incident, and share with the other services a responsibility to save life.

Specific police responsibilities include:

- prevention of escalation
- evacuation of casualties and those at risk
- traffic control
- maintenance of casualty records
- identification of the dead
- maintenance of public order
- prevention of crime (e.g. looting)
- criminal (forensic) investigation
- liaison with the media.

The police will establish co-operation with the other emergency services and set up cordons where appropriate, so as to control access to the scene.

The police are in overall control of the scene of a major incident.

Evacuation

The evacuation of uninjured survivors and those who would be at risk were the incident to escalate is a vital component of the police role. All apparently uninjured survivors must be recorded as they may be witnesses in any future hearing. In addition, some may subsequently deteriorate and require medical assistance; for this reason, and in order to avoid distress to relatives seeking information, all such people should initially remain together under medical and police supervision. This area is termed the survivor reception centre. If those evacuated from their homes for fear of escalation require temporary accommodation, this is the responsibility of the local authorities.

Control of traffic

The police are responsible for traffic control, and must ensure that emergency vehicles are able to gain access to the scene and leave without obstruction. Control of vehicles belonging to the media and bystanders will also be necessary.

Maintenance of casualty records

The police will establish a casualty bureau as a central point for the collation of accurate information regarding all those who have been involved in the incident. Police documentation teams made up of members of the bureau will be allocated to each of the receiving hospitals, the survivor reception centre and the mortuary. The role of police documentation teams is to build up a detailed and accurate picture not only of who has been killed or injured, but of the nature of people's injuries and the hospital to which they have been taken. The casualty bureau acts as a single focus for enquiries from the general public via a telephone number released through the media.

Identification of the dead

The police are responsible for dealing with the dead. A police identification commission will be established under the authority of the police incident officer and is responsible for this aspect of major incident management. Only a doctor can certify death, and this must take place in the presence of a police officer. In some circumstances, members of the ambulance service may be able to pronounce 'life extinct'. Dead bodies must be clearly labelled as such (to prevent time being wasted in further fruitless assessment and treatment), including the identification of the police officer.

At the scene of the incident, bodies are kept together in a holding area before being removed to a temporary mortuary. In order to facilitate forensic examination, there are only two situations in which a body can be moved before such investigations are complete: when the body is at risk of damage by fire, chemicals or an other agent, or when it is necessary in order to reach a live casualty.

Maintenance of public order and crime prevention

The police are responsible for the prevention of crime and maintenance of public order at the scene of a major incident. This includes the protection of property and possessions, the prevention of looting and criminal damage, and prevention of illegal access to the scene of a possible crime. In addition, the police are responsible for the prevention and control of rioting.

Criminal investigation

As discussed above, the police are responsible for forensic aspects of a major incident. In every case, whether crime is suspected or not, a full enquiry will subsequently be held. The police must therefore ensure that evidence is not lost or damaged or interfered with so that a thorough investigation can be carried out.

Media liaison

The police are responsible for liaison with the media and will appoint a press liaison officer to carry out this role. A media liaison point situated outside the outer cordon will be established.

Specialist police forces

The British Transport Police are in control at any major incident involving the railways, although this responsibility will normally be shared with the conventional police forces owing to lack of manpower. The Ministry of Defence, Atomic Energy Authority and Royal Parks Police may be involved in incidents that fall within their jurisdiction.

THE AMBULANCE SERVICE

Like the police, the ambulance services have a number of specified roles at the scene of a major incident. The medical incident officer works most closely with the ambulance incident officer, and together they are responsible for the health services' response at scene. The main ambulance service responsibilities are as follows:

- establishment of a casualty clearing station
- provision of communications
- triage
- patient evacuation.

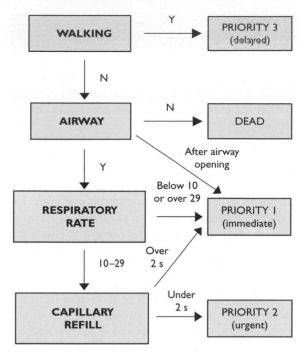

Figure 42.9: The triage sieve.

Casualty clearing station

The ambulance service will establish a casualty clearing station in the silver area. Use may be made of an appropriate permanent building, or a temporary shelter erected. A rapid triage of patients will have been made in the bronze area using the triage sieve (Fig. 42.9). On arrival at the casualty clearing station the patients are retriaged using the triage sort. Following this, treatment can be organized according to priority. This will be performed by medical personnel and ambulance staff. A senior doctor will be in overall control of the casualty clearing station and another responsible for triage. In some circumstances, P3 patients may bypass treatment at the casualty clearing station and be taken direct to hospital, although they should normally be taken to a hospital further from the incident in order to leave the primary receiving hospitals free to deal with the more seriously injured.

Provision of communications

The ambulance services are responsible for the provision of communications for ambulance personnel, doctors, nurses and associated workers.

Triage

The triage of patients is an ambulance service responsibility. Initial triage using the triage sieve is carried out by the forward triage officer in the bronze area. The retriage at the casualty clearing station is carried out by the secondary triage officer.

Patient evacuation

In order to produce the optimum outcome for patients, efficient evacuation to the most appropriate hospital for each patient is necessary. This is the responsibility of the ambulance service, acting on advice from medical staff in the casualty clearing station.

Most of the patients will be evacuated from the scene of the incident by ambulance. The ambulance loading officer is responsible for this and for recording the destinations of all patients in order to ensure that patients are not 'lost'. If there are large numbers of patients with minor injuries, however, they may be evacuated by other means, such as by bus. In addition to appointing an ambulance loading officer, the ambulance incident officer will also appoint an ambulance parking officer.

THE FIRE SERVICE

Fire service staff are under the overall command of the fire incident officer. Personnel working in the bronze area report initially to the forward fire officer. Fire service rank markings are given in Figure 42.10. The main fire service responsibilities are:

- fire fighting
- victim extrication
- safety.

The fire service, like all the emergency services, is responsible for saving life and preventing injury and incident escalation. The fire service has a number of responsibilities apart from fighting fire. The most important of these are overall responsibility for safety, of both victims and rescue workers (from fire, building collapse or chemical contamination), and patient extrication.

OTHER AGENCIES

In addition to the police, fire and ambulance services, the following agencies may be involved in the management of a major incident:

- Her Majesty's Coastguard
- Voluntary ambulance services
- Women's Royal Voluntary Service
- Salvation Army
- Local authorities
- Government agencies
- Armed forces.

Her Majesty's Coastguard

The coastguard service has a co-ordinating role in incidents that occur off-shore, such as ferry disasters and oil-rig incidents.

The Voluntary Ambulance Societies

The voluntary ambulance societies, St John Ambulance Service, St Andrew Ambulance Service (in Scotland) and the British Red Cross Society, can all assist with patient treatment and transport.

The Women's Royal Voluntary Service and the Salvation Army

Both these organizations have a long tradition of service, and in the context of a major incident can provide comforts such as food and blankets as well as encouragement and support to rescuers and victims. Both organizations contain trained personnel able to respond to a major incident and provide local contact points for use should such an occasion arise.

DEBRIEFING

Major incidents are stressful events for hospital staff and emergency services personnel as well as victims. Members of hospital staff in particular will probably have been exposed to more horrific sights and more injured people than normal. It is not surprising, therefore, that acute stress reactions

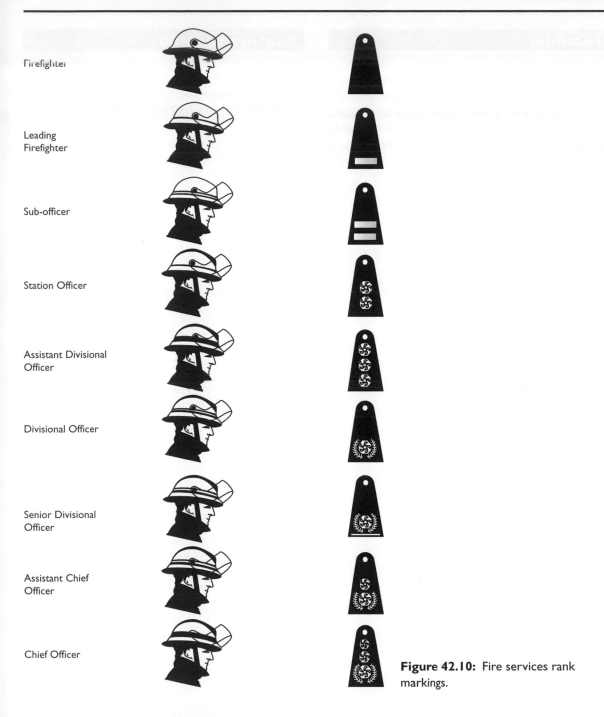

Firefighter

Leading
Firefighter

Sub-officer

Station Officer

Assistant Divisional
Officer

Divisional Officer

Senior Divisional
Officer

Assistant Chief
Officer

Chief Officer

Figure 42.10: Fire services rank markings.

occur. Every conceivable step should be taken, therefore, to prevent the onset of long-term psychological consequences. Immediately after the incident, senior staff and officers should hold a 'hot debrief' of personnel to thank them, tell them what they have achieved, and deal with any immediate concerns (could we have done more? What if … ?).

Shortly after the incident, more formal debriefing should be offered to all, and everyone should be on the look-out for colleagues who may be behaving in an unusual or unexpected manner. The debriefing is also an opportunity to establish areas of the major incident plan that will need revision in the light of events.

TRAINING

All doctors should be aware of their role in the hospital major incident plan. When possible, involvement in a major incident exercise is a valuable experience. All those who are likely to be called upon to work at the scene of a major incident should attend a major incident medical management and support (MIMMS) course.

FURTHER READING

The Advanced Life Support Group (2002) *Major Incident Medical Management and Support: The Practical Approach*, 2nd edn. BMJ Books, London.

INDEX

Note: page numbers in *italics* refer to tables, page numbers in **bold** refer to figures.